D0021797

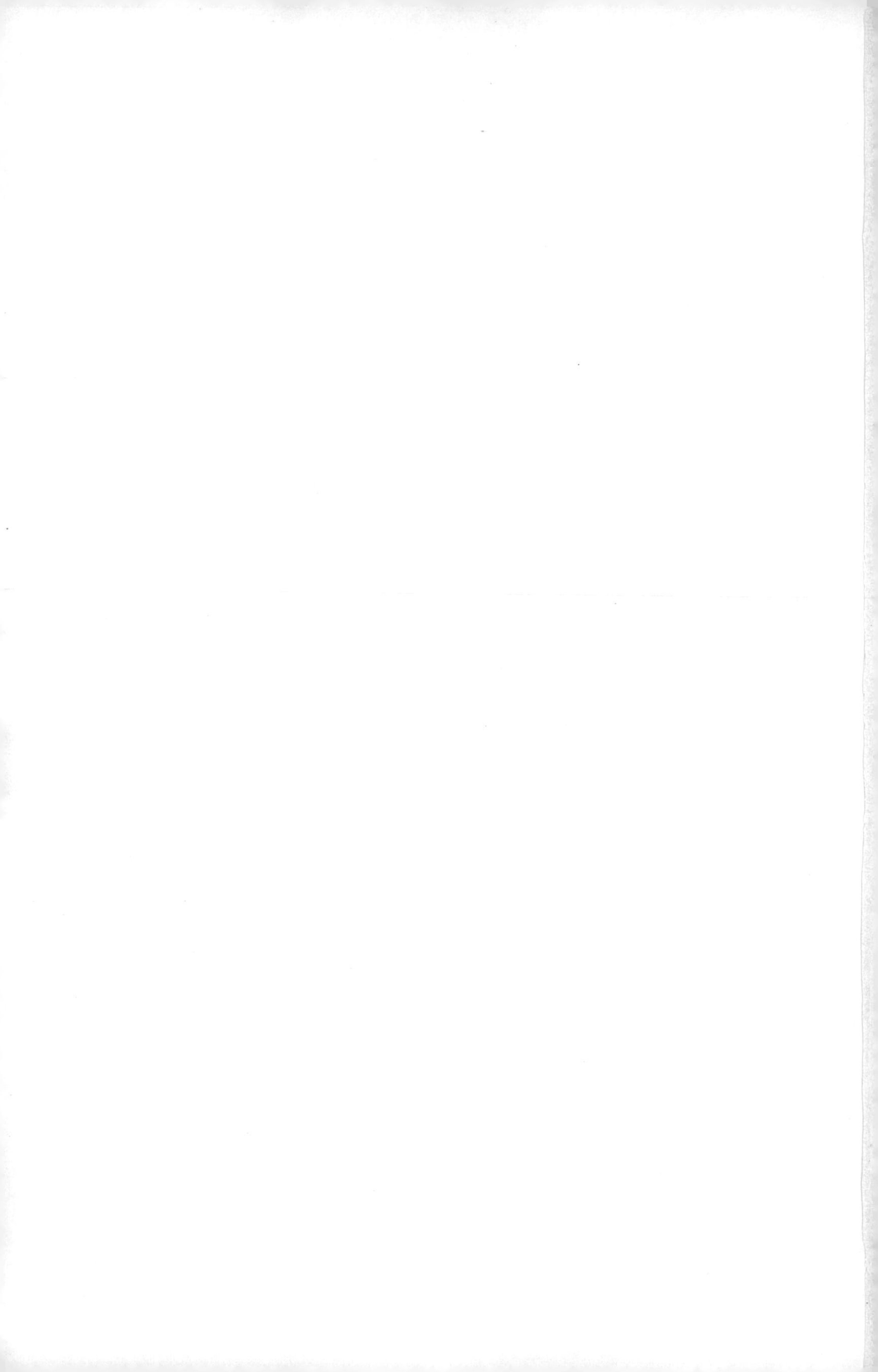

BIOGENESIS
an evolution of fitness and regeneration of youth

by Frank Campitelli and David Dearth

Printed in the United States of America.

IMPORTANT HEALTH INFORMATION

The information contained in this book is intended to help you make informed decisions about your diet and health, not to substitute for any treatment that may have been prescribed by your physician. If you suspect that you have a medical problem, we urge you to seek competent medical help. Keep in mind that nutritional needs vary from person to person, depending on age, sex, health status and total diet. Anyone considering a weight management or exercise program should obtain approval from their health care provider before beginning such a program. Because there may be some individual risk involved, the publisher and researchers are not responsible for any adverse effects or consequences resulting from the use or misuse of any of the suggestions, preparations, procedures or other content in this book.

TABLE OF CONTENTS

ABOUT THE AUTHORS

FRANK CAMPITELLI (Personal Trainer)

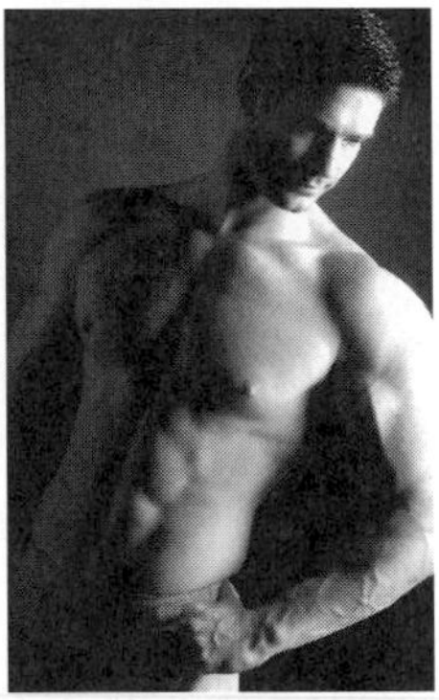

I grew up in the rural lakeside community of Lake Mohawk near Canton, Ohio. As a youngster I developed a love for sports and the outdoors that I enthusiastically maintain today. I became interested in fitness by watching my older brother lift weights. At the age of fourteen I started my first weight lifting program. My goal? Impress girls and increase his performance in sports.

I did not experience immediate muscle growth and success. My mother often wondered why I did not develop like my older brother and began supplementing my diet with large amounts of vitamins, minerals, and other food products from bee pollen to brewer's yeast. At the age of fourteen I was roughly 80 pounds in body weight and just over five feet tall. In the eighth grade I did not have to drop any weight to make the lowest weight class in my school's wrestling program. Over the next four years I took as many Home Economic classes in high school as possible. My goal? Learn about nutrition and talk to girls.

I finally started growing taller and adding muscle at the age of seventeen. Considering that my mother is 5' 3" and my father is 5' 10", and now I am a muscular 6'2", I optimized my genetic potential through nutrition.

Ohio University was my next step in education. I continued to learn new fitness ideas while continually working on my own fitness goals. I graduated in 1990 with a Bachelor of Science degree in Nutrition and Home Economics. I decided not to become a registered dietician, but instead chose to pass on my knowledge of nutrition and fitness to those who really wanted to learn about these topics. I became a personal trainer.

Developing a clientele was easy because of my straightforward approach to diet, weight loss, and a good workout ethic. Within the Canton area I was known to get results like no other trainer could. The majority of my results come from my education and application of nutrition designed around the way each person exercises. I believe that you should match the diet to the output and requirements of each person's exercise program.

My successful methods have translated into a successful series of books and infomercials. I have coauthored three books and eight videotapes, and have been certified through several personal training programs. My quest and thirst for knowledge to be passed on to others has turned a one time hobby into a full-fledged occupation.

"There is nothing like reading about a piece of particular training or nutrition information and experimenting and applying this information to myself first, and then to my clients, which improves their quality of life," Frank says.

As a trainer I put emphasis on results that relate to the real world, like activities and sports. I am very involved with many athletes and appreciate the time involved with training for events. The emphasis in my own personal training and diet program is geared for sport performance that encompasses many sports and hobbies.

Depending on the season, you will find me still involved in outdoor activities; from snowboarding, snowmobiling, and ice skating, to riding motocross bikes, mountain biking, jet skiing, rollerblading, skateboarding, swimming, scuba diving, and playing beach volleyball. My weight training program varies during the season but is never absent from my training schedule.

"Doing all of these activities takes some type of resistance training to stay in shape in order to perform at a high level. I like to be able to do an activity or sport with above average ability and I don't have time to make that particular activity my workout because I have so many different things I love to do," Frank says.

I relax by cooking, constantly reading about training and diet, and working as a mechanic on my toys.

In 1997 I was introduced to David Dearth whom I used as a model for a workout videotape. I had seen Dave grace the cover of numerous bodybuilding magazines and we have the same approach to creating and recreating clients' bodies. Since then we have collaborated on many fitness and diet projects. Weight loss, weight gain, shaping, toning, athletic sports performance, we have all the information and motivation to provide our clients with real world applications to diet and exercise. The fundamentals of the Biogenesis program are a philosophy that we truly believe in and want to pass along to you.

DAVID DEARTH (Professional bodybuilder and personal trainer)

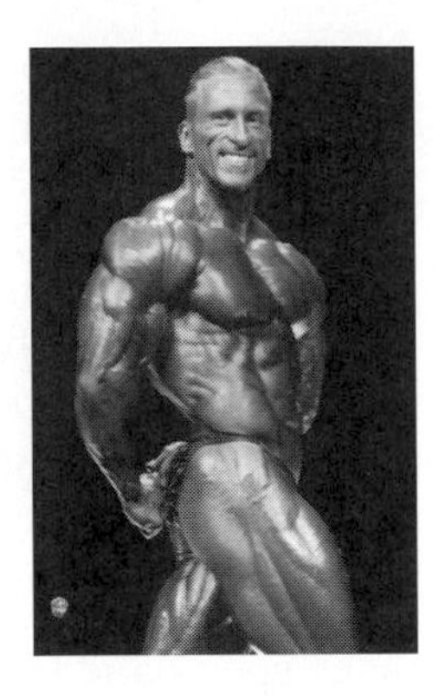

In high school I played all of the sports, but my small stature really kept me from excelling at any one sport in particular. At 5' 7" and 145 pounds there were not many college football scouts looking to recruit me. I was picked on a lot and came from a tough neighborhood where I learned that you have to stand up and defend yourself. During my senior year in high school, I was badly injured during our football season opener. My knee was completely destroyed along with any hopes of a collegiate athletic career. It was a very depressing time for me.

I began weight lifting for the first time for rehabilitation purposes and I hated it. I kept on exercising and before long my legs began to get stronger. I remember one day looking at the scar on my leg in the mirror and I noticed my quadricep muscles had a cool new shape. I started to train my arms and in just a few weeks I started to get more attention from the girls. That was the deciding factor on whether or not I was going to keep working out. The bigger and stronger I became, the more confident I felt.

These may sound like superficial reasons to work out. Well, actually they are. But, it's twenty years later and I am still working out. I enjoy it now as much, if not more, then ever before. My reasons for working out have changed since those days of training to pick up girls. There have been many points in my life where if it were not for my training, I don't know how I would have made it through. My reasons for working out and gaining knowledge on the biodynamics of the human anatomy were purely selfish in the beginning.

I wanted to be Mr. America. I ate, drank, and slept bodybuilding twenty-four hours a day. I spent three hours a day on the treadmill, two hours a day hitting the weights and the rest of the day talking with the renowned experts in the fitness industry. I wanted to know what the best sources of protein were, what supplements could bring my body fat to the lowest possible percentage and what exercises could give me maximum results with minimum wasted energy. If there was something to learn about gaining muscle and losing fat I was not only going to learn it, but I was also going to apply that knowledge toward creating a body for myself.

Winning the Mr.America contest was great but the benefits I have received over the years from training have far outweighed my ten-year-old trophy. The one thing I can tell you about being in this industry for so long is that I have seen it all! I have seen many fads come and go; but the one fitness commandment that has stood the test of time is resistance training. Today, more than ever before, resistance training is the backbone in nearly every aspect of fitness for either health or appearance. Knowing all of the wonderful benefits that exercise has brought to my life, I feel obligated to give my knowledge back to the sport.

I have been a personal trainer for many years and have had the awesome experience of bringing new joy into peoples' lives through exercise. When I met Frank, it was my intention to acquire knowledge on his "state of the art" nutritional programs. I was in California and he was in Ohio and his research was considered to be on the cutting edge in the fitness industry. Frank and I had quite a lot in common, including a shared desire to reach the masses with the ultimate complete fitness program. It has taken us two years but we did it. Frank and I, along with the Biotech Research staff, developed Biogenesis.

During the early stages of Biogenesis development we created a theory on why we have had so much success with ourselves and with our thousands of clients. We suggest that you read this carefully and hopefully one or more of these reasons will be something you can relate to and grab onto as your own personal reason for continuing the Biogenesis program for the rest of your life.

Number one. We realize that there is no one simple solution. Everybody is different and everybody has different needs for exercising. By realizing this, Biogenesis does not offer one program for everyone. There are four different phases to Biogenesis which will help you no matter where you are at in your life. Whether you have never exercised before or if you are a fitness enthusiast, there is a phase in Biogenesis for you.

Number two. We understand that we are three-part beings; consisting of a mind, a body, and a spirit. We understand that we could not truly offer you a legitimate, complete, fitness program if we did not help you achieve maximum efficiency in each of these areas. We educate your mind with all of the knowledge you will ever need regarding exercise, nutrition and supplements. We lift your spirit by making your exercise program fun, effective and practical. And of course we give you the body that you always dreamed of having.

Number three is that we believe that addiction is one of the main reasons Americans are so out of shape. You don't have to be addicted to drugs or alcohol to be an addict. You can be addicted to work or to food. For many of us, overeating relates to having an addictive personality. When we are bored, we eat. When we are depressed, we eat. Our poor choices lead to poor habits and our poor habits often lead to certain addictions, such as food. We have done extensive studies on people with addictions. The number one way we found to break the pattern of addiction is to replace the addiction with other activities that are more productive and positive. You can't be expected to live a certain way for all of your life and then just change. The change has to come at a pacc that is comfortable for each individual. Biogenesis, slowly through each phase, adds new dimensions toward your progression in health and fitness.

PREFACE

Over the last 100 years our society has made tremendous progress. Our knowledge in the fields of science and medicine make the United States a world leader. Americans' have every modern convenience that our high tech society can offer. Our work is less labor intensive thanks to automation. Cleaning our homes and cooking our meals has become easier and more convenient. Today information is at our fingertips thanks to satellite television and the Internet.

However, these technological advances have come with a price. The percentage of American adults classified as "obese" has increased dramatically. The increase in pre adult obesity is even more dramatic. Scientists have a greater understanding of the human body and nutrition. Yet more Americans are out of shape than ever before.

Readers of this book must understand a simple formula. Proper nutrition and proper exercise combines to make a healthy body. There is no "quick fix" pill or diet plan. You must combine exercise and diet to maintain a healthy body. As adults we set examples for our children with our eating and exercise habits.

Biogenesis is a complete fitness and nutrition program. One of the four exercise programs will work for you if you follow the nutritional guidelines. This is the Biogenesis guarantee! Remember to consult your physician before starting any new fitness program.

1

Introduction

Biotech Research is a research center located in Canton, Ohio. Biotech's primary functions are to research and develop ways for people to live longer and to look and feel better through proper exercise and nutrition. Biotech has been a leader in the fitness industry for more than thirty years and has been a pioneer in the development of many of the exercise programs and principles used today.

The Biogenesis program was developed by the Biotech research staff along with Frank Campitelli and David Dearth.

Frank is a born and raised Ohio native who has more than fifteen years servicing the fitness industry. He has appeared in nearly every major newspaper in the country and has had incredible success with his exercise programs. His last book was a best seller and his services have been in great demand from many large corporations throughout North America. Frank goes into their work place and develops exercise programs for their workers. These programs have greatly improved productivity, lowered absenteeism as well as lowered the cost of health insurance for these companies. Frank's extensive education in nutrition has served him well, as he is a major contributor in the development of many of the nutritional supplements you see on the market today.

David was also born in Ohio, but has spent the most part of his thirty-five years in southern California. David is one of the best bodybuilders in the world and has dedicated the latter part of his career to personally training many of Hollywood's elite movie stars and musicians. He would earn as much as five hundred dollars an hour training these celebrities. He has appeared on the cover of nearly every exercise or fitness magazine in the United States and Europe.

Until recently, to get Campitelli or Dearth as personal trainers or fitness programmers would have been nearly impossible. In 1994, Biotech Research hired Frank to organize its health and fitness development division. In 1998, Biotech completed its elite staff with a person with the most credible "hands on" experience in the fitness industry, David Dearth. And now with three of the leading sources all working together for the first time, the bible of fitness has been created – Biogenesis.

WHAT IS BIOGENESIS?

Now that you know a little bit about who created Biogenesis, let's find out exactly what it is. Biogenesis is nothing more than a new way of life. It's a new way of thinking and feeling, of being more healthy and alive. So many of us have gotten lost in the shuffle and became caught up in the rat race of everyday living. The things we enjoyed as children, like the joy of being full of energy, have been replaced with stress and aggravation that can be brought on without any warning at all. You are all grown-up now and have too many responsibilities to be able to take the proper time and effort to get and maintain a healthy and vigorous body and life style. Right?

Not anymore. For the majority of overweight or out of shape Americans, it all boils down to one simple factor. Time.

It seems the more time we spend on this planet the less time we actually have for ourselves. We get jobs, get married, have children, and the responsibilities of taking care of others' needs, whether it is our family or our bosses, take priority in our lives. Before we know it, the good old days of living healthy, carefree lifestyles are just memories we reminisce about. Usually by the time we say enough is enough, we have to do something to get back in shape and we have no idea how to do it.

We hear all the time our friends, or perhaps ourselves, stating, "I have never been this out of shape." For many it may be that you are not overweight at all; you just need to tone up what was once firm and solid and is now a little soft or flabby. Then there are those of you who long to lose the few extra pounds you have put on over the last couple of years. "I would just like to get back to the way I looked in high school or college," is a statement we hear often. There are also people who have never been in great shape. You may just be sick and tired of having no energy and not looking the way you've always wanted to. Or, maybe you've decided, "I don't want to die young from a heart attack or clogged arteries."

As you can see, there are many different levels to being either "in" or "out" of shape. How can any one program be designed to accommodate a person that is five pounds overweight and a person who is two hundred pounds overweight? Is it going be safe for someone in relatively good shape as well as an individual who has a medical condition? If I am a woman, am I supposed to follow the same nutritional program or diet that a man would? Is the same exercise program for a twenty-year-old appropriate for someone who is in their seventies? As preposterous as this sounds, this is exactly the way most exercise and nutritional programs have been set up. We are destined to fail with these programs before we even begin them.

Unfortunately, the fitness industry has capitalized on Americans' desires to lose weight and get into shape by selling them pills, shakes, prepackaged meals, grapefruit diets, all protein diets, butt blasters and ab masters; we could go on and on with these ridiculous quick fixes. We are personally outraged and offended at the way many of the supplement companies and weight loss organizations abuse the misfortune of a person trying to lose weight and get in shape.

This is the reason for Biogenesis. Biogenesis isn't just one diet to meet the needs of over 100 million overweight or out of shape Americans. We are not a company trying to convince you that if you take one of our special pills that block fat, you can go ahead and eat whatever you want and lose weight and look great. Wouldn't it be nice if that were possible though? We don't belittle you by asking you to believe that getting into great shape is simple and fun. Biogenesis is a total way of living. Biogenesis was scientifically designed to create opportunities for individuals with a sincere desire to change not only their appearance but their lives.

Given the option of being in great shape, healthy and full of energy or overweight, flabby and tired, we all would choose the first. So why are so many people out of shape? We've discussed the fact that most of us got out of shape by not having or no longer taking the time to give our bodies the maintenance required to look and function at optimal levels. But there are other factors as well.

Stress in a person's life has been shown not only to be detrimental to your health but has also been linked to obesity. Depression, addictions and other mental states are also major contributors to the overall health and weight problems of our society. And then there are the subjects that most weight loss or fitness programs are afraid to address. Just plain and simple laziness. With every passing year, everything becomes more convenient for us to do with less energy. It becomes more and more acceptable for Americans to have higher body fat percentages and to walk around huffing and puffing if we have to walk up a flight of stairs. We allow our children to replace gym class with computer class. We take no concern with what they are eating in school and we ourselves would rather pick up fast food for our family dinner then take the time to prepare a meal. With so many variables to address, we believe that Biogenesis is truly the ultimate in a complete guide to living a more well rounded, healthy, long life.

You may not agree with some of our principles or techniques. In fact, some of you may even take offense to our blatant honesty. Biogenesis is not a socially accepted way of living. But it should be! This is our theory to helping you to achieve the physique you have always dreamed of and to be able to fully enjoy all that life has to offer.

HOW DOES BIOGENESIS WORK?

Biogenesis is unique from all of the other exercise and diet programs on the market for many different reasons. In this next section we will be discussing why you are reading this book. You are reading Biogenesis for one of two reasons. Either you have never been on a diet and exercise program before or the programs you have tried in the past have fallen short of your expectations, or just outright failed you completely.

Do not despair. It may not have been in your control at all. Let us give you a common case scenario and let's see how many of you this has happened to. You make the decision to begin an exercise program or a diet. You ask your friends who have lost weight on a certain program what they are doing to lose their weight. Whatever the current fad diet is at the time, whether it is an all grapefruit diet or the ever popular all protein diet, or maybe even the drink a shake for breakfast and a shake for lunch, then eat whatever you want for dinner diet, your friends rave about the awesome results they are getting, and they look like they are losing weight so you make the decision to go for it.

In the beginning the pounds seem to melt off and you are very happy with what you see. Then things start to slow down. The pounds aren't coming off at the rate they were a couple of weeks ago; on top of that, your energy is starting to drop off. What's happening? Maybe if you reduce your calorie intake a little more that will accelerate your weight loss back to what it was. Didn't work, did it? In fact, the friend that got you started on the diet in the first place has since gone off of the diet and has a convenient excuse for doing so. They have probably put all of the weight that they had lost back on and probably even added a few pounds extra.

Well that could be depressing. It's probably not going to be much motivation for you to continue on that diet especially if the gains you had previously been making had slowed down considerably or maybe even stopped all together. Thus, another failed attempt to lose weight and keep it off. Trust us, for many Americans having one after another after another failed diets will soon leave a person very depressed and skeptical of their next dieting venture. That's if they even will try another one. This is something we deal with on a daily basis and, trust us, it is no easy task trying to convince a person who has failed time and time again that they won't fail this time.

Being in great shape is no easy task; if it were we would have no out of shape Americans at all. If a great body came in a bottle, or a pill, or by wrapping yourself up in cellophane, what would be the need for a gym or a health club? Yet everywhere you look, there's a new supplement company trying to sell you some ridiculous program with outrageous claims to "a new scientific discovery" that will give you the body you have always wanted. This infuriates us to no end! As professionals who have been in the fitness field for more than twenty years and trained thousands of people, to see companies, clinics, and in many cases doctors take advantage of unsuspecting overweight or out of shape people the way that they do . . . it's just plain wrong.

Everybody cannot be educated in every area of life. There are certain professions that are trusted professions. So if we are a person looking for a diet or exercise program and we see one that has been created by a person with a "doctor" in front of his name, we like to assume that he knows what he is talking about!

Do you want to know if a program works? There are several things to look for. We want to know what the person looks like that created the program. Secondly, do they look that way because they follow that program themselves, or did they get in shape by another means and sell tapes saying that if you follow a program where you do martial arts moves to music that you can get a body that they created for themselves through training with weights? The next thing to look for is on what do they base their claims of success? University studies? Actual documented proven theories that have stood the test of time? We implore you, who on earth thinks of some of these diets? Grapefruit? All protein?

Biogenesis is not a program. Biogenesis is combination of programs that work together to create an opportunity for a person with a sincere desire to better themselves physically, mentally and spiritually. Biogenesis provides a detailed plan of action to accomplish this through different levels of diet, exercise and nutritional supplementation. We have an entirely different approach to fitness than any other company or program out there. We actually help the individual to prepare themselves mentally in order to be able to focus properly on their exercise program.

WHY DOES BIOGENESIS WORK?

Biogenesis cannot work without the most important element – You! There are several important things that are going to be required from you and will be completely out of our hands. The first and most important is going to be an intense desire from you to succeed at this program. Just hoping or wishing for a great body obviously doesn't work. Like anything that is good and has a high value to it, getting in shape will require the same effort.

As human beings most people will agree that we are a three-part being, composed of a mind, a body, and a spirit. If one part of us is out of wack, then it makes it very difficult for us to be happy. For example, if our spirit is down and always depressed then our bodies, as well as the way we think about or look at things, are usually affected in a negative way. On the counter side to that, if our spirit is up and positive then it is much easier for us to think clearly and be more positive.

By using the Biogenesis program you will improve your entire way of living. By learning how your body works and understanding the importance of exercise and nutrition, you will begin to develop a completely new way of living. We take you step by step through every phase. There are four phases to our program. Our first phase is designed for a person who has not exercised for a while, or maybe has never even exercised at all. We teach you basic anatomy and take you through five very specially designed workouts. Even though the workouts only take ten minutes per day, the results are amazing! In Phase One the exercise movements are done with no weights or equipment and are very low impact. This means ANYONE can do it. As you progress through your workouts, they become easier and easier to do. Once you get to the point of being able to complete an entire week with relative ease then it is time for you to move onto the next phase.

In Phase Two we take many of the same movements and exercises that you used in the first phase and incorporate weights for resistance. We limit the weights you use to dumbbells. As in Phase One, you are exercising the entire time so we are still able to keep each workout to only ten minutes. Phase Two is a very exciting phase for many people because we have made weight training so extremely easy. Even though all of the latest research has indicated resistance training to be as much as five hundred percent more effective then aerobic training, most people still think that it would be much easier and far more practical to walk on a treadmill or ride a stationary bike than it would be to learn how to exercise with weights. Well, if you have completed Phase One and are able to do those exercises then you will certainly be able to do the exercises in Phase Two.

In Phase Two of the Biogenesis 10 minute workout, Frank and David pick up the intensity with a series of short but effective workouts using dumbbells and an adjustable bench. It won't take long before you start to see the similarities in the movements used in the first phase. As the weeks pass and you begin to master the second phase you will be overwhelmed with the changes your body makes. With each body part receiving equal attention, your physique will take on a pleasing symmetrical and streamlined look with separation between each muscle group. Depending on your own personal desires for your physical appearance, the Phase Two 10 minute workout may be where you would like to stay. However, if you are like most of our clients, you have just watched your body transform to a level you had not previously thought possible for yourself. At this point you should have enough confidence in both the Biogenesis program and your own abilities to move on to Phase Three, The Star and Model Look.

When asked the question, "What would you like your physique to ultimately look like when you reach your goals?" The most common answer we get is, "I would like to look like one of those Hollywood movie stars or models." Well grab a pen and get ready for some autograph signing because Phase Three is all about obtaining a toned, firm, sexy physique that many movie stars and models display.

As you might have guessed this phase is more strenuous. Dave has spent the majority of his adult life living in Venice Beach, California (where else would Mr. America live?) where he made his living not only by competing in bodybuilding shows, but also by earning the better part of his income through personal training. Most of his clientele being, you guessed it, stars and models. David charged as much as five hundred dollars per hour for his services and you can rest assured that he was in great demand as a personal trainer. In Phase Three, Dave took the exercise program that he had been using in California and, with Frank's added expertise, created the Phase Three Star Model Program.

We make this program so easy to learn and understand that you will wish you had acquired the Biogenesis program years ago. Frank and David are very serious about every single one of their clients obtaining their goals. Both men take it very personally and are extremely articulate in each phase making sure to cover every last detail of the program.

The Star and Model program is no exception. You are not going to be sugar-coated and led to believe you can obtain the body of a Hollywood movie star by doing some halfhearted exercises along with some magic pill. There is no magic pill and this workout is not easy. But if you have made it through Phase One and Phase Two then we are sure you are looking forward to conquering this phase as well. Wether you use the Star and Model tape series or if you follow the program in this book, we are sure that you will become a changed person for the rest of your life.

Each Biogenesis phase progressively gets more in depth as you learn more and more about protein, carbohydrates and fats and exactly what roles each of them play in your progress. You will gain an understanding of vitamins and nutrients. You will become more knowledgeable of not only what foods you should eat but when you should eat. You advance from phase to phase at a pace that is comfortable for you. We do recommend that you don't get too comfortable though, because for most of us getting too comfortable was how we got out of shape in the first place. We do ask you to push yourselves. It's supposed to hurt. It's work. Is work fun? It can be, but most of us work for the rewards and benefits that come from it. As with most things in life, the harder you work, the greater the rewards.

By the time you reach Phase Four you will look unbelievably improved. You will know more then ninety percent of America about diet and exercise. Dieting will be easy for you because you slowly changed your body back to utilizing all of the food you eat for energy. No more stored fat. No more being tired all of the time. You will be a physically, spiritually and mentally changed person for the rest of your life.

Phase Four is hard core. Some of you may never get here. Some of you may never want to get here. In Phase Four Frank and Dave take it to the extreme. We teach you how to bring your body fat to its all time low. At the same time you learn how to be able to walk into any gym or health club and get a fantastic workout using whatever weights and equipment available to you. Even though this phase is the most difficult, it is also the most rewarding. You've learned your own body so well by this point that many of the movements will be second nature to you. By not having to learn new movements, you will be totally free to concentrate on the intensity of your workout. Great intensity brings great results. You will see changes almost daily in this phase.

We must emphasize, if you are not sure which phase you should be in then Phase One is highly recommended. Phase One is the foundation for the rest of the Biogenesis program.

2

MENTAL ASPECTS

These next few pages deal with turning your "wanting" to get in shape into a need that you desire for yourself.

Desire is described in Webster's dictionary as 1. To wish or long for; want strongly [to desire fame]. 2. to ask for; request [the principal desires to see you in her office]. Desired, desiring 1. Strong wish. 2. the thing wished for.

The definition for want. Want 1. To feel that one would like to have, do, or get. A synonym for want is desire. To change a want to a desire you must create a need. Need: something that one wants or must have.

Most of us accomplish nothing of any value in our lives without first wanting it. However, wanting to have something is rarely going to be enough to acquire it. To make a "want" become a reality you will have to create a "need" for what you are wanting. Once the need has been established you will then have to apply your "desire" to complete your goal.

A person with a strong desire to accomplish a particular goal will apply all of their knowledge and effort toward creating a means of successfully fulfilling their needs. An example to what you have just read could be this. A person sees a car that they want. The car is very nice and very expensive. By just wanting the car, the person makes little or no effort to actually make the car theirs since the car is more than the money they have. But if the individual's car that they currently own is destroyed in an accident then the person now has an immediate "need" for a new source of transportation. The need for transportation alone is not going to be enough for this person to purchase the nice car. But by applying a desire to drive a nice car with the need for transportation, I now have the proper formula for taking the correct steps in order to get that car.

Wanting to lose weight or shape up is the first step, but it is not nearly enough to make it happen. If wanting to look great was all it took, then we would have no out of shape or overweight people in the world. We have yet to talk to a single person who wants to be fat and flabby with no energy.

Desiring to lose weight or shape up is the only way you will accomplish your goal. Only when you get to the point of desiring to lose weight or shape up will you be in a position to learn and understand what will be involved and what you will need to know in achieving your specific needs for health and fitness. The desire to better yourself will keep you focused on your program. Desire usually doesn't come to us just by saying I desire this or I desire that. It is very hard to desire something we do not believe we have any chance of achieving.

Now that you know having a desire to change your physique is necessary, you are probably wondering if indeed it is a desire for you. Do not feel bad if it is not. When a person is unsure of how to do something or has tried their best in the past only to come up short, it then becomes more and more difficult to believe you could do it this time. With so many people wanting to lose weight and get in shape a market for almost anything that claims to cause weight loss has been created. We want to lose weight but at the same time can't drastically alter our current way of living.

Some supplement companies and weight loss centers have decided to capitalize on this dilemma. Hence, lose thirty pounds in thirty days, take one pill before each meal and you can eat any foods you want including pizza and ice cream, and so on and so on. If you have been sucked into one of these quick fix forms of weight loss don't feel bad, so have millions of other people. They had no better luck or success then you have with these outrageous claims to weight loss. The reason these programs do not succeed is that there is no sustenance to their claims. They make their claims off of short term studies and use one specific type of group to study. If you have thought in the past that you have had a desire to lose weight, then gone out and purchased a program that had you taking a bunch of pills or shakes, or gone on an all protein diet and expected to lose weight and shape up, we have got bad news for you. That is not desire. That is hoping for a miracle. You may have lost a little weight, but did you keep it off? No, you didn't. And did you get into great shape? Probably not. What these bogus companies do not tell you is that you HAVE TO EXERCISE to shape your body. Dieting alone will not shape your body. It is impossible.

We understand the apprehensiveness most people have regarding starting a new exercise and nutritional program. Most people have been lied to or scammed so many times that it is difficult for them to allow themselves to jump full force into another program with expectations of finally realizing their weight loss or fitness goals. By not jumping directly into another program you are using good common sense. Before starting any new program, you should really study it. The old saying "if it sounds too good to be true, then it probably is," still holds true.

There are two important questions to ask yourself. How long has the company been around? Biogenesis has been around for more than thirty years. What are some of the bases on which these other programs have made their claims? Our claims are based on university studies, doctor studies, and the combined thirty-two years of having a nearly one hundred percent success rate with our clients.

If a program is making the claim of being able to help you shape up, does it include resistance training? Although Biogenesis is not against aerobic exercise, we use resistance training for our means of exercise. Resistance training has been proven to be several hundred percent faster and a more effective form of weight loss than any other form of exercise. Does their program provide a safe and effective way for you to lose weight and keep the weight off for good? Biogenesis's source for weight loss comes not only from diet but also from exercise. And since both, the exercise and the nutritional programs, are constantly changing, your body never has a chance to adjust or grow stagnant.

Would your doctor approve of their program? If you are wondering if your doctor would approve of our program, don't take our word that he would; ask him. We already know that the chances are very good he will give you his blessings. How a person looks depends on the phase of Biogenesis in which they are involved. Regardless of the phase you are in, you look much better then when you started.

If you have gotten this far in the Biogenesis book then we are inclined to believe you now have the desire to get in shape. Follow whatever phase of Biogenesis that you start in as close to the book as possible. Have a sincere expectation to see results. Learn as much from each chapter as you can. The more you understand the way weight loss and body shaping work the better chance you have of making it work for you. You did not get out of shape overnight nor will you get in shape overnight. With the Biogenesis program, however, you will get into the best shape that you have ever been in your entire life faster then ever imagined. This is a fact. And this is guaranteed. There is no program in the world that is more complete and effective than Biogenesis. Getting into great shape is within your reach. You now have all of the tools and knowledge you will ever need to have a trim, firm and healthy body for the rest of your life right in this book.

Remember, work each program as it is written; follow the nutritional programs, use the Biogenesis Ultrabody supplements and you will begin to truly enjoy life.

GOAL SETTING

An important step toward obtaining success is to have goals. It is much easier for us to strive toward something if we know what we are striving for. To say "I want to lose a lot of weight as soon as possible," is a very broad statement. Furthermore, chances of the weight loss happening are not very good because you have not set a time frame for yourself. When given an open time frame we fail to create a sense of urgency on what we are trying to accomplish. Now, if you were to say, "I would like to lose thirty pound in three months." You have set a deadline for yourself on when you would like to see thirty pounds gone. This is now your goal.

There are two different types of goals, short range goals and long range goals. We always recommend writing your goals down. Start by trying to figure out what you would like to see as an end result from the Biogenesis program. For example, "At the end of one year on the Biogenesis program I want to be 85 pounds lighter and look like one of those models in a magazine." This would be your long range goal.

Once you have established your long range goal it is very important to identify several short range goals which, once accomplished, will bring you closer to your ultimate goal. A short range goal in this case may be, "I want to complete Phase One in three months and I want to lose 30 pounds." A second short range goal could be to lose another 20 pounds by the end of Phase Two and take ten weeks to do so.

The advantage of setting short range goals is very apparent in this example. When you look at losing 85 pounds over more than a one year period, that seems like a lot of weight and a long time before you will ever see your goal accomplished. But by having short range goals and accomplishing them, you are able to make what was once seemingly out of reach much closer. The first short range goal was to lose 30 pounds and the second one was to lose 20 pounds; you have now knocked 50 pounds off of your overall goal. At this point, if we were to tell you your long range goal it would only be 35 more pounds until you are at your ideal weight. This seems much more accessible. And if we take these next 35 pounds and create short term goals toward losing them, it would seem like no time at all before you had achieved your ultimate goal.

Short term goals are good for another reason and this is positive reinforcement. You feel like you have done something special each time you reach one of these goals and that's a great feeling. It keeps you motivated to continue doing what you have to in order to make your dream a reality. It also lets you know that what you are doing is working. If it's not broke, don't fix it.

Hang your goals in plain view for yourself for motivation. Place your goals on the refrigerator, at the office, or wherever you may need reminded that you are on a mission. Without any goals you don't have much of anything. Goals are what drive us. The bigger your goals, the harder you work; the harder you work, the more success you will have. Don't be afraid to dream big and have great goals. Biogenesis is more than capable of giving you all you will need to know how to fulfill your fitness goals. Good luck!

IS THIS NORMAL

Normal; adjective, 1. Agreeing with a standard or norm; natural; usual; regular; average. {it is normal to make a mistake sometimes} 2. In good health; not ill or diseased. What is normal; the usual conditions; amount, level etc. [His blood pressure is above normal]

To determine what is normal you must examine your project in a very controlled environment. Unfortunately, determining a norm for being fit would be virtually impossible considering how broadly the definition for being fit has become. An example of what we are saying is that being fit for one person may be viewed as very out of shape for another.

Most of your confusion will occur during Phase One of Biogenesis. Since Phase One Bio Speed Shape is an entry level program, most people don't know what to expect. Some of the claims we make for Bio Speed Shape are: more energy, loss of weight, lowering of blood pressure and cholesterol, and feeling better overall than you ever have before. Although the claims are self explanatory, many of the words and phrases used to guide you through this program will be anything but normal to you. Please do not get discouraged if you don't see things happen as quickly or in the exact manner you expect them to.

It is important for you to understand that there is absolutely no better entry level fitness program in the world than Bio Speed Shape! Bio Speed Shape has been rated the number one entry level fitness program of all time. If you did not previously know this, you do now. It is virtually impossible for someone to follow the Bio Speed Shape program and not see dramatic results. We are not bragging (well, maybe we are a little); we are simply trying to encourage you to have faith and stick with the program as close as you can for a minimum of two weeks and you will be hooked.

Some reasons you may feel like quitting are that you may not feel or see improvement. We promised you more energy. The reason you have no energy now is that you are not active enough in a physical manner to create a mode of building more fuel for your body. Chances are very good that during the first week or two that you may feel a little run down or exhausted. Think about it for a minute. You are going from eating foods that cause you to be fat and sluggish. You also have little or no exercise in your daily routines (and walking is not exercise). And now you are eating healthy and exercising for ten minutes five times a week. Although ten minutes a day sounds easy enough, there is still a good chance that it is a more exercise then you are currently doing. And trust us, you are exercising the entire ten minutes straight.

Associate this with the first time you ever jogged around the block. Your lungs burned, your legs were wobbly and you probably felt like you were about to have a heart attack. But after a week or two, jogging that block becomes much easier and the easier it gets, the more energy you have throughout the day. The same principles apply here. The key is to know that you may encounter being a little more tired at first and that this feeling is NORMAL. Push your self through this period and you will be amazed at the difference Bio Speed Shape will make in your energy levels.

"Having more energy is great but why haven't I lost any weight yet?" This is a simple question with a rather complex answer. Let's first set you straight on our feelings regarding "weight" loss. Weight loss in and of itself is not necessarily a good thing. You can be losing weight and actually be getting fatter. Confused? Don't be. Most people think that as long as they are losing weight then they are on a successful fitness program. This is not always true. In fact, if you are on a program in which you are losing weight at a rate of more then 2-3 pounds a week you are doomed for failure. And if you are on solely a diet to lose weight with no exercise involved, forget about it. You will soon gain your weight back and probably a few extra pounds with it. This is not something that might happen. This is something that will happen. Believe it or not, losing weight on a diet and gaining the weight back has become NORMAL. The reason for so many people failing at their diets and becoming totally frustrated is not usually the individual's fault for lack of effort.

How many times have you or perhaps a friend said, "I seem to be at a sticking point. I'm only eating a small salad and a little bit of fruit and I can't seem to lose any more weight." It takes an extreme amount of effort and will power to be able to make it through day after day eating only salads and fruit. Even the most dedicated dieter will eventually breakdown and pig out. Here is the reason that most people don't just gain the weight they initially lost back, but also additional poundage. During all of that time that you spent eating salads, you deprived your body of crucial protein and amino acids that are needed to maintain muscle. Even though you were losing weight on this diet you were also losing muscle. The more muscle your body has the more calories your body requires to function. By losing some of your muscle on the salad and fruit diet you caused your body to require fewer calories then previously needed. If you were eating 1,500 calories a day and went on a low protein diet, such as salads and fruit, you would initially lose weight. Since protein is what your muscles are comprised of, the weight you were losing was muscle. Now that your body has lost muscle, it needs fewer calories to function. So when you finally break down and go off your diet and go back to eating the way you were before you ever started dieting, you are now overeating more than ever. You no longer have the muscle to require 1,500 calories. Now your body may only have enough muscle to require 1,000 calories.

You can see that by dieting like this over and over you will eventually slow your body's metabolism down to the point that all you have to do is smell a pizza and you'll gain five pounds. Hopefully you now see that no matter what you may have been lead to believe in the past, exercise in the form of resistance training is an absolute must if you are looking to keep those unwanted pounds off for good. The second absolute to remember is that any diet low in protein is just plain stupid. Whoever is inventing these all juice diets or these grapefruit diets have the nutritional knowledge of a monkey. It's very normal to feel frustrated and unmotivated when it comes to starting a new fitness program. It is also normal for you to be prepared for your new program not to work. What we are doing is asking you to be a little abnormal. You should also remember this, muscle weighs more than fat.

When starting the Bio Speed Shape program you are doing two things you probably have not been doing. First, you are now eating enough protein for your body to maintain and even build up a little muscle. Secondly, you are exercising using resistance. Not only is this a great combination for losing fat and shaping and toning your body, it is also the ONLY way. Our suggestion is you weigh and measure yourself before starting the program then hide your scale. Use how you look in the mirror, how you feel and what the tape measure says for determining whether or not Bio Speed Shape is working for you.

Finally consider this. Would you rather lose ten pounds in two weeks and still look fat and flabby, or would you rather lose only five pounds in two weeks but drop a couple inches off of your waist and a couple pant or dress sizes and have the five pound weight loss look more like a fifteen pound weight loss because of the more toned and conditioned muscle? It is much nicer eating four or five meals a day and still losing weight then it is eating a salad and some fruit and be starving all day.

There are no set times or specific numbers we have to give you to indicate normal progress. This is left entirely up to the individual. The more you apply yourself and the closer you follow the instruction of each phase of the Biogenesis program, the faster you will see the results. We provide all of the information and tools you will need but it is up to you to apply them toward your life. The current statistic for the normal American is that he is 15.2 pounds overweight. For the normal female it is 22 pounds. We don't know about you, but this is one area in which we don't mind not being normal.

DEVELOPING A PLAN OF ACTION

In this section we will teach you how to develop a plan of action. A plan of action is crucial if you are to be successful in getting and maintaining your ultimate physique. Dave, as a professional bodybuilder, learned over the years that if he did not have his entire contest preparation written down, then it left too many ways for him to make mistakes. He would have two separate notebooks.

The first notebook would be his plan of action notebook. Before each show he would write down everything that he hoped to accomplish and exactly how he intended to go about doing so. The second notebook would be his log. The log would include all of his daily notes regarding contest preparation. The ideal goal would be to have his plan of action notebook be identical to his log. Although this rarely happened, the two of them usually ended up looking close to one another.

Here is the way you should set up your plan of action. We have already discussed the importance of goal setting. So with this in mind we will start of by writing all of your statistics as they currently read. This should include your current weight and measurements. There are five areas that we recommend you take measurements from: 1)Chest, 2)Arm, 3)Waist, 4)Hips, 5)Thighs.

Start with your chest. Measure directly underneath the armpit around the largest part of the chest and back. The next measurement is the arm. With your arm completely relaxed and hanging to your side you will again measure around the largest part of the arm. Next we will measure the waist. Find the smallest part of your midsection and measure at that point. You want to stand relaxed and not suck in or push out the stomach. Now take the tape measure and measure seven inches down from where you just measured your waist. Seven inches down from your waist is where you measure your hips. Lastly, you measure your thigh at the point where your glutes and hamstrings join. More simply put, you measure your thigh around the largest part, which is usually right beneath your buttocks.

Refer to the illustration to help you locate the exact areas you will be measuring. Remember that it is very important to consistently measure in the exact same spots from week to week in order to get the most accurate measurements. Now that you have your current weight and measurements documented, it is time to write down your goals. Below is a sample of how the first page in your plan of action should look.

Mary Jones	January 1, 2000
Weight: 180 lbs	
Chest	42 1/4 inches
Arm	14 1/4 inches
Waist	36 inches
Hips	46 inches
Thigh	29 3/4 inches

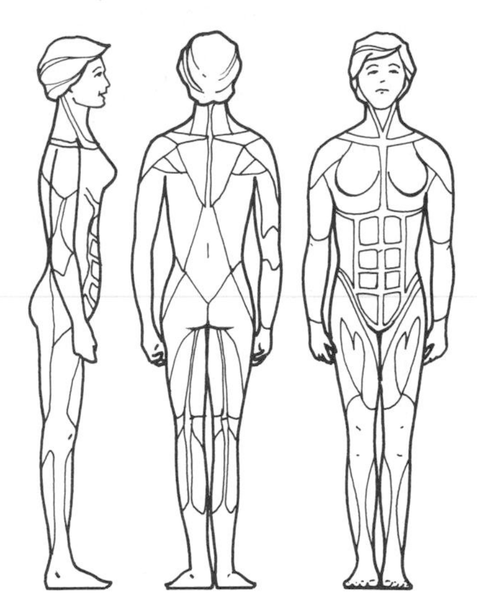

Additional figures you may want to include here are current pant or dress sizes. A man would measure the same areas as a woman, although some men even like to take it a step further and measure body parts such as calves and forearms. For many men, having a potbelly is a major issue so measuring around the belly as opposed to the waist is also an option.

Once you have your current weight and measurements documented then it is time to write down your goals. We'll use Mary Jones as an example again.

Mary Jones	3 month goal	6 month goal	1 year goal
Weight: 180 lbs	160 lbs	140 lbs	125 lbs

One thing that must be emphasized is that your weight and measurements should be viewed as reference points only. That is to say, you should not judge wether or not you are successful with this program by your weight. One of the most common problems we run into while training someone using resistance movements is their infatuation with immediate weight loss. This is probably the single biggest mistake a person could make.

Now that we have your current data along with your goals written down we need to map out your means of execution. If you were building a house and had all of the tools and supplies you would need, constructing your house would still be impossible without blueprints. Blueprints tell you what goes where and why. As you develop a greater understanding of what is involved in building a house you soon realize that without your blueprints, or plan of action, you might as well just rent an apartment. With building such a complex structure as a house you had better know exactly what you are doing and if you don't know anything about electricity then you had better hire an electrician. The same goes for plumbing, roofing and so on.

As complicated as constructing a home is, it pales in comparison to the complexity of the human anatomy. Our bodies are the most amazingly simple and yet complex things in the world. Although we may never know everything there is about the physiological make up of our anatomy, we have made tremendous advancements over the last ten years as far as safe and effective ways to achieve and maintain a more beautiful, healthy physique. As far as we have come, we are still not to the point of being able to lose weight and get into shape without proper diet and exercise, despite what many companies would like you to believe.

However, advancements in vitamins, supplements, and new exercise techniques have made losing weight and shaping up faster and easier than before. Biogenesis is far and away the most advanced and complete fitness program ever. We have gone to great lengths to provide you with all of the very best in every aspect of your fitness needs. We have made it virtually impossible for you to fail if you follow the steps of each phase as closely as you can.

In your plan of action notebook you will need to include steps and items that will ensure your success. Here are some, but not all of, the things you may want to include.

1. The time of day in which you intend on training.
2. Which phase of the Biogenesis program you will start with and when you hope to have advanced to the next level.
3. The foods you will need to buy for the weeks that are included on your diet.
4. The vitamins and supplements you are going to need.
5. Which day of the week you are going to take your weight and measurements.

The following is an actual page from David Dearth's plan of action that he used in preparing for one of his professional bodybuilding contest.

David Dearth

Plan of action for the Arnold Classic bodybuilding contest

Current		Contest goals	
April 1st, 1994		Contest on March 03, 1995	
Weight 240 lbs		Weight 215 lbs	
Body fat:	11%	Body fat:	2.5 %
Chest:	50"	Chest:	50"
Waist:	34"	Waist:	30"
Arm:	20"	Arm:	20"
Quad:	31"	Quads:	29"

Calves:	20"	Calves:	20"

Week 1

Start diet this week. Make sure I get 5 meals in per day. I need to have a protein intake of no less then 300 grams of protein per day, so around 60 grams of protein per meal. This week I will also start my Ultrabody protein powder.

Monday 4/1/94	Weight 240 lbs.
6:00 a.m.	Get up. Coffee and vitamins
6:30 a.m.	Treadmill 30 minutes
7:30 a.m.	Meal #1
	12 egg whites
	6 oz. chicken breast
	1 bagel with fat-free cream cheese and jelly
8:30 a.m.	Leave for work
10:00 a.m.	Protein shake and fat burners
12:00 P.M.	4 cans of water packed tuna
	Supplements
	Broccoli and 1 small potato
2:00 P.M.	Tanning bed 30 minutes
3:00 P.M.	Protein shake
	Fat burners, aminos, energy drink
5:00 P.M.	Leave for home
5:30 P.M.	12 oz. Chicken breast
	1 serving rice
7:00 P.M.	Treadmill 30 min.
7:30 P.M.	Train chest, shoulders and triceps
9:00 P.M.	12 oz. Lean steak
	Fat burners, and supplements
11:00 P.M.	Protein shake
11:30 P.M.	Bed

Things to do today;

01. Call Wayne Demillia to have him mail my contest entry form.
02. Call travel agent to check on flights to New York
03. Pay phone bill and cable bill

04. Try to set up photo shoot for sometime in June with Muscle and Fitness

05. Make out grocery list for the next two weeks

As you can see, David has nearly every minute of his day preplanned. We don't necessarily recommend that you go to this extreme, but if you could put your day into some sort of order it will teach you to become more disciplined and will also help you to incorporate your new fitness program into your life. It seems most people function at a higher level of efficiency when they have their days and weeks mapped out. Remember you can make your plan of action as basic or as detailed as you wish. The important thing is to figure out some sort of way for you to be able to regiment all of the things you learn in each phase of Biogenesis. This will ensure you a solid plan toward achieving your fitness goals.

WHEN WILL I BEGIN TO SEE RESULTS

It would be a contradiction to say everyone will see the same results in the same amount of time. Factors such as what kind of condition you are in when you begin the program and if you have ever done an exercise program before are going to contribute to the time it takes to see results. The amount of intensity that is applied to each workout and how close you follow the nutritional program are also keys.

However, within the first week of starting the Biogenesis program, you should begin to feel better. If you continue to follow your program closely, by the end of the second week, you should have already dropped one size in your jeans or dress. Each week you will continue to see similar results.

When the results begin to slow down one of two things is happening. The first factor could be that you need to increase the intensity level of your exercising. If you are already exercising very hard then it may be time for you to advance to the next phase. Results will come to you in stages. One week you may train very hard and follow your diet precisely and may not lose any weight at all. The next week, doing the exact same thing, you discover that you have lost three pounds and three inches. This is where we emphasize consistency.

Please do not get frustrated if you have one of those weeks where you worked hard and didn't lose anything. It could be one of a hundred different things from stress, to depression, to menstruation. Remember, it is impossible for you to eat right, get the right amount of sleep and exercise correctly without losing weight or shaping up. Don't let one bad week dictate the success or failure of your program. People cheat on their diet for a meal and just blow the whole day off as a failure and continue to eat whatever they want all day long. Using that logic would this same person flatten three tires on their car if they discovered one flat?

Remember that Biogenesis is designed in four phases. You start with the program that is correct for your current physical condition. The Biogenesis diets and supplements are designed to allow you to eat normal, delicious, and healthy food. Our files are overflowing with testimonials from average Americans who tried other diets and workouts and failed. Most of these people initially succeeded on their fad diets, but found themselves in what Frank and Dave call the "Yo-Yo" syndrome. This means they would lose weight and then gain it back as they moved from one fad diet to another.

Biogenesis is designed to stop the "Yo-Yo" syndrome and transform you mentally and physically into a healthy and happy lifestyle.

3

FREQUENTLY ASKED QUESTIONS

1. What kind of exercises do I have to do on the Biogenesis program?

You start at Phase One, called Bio Speed Shape, and do simple resistance exercises that use body weight instead of weight equipment. These exercises include: push-ups, squats, lunges, and crunches. Isometrics also play a part in Bio Speed Shape. There is no fast moving, jumping, or dance choreography to learn.

Phases Two and Three add simple home gym equipment as the exercise intensity increases as do your results. Phase Four is a weight and exercise machine program to be used at a gym or health club.

2. Why do I have to work out on the Phase One, Phase Two, and Phase Three programs everyday?

Many things affect the way our body is shaped and the more times we do them the more likely the change. Duration of exercising does not seem to have as much effect as frequency when we compare both to accumulative time. If we can stimulate our hormonal output everyday in a positive way that makes weight loss occur, weight loss is more successful. This type of frequency develops a behavior pattern which then becomes a habit. When this becomes a habit, working out becomes less of a burden on our daily schedule and then becomes more enjoyable. Also, we take in high levels of psychological and emotional stress every day, so we need to combat these with physical stress that we give off from working out.

3. Why is resistance training better than aerobics for weight loss?

Two reasons: the stronger you get the more work you are able to do, and resistance exercise promotes lean body tissue which, in turn, promotes our metabolism to higher levels. Weight loss occurs when we burn off more energy than we take in from foods, not only when we are exercising. So it makes sense to burn more calories all the time if we want our fat reserves to disappear. Here is something to think about when it comes to facts, every pound of muscle that we add to our bodies will burn roughly 30 calories every twenty-four hours while at rest. That is more than 10,000 calories a year, or the equivalent of 3 pounds of body fat.

4. How do you burn more calories at rest?

By raising our basal metabolic rate with a high protein, low fat diet and resistance training. Our bodies have a series of millions of chemical reactions going on all the time. Calories fuel these reactions and our diet and exercises stimulate the rate of these reactions.

5. Will I get big muscles from Phase One Bio Speed Shape?

No, you won't get big muscles from this program. You will get some muscle from this program, but not like a more intense program like Phases Two, Three, and Phase Four.

6. Do aerobics burn more fat than weight training?

When we compare the two by duration and post exercise calorie burning, the more intense the work load the more calories burned and the higher the post workout calories burning effect. Therefore, resistance training wins hands down.

7. I don't have weights. How do I get resistance with Phase One Bio Speed Shape?

You can get resistance from your own body weight and by opposing forces of other muscle groups. Isometrics are also a form of resistance training.

8. I have arthritis. Can I exercise with Phase One Bio Speed Shape?

Arthritic flare ups are a major concern when activity is introduced to a part of the body that has been known to have arthritis. In general, physical therapy is used quite extensively to combat the effects of arthritis, and a lot of the therapy is based in resistance training. This program is designed so there aren't any fast movements so that all types of people can participate. There are certain days that you can avoid the body part that is affected and still workout the rest of your body.

9. I already work out with weights. Should I do Phase One Bio Speed Shape?

If you are already working out with weights, you already know the powerful effects of this type of training. This is a great program for someone that understands the fundamentals of resistance exercise but sometimes doesn't have time to do their regular workout. If you believe you are experienced, start at a higher Biogenesis phase. Anyone, no matter what level of fitness, can do this program.

10. Am I too old to do Biogenesis?

No one is too old to do this program. Geriatric studies on resistance exercise show dramatic benefits from increased strength, stronger bones, improved circulation and better mental capacities.

11. I don't need to lose weight, can I still do Biogenesis?

Weight loss is only one of the benefits that come from Biogenesis. There are many other benefits that come from this program. Some of them are more energy, higher self-esteem, increased confidence and more strength and flexibility. Everyone can get something from this program, whether it is physical or mental.

12. I walk; should I do Biogenesis on the same day?

Yes, Biogenesis should be done at least five days a week. I would still walk because this program is not a substitute for aerobics; it should compliment aerobics, and the effects are even better when combined.

13. Why do the Phase One and Two programs take only 10 minutes?

There are several reasons. First, the entire body is not exercised every workout, only parts of it every day. Second, Phase One and Two are designed more as entry level programs. And third, exercise duration is not as important as focused intensity for resistance training. If it only takes several minutes to stimulate our bodies to make a physiological change, why do all the extra things that take up too much time and are not effective?

14. I only have fat on my legs. Why should I work my whole body?

If you have a V-8 engine in your car would you want it running only on four or five cylinders? Of course not; think of our muscular system as the engine for our bodies and we are trying to empty out our fuel tanks to make us lighter. The fat that covers muscle on any part of the body is not owned by those muscles alone, and your fat deposits are drained by all parts of your body when fuel is needed.

15. Why is the Fat Flush Diet recommended with Biogenesis?

The Fat Flush Diet is recommended because it supports the nutritional needs that a resistance training program induces. When we do resistance exercise, we are trying to change the composition of tissues that will turn our bodies into a fat burning machine. If we don't supply our bodies with the materials it needs to build and replace muscle tissue that resistance training demands, our metabolism will slow down to conform to the nutrient input levels.

Again, using the car as an example, we may have a V-8 engine in our car but the vehicle may not allow us to burn a great deal of fuel unless we give the car some space to run and the right type of fuel to make it run perfectly.

16. Do I need any special clothing to do Biogenesis?

Having the right clothing to keep you cool during the exercise portions of this program would be a good idea, but is not necessary. As you get into Phase Three and Four, you might want to consider a pair of gloves and maybe a weight training belt. These are merely to protect your hands and back from the repeated lifting and gripping of the equipment. Comfortable clothes and shoes that enable you to move freely while exercising will make the workout more enjoyable. By the time you get to Phase Four, you will probably be wearing very light clothing to show off those results that you are getting anyway!

17. Will I experience pain from this Biogenesis program?

There are several types of pain you may encounter during Biogenesis. Some are perceived and some can actually require medical attention. First, let's start out with the worst case scenario, like getting injured while training. Sprains, strains, and other connective tissue injuries usually happen as a result of trying to do to much of a good thing, or by just not paying attention to what you are doing. In cases like these, the injury could have been avoided if precautionary measures were taken and if safety in exercise execution was high.

The other types of pain, like a lactic acid build up, are actual measures of intensity generated; so the higher that this level is pushed, the higher your level of exertion. Eventually, repetitive exposure to these movements will elevate your pain tolerance and this will not bother you anymore. Then there is pain associated with hard work. This is perceived pain that doing something difficult seems like pain. We have lifted literally tons of steel in single workouts and when we analyzed it, we did not experience pain at all.

There is one last type of pain, and it is delayed muscle soreness. This is a direct result of the intensity of the workout, which causes muscles to be rebuilt and repaired. This can take up to 72 hours to go away. It is not terribly painful. It will actually make you feel good that you were able to control your body and make it change, and sometimes changes are painful.

18. How should I feel after a work out?

The post workout experience is one of the most peaceful times you will probably ever experience. You should eliminate every bit of psychological stress that you had taken in and turn it into physical stress and vent it off. This is a result of endorphins. These are hormones the body produces in response to physical stress. Learn to enjoy this high, or feeling of tranquility, after the workout. It is the short term reward for all your hard effort exercising.

Sometimes you can feel nauseated during the workout and this is a result of what is called "the pump." If large muscle groups are exercised, they will require large amounts of blood to pump away the chemical by-products of muscular contractions, like lactic acid. When this happens, the blood that circulates through the digestive tract will be directed to the muscles that are performing work. The stomach and digestive tract do not like this situation and they makes you nauseated so that digestion can continue and the blood will be returned to them. If this happens, slow the workout down, or rest until the condition is gone. Don't try to work through this situation and keep working out, unless you want to vomit during your workout, which is not advisable.

4

MACRONUTRIENTS

In this Chapter we will go into some detail on protein, carbohydrates, fat, and water; where they come from, how we use and store them in our bodies, and what their functions are. All foods that we eat have at least one of these four macronutrients. We call them macro nutrients because we ingest them in large quantities, sometimes in too many quantities compared to other nutrients like vitamins and minerals.

We eat food for three basic purposes, two of them are for sustaining life and one is for pleasure. Growth, repair, and fuel are the primary uses of food, but when we start using food for pleasure, it is then that we get ourselves into trouble. Food can taste good and stimulate the body into a "feel good state" that many people get satisfaction from that they can get from no other activity or drug. But this is a problem that can lead to abuse of this "feeling." The next thing you know is that it becomes a bad habit that develops into a life style which can then becomes a slow suicide. Eating can be fun and is normally combined with social activities such as going out with friends and family, but anything that is done to extremes can have detrimental effects on one's health.

Using food for its primary functions like development, as a child does to become an adult, and fueling the body to perform activity is why we need to eat. But, food can also create a "feel good state"that can have detrimental side effects of abuse. It is amazing that people will not give up their short term satisfaction derived from food for a longer, healthier, and more active life style. There is so much fun to be had in the world when you are in shape and healthy. To combat the rigors of everyday life, such as an occupation, family, relationships, bills, deadlines, illness, etc., we have to be healthy to get through all daily rigors. If you are not eating the right food, not getting the right nutrition, and not exercising off all of this social stress, you will live a short life, and that is guaranteed. Life is tough, and if you are strong, life will not be as big a burden on you. It all comes down to what you put into your body and what you make your body do that will increase the quality and quantity of life.

The amount of these four nutrient components that we take in will determine what we will look like, how we are shaped, and how we perform and interact with everyone and everything around us. In other parts of this book we discuss the workout sections of this program, and these are important, but what drives all of this activity and the results that you get from it is what goes into your body, and this is the important part of a good nutritional program. Before you start a good nutritional program you must understand why you should be eating correctly. You need to supply your body with the proper nutrients to create an environment for resistance exercise.

So many people are out there trying to lose weight and get in shape doing all of this work and have no nutritional program to support their workout. It is no wonder they get only marginal results. Why would you sabotage yourself after a workout with unhealthy fast food that has no nutritional value which, in effect, results in no progress to your goals of getting in shape? If you wanted to build a house made of bricks that can weather any storm, would you buy cheap materials made from straw and mud? Of course not. You would get the best bricks and mortar and build it with the best design that will last a lifetime. Your body is no different. Now do you understand why it is important to get the right nutritional components?

FAT

With all of that being said, lets look at each one of the macronutrients in detail. First, let's look at fat because of its role in getting you into the poor shape. Fat is a structure that is primarily used for long term fuel storage. For every gram of fat by weight there are nine calories of energy stored in it. We can oxidize protein, carbohydrates and fat for energy, but fat is the densest form of energy storage that we have. Back in the old days before 24 hour drive-thrus and convenient stores this was a good thing to have because it could be days before we ate again. If we could store a whole lot of energy from one meal, we could survive until the next time we ate. Now that we don't have this problem in the 21st century, our fat content does not have to be that high to combat life's necessity to find food. If you ingest high fat foods repetitively, you eventually become fat yourself. This makes sense to us, and it should to you as well. But let's face it, we like the taste of fat and it makes us feel satisfied from a meal. Don't worry, we believe this to be a genetic trait passed down from many thousands of years ago and this can be changed over time with the right food intake.

We also use fat for insulation of our internal organs and from the environmental elements. Fat cushions our internal organs like shock absorbers from impact and trauma. Our bodies can withstand cold and heat changes easier if we have a thicker fatty layer under our skin. This is another survival instinct that our bodies have; but now we have coats, shoes, hats, and heated homes with air conditioning to take care of this problem. So do we really need all of this fat now? Of course not. People that are overweight just don't know what to eat that does not make them fat. We are not saying that eating fat is the main culprit that makes us fat. There are many reasons that will be discussed. Is there any reason why we would want to become fat from purposely eating fatty foods? Not only is your appearance frowned upon by social standards when you are fat, but also your health is going to be affected directly by how much extra body fat that you carry and this has been documented and verified many times. If choosing the wrong foods can cause a premature death then why do we consistently do this? Having a bad diet is a risk factor that anyone can change; and if they knew a better way to eat they would.

So this leads us to finding fat in our food and trying to make better choices to avoid the excess fat. We do need fat in our diet because it has certain fat soluble nutrients in it; but the problem is that we take in way too much fat and cannot burn off the calories that the excess fat contains. We also take in too many carbohydrates that can be converted to fat, which makes us fat too. But we will get into that topic in the carbohydrates section.

There is fat in many foods and some of them are hidden because of our preconceived idea of what fatty foods look like. Obviously deep-fried foods have fat in them because of the way they are prepared. Another obvious food category that has fat in it is meat. You can visually identify the difference between the fat on the meat and the meat itself. Butter should also be an easy fat to spot. But when nuts and seeds are the topic, we would not think that most of the calories come from fat, but they do.

There exists the false notion that just because some fats are more healthy than others, such as saturated fats versus polyunsaturated fats, that it is okay to use them without any regard to the amount used. Dipping bread into olive oil at a restaurant for an appetizer is probably one of the worst things that you could possibly do; and it is not a good idea if weight loss is your goal. Most snack foods like potato chips, corn chips, cheese sticks, etc. look somewhat harmless, but if you read your labels, and you should, you will notice that there is an abundance of calories coming from fat. Not only are some of these foods fattening, but they also don't have any nutritional value when we take into consideration the amounts of vitamins and minerals that they do not have.

Getting enough fat in our diet does not seem to a problem in our present culture so we really don't worry about it. What we don't get enough of, when speaking of fat intake, are fats that are good for us and getting too much fat that is bad for us. The only ways to combat this situation are to stay away from deep-fried foods, foods prepared with lard or margarine in excessive quantities and, if you do cook with fat, try reducing the amount of fat used; use a non-stick spray with non-stick cookware. Also develop the habit of reading labels to educate yourself on what foods you are eating that might have the potential of being high in fat. Even fast food restaurants have nutritional information available. Take advantage of the information and become an educated consumer.

CARBOHYDRATES

If fats are for long term energy storage when we won't have food available, carbohydrates, a class of nutrients different in chemical structure, are used for immediate energy, such as intense exercise. Lately, the diet community has been attacking carbohydrates for being the reason that people are getting fat. This is only partially true. Too many calories of any type will add fat to our bodies, period. The problem with carbohydrates, and storing them, is the fact that your storage space is limited. If your carbohydrate storage capacity is full, additional "carbs" will be converted to fat and stored as fat.

Carbohydrates will not make you fat if you create a stimulus to deplete the reserves of carbohydrates in our body. Exercise is a good stimulus, but resistance exercise is the perfect stimulus. The more intense the exercise, the more you will use carbohydrates as a fuel to produce quick energy for muscular contractions. Then there is room for the intake of more carbohydrates for storage for another workout, without spilling over the carbohydrate storage capacity that will end up as stored fat.

Without carbohydrates our brains cannot function; this is a fact. You will also have zero energy to do physical work and feel tired and listless all the time if you do not take in carbohydrates. The latest diets that have no carbohydrate content and put you into keto-acidosis are some of the most ridiculous ideas that we have heard. Why would you put yourself into a dangerous physical state to lose weight? If weight loss is the objective, you want to give yourself the best nutritional and physical program your body can handle to burn off that extra fuel stored on your body, not put yourself into a potentially life threatening condition to lose weight. The best looking bodies on the planet are not using these dangerous methods, so why do you think that it would be okay for you to do them? These diet fads are actually creating more problems than they are curing.

There are many types of carbohydrates, and without trying to make this topic into rocket science and overwhelming you with technical information about the glycemic indexes of foods, monosaccharides, disaccharides, polysaccharides, and their different effects on storage of carbohydrates, insulin levels, blood sugar levels, fat conversion, and all the interactions between these factors, we are going to make this easy on you. The more processed the carbohydrate is, the more detrimental its effects are on our system. For example, table sugar, a bad glycemic index that causes blood sugars to spike really high, then really low once the body tries to regulate it, causes you to get hungry.

On the other hand, the more complex carbohydrate is better because your system can utilize the fuel and handle storage of it. For example, vegetable sources of carbohydrates, like rice and potatoes, give a nice, long, even stream of sugars into the blood stream without causing high levels of blood sugar that will eventually crash and make you tired and hungry. Keep these two things in mind when selecting your carbohydrate sources that will fuel your exercise and fitness program.

When taking these two points into consideration of carbohydrate selection, we also must look at the vitamin and mineral content of the foods that are in the highly processed group that is not good for you and the complex carbohydrate group that is good for you. It should be noted that the more refined and processed the carbohydrate is, such as simple sugars, the less vitamins and minerals you are going to get from your foods. This is a general rule of thumb and there will be some exceptions to the rule. Fruits will be an exception to some extent; but if given the choice between getting the carbohydrate content and nutrition from an orange or wild rice, we would choose the wild rice.

Remember, carbohydrates are important for a balanced diet. Diets or nutritional plans that eliminate any macronutrient are short term solutions and potentially dangerous. The Biogenesis program provides guidance for a healthy diet combined with resistance exercise.

WATER

Water is one of the most abundant and valuable resources on earth. Every single living thing on the planet uses water for one purpose or another. But people don't seem to get enough of this huge component of the body. Without it we cannot survive. Your brain is 35% water, your blood is 85% water; there is water to some extent in every living cell in your body.

The Biogenesis program advocates lots of water, especially if you are doing the Fat Flush Diet program. It has been recommended that as adults we should get six to 8, 8 ounce glasses of water a day. We believe this to be true for normal health conditions. However, if you incorporate resistance exercise, respiration and sweating are going to increase and so will water loss. Dehydration is a condition you should avoid at all costs. Water doesn't cost much and it won't hurt you to get the extra amount; it will only help.

When our metabolism is turned up from exercise and diet conditions, there is going to be a higher level of chemical reactions going on which will require water to cool the body and transport nutrients in and wastes out of the body. Water also has diuretic properties that will cause you to hold less water when you actually drink more. It even helps with digestion. Water can be very nutritive depending on its source and can have an abundance of trace elements that the body uses. Mineral water is highly nutritive, while distilled water doesn't have any minerals or trace elements in its contents.

Bottled water, filtered water, tap water, carbonated water, mineral water, sparkling water, flavored water, and distilled water – get plenty everyday. You will feel better, and live longer.

PROTEIN

The last macronutrient we will discuss is different in several ways. Protein can serve two purposes for the body and, if you understand its importance, you will be able to manipulate protein to make you lose weight, shape your body with the right curves, increase strength, and increase your ability to burn more calories at rest.

Protein can be used for energy. But its real use is to build the components of your body. Every part of the human body needs protein in one way or another. If "amino acids are the building blocks of life" then protein is the "building" or "structure" that becomes life. When amino acids are put into sequence, or linked together, they form a protein. There are 22 different amino acids that are the "building blocks" and we will discuss these individual amino acids in a later section. To make a simple analogy of the relationship between amino acids and proteins, think of a brick wall being protein and all the different bricks as the amino acids. Think of every structure in your body: skin, blood, brain, heart, muscles, tendons, hair, eyes, finger and toe nails all have protein in them. The only structures that are not made of protein are teeth and bones and they were made by protein. Are you getting the picture as to how important protein is now?

Even as we are developing as a children, we are constantly replacing and rebuilding our body. If we don't supply our body with the needed building materials we wear out, we believe we grow old faster. Some experts think if there are enough of the right nutrients the body needs to process proteins into rebuilding and replacing tissue, we can live to our potential genetic life span which is dictated by another protein, DNA.

Protein has become quite popular in the diet industry, but its importance is obviously more than a weight loss aid. There are several reasons why protein makes a good weight loss component. First, it only has four calories of energy per gram of protein, which is the same as carbohydrates, and half of the amount of fat. You would have to eat more than twice the amount of protein to get the same amount of calories that fat provides. It is inefficient to store extra proteins that we eat, so the body converts it into sugars. Then, if proteins can't be stored or used as sugar, they are converted to fats and stored. But during the conversion to fat, protein loses some of its caloric value. So if you started out with 100 calories of fat to store, it might be converted to only 60 calories of fat because of conversion losses. So by the time you totally convert protein, depending on the type of protein, to stored fat, one gram of protein that was originally worth four calories is now worth two calories of fat. This is one of the ways it will cause weight loss. If we do store it as protein, we normally store it as lean muscular tissue. This creates weight loss by creating muscle tissue that burns a lot of calories just to exist as living tissue. If a need is created to build more muscular tissue that burns more calories, our bodies will burn up its fatty fuel reserves if the fat is not replenished. Biogenesis uses resistance training to create a stimulus that requires the growth and repair of muscular tissue which will create a high rate of energy expenditure. If we don't use protein as fuel for energy, it is used for body structure, and this means that protein really does not have energy value. Remember, it can't be used for both body structure and fuel; it's one or the other. Let's say we eat 1500 calories a day in protein carbohydrates and fats, and 500 calories come from protein. We can expect that some of those protein calories will be made into body structure and not used for energy needs. We can assume that we really did not get to burn 1500 calories for energy needs. Let's say you performed a workout on that same day that requires 125 grams of protein to repair your muscles that were damaged as a result of the workout. You now only have 1000 calories for the energy system. This is the biggest reason why men can consume more calories than women and not get as fat. Men have more muscle than women of the same body weight in their natural state. But, if either men or women increase their muscular weight through resistance training, they will burn more calories and use more protein for body structure instead of energy.

There are a few other minor reasons why protein makes a good diet component but the three reasons that are mentioned here, energy conversion loss, highly metabolic tissue storage, and structure usage instead of energy usage, make up 90% of the reasons why it works so well. These are some of the main reasons that Biogenesis works so well.

The only problem that occurs with the high consumption of protein is the fat that usually is associated with the foods. There are many sources of protein and most of them are animal products. It seems that the protein rich foods available to us, and the ones that we prefer, tend to have higher amounts of fat in them. But, if you know where to look for good low fat sources of protein, you can make giant gains in changing your physique. Another option is to supplement your diet with high protein nutrition bars and protein shakes, like our Ultrabody line of supplements. The latter are the most efficient and effective way to do this without getting the fat with your protein.

If you go the route of lean or low fat foods that fit this bill, some of the best protein sources are: egg whites, chicken breast, fish, skim milk, and extra lean cuts of beef and pork. Another thing to consider when using these items is how you prepare them. If you use breading or deep-frying for taste you are going to increase the fat content dramatically and defeat the purpose of trying to reduce the fat. Baking, broiling, grilling, and pan frying with low fat cooking spray are the best ways to prepare these items without adding fat. Use the protein table to find the best protein sources.

Proteins, carbohydrates and fats all have their roles in metabolism. If you know how to manipulate these components with your selection of foods, you can make a big difference in how you look and feel immediately. If you use this information in conjunction with an exercise program, like the Biogenesis program, you will transform yourself into only what you thought others could do. Knowledge of nutrition and the application of that knowledge can be powerful tools that can radically change your lifestyle, health, and your quality of life. It has been proven over and over by many satisfied clients of the Biogenesis program, and you are next.

Foods ranked by least amount of calories and fat to get one ounce of protein

Column A	Column B	When you take in the amount of food in Column B you will take in this amount of calories, fat, carbohydrates and protein.			
To get 1 ounce (28.35 grams) of protein from this food	You need to eat this amount of this food	Calories	Fat	Carbohydrates	Protein
UltraBody Super-food Optimized Whey Protein	1.2 oz.	129.6	0.0 gms.	.3 gms.	1 oz.
Egg whites	8.4 oz.	133.0	0.0 gms.	1.5 gms.	1 oz.
Tuna in water	3.9 oz.	133.0	0.9 gms.	0.0 gms.	1 oz.
Broiled cod	4.3 oz.	133.0	.9 gms.	0.0 gms.	1 oz.
Orange roughy	5.3 oz.	133.0	1.4 gms.	0.0 gms.	1 oz.
Skinless chicken breast	3.2 oz.	136.0	3.2 gms.	0.0 gms.	1 oz.
Couscous	7.3 oz.	137.0	0.2 gms.	28.3 gms.	1 oz.
Skinless turkey breast	5.3 oz.	140.0	4.8 gms.	0.0 gms.	1 oz.
Crab	5.2 oz.	141.0	2.2 gms.	0.0 gms.	1 oz.
Designer Protein, the best protein powder sold in stores	1.3 oz.	155.0	2.1 gms.	5.2 gms.	1 oz.
Shrimp	4.9 oz.	147.0	2.5 gms.	1.3 gms.	1 oz.
Beef round steak	3.5 oz.	167.0	5.2 gms.	0.0 gms.	1 oz.
Lean veal	2.9 oz.	170.0	5.4 gms.	0.0 gms.	1 oz.
Turkey breast with skin	3.0 oz.	175.0	8.2 gms.	0.0 gms.	1 oz.
Beef sirloin steak	3.3 oz.	178.0	6.3 gms.	0.0 gms.	1 oz.
Chicken breast	3.3 oz.	187.0	7.3 gms.	1.5 gms.	1 oz.
Ham	5.2 oz.	192.0	7.6 gms.	6.0 gms.	1 oz.
Beef flank steak	3.4 oz.	198.0	9.7 gms.	0.0 gms.	1 oz.
Whey powder	2.0 oz.	202.0	1.7 gms.	18.1 gms.	1 oz.
Canadian bacon	4.2 oz.	216.0	9.8 gms.	1.5 gms.	1 oz.
Beef T-bone steak	3.6 oz.	216.0	10.5 gms.	0.0 gms.	1 oz.
Ham	4.4 oz.	223.0	11.3 gms.	0.0 gms.	1 oz.
Cottage Cheese	8.0 oz.	235.0	10.5 gms.	6.5 gms.	1 oz.
Lean pork	3.5 oz.	246.0	13.8 gms.	0.0 gms.	1 oz.
Lasagna	16.0 oz.	252.0	12.1 gms.	72.7 gms.	1 oz.
Tofu	6.3 oz.	260.0	8.4 gms.	3.2 gms.	1 oz.
Skim milk	29.2 oz.	261.0	1.4 gms.	40.1 gms.	1 oz.
Fried chicken	3.5 oz.	266.0	14.7 gms.	3.2 gms.	1 oz.
Sausage	4.7 oz.	268.0	16.8 gms.	0.8 gms.	1 oz.
Chicken breast with skin	4.0 oz.	275.0	17.3 gms.	0.0 gms.	1 oz.
Ground beef	3.9 oz.	285.0	18.2 gms.	0.0 gms.	1 oz.
Meatloaf	5.8 oz.	302.0	15.2 gms.	12.7 gms.	1 oz.
Turkey w/gravy	16.9 oz.	320.0	12.5 gms.	22.2 gms.	1 oz.
Chop suey	9.6 oz.	327.0	18.5 gms.	13.9 gms.	1 oz.
Pork chops	3.7 oz.	327.0	22.9 gms.	0.0 gms.	1 oz.
Scallops	5.5 oz.	339.0	17.2 gms.	15.7 gms.	1 oz.
Boiled egg	7.9 oz.	347.0	23.9 gms.	2.7 gms.	1 oz.
Low fat yogurt	20.6 oz.	361.0	10.3 gms.	38.7 gms.	1 oz.
Mushrooms	50.0 oz.	362.7	8.1 gms.	64.8 gms.	1 oz.
Beef stew	15.6 oz.	393.0	18.9 gms.	27.4 gms.	1 oz.
Chicken noodle	12.9 oz.	394.0	19.4 gms.	27.1 gms.	1 oz.
Salisbury steak	10.0 oz.	402.0	24.4 gms.	17.0 gms.	1 oz.
Beef veg. soup	51.4 oz.	405.0	12.9 gms.	44.4 gms.	1 oz.
Red kidney beans	11.4 oz.	414.0	1.7 gms.	74.4 gms.	1 oz.
Lima beans	12.8 oz.	418.8	1.4 gms.	75.8 gms.	1 oz.
Swiss cheese	4.5 oz.	420.0	31.1 gms.	5.9 gms.	1 oz.
Ham & cheese omelet	6.9 oz.	422.0	29.3 gms.	11.1 gms.	1 oz.

Foods ranked by least amount of calories and fat to get one ounce of protein

Column A	Column B	When you take in the amount of food in Column B you will take in this amount of calories, fat, carbohydrates and protein.			
To get 1 ounce (28.35 grams) of protein from this food	You need to eat this amount of this food	Calories	Fat	Carbohydrates	Protein
Stuffed green pepper	14.4 oz.	431.0	18.5 gms.	38.6 gms.	1 oz.
Roast beef sandwich	6.5 oz.	456.0	18.2 gms.	44.2 gms.	1 oz.
Navy beans	11.4 oz.	463.6	1.7 gms.	85.7 gms.	1 oz.
Chef salad	16.1 oz.	467.0	33.0 gms.	14.7 gms.	1 oz.
Pinto beans	12.1 oz.	474.7	1.6 gms.	88.6 gms.	1 oz.
Ham & cheese sand.	7.1 oz.	483.0	21.2 gms.	45.6 gms.	1 oz.
Refried beans	15.9 oz.	483.0	48.3 gms.	83.7 gms.	1 oz.
Chicken nuggets	6.0 oz.	486.0	29.7 gms.	26.0 gms.	1 oz.
Bran	7.0 oz.	496.0	7.0 gms.	155.9 gms.	1 oz.
Hamburger	6.1 oz.	504.0	28.9 gms.	32.1 gms.	1 oz.
Spaghetti w/meatballs	13.3 oz.	506.0	17.8 gms.	58.9 gms.	1 oz.
Taco	8.3 oz.	507.0	28.2 gms.	36.6 gms.	1 oz.
Cheeseburger	7.1 oz.	522.0	24.9 gms.	47.0 gms.	1 oz.
Peas	18.4 oz.	523.4	2.1 gms.	75.6 gms.	1 oz.
Bacon cheeseburger	6.0 oz.	524.0	30.8 gms.	32.9 gms.	1 oz.
Bacon	3.3 oz.	533.0	24.9 gms.	47.0 gms.	1 oz.
Sausage	5.1 oz.	535.0	44.9 gms.	1.6 gms.	1 oz.
Special K	5.0 oz.	557.0	0.5 gms.	107.8 gms.	1 oz.
Celery	133.3 oz.	567.0	9.4 gms.	283.5 gms.	1 oz.
Ham salad	10.6 oz.	567.0	34.0 gms.	22.7 gms.	1 oz.
Baked beans	19.3 oz.	580.0	8.4 gms.	109.5 gms.	1 oz.
Chicken sandwich	7.6 oz.	606.0	34.7 gms.	45.5 gms.	1 oz.
Slim Fast	31.2 oz.	625.0	8.5 gms.	114.0 gms.	1 oz.
Smoked sausage	7.0 oz.	631.0	53.9 gms.	4.9 gms.	1 oz.
Cucumber	173.3 oz.	661.5	9.4 gms.	141.7 gms.	1 oz.
Chicken salad	6.4 oz.	666.0	39.9 gms.	18.2 gms.	1 oz.
Power Bar	6.7 oz.	667.0	5.8 gms.	130.0 gms.	1 oz.
Peanut butter	4.1 oz.	674.0	57.4 gms.	23.7 gms.	1 oz.
Boost	24.1 oz.	683.0	11.6 gms.	116.6 gms.	1 oz.
Quaker oats	39.0 oz.	684.0	11.3 gms.	118.9 gms.	1 oz.
Peanuts	4.2 oz.	704.0	59.7 gms.	25.8 gms.	1 oz.
Wheat bread	10.4 oz.	720.0	12.9 gms.	134.6 gms.	1 oz.
Fried fish sandwich	9.3 oz.	723.0	38.2 gms.	68.8 gms.	1 oz.
Mac & cheese	11.9 oz.	726.0	37.5 gms.	67.8 gms.	1 oz.
Bologna	8.2 oz.	729.0	65.8 gms.	2.0 gms.	1 oz.
Whey	8.0 oz.	737.0	2.8 gms.	158.7 gms.	1 oz.
Beef salami	7.9 oz.	743.0	67.4 gms.	3.9 gms.	1 oz.
Vienna sausage	9.4 oz.	750.0	66.7 gms.	5.0 gms.	1 oz.
Enchilada	19.8 oz.	764.0	36.8 gms.	79.2 gms.	1 oz.
Bagel	9.1 oz.	770.0	6.6 gms.	146.0 gms.	1 oz.
Baked beans	18.0 oz.	772.0	26.2 gms.	109.2 gms.	1 oz.
Corn dog	10.4 oz.	776.0	31.9 gms.	94.1 gms.	1 oz.
Ensure	25.0 oz.	780.0	18.4 gms.	124.8 gms.	1. oz.
Oyster stew	114.8 oz.	797.0	51.3 gms.	55.3 gms.	1 oz.
Hot dog	8.8 oz.	800.0	72.8 gms.	6.7 gms.	1 oz.
English muffin	12.7 oz.	850.0	6.9 gms.	165.1 gms.	1 oz.
Chili	67.6 oz.	850.0	67.6 gms.	30.5 gms.	1 oz.
Scalloped potatoes	34.8 oz.	850.5	36.4 gms.	106.9 gms.	1 oz.
Egg/sausage biscuit	9.4 oz.	859.0	57.1 gms.	60.8 gms.	1 oz.
Rye bread	11.9 oz.	891.0	12.1 gms.	162.0 gms.	1 oz.

Foods ranked by least amount of calories and fat to get one ounce of protein

Column A	Column B	When you take in the amount of food in Column B you will take in this amount of calories, fat, carbohydrates and protein.			
To get 1 ounce (28.35 grams) of protein from this food	You need to eat this amount of this food	Calories	Fat	Carbohydrates	Protein
Sloppy Joes	18.0 oz.	897.0	63.7 gms.	54.3 gms.	1 oz.
White bread	12.0 oz.	904.0	12.8 gms.	165.8 gms.	1 oz.
Pancakes	17.9 oz.	910.0	11.9 gms.	181.5 gms.	1 oz.
Mountain trail mix	10.0 oz.	921.0	12.1 gms.	216.5 gms.	1 oz.
Shredded Wheat	9.0 oz.	932.0	0.5 gms.	206.5 gms.	1 oz.
Corn	30.3 oz.	934.5	11.5 gms.	216.3 gms.	1 oz.
Angel food cake	12.5 oz.	952.0	0.6 gms.	211.0 gms.	1 oz.
Pizza thin crust	16.8 oz.	955.0	13.7 gms.	179.1 gms.	1 oz.
Grape Nuts	9.0 oz.	960.0	0.9 gms.	211.1 gms.	1 oz.
Cream chick. soup	71.8 oz.	967.0	61.7 gms.	77.6 gms.	1 oz.
Cream of Wheat	64.8 oz.	977.0	3.9 gms.	203.2 gms.	1 oz.
French toast	13.1 oz.	979.0	51.7 gms.	99.1 gms.	1 oz.
Frozen mixed vegs.	34.9 oz.	991.9	1.0 gms.	129.7 gms.	1 oz.
Clam chowder	110.9 oz.	993.0	28.6 gms.	157.2 gms.	1 oz.
Waffles	10.9 oz.	1006.0	51.8 gms.	105.5 gms.	1 oz.
Almonds	6.1 oz.	1029.0	90.6 gms.	42.5 gms.	1 oz.
Chicken potpie	13.2 oz.	1040.0	68.0 gms.	73.7 gms.	1 oz.
Wheaties	10.4 oz.	1050.0	5.2 gms.	237.3 gms.	1 oz.
Cashews	6.4 oz.	1050.0	85.0 gms.	59.9 gms.	1 oz.
Granola	8.0 oz.	1118.0	62.3 gms.	126.3 gms.	1 oz.
Tomato soup	116.1 oz.	1161.0	25.6 gms.	224.1 gms.	1 oz.
Beef potpie	16.5 oz.	1204.0	77.9 gms.	92.0 gms.	1 oz.
Carrot	102.9 oz.	1255.5	4.0 gms.	295.6 gms.	1 oz.
Parmigiana	24.3 oz.	1297.9	80.6 gms.	114.2 gms.	1 oz.
Baked potato	42.9 oz.	1326.6	1.2 gms.	307.5 gms.	1 oz.
Stuffing	22.7 oz.	1340.0	82.4 gms.	126.9 gms.	1 oz.
Fried rice	29.0 oz.	1346.0	7.1 gms.	290.0 gms.	1 oz.
Pumpkin pie	24.8 oz.	1485.0	78.9 gms.	171.9 gms.	1 oz.
Blueberry muffin	16.7 oz.	1488.0	50.8 gms.	230.3 gms.	1 oz.
Coleslaw	75.0 oz.	1488.4	56.4 gms.	265.8 gms.	1 oz.
Potato salad	36.7 oz.	1492.8	85.9 gms.	116.7 gms.	1 oz.
White rice	41.1 oz.	1508.0	41.5 gms.	250.0 gms.	1 oz.
Mashed potatoes	52.4 oz.	1572.8	62.3 gms.	247.9 gms.	1 oz.
Cheesecake	18.5 oz.	1583.0	100.4 gms.	149.7 gms.	1 oz.
Vanilla ice cream	28.7 oz.	1628.0	90.0 gms.	191.1 gms.	1 oz.
Sugar coated almonds	12.7 oz.	1662.0	68.2 gms.	256.3 gms.	1 oz.
Baked potato w/sour cream	45.1 oz.	1667.0	94.4 gms.	211.6 gms.	1 oz.
Sweet potato	56.9 oz.	1672.0	1.4 gms.	392.5 gms.	1 oz.
Peanut brittle	13.3 oz.	1728.0	72.9 gms.	265.9 gms.	1 oz.
Hershey bar	12.6 oz.	1928.0	109.3 gms.	206.3 gms.	1 oz.
Onion rings	22.4 oz.	2107.0	118.7 gms.	239.8 gms.	1 oz.
M&M's candy	16.0 oz.	2164.0	100.1 gms.	309.0 gms.	1 oz.
French fries	24.9 oz.	2238.8	117.6 gms.	283.4 gms.	1 oz.
Hash browns	37.9 oz.	2253.0	137.3 gms.	241.7 gms.	1 oz.
Potato chips	15.6 oz.	2331.0	159.1 gms.	231.5 gms.	1 oz.
Raisins	25.0 oz.	2764.0	106.3 gms.	481.9 gms.	1 oz.
Peppermint patty	33.0 oz.	3250.0	85.0 gms.	732.8 gms.	1 oz.
Apple pie	51.1 oz.	3638.0	143.3 gms.	574.9 gms.	1 oz.
Chocolate fudge	56.7 oz.	6143.0	132.3 gms.	1275.7 gms.	1 oz.

5

MICRONUTRIENTS: VITAMINS AND MINERALS

Vitamins and minerals are micronutrients that the body uses every day for normal everyday functioning of the body. The human machine is a very complex organization of chemical reactions that use many different kinds of elements for ongoing life processes, and vitamins and minerals play a big part in these chemical reactions. If there is a deficiency in one or more of these vitamins or minerals some of the functions of the body can be halted, which can cause disease or some malfunction of bodily systems that can cause death or extreme sickness. It is understood that by replacing these nutrients through our diet and supplementation, we can restore our normal body functioning and keep our health at an optimum level.

Experts on health and fitness all agree that vitamins and minerals supplied by our diet and supplements will help prevent disease, but there is still some controversy as to how much of these nutrients we should have every day. Recommended Daily Allowance's (RDA's) were established many years ago and are still used today. Lately, there have been new thoughts on how much of these nutrients should be taken in depending on your life style, age, sex, health risk factors, and activity level. In our opinion they are like other resources the body uses and needs, the more you use up, the more you should take in.

If we think of the body as a car, it is made up of many components: an engine, tires, transmission, suspension, electrical system, etc. All of these parts rely on the others to make the car go, but these individual parts rely on smaller parts that make these individual units work. Tires need the correct amount of air, the engine needs the correct spark plugs and fuel, and the suspension has to have the right shocks. All of these components will work to some extent if worn out, but if replaced or renewed with the right calibration and adjustments the car works very efficiently and lasts a long time. Our bodies are really no different in this respect except that the human machine is extremely complex; to operate at the maximum it has to have vitamins and minerals on a continual basis.

There are 18 vitamins and 22 minerals that are recognized by nutritional experts as essential, and we have to have them for healthy body functions. Experts say that there are more than ninety elements the body uses. These elements include trace minerals, electrolytes, essential amino acids, fatty acids, etc. Suggested intakes are not established yet for some of these nutrients.

Vitamins differ from minerals in several ways. Plants, bacteria and other life forms make vitamins from combinations of different chemical elements and are considered organic because they contain at lest one carbon atom in their structure. With few exceptions, vitamins must be supplied by an outside source, and those exceptions that are made inside the body have components that are from an outside source. Each vitamin has its own disease or symptoms from deficiencies and can be corrected if replaced.

Minerals, on the other hand, are not considered organic and cannot be made by living systems. We do get our intake mostly from plants and animals that have a high intake of mineral rich plants like vitamins. Although the source is the same for vitamins and minerals, vitamins tend to have a fairly consistent content, whereas the content of minerals will vary upon the region the plant or animal came from because of the mineral content of the soil or environment.

Minerals work through a variety of mechanisms, from the basic parts of body structures like teeth and bones to the involvement of energy metabolism. Electrolyte minerals regulate water balance and are responsible for the transmission of electric impulses across cell membranes. Some minerals are needed in large quantities and are deemed essential for life. Some are needed in such small amounts that there is little scientific information as to what they actually do, but are still present in the body.

As you can see, vitamins and minerals play vital roles in our life systems that we take for granted. It only makes sense to make sure that we have adequate amounts of these nutrients at all times so that we can live our lives to their fullest extent. The thing to realize with this simple thought is that we get most of our intake of these substances from the foods we eat and if our diet is diminished in quantity, such as with traditional lower calorie diets, we should also expect to lower our nutritional intake as well. This poses a large problem that can lead to nutritional deficiencies that could cause health problems; and if weight loss, or fat loss, is our goal, our health will be compromised as a result. What most of us do not understand is that vitamin and mineral deficits will reduce our metabolism which, in turn, will make it harder to lose those unwanted pounds. This seems to be a catch twenty-two situation unless we do some sort of supplementation to our diet without adding the calories from our normal food intake that can lead to weight gain.

So what is the solution? There are several solutions to this problem of optimum nutrition for weight loss situations. First and foremost we should educate ourselves about our own nutritional habits and find out what foods are the most nutrient rich. Second, supplementation of our diet with a full spectrum of the known vitamin/mineral/trace mineral tablets, capsules or liquids is a good idea. This is not saying that a poor diet can be replaced by supplements alone because a poor diet lacks other things that are needed in the body that can only come from food. One thing to remember also when supplementing is that too much of anything can be bad; and mega-dosing with vitamins and minerals can lead to toxicity which can cause health problems and be expensive. Another option is prepackaged meals that are specifically designed for a nutritious diet, but anything that is already made for you tends to be expensive. The best solution is to educate and plan. Think of your diet in strategic terms of how can you get the most nutrition to make your body look the way you want it to. Plan what foods you are going to consume and plan what supplements you are going to take. Even the best diets in the world are deficient in the basic RDA's of some vitamins and minerals. If you think that you don't need supplements, have a registered dietician look at your meal plan for several days and they will show you otherwise.

VITAMINS

Vitamins are categorized as water-soluble or fat-soluble. This means that they dissolve either in water or fat. Water-soluble vitamins are B1(thiamin), B2 (riboflavin), B3 (niacin or nicotinic acid), B5 (pantothenic acid), B6 (pyridoxine), B12 (cyanocobalamin), B17 (laetrile nitrilosides) C (ascorbic acid), biotin, and folic acid. These vitamins are easily absorbed in the gastrointestinal tract and the blood stream and do not require any assistance from other substances for their absorption. They are not stored in large quantities in the circulating body fluids and excess are excreted through our urine.

Fat-soluble vitamins are A, D, E, and K. They are stored in our fatty tissues and need special carrier proteins to transfer them to areas of the body that need them. Absorption of fat soluble vitamins needs bile acids to help with transfer to the blood steam. These vitamins can accumulate very easily and can reach toxic levels because we cannot excrete them as easily as water soluble vitamins.

VITAMIN A (FAT-SOLUBLE)

Vitamin A establishes healthy skin and mucous membranes. Line of defense against invading toxins. Part of the powerful antioxidant group of nutrients. When grouped with beta-carotene can destroy carcinogens.

NATURAL SOURCES: Carrots, fish liver oils, liver, green leafy vegetables.

THERAPEUTIC USES: Acne, allergies, asthma, bronchitis, colds, diabetes and vision deterioration.

RDA: 5,000 I.U.

VITAMIN B1 (THIAMIN)

Should be consumed daily since this water-soluble vitamin leaves the body each day. Thiamin burns carbohydrates for energy.

NATURAL SOURCES: Whole grains, brewer's yeast, wheat germ, rice, seeds and milk.

THERAPEUTIC USES: Diabetes, heart disease, mental illness, nausea, stress.

RDA: 1.5 mg

VITAMIN B2 (RIBOFLAVIN)

Water-soluble Riboflavin helps the mitochondria of muscle cells to produce energy. Critical for weight management.

NATURAL SOURCES: Liver, cheese, fish, eggs, seeds and cooked leafy vegetables.

THERAPEUTIC USES: Baldness, hypoglycemia, nausea, stress, weight control.

RDA: 1.7 mg

VITAMIN B3 (NIACIN)

A water-soluble vitamin that works in the energy cycle and in tissue respiration. A dosage over 30mg may cause a "niacin flush" which is uncomfortable but not toxic. Some research suggests this technique can be used to break through migraine headaches.

NATURAL SOURCES: Meat, poultry, fish, eggs, rice and sunflower seeds.

THERAPEUTIC USES: Acne, diarrhea, leg cramps, migraines, poor circulation.

RDA: 19 mg

VITAMIN B5 (PANTOTHENIC ACID)

Used in energy metabolism. Produces brain neurotransmitters and natural body steroid hormones.

NATURAL SOURCES: Beef, eggs, vegetables, legumes, saltwater fish and whole wheat.

THERAPEUTIC USES: Arthritis, depression, fatigue, stress, migraines.

RDA: 6mg

VITAMIN B6 (PYRIDOXINE)

Used in the formation of body proteins and amino acid metabolism. Important for mucous membranes, the immune system, skin, red blood cells, and brain chemistry.

NATURAL SOURCES: Bananas, wheat germ, cantaloupe, eggs, beef and green leafy vegetables.

THERAPEUTIC USES: Allergies, anemia, bursitis, fatigue, insomnia, stress.

RDA: 2.0 mg

VITAMIN B9 (FOLIC ACID)

Critical in cellular division and DNA synthesis. Found to reduce birth defects and the U.S. Center for Disease Control recommends that all women of childbearing age supplement their diet with folic acid.

NATURAL SOURCES: Brewer's yeast, mushrooms, liver, broccoli, asparagus, lima beans and green leafy vegetables.

THERAPEUTIC USES: Baldness, constipation, heart disease.

RDA: 400 mcg

VITAMIN B12 (COBALAMIN)

Increases energy and promotes growth. Commonly deficient in elderly patients. Also regulates red blood cell formation.

NATURAL SOURCES: Comfrey leaves, bananas, peanuts, grapes, beef, pork and milk.

THERAPEUTIC USES: Arrhythmia, depression, eczema, leg cramps.

RDA: 2mcg

VITAMIN B17 (LAETRILE NITRILOSIDES)

Research suggests B17 has Cancer controlling and prevention capabilities.

NATURAL SOURCES: Peach and plum pits, lima beans, garbanzos, blackberries, millet and flaxseed.

THERAPEUTIC USES: Cancer

RDA: Not established.

BIOTIN

A B complex vitamin used to form enzymes. Research suggests a link between Biotin and hair and nail growth. Important for fat metabolism.

NATURAL SOURCES: Brewer's yeast, fruits, nuts, rice, egg yolk, milk and kidney.

THERAPEUTIC USES: alcoholism, heart trouble, high blood pressure.

RDA: 30 mcg to 100 mcg mg

CHOLINE

A fat metabolizer. Also improves your memory and is used to treat Alzheimer's.

NATURAL SOURCES: Wheat germ, egg yolk, liver, and green leafy vegetables.

THERAPEUTIC USES: Alcoholism, anemia, fatigue, stress.

RDA: Not established.

INOSITOL

Another fat metabolizer. Reduces cholesterol levels. Provides a calming effect.

NATURAL SOURCES: Beef brains, cabbage, citrus fruits, raisins, whole grains, lecithin and unrefined molasses.

THERAPEUTIC USES: Baldness, eczema, high blood pressure, high cholesterol.

RDA: Not established.

VITAMIN C (ASCORBIC ACID)

An antioxidant, minimizes oxidative damage to DNA. Also prevents cancer by neutralizing nitrates that are shown to cause cancer. Protects the heart muscle. Delays cataracts. Has been proven time and again to prevent numerous diseases.

NATURAL SOURCES: Citrus fruits, black currants, tomatoes, sweet potatoes, and green bell peppers.

THERAPEUTIC USES: Alcoholism, arthritis, colds, diabetes, hepatitis, stress, tooth decay.

RDA: 60 mg

VITAMIN D (ERGOSTEROL, FAT-SOLUBLE)

Maintains the nervous system. Induces normal blood clotting.

NATURAL SOURCES: Butter, egg yolks, fish liver oils, sardines, salmon, mushrooms and sunflower seeds.

THERAPEUTIC USES: Acne, allergies, cystitis, psoriasis.

RDA: 200 I.U. to 400 I.U.

VITAMIN E (TOCOPHEROL, FAT-SOLUBLE)

An antioxidant that prevents the oxidation of fats by free radicals. Fights heart disease, cancer and respiratory problems. Keeps skin moist and youthful. Used for anti-aging.

NATURAL SOURCES: Wheat germ, brussel sprouts, leafy greens, vegetable oils and eggs.

THERAPEUTIC USES: Allergies, blood clots, diabetes, migraines, myopia, stress, sterility, varicose veins, warts.

RDA: 10 I.U.

VITAMIN K (MENADIONE, FAT-SOLUBLE)

Vitamin K helps the liver deposit minerals into the bone matrix. Also helps prevent blood clots.

NATURAL SOURCES: Alfalfa, leafy green vegetables, kelp, fish liver oil and yogurt.

THERAPEUTIC USES: colitis, gall stones, menstrual problems, preparing women for childbirth.

RDA: 80 mcg

PABA

Helps protect your skin from sunburn and skin cancer. Assists in the formation of red blood cells.

NATURAL SOURCES: Kidney, liver, molasses, spinach and whole grain.

THERAPEUTIC USES: Skin disease, graying hair, nervousness.

RDA: Not established.

BIOFLAVONOIDS

Found in vegetables. This large family of compounds is grouped under vitamins but has yet to be formally identified.

NATURAL SOURCES: Buckwheat, cabbage, egg yolks, sesame seeds, sauerkraut, and the white skins and segment parts of all citrus fruits.

THERAPEUTIC USES: Asthma, colds, hemophilia, ulcers and varicose veins.

RDA: Not established

MINERALS

Minerals are different from vitamins in several ways such as coming from the earth, not being made by living systems, and their contribution to body parts for structures like bones and teeth. Another interesting thing about minerals is the differences in the mineral content in the plants themselves are not constant. The mineral content of the plant has more to do with the content of the soil it is grown in. So if the soil is rich or depleted, the mineral content of the plant will vary.

Of the 22 minerals listed in this chapter some have RDA's and others do not. This is because not all is known about some of the minerals and their functions, which makes it hard to determine how much is needed. In this part of the chapter the sources, functions, and deficiencies of minerals will be discussed.

Minerals are critical for your body. Vitamins and amino acids are useless without minerals which provide for all enzyme activities. Minerals maintain the cellular fluid balance, form bone and blood cells, and regulate muscle tone and activity. Primarily stored in your bone and muscle tissue, minerals also provide for electrochemical nerve activity.

BORON

NATURAL SOURCES: Cheese, dark leafy vegetables, sardines, salmon and sesame seeds.

FUNCTIONS: Essential for hormones in bone metabolism. Also balances estrogen and testosterone.

MEDICAL USES: Arthritis, fatigue, depression and migraine headaches.

RDA: Not established.

CALCIUM

NATURAL SOURCES: Cheese, dark leafy vegetables, sardines, salmon and sesame seeds.

FUNCTIONS: Critical for bone and tooth formation, heart rhythm, and muscle growth. Contained in bones, teeth, nails, blood, heart, and skin.

MEDICAL USES: Backache, insomnia, menopause, nervousness and rheumatism.

RDA: 1,200 mg

CHROMIUM

NATURAL SOURCES: Brewer's yeast, chicken, clams, corn oil, meat and shell fish.

FUNCTIONS: Assists in weight loss and increases lean body mass. Metabolizes glucose and insulin for energy.

MEDICAL USES: Acne, diabetes, hypoglycemia and weight loss.

RDA: 50 mcg to 200 mcg

COBALT

NATURAL SOURCES: Clams, green leafy vegetables, liver, milk, oysters and red meat.

FUNCTIONS: Important for hemoglobin formation in your blood.

MEDICAL USES: Anemia and retardation.

RDA: 3 mcg to 4 mcg

COPPER

NATURAL SOURCES: Almonds, beans, legumes, beef liver, green leafy vegetables, oysters and prunes.

FUNCTIONS: Important in building bones and making blood. Used in developing hair and skin color. Also important in the general healing process of the body.

MEDICAL USES: Arthritis, chronic fatigue and skin dryness.

RDA: 1.5 mg to 3.0 mg

FLUORIDE

NATURAL SOURCES: Carrots, fluoridated drinking water, garlic, milk and seafood.

FUNCTIONS: Reduces tooth decay and strengthens bones.

MEDICAL USES: Bone growth and tooth decay.

RDA: Not established.

GERMANIUM

NATURAL SOURCES: Aloe, comfrey, chorella, garlic, ginseng and watercress.

FUNCTIONS: The mineral Germanium carries oxygen to the cells. This process helps fight pain and flush the body of toxins.

MEDICAL USES: Anemia and arthritis.

RDA: Not established.

IODINE

NATURAL SOURCES: Citrus fruits, egg yolks, fish liver oils, garlic, kelp and seafood.

FUNCTIONS: Important in the construction of thyroid hormones. Assists in the metabolism of excess fat.

MEDICAL USES: Arteriosclerosis, goiter, hair problems, hypothyroidism.

RDA: 150 mcg

IRON

NATURAL SOURCES: Bananas, black molasses, kelp, lentils, liver, kidney, prunes, raisins, red meat and whole rye.

FUNCTIONS: Functions in your hemoglobin in red blood cells which transport oxygen from the lungs to the body's tissues (muscles, brain). Almost 50% of all women suffer from iron deficiency.

MEDICAL USES: Alcoholism, anemia, colitis, menstrual problems.

RDA: 15 mg

LITHIUM

NATURAL SOURCES: Dulse, kelp and seafood.

FUNCTIONS: Assists in the transportation of sodium metabolism to brain nerves and muscles.

MEDICAL USES: Paranoid schizophrenic.

RDA: Not established.

MAGNESIUM

NATURAL SOURCES: Molasses, nuts, fish and whole grains.

FUNCTIONS: Critical in numerous enzyme reactions in your body. Higher concentrations found in the brain, heart, liver and kidney. Important for bone building.

MEDICAL USES: Alcoholism, heart attack, kidney stones, tooth decay and overweight.

RDA: 350 mg

MANGANESE

NATURAL SOURCES: Brussel sprouts, beets, kelp and grains.

FUNCTIONS: Helps build and support strong bones in your body.

MEDICAL USES: Allergies, asthma, diabetes, fatigue.

RDA: 2.0 mg to 5.0 mg

MOLYBDENUM

NATURAL SOURCES: Buckwheat, brown rice, leafy vegetables, legumes, millet and whole cereals.

FUNCTIONS: Involved in the oxidation process, such as alcohol detoxification.

MEDICAL USES: Copper poisoning and improper carbohydrate metabolism.

RDA: 50 mcg to 250 mcg mg

PHOSPHOROUS

NATURAL SOURCES: Dairy products, eggs, fish, poultry, and whole grains.

FUNCTIONS: Assists in cell growth and repair and the metabolism of red blood cells.

MEDICAL USES: Arthritis, stress, stunting growth in children, and tooth and gum diseases.

RDA: Not established.

POTASSIUM

NATURAL SOURCES: Bananas, green leafy vegetables, tomatoes, watercress, and whole grains.

FUNCTIONS: An important electrolyte that interacts with sodium to conduct nerve impulses. Today many foods have a much higher sodium-potassium ratio resulting in an increase in high blood pressure.

MEDICAL USES: Acne, burns, high blood pressure and heart disease.

RDA: 3,500 mg

SELENIUM

NATURAL SOURCES: Bran, garlic, kelp, seafood, and wheat germ.

FUNCTIONS: An antioxidant that works with vitamin E to destroy hyper oxides and free radicals.

MEDICAL USES: Cardiovascular disease, heart attack and stroke.

RDA: 70 mcg

SILICON

NATURAL SOURCES: Apples, beets, flaxseed, oats, nuts, and seeds.

FUNCTIONS: The second most abundant element on earth. Important for proper bone growth.

MEDICAL USES: Hair loss, insomnia, irritations in mucous membranes and skin disorders.

RDA: Not established

SODIUM

NATURAL SOURCES: Carrots, kelp, kidney, sea salt, and shellfish.

FUNCTIONS: One of the three main electrolytes in the body.

MEDICAL USES: Heat prostration, mental apathy, muscular weakness and sun stroke.

RDA: 0.5g

SULFUR

NATURAL SOURCES: Kale, onions, radish, and watercress.

FUNCTIONS: A part of most proteins, sulfur is involved in most enzyme, antibody, and tissue functions.

MEDICAL USES: Arthritis, eczema, dermatitis and psoriasis.

RDA: Not established

VANADIUM

NATURAL SOURCES: Fish

FUNCTIONS: Essential to the body and improves insulin action.

MEDICAL USES: Arteriosclerosis, diabetes, heart attack prevention and high blood pressure.

RDA: 10 mcg to 60 mcg

ZINC

NATURAL SOURCES: Meat, poultry, liver, eggs, seafood (oysters) and whole grains.

FUNCTIONS: Important for immunity and strength.

MEDICAL USES: Arteriosclerosis, arthritis and high cholesterol.

NUTRIENTS

There are nutrients that fall into the category of vitamins as a chemical structure, and we know they are a part of our life systems, but don't fall into the two vitamin categories. Choline, inositol, PABA, and bioflavonoids are nutrients that don't have RDA's but have functions and deficiency symptoms like vitamins.

AMINO ACIDS

There is yet one more class of nutrients that is very similar in make up, the Amino acids. There are 22 known amino acids and eight of them cannot be made by the body, which classifies them as "essential." The other fourteen amino acids can be manufactured from other sources if the right nutrition is supplied. These structures are called "the building blocks of life" because they make up proteins when linked together. They perform a wide range of duties from building new tissue, to forming antibodies, enzymes and hormones. They build nucleo-proteins (DNA and RNA) and are a part of all muscular activity. We get protein from many sources and those sources have their own amino acid profiles.

ALANINE

Produces antibodies to strengthen your immune system. Important for the brain and central nervous system. Provides energy for muscle tissue and helps metabolize sugars and organic acids.

ARGININE

Will enhance your immune system by manufacturing T cells by stimulating the Thymus. Also used for insulin production and muscle metabolism. Thought to be effective in fighting bacteria, viruses and cancerous tumor cells. Helps maintain nitrogen balance in muscles. Component of collagen. Important for weight management.

ASPARAGINE

Balances the central nervous system. Produced almost entirely from meat sources. Thought to prevent anxiety.

ASPARTIC ACID

Protects circulatory system form ammonia. Thought to be a factor in chronic fatigue syndrome, a deficiency decreases cellular energy. Abundant in plants.

CARNITINE

Transports fat to the mitochondria. Thought to prevent diabetes and heart disease. Critical for weight loss.

CITRULLINE

Functions in liver as an ammonia detoxifier like Aspartic Acid. Enhances the immune system.

CYSTEINE

Collagen producers important in skin elasticity. Used for arthritis and burn recovery. Can be used in conjunction with cancer treatments. Thought to provide an anti-aging effect and assists in the treatment of respiratory conditions.

DIMETHYLGLYCINE (DMG)

Thought to be good for the heart. Lowers cholesterol and helps to normalize blood pressure.

GAMMA-AMINOBUTYRIC ACID (GABA)

Operates in the central nervous system. Helps relieve stress and anxiety. Used as a treatment for hypertension, epilepsy and ADD.

GLUTAMIC ACID

Detoxifies ammonia in the brain. Called "brain food." Used in the treatment of depression, alcoholism, epilepsy, and schizophrenia.

GLUTAMINE

Increases the amount of Glutamic Acid and GABA. Used as a supplement L-Glutamine for arthritis, impotency, schizophrenia and damaged tissue repair as a result of cancer radiation treatments.

GLUTATHIONE

Produced in the liver. Supplements taken for anti-aging. Caution should be used with the supplement. Possible to utilize cysteine, glutamic acid and glycine supplements to produce glutathione.

GLYCINE

Provides creatine to muscles. Constructs DNA and RNA. Functions in the central nervous system. Overuse of the supplement may cause fatigue.

HISTIDINE

Found in red and white blood cells. Used to treat ulcers, allergies and arthritis. Used to produce histamine.

ISOLEUCINE

A three-branched chain amino acid. Aids in muscle tissue repair. Increases endurance and enhances energy. Caution should be used when using with other three-branched chain amino acids (leucine and valine).

LEUCINE

Another three-branched chain amino acid. Also enhances energy and endurance. Thought to lower blood sugar levels and increases the production of growth hormones.

LYSINE

Critical for bone development in children. Helps produce antibodies, hormones, and enzymes.

METHIONINE

Produces sulfur. Thought to help lower cholesterol. Detoxifies the body of heavy metals.

ORNITHINE

Helps in the release of growth hormones and produces the metabolism of excess body fat.

PHENYLALANINE

Used in the brain to promote alertness and memory. Thought to reduce hunger and appetite.

PROLINE

Maintains collagen (skin protein). Obtained from meat sources. Also strengthens joints and connective tissue.

SERINE

A storage source for glucose. Strengthens the immune system by producing antibodies.

TAURINE

Thought to stabilize membrane excitability. Important in the controlling of epilepsy. Helps to clear free radical wastes. Used in treatments for hypertension and muscular dystrophy. Not found in vegetable proteins.

THREONINE

Thought to help prevent fat build up in the liver. Helps digestion.

TRYPTOPHAN

Thought to relieve insomnia, anxiety and depression. Reduces cholesterol levels along with lysine.

TYROSINE

Helps the thyroid, adrenal and pituitary glands. May reduce anxiety and depression. Suppresses appetite and reduces body fat.

VALINE

The last of the three-branched chain amino acids. Enhances energy and endurance. Aids in muscle tissue recovery and repair.

Sometimes certain dietary habits will provide inadequate profiles needed by the human body and deficiencies can occur. This seems to be the case with vegetarians because their protein sources are incomplete and they need a wide variety of plant sources to cover the human body's amino acid profile for their diet. This is a much debated subject, and vegetarians and non-vegetarians have their reasons for their dietary consumption. If one desires to be vegetarian, they should really look into the nutrition aspcct of their diet to see what nutrients are missing and find out what food they can add that will fill the holes in their dietary style.

When you read through each of these listed nutrients, you are probably wondering if you are deficient in some areas. It isn't uncommon to be deficient in a few, and you can usually get by for a while without getting your RDA and not notice that you are having symptoms. Just because you feel good does not mean your body is operating at its best condition. Most people that are somewhat fit or healthy and eat a good diet, or supplement their diet, tend to have fewer illnesses and heal much faster than those who don't. What is really important about these nutrients is their function. Most people would not want to compromise any of these functions if they want to maintain their health.

When we are looking for the best scenario for weight loss, it really makes sense to have our metabolism, our total chemical reaction systems, operating at full power. This ensures that we are repairing, replacing and restoring our bodies to their best conditions so that they can cope with everyday physical and psychological stress. If one's diet is sufficient in vitamins, minerals, and the other trace elements to process our macronutrients, protein, carbohydrates, and fats, then our calorie intake will be a match for our ability to utilize those calories. When this happens, our bodies don't have all their fat reserves backed up and growing. This is one reason, in our opinion, that many people are overweight. All we have to do is give the body what it needs to burn the excess fuel it has not burned yet. It sounds simple to do if you know what foods to eat to get these nutrients. But not everyone knows about all of these food nutrients and how to get them.

Today's food selections are based on convenience, cost and taste. These convenient "fast" foods are big contributors to most of the dietary problems that exist today. Obesity and malnutrition are very closely related if you look at it on a micronutrient basis. Just because someone is overweight, most would consider that they are getting plenty of vitamins and minerals because they are getting plenty of food. This is not the case. Many times the person who suffers from obesity doesn't really eat more than the average person. The problem lies in that they are consuming empty calorie foods which causes weight gain because of the lack of nutrients to burn the food.

In fact, you can observe the opposite effect with healthy, fit individuals. Take athletes for example. They consume large amounts of food. You would think they would be really obese if you looked at just calories consumed. Now, let's look at what they actually are eating for food. They eat four to six meals a day that are well balanced with a variety of foods, and they are taking supplements as well. You don't see professional athletes that are fat unless their sport calls for being large and heavy. Another thing to observe from athletes and their dietary practices is how much bigger, stronger and faster they are now compared to 25 years ago. Some of these athletes are still professionals well into their fifties, and are still competitive with younger athletes in their twenties. It is believed that supplementation and nutritional knowledge have had the biggest impact on this development.

Knowing more about your food selection can change your eating habits. This can lead to many improvements in the quality of one's health. I have never met anyone who would deliberately eat bad things so they would feel worse and increase their chances of illness, but people do it every day without caring or knowing they are doing it at all. Hopefully, the next time you put something into your mouth you will think about overall nutrition rather than taste.

TEN CRITICAL NUTRIENTS FOR FAT BURNING

In the quest for fat loss and fat metabolism there are now literally hundreds of products that claim to be "fat burners." Many of these are merely amphetamine or "speed" based products to make the user hypersensitive so they are more active. This makes you burn more calories because these products reduce laziness. These products also have drawbacks as any drugs do. Symptoms such as restlessness, poor sleeping cycles, reduced focus, jitters, stomach cramps, headaches and even nausea may result.

The Biogenesis program does not use these types of drugs to aid in weight loss because they are not healthy or long term. If you are currently using these types of weight loss aids, you may experience short term benefits. Long-lasting weight loss comes from an optimum nutrition program that can be supported by good food and supplements, like Biogenesis.

There is a misconception that these products increase your metabolism. The only ways that a person's metabolism can be increased is to either add more biologically active tissue to the body or to become more active. Neither of these two scenarios requires amphetamines. Your body requires adequate nutritional support. Fat needs the right combination of nutrients so that it can be processed into energy the body can use for metabolism. Metabolism is the total amount of chemical reactions the body produces to live.

There are several nutrients that are needed to process fat into energy. There are other nutrients that are responsible for the regulation of fat production from carbohydrates. These nutrients are constantly used up if there is an abundance of calories to be processed. If these nutrients run out, or are run down your ability to burn fat will go down, and you will start converting carbohydrates to fat when some of these nutrients are low.

Scientific studies have shown that there are many nutritional components that aid in fat loss and lean muscle gain. We at Biotech feel there are ten that are a must. These nutrients are:

Choline
Inositol
L-Methionine
L-Carnitine
Chromium
Biotin
Vitamin B-12
Vitamin B-6
Betaine Hcl
Pancreatin

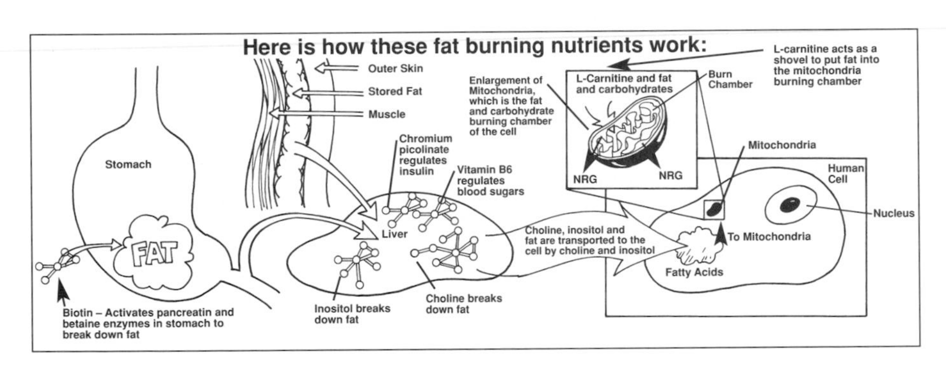

To make energy from fat there are numerous chemical pathways and stages that fat is taken through. In many of these stages key nutrients are needed as catalysts to break down fat into different components. These catalysts and chemical signals include the critical nutrients choline, inositol, biotin, and vitamin B6. Two critical enzymes are also needed to break down fat, which are pancreatin and betaine. Fat also needs to be transported to the fat burning chamber of the cell called the mitochondria. Once outside the mitochondria, fat is transported inside with the aid of L-carnitine and is converted to energy that the cell can use for other processes that the cell uses for life. Some of the other critical nutrients, such as chromium picolinate, help regulate and produce insulin; and insulin helps control hunger, regulates fat storage, and aids muscle building. These nutrients get used up in the process. Lack of these nutrients slows down fat metabolism. If we supplement our diet or eat the right foods that contain these critical nutrients, our fat metabolism will occur at a very high rate all the time.

Of these ten nutrients only Betaine Hcl and Pancreatin are not found elsewhere in this chapter. These two nutrients are not really nutrients at all. They are enzymes that help break down foods and aid in digestion so that the body systems can use them to process fats and proteins into energy. If all nutritional aspects for energy production are available, then fat loss can be maximized to its full 100% ability!

Biogenesis offers our line of nutritional supplements including our Ultrabody Lipotropic Metabolizers. These capsules can maximize fat loss when used with the Biogenesis program.

Fat Burning Nutrients	**Natural Sources**
Vitamin B-6	Bananas, wheat germ, cantaloupe, eggs, beef, green leafy vegetables
Vitamin B-12	Comfrey leaves, bananas, peanuts, grapes, beef, pork, milk
Betaine Hcl	Enzyme produced by your body. Available in supplements (Ultrabody Ultra-Lipotropic Fat Burners)
Biotin	Brewers yeast fruits, nuts, rice, egg yolk, milk, kidney
Choline	Wheat germ, egg yolk, liver, green leafy vegetables
Chromium	Brewers yeast, chicken, claims, corn oil, meat, shellfish
Inositol	Beef brains, cabbage, citrus fruits, raisins, whole grains, unrefined molasses
L-Carnitine	Produced by your body to aid in the transportation of fat. Available in supplements

6

SUPPLEMENTS AND FOOD

Protein has recently hit the main stream as the most important key to dietary weight control. We say weight control because for years athletes have known the importance of protein in regards to muscle building and strength gaining. What exactly is protein and what are the benefits of maintaining an ample supply of protein in your diet?

The technical definition of protein is: any of numerous naturally occurring, extremely complex combinations of amino acids that contain the elements carbon, hydrogen, nitrogen, oxygen, sulfur, and occasionally other elements such as iron. Proteins are essential constituents of all living cells, and are synthesized from raw materials by plants but assimilated as separate amino acids by animals.

So technically, protein probably doesn't mean much to you. So we will try and simplify the importance of high protein intake. If you have read the Fat-Flush Diet, (Chapter 7) then you know that your body is like a machine that never rests, constantly producing metabolic energy. Your body functions mainly through the use of glucose. Since your body's entire energy is supplied from glucose, everything you eat is processed and turned into this form of sugar. As long as your body has anything in it at all, it can be turned to glucose.

Food is consumed and your body then goes to work separating and processing the different elements. Absorption mainly takes place on the surface of the small intestines. Carbohydrates are absorbed as sugar, which they already are or can easily be converted into. Fats will be absorbed as glycerol and fatty acids, and finally from protein your body absorbs amino acids. You would think that by consuming large amounts of simple carbohydrates like sugar and fruit you would be full on energy all day long. The problem with this is when your blood sugar rises that fast your body compensates by determining how much energy you actually need right at that moment and then stores the unneeded calories for future use.

Storing calories is not a good thing. Whatever glucose cannot be used is then converted to glycogen. Glycogen is a starch that is stored in the muscles and the liver. If all of your glycogen stores are full, then insulin converts the excess to triglyceride, which is fatty tissue. So a key to weight fat loss is to control your insulin level. Since simple sugars as well as refined carbohydrates have an immediate effect on your insulin levels, avoiding these foods or at least lowering them will dramatically lower your fat production and storage levels. Protein takes a small amount of insulin to be processed and fats take little to no insulin for conversion. In short, carbohydrates produce high amounts of insulin. Because causing your body to convert carbohydrates to fat, insulin also produces more of the bad cholesterol LDL, and also causes water retention which, in turn, causes high blood pressure.

When dieting you want to lower your carbohydrates to the point of releasing ketones. When you are releasing ketones, or your body is in a state of ketosis, this means your body is dissolving fats. Fat dissolving is good. Since your muscles are comprised of amino acids and amino acids come from protein, this should be starting to make a little sense to you. So by using the Biogenesis workout and keeping a low carbohydrate, low fat and high protein diet, such as the Fat Flush Diet, you will be able to burn fat and gain muscle and understand how you are doing it.

We have mentioned that it is very difficult for protein to be converted to and stored as fat. So we know that by eating too much fat we will get fat and by eating too many carbohydrates we will get fat. What happens when we eat too much protein? Since protein is the last thing to be converted to glucose, it is not your source for immediate energy. Instead, protein is the building blocks for your muscles. The more you exercise, the more protein you can assimilate. Once the body has utilized all of the protein it needs at that time the remains are excreted as waste. Something very important to remember is that one pound of muscle takes approximately thirty calories to maintain where as a pound of fat may take as few as two. So by adding muscle to your body you are, in turn, creating an avenue for you to be able to consume more calories without getting fat, as long as the calories are quality calories such as chicken, fish, lean beef, etc.

The down side of this is that not all of the essential amino acids are available in all of the various foods we eat. A food could lack as few as one of the essential amino acids and become of far less value to you. This brings us to the importance of supplements.

Although exercise and nutrition are very important to our health and our appearance, there is yet another contributing factor – supplements. A supplement is anything we add to our nutritional intake that enhances the productivity of muscle building and fat burning by adding any nutrient that the food we eat would be missing. Supplements should not be used to replace food but rather only as a dietary enhancement. Good supplements help the foods we eat become complete, maximally efficient and effective. Supplements can play a major role in quickening your progress. Although some companies would like you to believe that you can drink one of their protein shakes and eat whatever you like the rest of the day and look great, this is definitely not true. In fact for many companies the exact opposite is true. Many protein powders contain high levels of sugar or fructose and we just learned how insulin levels can destroy our fat burning rhythm.

Biogenesis has developed our own supplement line called Ultrabody. Of course, Frank and Dave make sure the quality of all the Ultrabody supplements are grade A. They did this by not only keeping the company in the United States, but also right in their home state of Ohio. "By having our company only several hours away, David and I can easily take a better hands on approach to the way our products are made and handled," says Frank. "It cost us a little more to ensure that only the best ingredients are used, but we wanted to be able to say that there is not a single company out there with a better product then ours. That's what our goal was and we have accomplished it with Ultrabody." To learn more about all of our Ultrabody products you can write us for information at: Ultrabody, 7800 Whipple Ave., Canton, Ohio 44767-0003 or visit us at the Biogenesis Web site at www.biogenesis.net or at www.ultrabody.net, and click on the Ultrabody icon. Frank and David also have their own websites: www.frankcampitelli.com and www.daviddearth.com.

GROCERY LIST

If you need a grocery list for the fat-flush program and recipes, here are some of the items that you should include. These items are placed into two categories, but are in no particular order of importance.

PROTEIN SOURCES

eggs or egg beaters
skinless chicken breast
flank or round steak
lean ground beef
fish (your preference)
Fat-free cheese
canned tuna (water packed)
Fat-free turkey breast
skim milk

CARBOHYDRATE SOURCES

bagels
potatoes
bananas
broccoli
carrots
asparagus
tomatoes

rice
pasta
pretzels
rice cakes
strawberries
peanut butter
grapefruit
salad vegetables of preference
oatmeal
honey
apples
soy beans

These foods should make up the core of your grocery list when you take the trip to the super market. Look in the green, yellow, and red zone ranking, and the fat-flush diet section for extra foods that will fit the likes and needs of you and your body.

7

How To Quickly Drain Excess Fat From Your Body

You are going to see results on this program that you would never have believed possible. And, you're going to start seeing them very quickly, in a matter of weeks. In a matter of months, you will become almost unrecognizable.

To begin, we need to talk about the all-important nutrition program. Nutrition, as all qualified personal trainers know, is 75% of bodybuilding.

Therefore, you must follow this Advanced Nutrition Program carefully. The key things this nutrition program will show you are how to get the proper amount of protein, carbohydrates and fat intake.

Users of this breakthrough, advanced nutrition method have lost weight 100% to 200% faster than old style diets, even faster than on starvation diets or fasting. Some have lost up to 30 pounds in just eight weeks. Many of them also reached a remarkable 10% body fat for women and 5% body fat for men. The Fat Flush Nutrition Program drains excess fat from your body safely and with great eating pleasure.

On our new, advanced No-Hunger Fat-Flush Nutrition Program, you eat 5 times a day and 300% to 400% more and better-tasting food than you likely eat now.

Although the No-Hunger Fat-Flush Nutrition Program is new to the public, it has been time-tested in real life for safety and effectiveness. The origin of the No-Hunger Fat-Flush Nutrition Program is from the professional bodybuilding community. It was developed over a long period by certified personal trainers, certified nutritionists, physiologists, biologists and other scientists utilized by men and women champion professional bodybuilders.

Here is how this program works to drain fat from your body so rapidly and so painlessly.

Old style, fad diets don't work because they rely mainly on calorie counting or they have you eating limited types of food.

When you drop your calorie intake, your body is designed to perceive that it is being starved and turns on chemical systems to actually stop the loss of excess fat. Part of this results in lowering the body's metabolic rate, which is the rate of calorie and fat burning. Your body will actually start burning a great deal of your muscle. You will then lose very little fat, lose a great deal of muscle and be miserable because you are hungry all of the time.

If you go on a no-carbohydrate diet where you eat virtually all fat and protein with little or no carbohydrates, in a few weeks your body will actually become toxic. This is because you need carbohydrates to process protein. You will start losing muscle, start to damage your internal organs and even your brain cells. You will lose weight for a few weeks and then, since fat is so high in calories, you will again start gaining excess fat.

If you go on strictly a low-fat diet, your body is designed to store what it is getting the least in the way of nutrition. Therefore, it will try to store more fat and start burning your muscle for energy.

The No-Hunger Fat-Flush Nutrition Program, all safe and natural, ingeniously stops the body's mechanisms of lowering your metabolic rate, burning your muscle and preserving your fat. It then speeds up fat burning to an ultimate level. It does this, in part, through the Metabolic Confusion Technique. This is done by varying the amount of protein, carbohydrates and fat that you take in from day to day through a scientifically sequenced, ever-changing pattern. A great side benefit to this is that it also eliminates the boring diet and makes it into an exciting diet.

The No-Hunger Fat-Flush Nutrition Program also takes into account the fact that fat converts 100% to stored fat. Only 75% of carbohydrates can convert to stored fat because 25% is burned up in the process. And, less than 50% of protein can be converted to stored fat because protein goes through numerous conversions before it can be made into stored fat that eats up most of its calories.

And, very importantly, the No-Hunger Fat-Flush Nutrition Program works because of this. The foods are selected and put into combinations for many meals that take more calories to digest than the calories they contain. Also, nutrients are utilized that actually attach themselves to some of the fat molecules in the digestive process so they cannot be converted to stored fat and are drained harmlessly from your body.

And, last but not least, there is this important reason the No-Hunger Fat-Flush Nutrition Program works. You eat a lot of food on this diet. And it is not bland-tasting food. It is very delicious food. You eat 5 delicious meals a day. You never go hungry.

In fact, these meals are so delicious that people on this diet say they will never go back to their old bad eating habits again.

In layman's terms, to understand how the No-Hunger Fat-Flush Nutrition Program works, picture this. Picture a furnace. Below this furnace is a fuel tank. Feeding this fuel tank are three pipes: one from your digestive system, one from your muscle and one from your stored fat. At the end of these pipes, before they go into the fuel tank, is a fuel production mechanism which converts stored fat, muscle or digestive nutrition into fuel. Before the fuel from the fuel tank goes into the furnace there is a combustion chemical feed which brings in such chemicals as oxygen to burn the fuel. (See Figure 1.)

Your body is actually designed to keep at a minimum the production of fuel from stored fat. It would rather get the fuel from your digestive system first. But if the body thinks it is being starved, it is designed to protect stored fat because it believes it will need the stored fat for future energy. It then starts to burn muscle. And even worse, when it perceives it is being starved, it will lower the combustion chemicals, such as oxygen intake, so that the flames of the furnace are lowered.

To burn the maximum amount of excess fat, you need to first drain the fuel tank, reduce the calories that come in from the digestive tract by burning them up through digestion, shut off the muscle pipe valve and flush the maximum amount of stored fat into the fuel converter and into the fuel tank. You then need to open up the fuel-burning-chemical line wide to keep the furnace flame as high as possible. (See Figure 2.)

You will then have maximum fat burning and maximum fat drain to the point where you can lose 20 to 30 pounds in 8 weeks. And, under certain conditions, some people have lost 60 pounds in 8 weeks. Many average women on this program have lost a dress size in only 4 weeks and men have lost a pant size in 2 weeks.

Your objective, of course, is not only to take excess fat off, but to also keep it off. That is why with the No-Hunger Fat-Flush Nutrition Program there is also a Fat Prevention Diet which will maintain your desirable weight after you lose all your excess fat.

For the No-Hunger Fat-Flush Nutrition Program to work, you must get your proper protein first. When you're on an anaerobic exercise program, in order to build adequate muscle, you need to be taking in about 1-1/2 grams of protein per pound of muscle in your body. If you are at the proper fat level, about 1/2 of your body weight is muscle. We have provided you with protein intake charts on your enclosed nutrition program.

You will see that the average person who weighs 120 pounds with proper body fat has about 60 pounds of muscle. Sixty pounds of muscle times 1-1/2 grams gives you 90 grams of protein that you need to take in per day to get adequate muscle for body shaping and to maintain muscle. There are 28.35 grams in an ounce. Dividing 90 by 28.35 shows that you need 3.2 ounces of protein. But, you just can't go eat 3.2 ounces of steak or chicken. That's because only a third of steak or chicken is protein. Egg whites are another good source of protein and

OLD STYLE DIET BEFORE

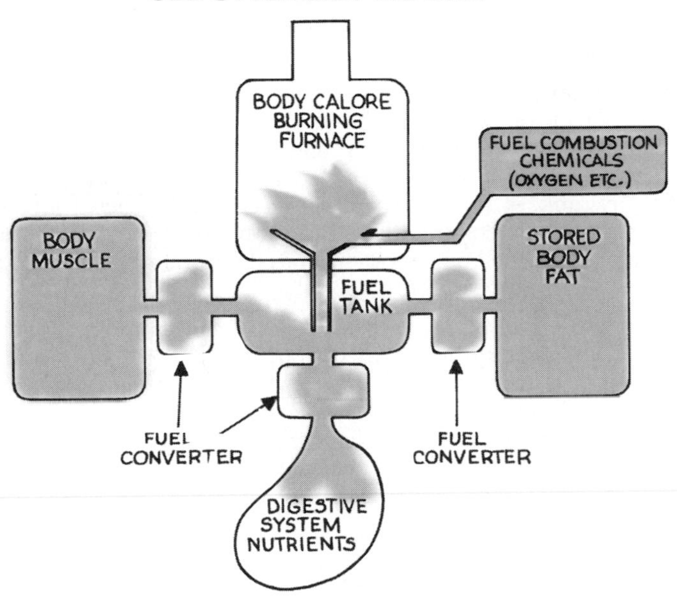

OLD STYLE DIET AFTER

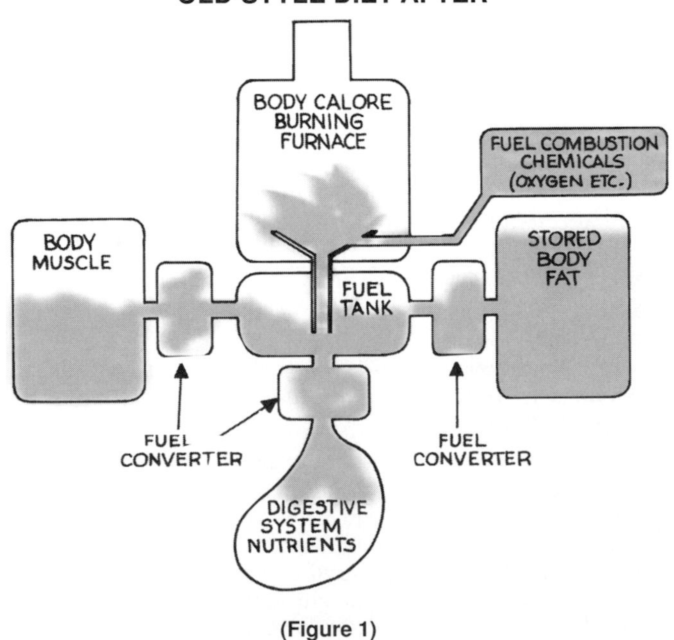

(Figure 1)

NO-HUNGER FAT-FLUSH DIET BEFORE

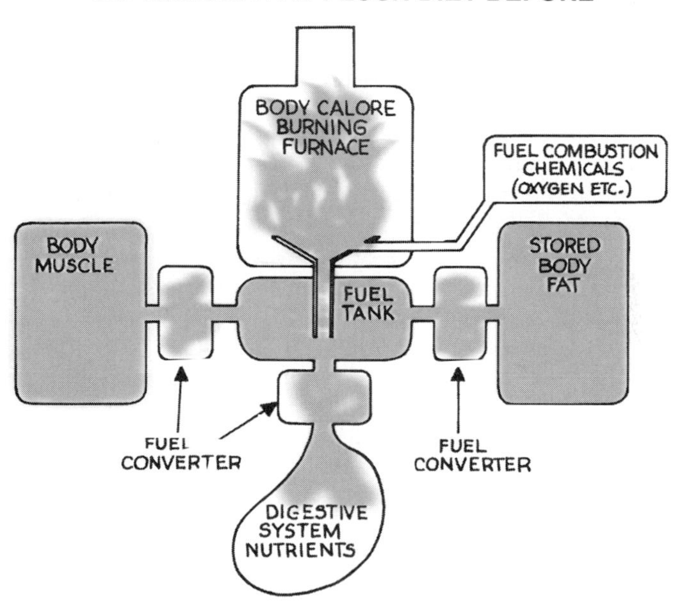

NO-HUNGER FAT-FLUSH DIET AFTER

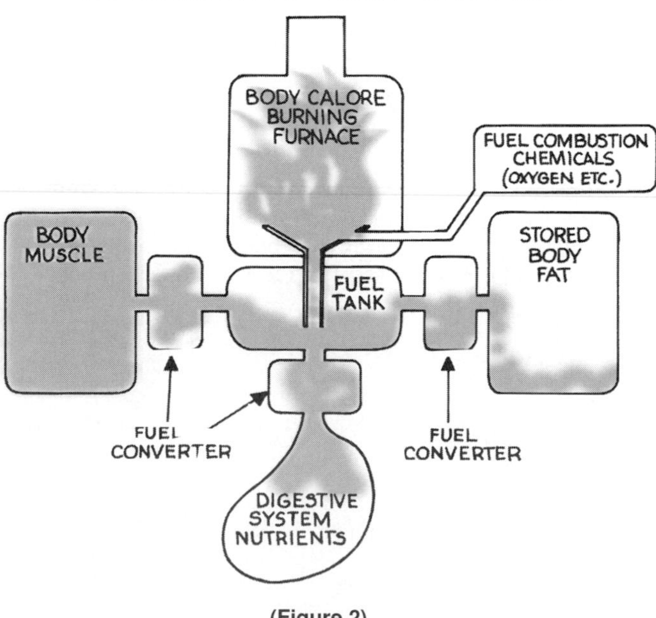

(Figure 2)

eggs are cheap (About 20% of egg whites are protein). Other protein sources like milk contain much less protein. Therefore, the average person who weighs 120 pounds would need to take in almost 10 ounces of steak, chicken or egg whites per day. If you weigh 160 pounds, you would need to eat about 13 ounces of steak or chicken and so on. Again, we have provided you with tables that show you how much protein intake you need and how much of each food you need to eat to get that adequate protein. (Refer to Chapter 4 Macronutrients)

Your body is mostly made up of protein, carbohydrates and fat. For a healthy diet, you need to have all three. For a normal, healthy maintenance diet, the calories you take in should be 55% carbohydrate, 30% protein and 15% fat. But, if you want to lose weight and shape your body, your average calorie intake should be 50% protein, 40% carbohydrate and only 10% fat. But, you must vary these amounts coming out to these averages to create the Metabolic Confusion Technique.

Most people take in entirely too much fat. Many people take in 3 to 4 times the amount of fat that they need. Excess fat intake is a big part of putting excess fat on the body.

For the average person, a 15% fat intake amounts to about 45 grams of fat per day; and a 10% fat intake amounts to about 30 grams of fat per day.

Now for most people, 30 grams of fat is hard to visualize. So, we have set up this demonstration which will help you understand what fat means in grams and how excess fat intake is not only bad by causing obesity, but is also bad for your health.

So let's convert these grams into something you can understand. There are 28.35 grams in an ounce. This shot glass has 28.35 grams of fat, or one ounce. For a healthy maintenance diet, you should only take in one and a half of these shot glasses of fat. To lose excess fat, you should only be taking in just 1 shot glass of fat per day. (See Figure 3.)

But most people take in 4 to 5 ounces of fat per day and some even more. So when you do that, picture yourself drinking down 4 to 5 of these shot glasses full of fat. Now a little over 1 of these is all your body really needs and utilizes. When you also take in more calories than you need a day, this extra fat intake is convert-

28.35 grams of fat is one ounce and will fill one shot glass.

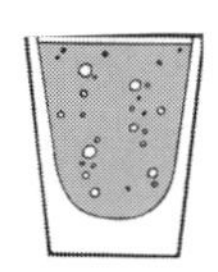

(Figure 3)

Hamburger and french fries =

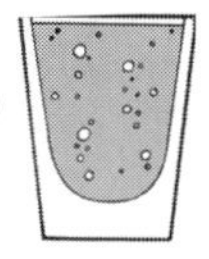
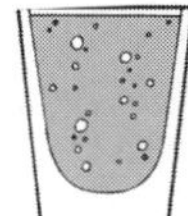
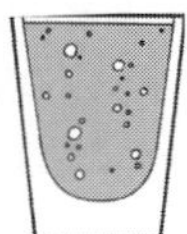
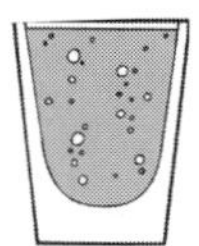

1/2 bag potato chips with dip =

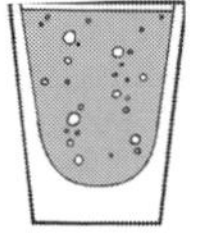
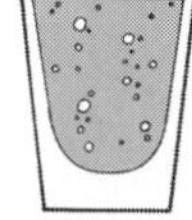
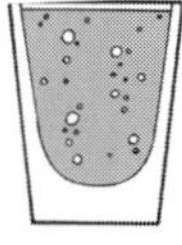
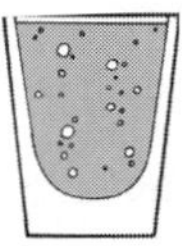

(Figure 4)

ed to excess fat storage in your body. And, 100% of it is converted to excess fat storage! This puts on 3 ounces of stored fat on your body. (See Figure 4.)

This excess fat storage on men mostly goes to the abdominal and waist areas. On women it mostly goes on the buttocks and thighs and a significant amount goes in the abdomen and the backs of the arms.

So when you're taking in those extra 3 or more shot glasses full of fat and too many calories, just think of them going right to your waist, buttocks, thighs and backs of the arms.

Now when you're taking on those 3 or more ounces of extra fat per day, remember there are only 16 ounces in a pound. That means in a little over 5 days you're putting on a pound or more of fat which will go to your waist, buttocks, thighs and backs of arms. And, in 10 days, you'll put on 2 pounds of fat, which is about what is contained in a quart bottle of salad oil. So picture this whole bottle of salad oil being turned into solid stored fat and put on your abdomen, waist, buttocks and backs of your arms. Not a pleasant thought is it?

We will give you a first-ever effective tool to cut your excess fat intake in this nutrition program. We have provided a first-ever ranking of foods, first by fat content and then by calories. This ranking is designated by Zone A for foods that you can eat a lot of, Zone B for foods you can eat in moderation, and Zone C for foods that you must stay away from or eat minimal amounts because of their very high fat content. It is important that you study this table so you will know which foods are bad regarding fat content. (See Appendix A)

This table ranks the fat content foods by giving you the amount of fat grams in every 8 ounces of the food. You will see on the worst end of the table that the highest content of fat foods are the oils, like Crisco oil and corn oil, which are virtually all fat. You will then go to peanut oil, olive oil, lard, chicken fat, butter, etc. which are almost 90% fat. You'll then see the other super-fat content items which are about 70% fat such as nuts. For instance, if you ate 8 ounces of macadamia nuts, pecans or even dry roasted mixed nuts, you would be taking in 5 to 6 ounces of fat, which is like drinking 5 to 6 shot glasses full of fat - which again goes right to your belly, buttocks, thighs and arms. Then you see, when you start taking in 8 ounces of things like chocolate, peanut butter and mayonnaise or salad dressing, for every 8 ounces you eat about 4 ounces of pure fat, or 4 of these full shot glasses goes to fat on your body. When you eat 8 ounces of sausage, potato chips, Fritos, or hot dogs, you'll be taking in 2-1/2 shot glasses full of fat . So if, for example, you are sitting around at night eating chips and chip dip while watching TV, it's not too hard to eat half a bag of chips, which is 8 ounces of chips and 8 ounces of chip dip. In the 8 ounces of chips you'll get 80 grams of fat and in the 8 ounces of sour cream chip dip you'll get 48 grams of fat for a total of 128 grams of fat, which means 4-1/2 ounces of fat. It'll be like drinking 4-1/2 of these shot glasses full of fat in one sitting. It's like taking 4-1/2 ounces of fat, over a 1/4-pound, and just painting it on your butt.

It is very important to broil or stir-fry foods rather than frying them in oils.

Broiled foods can be very delicious. We recommend that you also get a tabletop electric broiler and an electric wok. These give you delicious, high-protein food. The electric broiler gives you food that is hot with each bite. It extends the eating time for more satisfaction and enjoyment.

This tabletop electric grill will bring you many benefits. Now remember when we told you would be eating 300% to 400% more food and still lose weight?

People who are putting on weight eat a typical meal that consists of fattening foods that are high in fat and calories. One of the favorite meals of overweight people is hamburgers and French fries or hamburgers and potato chips. If you ate 8 ounces of potato chips or French fries and 8 ounces of hamburger, you would be taking in 82 grams of fat and over 1,900 calories. With this electric grill meal, if you ate 4 ounces of chicken and 4 ounces of beef for a total of 8 ounces of meat, these 8 ounces of meat would only come to 4-1/2 grams of fat and only 298 calories. The 8 ounces of delicious vegetables that are seasoned with a special seasoning come to zero (0) grams of fat and only 35 calories. Therefore, your total meal of 1 pound of food would only be 333 calories. That is 1/6th of your one-pound meal of hamburger and fries or potato chips. So therefore, you could eat 600% more of this meal than the other one for the same amount of calories. Now if you wanted to lose weight, you could simply cut that in half for over 900 calories and you would be eating 300% more food and cut your calories in half. Also, this chicken/beef and vegetables tastes super delicious. Also, meals like burgers and fries get cold quickly so you eat them quickly before they get cold. Usually you're done eating those 1900 calories in about 15 minutes. With this delicious meal on this grill, since you only put on one piece of meat at a time, every bite is hot and you could string this meal out for an hour and a half if you wanted to and watch a full-length movie while you're eating. You could eat a pound and a half of meat and a pound and a half of vegetables and still cut calories in 1/2 and reduce your fat intake by 8 times less.

In summary, we're going to tell you the two biggest things you can do nutrition wise to lose all your excess fat and never put on excess fat again.

We surveyed overweight people in a way that they told us the truth about why they were overweight. In most surveys, people will not tell surveyors the truth because they are face to face with the surveyor and do not want to be embarrassed. We did it in a confessional style where the person remained anonymous. They were on the phone with the surveyor in another room and the surveyor did not know who they were.

Besides not exercising, we found that the worst nutrition habit of overweight people that contributes to 50% of their excess fat was this. They snack between meals and after dinner at night before they go to bed on super high-fat foods - mainly deep-fried snack foods and/or chocolate and/or nuts and/or cheese. Most eat potato chips and many of these eat potato chips with sour cream chip dip. Many others eat chocolate candy and worse, chocolate candy with nuts.

Many people will snack between meals during the day and after dinner at night. Some would not snack during the day, but all did snack after dinner in the evening. Therefore, the number one problem was the snack after dinner at night while watching television. It was found that during this time they consumed mass quantities of calories and fat because they had a lot of time to do it and they were in the privacy of their own homes.

We found people eating a half bag to a full bag of chips and some with a full tub of chip dip. These people consumed 4 to 7 ounces of fat and 1,200 to 2,500 calories. Therefore, in just this one sitting they consumed more calories than they could burn in a day and took in 4 to 6 times the amount of fat that the body could use in a day. They took in over a quarter pound of fat in one sitting.

In another case, we found a typical candy and nuts eating person who ate Hershey's chocolate kisses with almonds. She told us she usually ate over half of a 12 ounce bag, about 8 ounces. This came to over 4 ounces of fat and over 1,200 calories.

The other thing we found in this survey was the 10 most popular foods eaten by overweight people. These 10 foods were super calorie and fat laden. This contributed to the other 50% of their excess fat.

These top 10 excess fat producing foods were: 1) potato chips, 2) ground beef, 3) French fries, 4) oil-based salad dressings, 5) pizza, 6) chocolate, 7) nuts, 8) butter, 9) sour cream, and 10) milk with fat. Other milk products like cheese and ice cream also contributed a great deal of fat and calories.

Here is what you can do to overcome these 2 top contributors to excess fat.

VERY IMPORTANT

For problem one, push the time you eat your dinner to as late as possible so you only have about one hour left before you go to bed so you don't have time to get hungry again. And, include a lot of protein in these meals. This later dinner will overcome the psychological problem of not wanting to go to bed hungry. Do other activities early in the evening such as hobbies or athletic activities. Or have some beer or wine in moderation and boost your education by reading in the early evening. Remember, it is easier to put off eating when you know you have a good meal coming than it is to put off eating when you know you will not have anything to eat the rest of the day.

If you have favorite shows you like to watch at night while you are snacking, have your late dinner while you are watching your favorite shows. Set up a card table with your meal in front of the TV and have your dinner. The most ideal meal for this is the tabletop electric grill meal that we showed you earlier.

These tabletop electric grill meals taste great, take a long time to eat, and they're high in protein and low in fat and calories.

If you cannot push your dinners back, then substitute the high-fat calorie food with other delicious snacks that we will tell you about next.

Now here is what you can do about problem 2, the top 10 worst food contributors to excess fat. Replace these bad foods with good foods that do not produce excess fat. Here are the good food for bad food substitutions:

1) For potato chips and other deep-fried snack foods, replace them with air-popped popcorn or low-fat popcorn like Orville Redenbacher's Smart Pop which contains only 6 grams of fat per bag; or eat fat-free pretzels and/or baked potato chips and other baked snacks etc.

2) For the ground beef bad foods, do this. Store-bought ground beef and ground beef used by most restaurants, especially fast-food restaurants, contains 30 grams of fat and over 350 calories for every 1/4 pound. When you go to the supermarket, buy a lean chuck roast or lean round steak and tell the meat department to cut off all the fat and bone and grind the meat for you. Do not buy the so-called lean ground beef and ground chuck and ground round that is in the meat case. Those are not much lower in fat than the regular ground beef. When you have your lean chuck or round steak ground for you, you will immediately reduce the fat and calories per quarter pound to only 2-1/2 grams of fat and 100 calories. Also, in place of ground beef, eat ground turkey or veggie burgers instead. When you are eating out, get roast beef sandwiches instead of hamburgers. And remember, other ground red meat is just as bad, such as ground pork used in sausage. And best, replace ground beef with the lean beef and chicken and electric grill them.

3) Replace French fries with baked potatoes and other non-fried potato recipes that you will find in the nutrition program. There are also fat-free frozen French fries at your supermarket. And best, replace them with low starch, low calorie vegetables like tomatoes, onions, mushrooms, green peppers and other green and yellow vegetables.

4) Replace oil-based salad dressings with fat-free salad dressings.

5) Replace regular pizza with Chef Valente's pizza that you will find in our nutrition program or low-fat pizza that you find in the frozen food section at stores.

6) Replace chocolate with other chocolate-tasting desserts from Ed Valente in our nutrition program.

7) Replace nuts with vegetables and fat-free dip.

8) Don't use butter on bread or other items. You won't miss it.

9) Replace regular sour cream with fat-free sour cream.

10) And, replace whole milk with fat with fat-free skim milk; eat fat-free cheese instead of regular cheese and fat-free yogurt instead of ice cream.

And, if you overeat because of psychological problem such as depression, tension and boredom, consider this. Overeating and not exercising will make you fatter, feel worse and more depressed, tense and bored. Exercise and proper diet can bring you out of depression, eliminate tension and eliminate boredom as we will discuss shortly.

But, you cannot go overboard on carbohydrates and protein. They both contain calories. And excess calories can be turned into stored fat.

We have provided you with diets in the nutrition program to lose weight which give you the proper protein, carbohydrates and fat as well as total calories.

After you start this program, you are going to lose inches in the right places and gain inches in the right places. You'll lose inches where fat is stored such as in the waist and other lower body areas and you'll gain inches in the right places such as the chest and shoulders. So, when you are checking your progress, don't worry about the scales - check the fit of your clothes and use a tape measure to measure your progress. Muscle is denser than fat and, therefore, weighs more per cubic inch. But, a pound of muscle takes up a lot less space than a pound of fat. So when you're putting on muscle in the right places and losing fat in the right places, you might not necessarily lose pounds on the scale. If you have a lot of excess body fat, you will eventually lose a lot of pounds also, but not necessarily at the beginning. But you will certainly lose a lot of inches at the beginning and that's what matters.

Progress women will see on this advanced program.

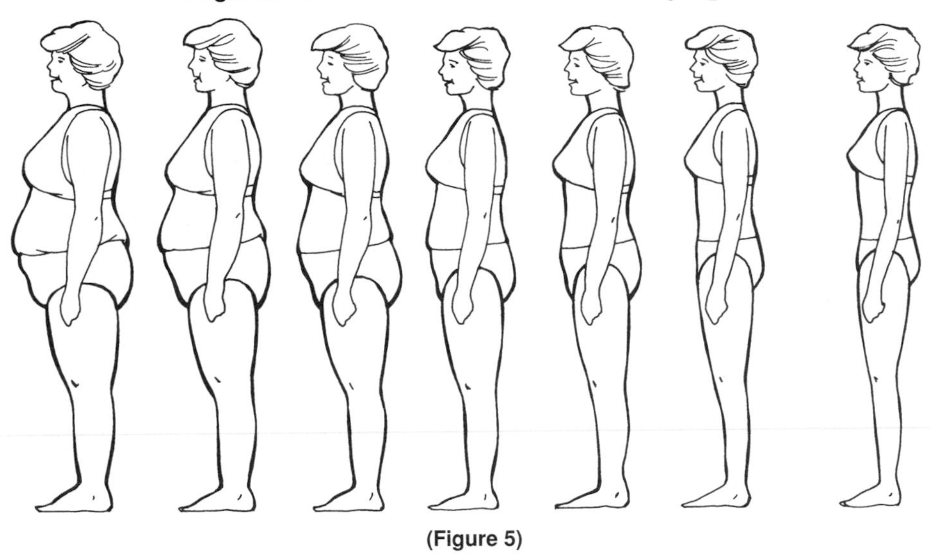

(Figure 5)

Progress men will see on this advanced program.

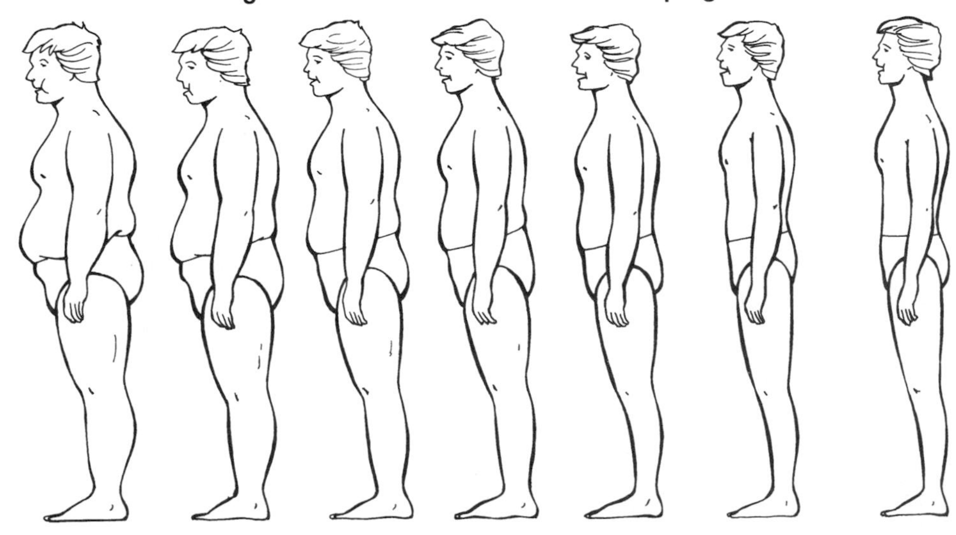

(Figure 6)

8

The No-Hunger Fat-Flush Nutrition Program

The No-Hunger Fat-Flush program uses a number of tested technologies including the Metabolic Confusion Technique. The basics of this technique are outlined below.

The human body is designed to be an efficient working machine. The body adapts to new work loads in a relatively short period of time. That's why the old style method of weight training doesn't produce nearly the results of the Muscle Confusion Method that we teach. Thus, during this phase we will need to reprogram our bodies into utilizing stored carbohydrates (note: unused carbohydrates get converted and stored as fat).

We've applied the body's ability to change and adapt to a nutrition and metabolic plan. Living, breathing, walking, sitting in a chair and the like all use up energy, and the body must provide it from somewhere. Simply stated, the body will always seek the most readily available source of fuel to use as energy for all these bodily functions.

The first source for energy is carbohydrates. There are two basic forms of carbohydrates, simple and complex. Simple carbohydrates consist of all sugars, including fructose. It is very easy for the body to utilize simple carbohydrates for energy. Keep in mind that all foods, not just carbohydrates, are converted into sugar or glucose because this is actually your body's way of generating energy. Complex carbohydrates, such as breads, pastas, rice and potatoes, are more difficult to convert to energy. But these complex carbohydrates are still easier to convert than protein or fat.

When our bodies see that they have an ample supply of carbohydrates, they will take the extra ones we consume, convert them to fat, and store them for future use. Our bodies understand the importance of carbohydrates as fuel for every single thing that keeps us alive. Unlike protein, most of the excess carbohydrates we take in are not excreted as waste, but are stored. Where do we store this extra energy? How about on the back of our thighs, or maybe our love handles, or our gluteus maximus. From this we see that if we do not use all of the carbohydrates we eat, we are going to get fat.

The second easiest food group to convert to energy is fat. Fats can be tricky because even though they make us look soft and overweight, they are important for keeping us alive. Besides providing the cushioning our vital organs need to keep from banging around on our bones, fats are also a standby energy supply in case our body ever runs low on carbohydrates.

The body will choose to burn ingested carbohydrates and fats, in that order, for fuel. An important point to remember is that it is difficult for the body to use stored carbohydrates for fuel. And it's even harder for the body to use protein for fuel since it must go through a long conversion process. So, since the body always seek to be as efficient as it can, it only burns stored carbohydrates or protein for fuel as a last resort.

The first place the body looks for calories is foods that have been eaten and are in the process of being digested. It looks for carbohydrates first. If it can't find carbohydrates, it looks for fats. If it can't find ingested fats, it will look for carbohydrates and fats that it has converted and stored away, in the form of stored fat. The Metabolic Confusion Technique continually changes what the body uses for fuel. This is the most efficient way to burn up stored fat and lose weight.

All of this adds up to the reason that most of us have had a difficult time losing "fat weight." By cutting calories below what we need to use for our daily energy output, almost anyone can lose weight. But losing weight does not mean that we are losing fat. And if our body isn't running efficiently, our metabolism slows down and our body goes into a form of nutritional shock.

Anytime the body is in a state of shock it kicks into survival mode. When a person is trying to survive, their body will collect any calories needed and store them or, at best, use them slowly. The body's not sure if, or when, it will get a fresh supply of food needed to survive. But when the body has an abundance of calories, then it's free to use up what it has without fear of running out.

Since our bodies are the most intense surviving machines in the world, they adjust very quickly to almost anything we do. This poses a problem. How do we get our bodies to switch to burning stored carbs for fuel without letting them lapse into survival mode? This would cause the body to slow down and store food for later use.

Your body's secondary source for energy is fat. With that in mind, here is why our No-Hunger Fat-Flush diet works. We never let our bodies adapt or become efficient at storing fat. And since our bodies adapt very quickly (usually within 48 hours to minor things), most of us take in an ample amount of carbohydrates per day for our bodies to function optimally. So we have never had a need to utilize our stored energy - fat. So, for the first two weeks of your fat-flush diet, you are manipulating your carbohydrates in such a way that it forces your body to start using fat as energy.

Here's how it works. On Monday and Tuesday, you eat protein and low-fat, but no carbohydrates. When the body needs fuel, it looks for ingested carbohydrates. Since it can't find any, it then looks for ingested fat. Finding some of this, it burns it up. But there's not enough to satisfy the body's demand for energy. So, it says "There's no carbs and no more ingested fat, but I need energy. I guess I'll just have to burn up some stored fat and use it." As a result, weight loss occurs.

By Wednesday, the body only sees ingested protein and low fat, so it's adapting to using stored fat for energy. Now it's looking for fat to use for energy.

On Thursday and Friday, we switch the foods to confuse the body again. The food plan switches to protein and some carbohydrates. The body has been looking for stored fat for fuel. Now some carbohydrates show up. All of a sudden, there's no ingested fat but some carbohydrates. It's still thinking that fat is what needs to be used for future energy. So, this frees the body up to use the ingested carbohydrates for fuel. Again, there aren't enough ingested carbohydrates for fuel, so it looks for ingested fats. Not finding any of those, the body once again resorts to burning stored fat for energy. The advantage of the Thursday and Friday plan is that while it gives the body fuel and keeps the body looking for fuel from various sources, it also provides us with a nice mix of "comfort food carbohydrates" so we don't feel deprived as on other "diets."

On Saturday, we switch food mixes to confuse the body again. You eat protein, low-fat and low carbohydrates. The body burns up the ingested carbs, then the ingested fat, and for any other energy needs, it must again resort to burning up stored fat. By now the body had adapted to not having any favorite food group for energy. This sets the stage to allow us to eat ANYTHING we want on Sunday.

The really wonderful part of the No-Hunger Fat-Flush plan is Sunday. On Sundays, we can eat whatever foods we want in any mix or portion size, as long as we stay under 2,000 calories for the day. Now the body gets a whole load of stuff for fuel. Now the body is really confused. It doesn't know what to look for to burn for fuel, so it takes the carbohydrates and fats from the food we eat, and only needs to dip into the fat stores for fuel if we have a lot of muscle mass to feed, if we're big-boned and tall or very physically active. The body's been working hard all week to find fuel to burn from stored fat and now it gets to rest a bit. Sunday also slightly "retrains" the body to look for ingested carbs and fats for fuel.

But guess what happens Monday morning. We "shock" the body again by depriving it of carbohydrates and making it work hard to find fuel.

It's this continual changing of fuel sources that makes the No-Hunger Fat-Flush program work. What we are doing is a type of manual override to teach our bodies how to function at an optimum level of efficiency using carbohydrates, fats and proteins. Adding resistance exercise to the program only accelerates the weight loss process. Adding muscle burns up many more calories and uptakes most of the ingested protein for muscle building and repair. The fat-flush diet is formulated to work with the expenditure of energy. Anaerobic exercise is the number one form of using energy. We all know how good we feel when we are full of energy. We all know how rotten we feel when we are low on energy. Since carbohydrates and fat are used as fuel, we need to know what they fuel. Besides energy for all our vital organs, they also fuel our bodies' movements. What moves our bodies? Muscles do. And muscles are made of protein. The more muscle you have, the more fuel your body requires.

Professional athletes and bodybuilders have used these same No-Hunger Fat-Flush principles to rise to the top of their sports. Dave Dearth has consistently achieved a body fat percentage as low as 1.9% every year for the last fifteen years in preparation for his tournaments. This is extremely low, and not too many of us can hope to go that low, but we can go from the American norm of 30% body fat into the low 20's and even teens and be healthier and stronger because of it. Let's get started.

The No-Hunger Fat-Flush Diet is very simple to follow. Each day's meals are outlined below. It is important to follow them exactly and not make substitutions. Begin the No-Hunger Fat-Flush Diet on a Monday and follow it exactly for 6 days. On Sunday, eat whatever you like as long as you stay under your calorie limit. This information is located on day 7 of your diet plan. Then, on Monday, begin the 6 day No-Hunger Fat-Flush Plan again.

Each day you will eat 5 meals. For each meal, you have several different selections that you may make. Simply pick the selection (A, B, C, D or E) for each meal based on your likes and dislikes. Prepare that meal, eat and enjoy.

There are six different meal plans included here: 3 for men, and 3 for women. Find the plan for you according to your gender and height. The proportions of those meals have been designed for weight loss under the No-Hunger Fat-Flush Program.

At the end of the 2 week No-Hunger Fat-Flush Program, if you have more weight to lose, you can continue the same eating program for another 2 weeks.

NO-HUNGER FAT-FLUSH MEAL PLAN

FIRST 2 WEEKS NO-HUNGER FAT-FLUSH DIET FOR MEN 5'2"- 5'6"

DAY #1 AND DAY #2 FIRST 2 WEEKS HIGH PROTEIN, LOW FAT, LOW CARBOHYDRATES

MEAL #1

A.	B.	C.
1 whole egg	Protein shake	4 oz. skinless chicken breast
3 egg whites	or protein bar	2 slices tomato
1-1/2 slices turkey bacon		

*Protein bars and shakes should contain at least 16 grams of protein and no more than 10 grams of fat.

It is hard to do a lot with these meals, but here are a few suggestions we have to flavor them up. Catsup, mustard, salt, pepper, Equal or Sweet and Low, barbecue sauce and fat-free salad dressings are fine if used sparingly.

MEAL #2

A.	B.	C.
4 oz. skinless chicken breast	3 oz. flank steak	Protein shake
1 small baked potato	1/4 C rice	1/4 C pasta
	1 C broccoli or cauliflower	Salad

On your salads you may use vinegar or three tablespoons of your favorite fat-free salad dressing. When weighing your food, it should be weighed before cooking. When cooking chicken, fish or beef, they are to be baked, broiled or barbecued. If you use a skillet or pan, use non-fat cooking spray.

MEAL #3

A.	B.	C.
A small bag of pretzels	3 rice cakes	1-1/4 oz. popcorn – air-popped

MEAL #4

A.	B.	C.
4 egg whites	Protein shake with banana and strawberries	4 oz. chicken
2 oz. ground beef		1 small baked potato
1-1/2 oz. fat-free cheese		Salad
1/4 C pasta		

MEAL #5

A.	B.	C.	D.
4 oz. lean ground beef	5 egg whites	4 oz. chicken	6 oz. fish
2 C broccoli	2 C broccoli	2 C broccoli	2 C broccoli

Drink plenty of liquids throughout the day.

DAY #3 OF YOUR FIRST 2 WEEKS NO-HUNGER FAT-FLUSH DIET

MEAL #1

A.	B.	C.
2 whole eggs 2 egg whites 2 oz. ham	2 whole eggs 4 oz. flank steak	4 oz. skinless chicken breast 2 slices turkey bacon
D.	E.	
Protein shake with 1 T peanut butter	Protein bar	

Make sure you drink plenty of fluids today due to the high amounts of protein and fat. This will help in the transport of excess protein as waste.

MEAL #2

A.	B.	C.
Protein bar or protein shake 1,000 mg. L-carnitine (OPTIONAL)	2 whole eggs 2 egg whites	4 oz. lean ground beef

MEAL #3

A.	B.	C.
4 oz. skinless chicken breast Salad	3 oz. tuna in water Salad (add all you can eat veggies)	Protein shake Salad (add all you can eat veggies)

MEAL #4

A.	B.	C.	D.
3 oz. steak 1 egg white Salad	3 oz. tuna 1 whole egg Salad	4 oz. chicken 2 whole eggs Salad	Protein shake 1 tsp. peanut butter (OPTIONAL)

Salad ideas for this day can include hard boiling the eggs and adding them along with your meat with some veggies and vinegar or 3 tablespoons of fat-free salad dressing.

(Meal 5 optional, choose any of the above)

DAY #4 OF YOUR FIRST 2 WEEKS NO-HUNGER FAT-FLUSH DIET

MEAL #1

A.	B.	C.	D.
3 egg whites 1/4 C oatmeal 1/2 bagel 6 oz. juice	4 oz. chicken 1/2 piece of fruit 1/2 English muffin 6 oz. juice	4 oz. turkey 1/4 C grape nuts 1/2 C skim milk 6 oz. juice	Protein shake Add fruit. Banana or other fruit

MEAL #2

A.	B.	C.	D.
Breakfast cereal bar	1 piece of fruit	1 small bag of pretzels	Fat-free muffin

MEAL #3

A.	B.	C.	D.
Chicken salad on pita	Turkey on bagel	Protein shake Add fruit	6 oz. chicken Breakfast bar

MEAL #4

A.	B.	C.	D.
4 oz. steak on a salad (all veggies okay, fat free dressing too) 1 small baked potato	4 oz. chicken Dinner salad 1/4 C rice	4 oz. fish 1/2 C pasta Salad	4 oz. turkey 1/4 C rice Salad

MEAL #5 (this meal is optional)

A.	B.	C.	D.
Protein shake	4 egg whites	5 oz. chicken	Protein bar

DAY #5 AND DAY #6 OF YOUR FIRST 2 WEEKS NO-HUNGER FAT-FLUSH DIET

MEAL #1

A.	B.	C.
3 egg whites 1/2 C oatmeal 6 oz. juice	4 oz. chicken 1/2 grapefruit 1 bagel (with fat free cream cheese or fruit spread)	1 protein drink Breakfast cereal bar Banana

MEAL #2

A.	B.	C.	D.
Breakfast cereal bar	Bagel	Small bag of pretzels	1 piece of fruit

MEAL #3

A.	B.	C.
Chicken salad pita (4 oz. chicken, add celery, lettuce, tomato, fat-free mayo, onion)	Turkey bagel sandwich (lettuce, onion, tomato, fat-free mayo)	Protein bar 1 piece of fruit

D.
Protein shake with 1 banana

MEAL #4

A.	B.	C.
4 oz. fish	3 oz. steak	4 oz. chicken
1 baked potato	1/4 C rice	1 baked potato
Dinner salad	Dinner salad	Dinner salad

D.	E.
4 oz. lean ground beef	4 oz. turkey
1/4 C rice	3 oz. pasta
Dinner salad	Dinner salad

MEAL #5

A.	B.	C.	D.
4 C air-popped popcorn	1 piece of fruit	1 bagel (with fat frcc crcam chccsc or fruit spread)	1 bag pretzels

DAY #7 OF YOUR FIRST 2 WEEKS NO-HUNGER FAT-FLUSH DIET

Today you can eat whatever you want, up to 2,000 calories total for the day. Divide up the 2,000 calories over 3-5 meals today to keep your metabolism stoked.

FIRST 2 WEEKS NO-HUNGER FAT-FLUSH DIET FOR MEN 5'7" - 5'10"

DAY #1 AND DAY #2 FIRST 2 WEEKS HIGH PROTEIN, LOW FAT, LOW CARBOHYDRATES

MEAL #1

A.	B.	C.
1 whole egg	Protein shake or protein bar	6 oz. skinless chicken breast
3 egg whites		2 slices tomato
1-1/2 slices turkey bacon		

*Protein bars and shakes should contain at least 16 grams of protein and no more than 10 grams of fat.

It is hard to do a lot with these meals, but here are a few suggestions we have to flavor them up. Catsup, mustard, salt, pepper, Equal or Sweet and Low, barbecue sauce and fat-free salad dressings all are fine if used sparingly.

MEAL #2

A.	B.	C.
7 oz. skinless chicken breast	3 oz. flank steak	Protein shake
1 small baked potato	1/4 C rice	1/4 C pasta
	1 C broccoli or cauliflower	Salad

On your salads you may use vinegar or three tablespoons of your favorite fat-free salad dressing. When weighing your food, it should be weighed <u>before</u> cooking.

When cooking chicken, fish or beef, they are to be baked, broiled or barbecued. If you use a skillet or pan, use non-fat cooking spray.

MEAL #3

A.
A small bag of pretzels

B.
3 rice cakes

C.
1-1/4 oz. popcorn – air-popped

MEAL #4

A.
4 egg whites
3 oz. ground beef
1-1/2 oz. fat-free cheese
1/4 C pasta

B.
Protein shake with banana and strawberries

C.
6 oz. chicken
1 small baked potato
Salad

MEAL #5

A.
5 oz. lean ground beef
2 C broccoli

B.
6 egg whites
2 C broccoli

C.
5 oz. chicken
2 C broccoli

D.
6 oz. fish
2 C broccoli

Drink plenty of liquids throughout the day.

DAY #3 OF YOUR FIRST 2 WEEKS NO-HUNGER FAT-FLUSH DIET

MEAL #1

A.
2 whole eggs
2 egg whites
3 oz. ham

B.
2 whole eggs
4 oz. flank steak

C.
6 oz. skinless chicken breast
2 slices turkey bacon

D.
Protein shake with 1 T peanut butter

E.
Protein bar

Make sure you drink plenty of fluids today due to the high amounts of protein and fat. This will help in the transport of excess protein as waste.

MEAL #2

A.
Protein bar or protein shake
1,000 mg. L-carnitine (OPTIONAL)

B.
2 whole eggs
2 egg whites

C.
4 oz. lean ground beef

MEAL #3

A.
4 oz. skinless chicken breast
Salad

B.
3 oz. tuna in water
Salad (add all you can eat veggies)

C.
Protein shake
Salad (add all you can eat veggies)

MEAL #4

A.	B.	C.	D.
4 oz. steak	3 oz. tuna	4 oz. chicken	Protein shake
1 whole egg	2 whole eggs	2 whole eggs	1 tsp. peanut butter
Salad	Salad	Salad	(OPTIONAL)

Salad ideas for this day can include hard boiling the eggs and adding them along with your meat with some veggies and vinegar or 3 tablespoons of fat-free salad dressing.

(Meal 5 is optional, choose any of the above)

DAY #4 OF YOUR FIRST 2 WEEKS NO-HUNGER FAT-FLUSH DIET

MEAL #1

A.	B.	C.	D.
3 egg whites	4 oz. chicken	4 oz. turkey	Protein shake
1/2 C oatmeal	1/2 piece of fruit	1/4 C grape nuts	Add fruit.
1/2 bagel	1/2 English muffin	1/2 C skim milk	Banana or
6 oz. juice	1 C juice	6 oz. juice	other fruit

MEAL #2

A.	B.	C.	D.
Breakfast cereal bar	1 piece of fruit	1 small bag of pretzels	Fat free muffin

MEAL #3

A.	B.	C.	D.
Chicken salad	Turkey on bagel	Protein shake	6 oz. chicken
on pita		Add fruit	Breakfast bar

MEAL #4

A.	B.	C.	D.
5 oz. steak on a	5 oz. chicken	5 oz. fish	5 oz. turkey
salad (all veggies	Dinner salad	1/2 C pasta	1/4 C rice
okay, fat free	1/4 C rice	Salad	Salad
dressing too)			
1 small baked potato			

MEAL #5 (this meal is optional)

A.	B.	C.	D.
Protein shake	4 egg whites	5 oz. chicken	Protein bar

DAY #5 AND DAY #6 OF YOUR FIRST 2 WEEKS NO-HUNGER FAT-FLUSH DIET

MEAL #1

A.	B.	C.
3 egg whites	6 oz. chicken	1 protein drink

1 C oatmeal
6 oz. juice

1/2 grapefruit
1 bagel (with fat free cream cheese or fruit spread)

Breakfast cereal bar
Banana

MEAL #2

A.
Breakfast cereal bar

B.
Bagel

C.
Small bag of pretzels

D.
1 piece of fruit

MEAL #3

A.
Chicken salad pita (5 oz. chicken, add celery, lettuce, tomato, fat-free mayo, onion)

B.
Turkey bagel sandwich (lettuce, onion, tomato, fat-free mayo)

C.
Protein bar
1 piece of fruit

D.
Protein shake with 1 banana

MEAL #4

A.
6 oz. fish
1 baked potato
Dinner salad

B.
3 oz. steak
1/4 C rice
Dinner salad

C.
6 oz. chicken
Potato
Dinner salad

D.
4 oz. lean ground beef
1/4 C rice
Dinner salad

E.
5 oz. turkey
3 oz. pasta
Dinner salad

MEAL #5

A.
4 C air-popped popcorn

B.
1 piece of fruit

C.
1 bagel (with fat free cream cheese or fruit spread)

D.
1 small bag of pretzels

DAY #7 OF YOUR FIRST 2 WEEKS NO-HUNGER FAT-FLUSH DIET

Today you can eat whatever you want, up to 1,800 calories total for the day. Divide up the 1,800 calories over 3-5 meals today to keep your metabolism stoked.

FIRST 2 WEEKS NO-HUNGER FAT-FLUSH DIET FOR MEN 5'11" AND TALLER

DAY #1 AND DAY #2 FIRST 2 WEEKS HIGH PROTEIN, LOW FAT, LOW CARBOHYDRATES

MEAL #1

A.	B.	C.
1 whole egg	Protein shake	8 oz. skinless chicken breast
3 egg whites	or protein bar	2 slices tomato
2 slices turkey bacon		

*Protein bars and shakes should contain at least 16 grams of protein and no more than 10 grams of fat.

It is hard to do a lot with these meals, but here are a few suggestions we have to flavor them up. Catsup, mustard, salt, pepper, Equal or Sweet and Low, barbecue sauce and fat-free salad dressings all are fine if used sparingly.

MEAL #2

A.	B.	C.
6-8 oz. skinless chicken breast	3 oz. flank steak	Protein shake
	1/4 C rice	1/4 C pasta
1 small baked potato	1 C broccoli or cauliflower	Salad

On your salads you may use vinegar or three tablespoons of your favorite fat-free salad dressing. When weighing your food, it should be weighed <u>before</u> cooking. When cooking chicken, fish or beef, they are to be baked, broiled or barbecued. If you use a skillet or pan, use non-fat cooking spray.

MEAL #3

A.	B.	C.
A small bag of pretzels	3 rice cakes	1-1/4 oz. popcorn – air-popped

MEAL #4

A.	B.	C.
4 egg whites	Protein shake with banana and strawberries	8 oz. chicken
4 oz. ground beef		1 small baked potato
2 oz. fat-free cheese		Salad
2 oz. pasta		

MEAL #5

A.	B.	C.	D.
6 oz. lean ground beef	6 egg whites	6 oz. chicken	8 oz. fish
2 C broccoli	2 C broccoli	2 C broccoli	2 C broccoli

Drink plenty of liquids throughout the day.

DAY #3 OF YOUR FIRST 2 WEEKS NO-HUNGER FAT-FLUSH DIET

MEAL #1

A.	B.	C.
2 whole eggs	2 whole eggs	8 oz. skinless chicken breast
2 egg whites	6 oz. flank steak	2 slices turkey bacon
4 oz. ham		

D.	E.
Protein shake with 1 T peanut butter	Protein bar

Make sure you drink plenty of fluids today due to the high amounts of protein and fat. This will help in the transport of excess protein as waste.

MEAL #2

A.	B.	C.
Protein bar or protein shake 1,000 mg. L-carnitine (OPTIONAL)	2 whole eggs 2 egg whites	4 oz. lean ground beef

MEAL #3

A.	B.	C.
5 oz. skinless chicken breast Salad	4 oz. tuna in water Salad (add all you can eat veggies)	Protein shake Salad (add all you can eat veggies)

MEAL #4

A.	B.	C.	D.
4 oz. steak 1 whole egg Salad	4 oz. tuna 2 whole eggs Salad	4 oz. chicken 2 whole eggs Salad	Protein shake 1 tsp. peanut butter (OPTIONAL)

Salad ideas for this day can include hard boiling the eggs and adding them along with your meat with some veggies and vinegar or 3 tablespoons of fat-free salad dressing.

(Meal 5 optional, choose any of the above)

DAY #4 OF YOUR FIRST 2 WEEKS NO-HUNGER FAT-FLUSH DIET

MEAL #1

A.	B.	C.	D.
3 egg whites 1 serving oatmeal 1/2 bagel 1 C juice	4 oz. chicken 1 piece of fruit 1/2 English muffin 1 C juice	4 oz. turkey 1/4 C grape nuts 1/2 C skim milk 1 C juice	Protein shake Add fruit. Banana or other fruit

MEAL #2

A.	B.	C.	D.
Breakfast cereal bar	1 piece of fruit	1 small bag of pretzels	Fat-free muffin

MEAL #3

A.	B.	C.	D.
Chicken salad on pita	Turkey on bagel	Protein shake Add fruit	6 oz. chicken Breakfast bar

MEAL #4

A.
6 oz. steak on a salad (all veggies okay, fat-free dressing too)
1 small baked potato

B.
6 oz. chicken
Dinner salad
1/4 C rice

C.
6 oz. fish
1/2 C pasta
Salad

D.
6 oz. turkey
1/4 C rice
Salad

MEAL #5 (this meal is optional)

A.
Protein shake

B.
4 egg whites

C.
5 oz. chicken

D.
Protein bar

DAY #5 AND DAY #6 OF YOUR FIRST 2 WEEKS NO-HUNGER FAT-FLUSH DIET

MEAL #1

A.
3 egg whites
1 serving oatmeal
1 C juice

B.
7 oz. chicken
1/2 grapefruit
1 bagel (with fat free cream cheese or fruit spread)

C.
1 protein drink
Breakfast cereal bar
Banana

MEAL #2

A.
Breakfast cereal bar

B.
Bagel

C.
Small bag of pretzels

D.
1 piece of fruit

MEAL #3

A.
Chicken salad pita (6 oz. chicken, add celery, lettuce, tomato, fat-free mayo, onion)

B.
Turkey bagel sandwich (lettuce, onion, tomato, fat-free mayo)

C.
Protein bar
1 piece of fruit

D.
Protein shake with 1 banana

MEAL #4

A.
8 oz. fish
1 baked potato
Dinner salad

B.
3 oz. steak
1/4 C rice
Dinner salad

C.
7 oz. chicken
Potato
Dinner salad

D.
4 oz. lean ground beef
1/4 C rice
Dinner salad

E.
6 oz. turkey
3 oz. pasta
Dinner salad

MEAL #5

A.	B.	C.	D.
4 C air-popped popcorn	1 piece of fruit	1 bagel (with fat free cream cheese or fruit spread)	1 bag pretzels

DAY #7 OF YOUR FIRST 2 WEEKS NO-HUNGER FAT-FLUSH DIET

Today you can eat whatever you want, up to 2,000 calories total for the day. Divide up the 2,000 calories over 3-5 meals today to keep your metabolism stoked.

FIRST 2 WEEKS NO-HUNGER FAT-FLUSH DIET FOR WOMEN 4'10" - 5'1"

DAY #1 AND DAY #2 FIRST 2 WEEKS HIGH PROTEIN, LOW FAT, LOW CARBOHYDRATES

MEAL #1

A.	B.	C.
1 whole egg 2 egg whites 1 slice turkey bacon	Protein shake or protein bar	3 oz. skinless chicken breast 2 slices tomato

*Protein bars and shakes should contain at least 16 grams of protein and no more than 10 grams of fat.

It is hard to do a lot with these meals, but here are a few suggestions we have to flavor them up. Catsup, mustard, salt, pepper, Equal or Sweet and Low, barbecue sauce and fat-free salad dressings all are fine if used sparingly.

MEAL #2

A.	B.	C.
2 oz. skinless chicken breast 1 small baked potato Salad	3 oz. flank steak 1/4 C rice 1 C broccoli or cauliflower	Protein shake 1/4 C pasta Salad

On your salads you may use vinegar or three tablespoons of your favorite fat-free salad dressing. When weighing your food, it should be weighed before cooking. When cooking chicken, fish or beef, they are to be baked, broiled or barbecued. If you use a skillet or pan, use non-fat cooking spray.

MEAL #3

A.	B.	C.
A small bag of pretzels	2 rice cakes	1-1/4 oz. popcorn – air-popped

MEAL #4

A.	B.	C.
3 egg whites 2 oz. ground beef	Protein shake with banana and strawberries	3 oz. chicken 1 small baked potato

1 oz. fat-free cheese 1/4 C pasta		Salad	

MEAL #5

A.	B.	C.	D.
3 oz. lean ground beef 1-1/2 C broccoli	4 egg whites 1-1/2 C broccoli	3 oz. chicken 1-1/2 C broccoli	4 oz. fish 1-1/2 C broccoli

Drink plenty of liquids throughout the day.

DAY #3 OF YOUR FIRST 2 WEEKS NO-HUNGER FAT-FLUSH DIET

MEAL #1

A.	B.	C.
1 whole egg 2 egg whites 2 oz. ham	1 whole egg 1 egg white 3 oz. flank steak	3 oz. skinless chicken breast 1 slice turkey bacon
D.	**E.**	
Protein shake with 1 T peanut butter	Protein bar	

Make sure you drink plenty of fluids today due to the high amounts of protein and fat. This will help in the transport of excess protein as waste.

MEAL #2

A.	B.	C.
Protein bar or protein shake 1,000 mg. L-carnitine (OPTIONAL)	1 whole egg 3 egg whites	3 oz. lean ground beef

MEAL #3

A.	B.	C.
2 oz. skinless chicken breast Salad	2 oz. tuna in water Salad (add all you can eat veggies)	Protein shake Salad (add all you can eat veggies)

MEAL #4

A.	B.	C.	D.
2 oz. steak 1 egg white Salad	2 oz. tuna 1 whole egg 1 egg white Salad	3 oz. chicken 1 whole egg 1 egg white Salad	Protein shake 1 tsp. peanut butter (OPTIONAL)

Salad ideas for this day can include hard boiling the eggs and adding them along with your meat with some veggies and vinegar or 3 tablespoons of fat-free salad dressing.

(Meal 5 optional, choose any of the above)

DAY #4 OF YOUR FIRST 2 WEEKS NO-HUNGER FAT-FLUSH DIET

MEAL #1

A.	B.	C.	D.
2 egg whites 1/4 C oatmeal 1/2 bagel 6 oz. juice	2 oz. chicken 1/2 piece of fruit 1/2 English muffin 6 oz. juice	2 oz. turkey 1/4 C grape nuts 1/2 C skim milk 6 oz. juice	Protein shake Add fruit. Banana or other fruit

MEAL #2

A.	B.	C.	D.
Breakfast cereal bar	1 piece of fruit	1 small bag of pretzels	Fat-free muffin

MEAL #3

A.	B.	C.	D.
Chicken salad on pita	Turkey on bagel	Protein shake Add fruit	3 oz. chicken Breakfast bar

MEAL #4

A.	B.	C.	D.
2 oz. steak on a salad (all veggies okay, fat free dressing too) 1 small baked potato	2 oz. chicken Dinner salad 1/4 C rice	2 oz. fish 1/4 C pasta Salad	2 oz. turkey 1/4 C rice Salad

MEAL #5 (this meal is optional)

A.	B.	C.	D.
Protein shake	4 egg whites	3 oz. chicken	Protein bar

DAY #5 AND DAY #6 OF YOUR FIRST 2 WEEKS NO-HUNGER FAT-FLUSH DIET

MEAL #1

A.	B.	C.
2 egg whites 1/2 C oatmeal 6 oz. juice	2 oz. chicken 1/2 grapefruit 1 bagel (with fat free cream cheese or fruit spread)	1 protein drink Breakfast cereal bar Banana

MEAL #2

A.	B.	C.	D.
Breakfast cereal bar	Bagel	Small bag of pretzels	1 piece of fruit

MEAL #3

A.	B.	C.
Chicken salad pita (2 oz. chicken, add	Turkey bagel sandwich (lettuce, onion,	Protein bar 1 piece of fruit

celery, lettuce, tomato, fat-free mayo, onion)

tomato, fat-free mayo)

D.
Protein shake with
1 banana

MEAL #4

A.
3 oz. fish
1 baked potato
Dinner salad

B.
2 oz. steak
1/4 C rice
Dinner salad

C.
2 oz. chicken
Potato
Dinner salad

D.
2 oz. lean ground beef
1/4 C rice
Dinner salad

E.
2 oz. turkey
1/4 C pasta
Dinner salad

MEAL #5

A.
2 C air-popped popcorn

B.
1 piece of fruit

C.
1 bagel (with fat free cream cheese or fruit spread)

D.
1 small bag of pretzels

DAY #7 OF YOUR FIRST 2 WEEKS NO-HUNGER FAT-FLUSH DIET

Today you can eat whatever you want, up to 1,200 calories total for the day. Divide up the 1,200 calories over 3-5 meals today to keep your metabolism stoked.

FIRST 2 WEEKS NO-HUNGER FAT-FLUSH DIET FOR WOMEN 5'2" - 5'7"

DAY #1 AND DAY #2 FIRST 2 WEEKS HIGH PROTEIN, LOW FAT, LOW CARBOHYDRATES

MEAL #1

A.
1 whole egg
3 egg whites
1-1/2 slices turkey bacon

B.
Protein shake
or protein bar

C.
4 oz. skinless chicken breast
2 slices tomato

*Protein bars and shakes should contain at least 16 grams of protein and no more than 10 grams of fat.

It is hard to do a lot with these meals, but here are a few suggestions we have to flavor them up. Catsup, mustard, salt, pepper, Equal or Sweet and Low, barbecue sauce and fat-free salad dressings all are fine if used sparingly.

MEAL #2

A.	B.	C.
4 oz. skinless chicken breast	3 oz. flank steak	Protein shake
1 small baked potato	1/4 C rice	1/4 C pasta
	1 C broccoli or cauliflower	Salad

On your salads you may use vinegar or three tablespoons of your favorite fat-free salad dressing. When weighing your food, it should be weighed before cooking. When cooking chicken, fish or beef, they are to be baked, broiled or barbecued. If you use a skillet or pan, use non-fat cooking spray.

MEAL #3

A.	B.	C.
A small bag of pretzels	3 rice cakes	1-1/4 oz. popcorn – air-popped

MEAL #4

A.	B.	C.
4 egg whites	Protein shake with banana and strawberries	4 oz. chicken
2 oz. ground beef		1 small baked potato
1-1/2 oz. fat-free cheese		Salad
1/4 C. pasta		

MEAL #5

A.	B.	C.	D.
4 oz. lean ground beef	5 egg whites	4 oz. chicken	6 oz. fish
2 C broccoli	2 C broccoli	2 C broccoli	2 C broccoli

Drink plenty of liquids throughout the day.

DAY #3 OF YOUR FIRST 2 WEEKS NO-HUNGER FAT-FLUSH DIET

MEAL #1

A.	B.	C.
2 whole eggs	2 whole eggs	4 oz. skinless chicken breast
2 egg whites	4-6 oz. flank steak	2 slices turkey bacon
2 oz. ham		

D.	E.
Protein shake with 1 T peanut butter	Protein bar

Make sure you drink plenty of fluids today due to the high amounts of protein and fat. This will help in the transport of excess protein as waste.

MEAL #2

A.	B.	C.
Protein bar or protein shake	2 whole eggs	4 oz. lean ground beef
1,000 mg. L-carnitine (OPTIONAL)	2 egg whites	

MEAL #3

A.	B.	C.
4 oz. skinless chicken breast Salad	3 oz. tuna in water Salad (add all you can eat veggies)	Protein shake Salad (add all you can eat veggies)

MEAL #4

A.	B.	C.	D.
3 oz. steak 1 egg white Salad	3 oz. tuna 1 whole egg Salad	4 oz. chicken 1 whole egg Salad	Protein shake 1 tsp. peanut butter (OPTIONAL)

Salad ideas for this day can include hard boiling the eggs and adding them along with your meat with some veggies and vinegar or 3 tablespoons of fat-free salad dressing.

(Meal 5 optional, choose any of the above)

DAY #4 OF YOUR FIRST 2 WEEKS NO-HUNGER FAT-FLUSH DIET

MEAL #1

A.	B.	C.	D.
3 egg whites 1/4 C oatmeal 1/2 bagel 6 oz. juice	4 oz. chicken 1/2 piece of fruit 1/2 English muffin 6 oz. juice	4 oz. turkey 1/4 C grape nuts 1/2 C skim milk 6 oz. juice	Protein shake Add fruit. Banana or other fruit

MEAL #2

A.	B.	C.	D.
Breakfast cereal bar	1 piece of fruit	1 small bag of pretzels	Fat-free muffin

MEAL #3

A.	B.	C.	D.
Chicken salad on pita	Turkey on bagel	Protein shake Add fruit	6 oz. chicken Breakfast bar

MEAL #4

A.	B.	C.	D.
4 oz. steak on a salad (all veggies okay, fat free dressing too) 1 small baked potato	4 oz. chicken Dinner salad 1/4 C rice	4 oz. fish 1/2 C pasta Salad	4 oz. turkey 1/4 C rice Salad

MEAL #5 (this meal is optional)

A.	B.	C.	D.
Protein shake	4 egg whites	5 oz. chicken	Protein bar

DAY #5 AND DAY #6 OF YOUR FIRST 2 WEEKS NO-HUNGER FAT-FLUSH DIET

MEAL #1

A.
3 egg whites
1/2 C oatmeal
6 oz. juice

B.
4 oz. chicken
1/2 grapefruit
1 bagel (with fat free cream cheese or fruit spread)

C.
1 protein drink
Breakfast cereal bar
Banana

MEAL #2

A.
Breakfast cereal bar

B.
Bagel

C.
Small bag of pretzels

D.
1 piece of fruit

MEAL #3

A.
Chicken salad pita (4 oz. chicken, add celery, lettuce, tomato, fat-free mayo, onion)

B.
Turkey bagel sandwich (lettuce, onion, tomato, fat-free mayo)

C.
Protein bar
1 piece of fruit

D.
Protein shake with 1 banana

MEAL #4

A.
4 oz. fish
1 baked potato
Dinner salad

B.
3 oz. steak
1/4 C rice
Dinner salad

C.
4 oz. chicken
Potato
Dinner salad

D.
4 oz. lean ground beef
1/4 C rice
Dinner salad

E.
4 oz. turkey
3 oz. pasta
Dinner salad

MEAL #5

A.
4 C air-popped popcorn

B.
1 piece of fruit

C.
1 bagel (with fat free cream cheese or fruit spread)

D.
1 small bag of pretzels

DAY #7 OF YOUR FIRST 2 WEEKS NO-HUNGER FAT-FLUSH DIET

Today you can eat whatever you want, up to 1,400 calories total for the day. Divide up the 1,400 calories over 3-5 meals today to keep your metabolism stoked.

FIRST 2 WEEKS NO-HUNGER FAT-FLUSH DIET FOR WOMEN 5'8" AND TALLER

DAY #1 AND DAY #2 FIRST 2 WEEKS HIGH PROTEIN, LOW FAT, LOW CARBOHYDRATES

MEAL #1

A.	B.	C.
1 whole egg 3 egg whites 1-1/2 slices turkey bacon	Protein shake or protein bar	6 oz. skinless chicken breast 2 slices tomato

*Protein bars and shakes should contain at least 16 grams of protein and no more than 10 grams of fat.

It is hard to do a lot with these meals, but here are a few suggestions we have to flavor them up. Catsup, mustard, salt, pepper, Equal or Sweet and Low, barbecue sauce and fat-free salad dressings all are fine if used sparingly.

MEAL #2

A.	B.	C.
5 oz. skinless chicken breast 1 small baked potato	3 oz. flank steak 1/4 C rice 1 C broccoli or cauliflower	Protein shake 1/4 C pasta Salad

On your salads you may use vinegar or three tablespoons of your favorite fat-free salad dressing. When weighing your food, it should be weighed <u>before</u> cooking. When cooking chicken, fish or beef, they are to be baked, broiled or barbecued. If you use a skillet or pan, use non-fat cooking spray.

MEAL #3

A.	B.	C.
A small bag of pretzels	3 rice cakes	1-1/4 oz. popcorn – air-popped

MEAL #4

A.	B.	C.
4 egg whites 3 oz. ground beef 1-1/2 oz. fat-free cheese 1/4 C pasta	Protein shake with banana and strawberries	6 oz. chicken 1 small baked potato Salad

MEAL #5

A.	B.	C.	D.
5 oz. lean ground beef 2 C broccoli	6 egg whites 2 C broccoli	5 oz. chicken 2 C broccoli	6 oz. fish 2 C broccoli

Drink plenty of liquids throughout the day.

DAY #3 OF YOUR FIRST 2 WEEKS NO-HUNGER FAT-FLUSH DIET

MEAL #1

A.	B.	C.
2 whole eggs 2 egg whites 3 oz. ham	2 whole eggs 4 oz. flank steak	6 oz.skinless chicken breast 2 slices turkey bacon

D.	E.
Protein shake with 1 T peanut butter	Protein bar

Make sure you drink plenty of fluids today due to the high amounts of protein and fat. This will help in the transport of excess protein as waste.

MEAL #2

A.	B.	C.
Protein bar or protein shake 1,000 mg. L-carnitine (OPTIONAL)	2 whole eggs 2 egg whites	4 oz. lean ground beef

MEAL #3

A.	B.	C.
4 oz. skinless chicken breast Salad	3 oz. tuna in water Salad (add all you can eat veggies)	Protein shake Salad (add all you can eat veggies)

MEAL #4

A.	B.	C.	D.
4 oz. steak 1 whole egg Salad	3 oz. tuna 2 whole eggs Salad	4 oz. chicken 2 whole eggs Salad	Protein shake 1 tsp. peanut butter (OPTIONAL)

Salad ideas for this day can include hard boiling the eggs and adding them along with your meat with some veggies and vinegar or 3 tablespoons of fat-free salad dressing.

(Meal 5 optional, choose any of the above)

DAY #4 OF YOUR FIRST 2 WEEKS NO-HUNGER FAT-FLUSH DIET

MEAL #1

A.	B.	C.	D.
3 egg whites 1/2 C oatmeal 1/2 bagel 6 oz. juice	4 oz. chicken 1/2 piece of fruit 1/2 English muffin 1 C juice	4 oz. turkey 1/4 C grape nuts 1/2 C skim milk 6 oz. juice	Protein shake Add fruit. Banana or other fruit

MEAL #2

A.	B.	C.	D.
Breakfast cereal bar	1 piece of fruit	1 small bag of pretzels	Fat-free muffin

MEAL #3

A.	B.	C.	D.
Chicken salad on pita	Turkey on bagel	Protein shake Add fruit	6 oz. chicken Breakfast bar

MEAL #4

A.	B.	C.	D.
5 oz. steak on a salad (all veggies okay, fat free dressing too) 1 small baked potato	5 oz. chicken Dinner salad 1/4 C rice	5 oz. fish 1/2 C pasta Salad	5 oz. turkey 1/4 C rice Salad

MEAL #5 (this meal is optional)

A.	B.	C.	D.
Protein shake	4 egg whites	5 oz. chicken	Protein bar

DAY #5 AND DAY #6 OF YOUR FIRST 2 WEEKS NO-HUNGER FAT-FLUSH DIET

MEAL #1

A.	B.	C.
3 egg whites 1 C oatmeal 6 oz. juice	6 oz. chicken 1/2 grapefruit 1 bagel (with fat-free cream cheese or fruit spread)	1 protein drink Breakfast cereal bar Banana

MEAL #2

A.	B.	C.	D.
Breakfast cereal bar	Bagel	Small bag of pretzels	1 piece of fruit

MEAL #3

A.	B.	C.
Chicken salad pita (5 oz. chicken, add celery, lettuce, tomato, fat-free mayo, onion)	Turkey bagel sandwich (lettuce, onion, tomato, fat-free mayo)	Protein bar 1 piece of fruit

D.
Protein shake with
1 banana

MEAL #4

A.	B.	C.
6 oz. fish	3 oz. steak	6 oz. chicken
1 baked potato	1/4 C rice	Potato
Dinner salad	Dinner salad	Dinner salad

D.	E.
4 oz. lean ground beef	5 oz. turkey
1/4 C rice	3 oz. pasta
Dinner salad	Dinner salad

MEAL #5

A.	B.	C.	D.
4 C air-popped popcorn	1 piece of fruit	1 bagel (with fat-free cream cheese or fruit spread)	1 bag pretzels

DAY #7 OF YOUR FIRST 2 WEEKS NO-HUNGER FAT-FLUSH DIET

Today you can eat whatever you want, up to 1,600 calories total for the day. Divide up the 1,600 calories over 3-5 meals today to keep your metabolism stoked.

NO-HUNGER FAT-FLUSH PROGRAM HINTS, TIPS AND GUIDELINES

1. All salad dressings need to be low-fat or fat-free. This includes mayonnaise and cheese too.

2. Protein shakes or bars need to contain close to 16 grams of protein, around 150 calories, and be low in fat. We recommend our UltraBody bars which provide 20 grams of protein and only 3 grams of fat.

3. Drink as much fluid as possible: water, coffee, tea, diet soda, flavored water beverages, unsweetened tea, etc.

4. Choose beverages drunk with meals from the following: 8 oz. skim milk, 6 oz. juice, or any beverage from #3 above.

5. If the desire to eat becomes overwhelming, try to occupy your time until the next meal, or, if you must, eat veggies or drink a flavored non-caloric fluid.

6. Replace oils and butter with a low-fat cooking spray.

7. Use spices as liberally as you desire: salt, seasoned salt, pepper, garlic, onion powder, paprika, herbs, dried peppers, ketchup, mustard, barbecue sauce, fat-free marinades, etc.

8. On salads, you can use fat-free salad dressing. Most grocery stores also carry the wonderful new vinaigrettes in various flavors, or you can make your own. These make salads really delightful.

9. When cooking meat, only bake, broil or barbecue. Pan-frying doesn't allow the fat in the meat to drain off. You can pan-fry once in awhile if you have to, but be sure to use a non-fat cooking spray.

10. Since this plan is high in protein, be sure to drink plenty of fluids. This helps in the transport of excess protein as waste.

11. For some of the meals with salad and a meat entree, you can combine these together for a scrumptious chicken or steak salad. You can even save some of your egg allowance and add this as hard boiled eggs to your salad.

12. Be sure not to have 2 protein bars or drinks in a row on any given day. Eat some food for fiber and nutrients as well as appetite satisfaction.

13. If you do not like broccoli, you may substitute with any other vegetable except peas, lima beans or corn.

14. If you don't like beef, substitute with lean pork, fish, chicken or turkey. Do not eat cold cuts or hot dogs. They are very high in fat and sodium, even some of the turkey-based products. Read the food labels first!

9

DINING OUT THE BIOGENESIS WAY

Cutting down on fat intake doesn't mean you can't eat out — either in your favorite "white tablecloth" establishment or at the local fast food restaurant.

Throughout this book, you've been given hints, tips, recipes and ideas on how to cut down on your fat intake. Most of those tips easily apply to dining out in your favorite sit-down restaurant. Remember — ask to have your food boiled, broiled or poached without oils, instead of sautéed, deep-fat fried or topped with butter or other high-fat sauces. Stick to salads, vegetables, complex carbohydrates and small portions of protein foods.

For your convenience, we've prepared the following chart to help you eat low-fat when you dine out.

HOW GOOD ARE FAST FOODS, A.K.A. "JUNK FOODS"?

Today, it is rare to find a community without a conglomeration of fast food establishments. A recent Gallup survey found that 42% of meals were eaten away from home, with Americans spending $43 billion on the fast food segment.

It was only ten years ago that the expression "junk food" became a part of our vocabulary. Foods cited as "junk" traditionally include pizza, candy, hamburgers, french fries, milkshakes, soft drinks, etc.

Fast foods are typically high in sugar, fat, calories and salt. Rarely is it mentioned that fast food refers to the way in which food is prepared, as well as the speed with which it is served.

TIPS TO DINING OUT IN RESTAURANTS

1. Choose seafood, poultry and lean meat.
2. Watch for processed foods. They are usually high in fat content.
3. Choose low-fat or fat-free yogurts.
4. Ask what type of oil, if any, is used for cooking.
5. Request skim milk if it's available.
6. Limit consumption of processed cheese foods. Ask for low-fat cottage cheese or cheese made with part skim milk.
7. Choose more fruits, vegetables and grains instead of foods high in fat content.
8. Order fat-free or low-fat salad dressings.
9. Use condiments such as mustard, chutneys or relishes instead of mayonnaise.
10. Eliminate fried foods. Ask for your foods to be poached or broiled. Do not be intimidated. You're the customer, so ask for what you want.
11. Ask if there is a special low-fat menu.
12. Order all sauces and dressings, if any, on the side.
13. Avoid baked goods made with palm oil, coconut oil or lard.
14. If ordering any meat, request that all visible fat be cut off your portion prior to cooking.
15. Avoid butter, sautéed, fried or crispy foods, hollandaise sauces, casseroles, escalloped, augratin, stewed or pan-fried foods.

Opinions on what foods are "junk" vary. Whether you consider a food nutritious or "junk" probably lies within the context of the rest of your diet. That is to say, the total diet, not the individual foods, should be assessed. Any food can find its place in the diet with proper nutrition education. Yes, even the occasional splurge of a burger and fries can be handled by your body if you eat well the rest of the time.

The fast food industry has been responsive to consumer interest in the nutritive value of its foods. Many of the fast food chains now provide nutrient analyses of their foods. As an example, consumers said they wanted more chicken and fish and less beef. Fast food chains were delighted. After all, chicken and fish are cheaper than beef. The problem lies in the fact that most of these new chicken and fish dishes come battered, breaded and deep-fat fried, making them high in fat content.

On the other hand, salad bars are now available at many of the chains. But remember — if you eat your salad with a high-fat dressing, you may have defeated your purpose. (One ladle of fat-based dressing can add 200 calories or more.)

The bottom line for good nutrition rests with the consumer. Fast foods are still food, and no food should be considered totally worthless. True, some are of limited nutritional value, but better food choices, both at home and away from home, are the answer.

Eating low-fat at the local fast food restaurant requires a bit more work. You usually cannot specify changes in the menu or the cooking method. And many of us at least occasionally eat fast food due to our hectic lifestyles. Thankfully, many fast food restaurants are now providing lower calorie foods, some low-fat cooking methods, as well as detailed nutritional information on their products.

It is possible to eat a relatively low-fat meal at a fast food restaurant. Here are tips that we've found to be the most important:

- Augment a fast food sandwich with fruit, salads or vegetables.
- Watch out for batter-fried foods — they're loaded with fat.
- Skip the fat-laden special sauces and toppings. Stay with mustard and ketchup instead.
- Say "NO" to greasy french fries - get a healthy side dish instead. Many restaurants now offer a variety of salads, cole slaw, vegetables, rice, baked potatoes and other foods which are low in fat.

To help you make educated food choices, we've included the following guide to help you eat the Biogenesis Low-Fat Way even in fast food restaurants. Enjoy!

Arby's

	Calories	FAT g	Sodium g
Entrees			
Beef 'n Cheddar (7 oz.)	455	27	955
Junior Roast Beef (3 oz.)	218	8	345
King Roast Beef (6.75 oz.)	467	19	766
Regular Roast Beef (5.2 oz.)	353	15	588
Super Roast Beef (8.25 oz.)	501	22	798

Burger King

	Calories	FAT g	Sodium g
Breakfast Items			
Breakfast Bagel Sandwich	387	14	780
Breakfast Bagel Sandwich with Bacon	438	19	905
Breakfast Bagel Sandwich with Ham	418	15	1130

Breakfast Bagel Sandwich with Sausage	621	36	1185
Breakfast Croissanwich	304	19	637
Breakfast Croissanwich with Bacon	355	24	762
Breakfast Croissanwich with Ham	335	20	987
Breakfast Croissanwich with Sausage	538	41	1,042
French Toast Sticks	499	29	498
Great Danish	500	36	288
Scrambled Egg Platter	468	30	808
Scrambled Egg Platter with Bacon	536	36	975
Scrambled Egg Platter with Sausage	702	52	1,213
Entrees			
Bacon Double Cheeseburger	510	31	728
Cheeseburger	317	15	651
Chicken Specialty Sandwich	688	40	1,423
Chicken Tenders (6 pieces)	204	10	636
Ham & Cheese Specialty Sandwich	471	23	1534
Hamburger	275	12	509
Whaler	488	27	592
Whopper	628	36	880
Whopper with Cheese	711	43	1,164
Whopper Junior	322	17	486
Whopper Junior with Cheese	364	20	628
Side Dishes			
French Fries, Regular	227	13	160
Onion Rings, Regular	274	16	665
Desserts			
Apple Pie	305	12	412
Beverages			
Coffee, (regular)	2	0	2
Diet Pepsi®, (regular)	1	0	*
Milk, 2% Lowfat	121	5	122
Milk, Whole	157	9	119
Orange Juice	82	0	2
Pepsi Cola®, (regular)	159	0	*
7up®	144	0	*
Shake, Chocolate Medium	320	12	202
Shake, Vanilla Medium	321	10	205
Salads			
Chef Salad	180	9	570
Chicken Salad	140	4	440
Garden Salad	90	5	125
Side Salad	20	0	20
Toppings (packets)			
Bacon Bits	16	1	1
Blue Cheese dressing	300	31	600
Croutons	29	1	88
French dressing	280	23	690

House dressing	260	26	530
1000 Island dressing	240	23	470
Reduced Calorie Italian dressing	30	2	870

* Indicates that information for this nutrient has not been analyzed or is not available.

Domino's Pizza

	Calories	FAT g	Sodium g
Entrees			
Cheese Pizza, Large (16"), 2 slices	376	10	483
Deluxe Pizza, Large (16"), 2 slices	498	20	954
Double Cheese/Pepperoni Pizza, Large (16"), 2 slices	545	25	1,042
Ham Pizza, Large (16"), 2 slices	417	11	805
Pepperoni Pizza, Large (16"), 2 slices	460	18	825
Sausage/Mushroom Pizza, Large (16"), 2 slices	430	16	552
Veggie Pizza, Large (16"), 2 slices	498	19	1035

Kentucky Fried Chicken

	Calories	FAT g	Sodium g
Entrees			
"Chicken Littles" Sandwich	169	10	331
Extra Crispy Chicken			
Center Breast	353	21	842
Drumstick	173	11	346
Side Breast	354	24	797
Thigh	371	26	766
Wing	218	16	437
Original Recipe Chicken			
Center Breast	283	15	672
Drumstick	146	8	275
Side Breast	267	16	735
Thigh	294	20	619
Wing	178	12	372
"Kentucky Nuggets" 6 pieces	276	17	840
"Kentucky Nuggets" Sauces			
Barbeque	35	<1	450
Honey	49	<1	<15
Mustard	36	<1	346
Sweet and Sour	58	<1	148
Side Dishes			
Buttermilk Biscuit	232	12	539
Cole Slaw	119	7	197
Corn-on-the-Cob	176	3	<21
French Fries (regular)	244	12	139
Mashed Potatoes with Gravy	71	2	342

McDonald's

	Calories	FAT g	Sodium g
Breakfast Items			
Biscuit with spread	260	13	730
Biscuit with Bacon, Egg & Cheese	440	26	1,230
Biscuit with Sausage	440	29	1,080
Biscuit with Sausage & Egg	520	34	1,250
Danish, Apple	390	18	370
Danish, Cinnamon Raisin	440	21	430
Danish, Iced Cheese	390	22	420
Danish, Raspberry	410	16	310
Egg McMuffin	290	11	740
English Muffin with Butter	170	5	270
Hash Brown Potatoes	130	7	330
Hot Cakes with Butter, Syrup	410	9	640
Pork Sausage	180	16	350
Sausage McMuffin	370	22	830
Sausage McMuffin with Egg	440	27	980
Scrambled Eggs	140	10	290
Entrees			
Big Mac	560	32	950
Cheeseburger	310	14	750
Chicken McNuggets (6 pieces)	290	16	520
Barbeque Sauce	50	<1	340
Honey	45	0	0
Hot Mustard Sauce	70	4	250
Sweet and Sour Sauce	60	<1	190
Filet-O-Fish	440	26	1,030
Hamburger	260	10	500
McChicken	490	29	780
Mc D.L.T.	580	37	990
Quarter Pounder	410	21	660
Quarter Pounder with Cheese	520	29	1,150
Side Dishes			
French Fries, Large	400	22	200
French Fries, Medium	320	17	150
French Fries, Small	220	12	110
Shakes and Desserts			
Apple Pie	260	15	240
Chocolaty Chip Cookies	330	16	280
Cone	140	4	70
McDonaldland Cookies	290	9	300
Shake, Chocolate	390	11	240
Shake, Strawberry	380	10	170
Shake, Vanilla	350	10	170
Soft Serve Sundae, Hot Caramel	340	9	160

Soft Serve Sundae, Hot Fudge	310	9	160
Soft Serve Sundae, Strawberry	280	7	80
Salads			
Chef Salad	230	13	490
Chicken Salad Oriental	140	3	230
Garden Salad	110	7	160
Side Salad	60	3	85
Blue Cheese dressing (½ ounce)	70	7	150
Caesar dressing (½ ounce)	60	6	170
French dressing (½ ounce)	58	5	180
Lite Vinaigrette dressing (½ ounce)	15	<1	75
1000 Island dressing (½ ounce)	78	8	100
Oriental dressing (½ ounce)	24	<1	180
Peppercorn dressing (½ ounce)	80	9	85
Ranch dressing (½ ounce)	83	9	130
Red French Reduced Calorie dressing (½ ounce)	40	2	110
Beverages			
Coca-Cola Classic (16 ounces with ice)	190	*	20
Diet Coke (16 ounces with ice)	1	*	40
Grapefruit Juice (6 ounces)	80	0	0
Orange Drink (16 ounces with ice)	180	*	15
Orange Juice (6 ounces)	80	0	0
Sprite (16 ounces with ice)	190	*	20
2% Milk (8 ounces)	120	5	130

* Indicates that information for this nutrient has not been analyzed or is not available.

Pizza Hut

	Calories	FAT g	Sodium g
Pan Pizza			
Cheese, Medium, 2 slices	492	18	940
Pepperoni, Medium, 2 slices	540	22	1,127
Supreme, Medium, 2 slices	589	30	1,363
Super Supreme, Medium, 2 slices	563	26	1,447
"Thin 'n Crispy" Pizza			
Cheese, Medium, 2 slices	398	17	867
Pepperoni, Medium, 2 slices	413	20	986
Supreme, Medium, 2 slices	459	22	1,328
Hand-Tossed			
Cheese, Medium, 2 slices	518	20	1,276
Pepperoni, Medium, 2 slices	500	23	1,267
Supreme, Medium, 2 slices	540	26	1,470
Super Supreme, Medium, 2 slices	556	25	1,648
"Personal Pan Pizza"			
Pepperoni, whole pizza	675	29	1335
Supreme, whole pizza	647	28	1313

Ponderosa

	Calories	FAT g	Sodium g
Entrees			
Chicken Breast (5.5 oz.)[1]	98	2	400
Chicken Wings, 2 pieces	213	9	610
Chopped Steak (4 oz.)[1]	225	16	150
Chopped Steak (5.3 oz.)[1]	296	22	296
Fish, Baked			
Bake 'N Broil (5.2 oz.)	230	13	330
Baked Scrod (7 oz.)	120	1	80
Fish, Broiled			
Halibut (6 oz.)	170	2	68
Roughy (5 oz.)	139	5	88
Salmon (6 oz.)	192	3	72
Swordfish (5.9 oz.)	271	9	*
Trout (5 oz.)	228	4	51
Fish, Fried (3.2 oz.)	190	9	170
Fish Nuggets, 1 piece	31	2	52
Hot Dog, (1.6)[1]	144	13	460
Kansas City Strip (5 oz.)[1]	138	6	850
New York Strip, Choice (10 oz.)[1]	314	14	1,420
New York Strip, Choice (8 oz.)[1]	236	10	570
Porterhouse, Choice (16 oz.)[1]	640	31	1,130
Ribeye, Choice (6 oz.)[1]	282	14	570
Sandwich steak (4 oz.)	408	11	850
Sirloin, Choice (7 oz.)[1]	241	11	570
Sirloin Tips, Choice (5 oz.)[1]	473	8	280
Steak Kabobs, Meat only (3 oz.)[1]	153	5	280
Teriyaki Steak (5 oz.)[1]	174	3	1,420
T-Bone, Choice (10 oz.)[1]	444	18	850
Side Dishes			
Macaroni and Cheese, (1 oz.)	17	<1	80
Potatoes,			
Baked	145	<1	6
French Fried, (3 oz.)	120	4	39
Mashed, (4 oz.)	62	<1	191
Wedges, (3.5 oz.)	130	6	171
Rice Pilaf (4 oz.)	160	4	450
Rolls, Dinner	184	3	311
Rolls, Sourdough	110	1	230
Salad Dressings			
Blue Cheese, (1 oz.)	130	13	266
Creamy Italian, (1 oz.)	103	10	373
Parmesan Pepper, (1 oz.)	150	15	282
Ranch, (1 oz.)	147	15	298
Reduced Cal. Cucumber, (1 oz.)	69	6	316

Reduced Cal. Italian, (1 oz.)	31	3	371
Sour Cream, 1 Tbsp.	26	2	6
Sweet-n-Tangy	122	9	347
Thousand Island, (1 oz.)	113	10	405
Desserts			
Gelatin, Plain, (4 oz.)	152	3	70
Ice Milk, Chocolate (3.5 oz.)	71	0	73
Ice Milk, Vanilla (3.5 oz.)	150	3	58
Mousse, Chocolate (1 oz.)	80	4	18
Mousse, Strawberry (1 oz.)	74	5	17
Toppings, Caramel (1 oz.)	100	<1	72
Chocolate (1 oz.)	89	<1	37
Strawberry (1 oz.)	71	<1	29
Whipped (1 oz.)	80	6	16
Beverages			
Caffeine Free Diet Coke, (6 oz.)	<1	0	8
Cherry Coke (6 oz.)	77	0	4
Coca-Cola (6 oz.)	72	0	7
Coffee (6 oz.)	2	0	26
Diet Coke (6 oz.)	<1	0	8
Diet Sprite (6 oz.)	2	0	4
Dr. Pepper (6 oz.)	72	0	14
Lemonade (6 oz.)	68	0	50
Milk, Chocolate (8 oz.)	208	8	149
White (8 oz.)	159	9	122
Mr. Pibb® (6 oz.)	71	0	10
Orange (6 oz.)	82	0	0
Root Beer (6 oz.)	80	0	9
Sprite (6 oz.)	72	0	16

[1] Pre-cooked weight. Nutritive value calculated on cooked weight.

* Indicates that information for this nutrient has not been analyzed or is not available.

Rax

	Calories	FAT g	Sodium g
Entrees			
BBC (Beef, Bacon and Cheddar Sandwich)	720	49	1,873
BBQ Sandwich	420	14	1,343
Fish Sandwich	460	17	935
Ham and Swiss Sandwich	430	23	1,737
Philly Beef and Cheese Sandwich	480	22	1,346
Roast Beef Sandwich, Large	570	35	1,169
Roast Beef Sandwich, Regular	320	11	969
Small Roast Beef Sandwich (Uncle Al)	260	14	562
Turkey Bacon Club	670	43	1,878
BBQ Potato (2 oz. cheese)	730	24	1,071

Cheese (3 oz.) and Bacon Potato	780	28	910
Cheese (3 oz.) and Broccoli Potato	760	26	489
Chili and Cheese (2 oz.) Potato	700	23	599
French Fries, Large (Salted)	390	20	104
French Fries, Regular (Salted)	260	13	69
Plain Potato	270	<1	70
Plain Potato with Margarine	370	11	170
Sour Topping Potato	400	11	149
Drive-thru Salads			
Chef Salad (without dressing)	230	14	1,048
Garden Salad (without dressing)	160	11	362
Salad Bar			
Blue Cheese dressing (1 Tbsp.)	50	5	110
Cole Slaw (3.5 oz.)	70	4	187
French dressing (1 Tbsp.)	60	<4	140
Gelatin, Lime (½ cup)	90	<1	90
Gelatin, Strawberry (½ cup)	90	<1	90
Italian dressing (1 Tbsp.)	50	4	159
Lite Blue Cheese dressing (1 Tbsp.)	35	3	240
Lite French dressing (1 Tbsp.)	40	2	122
Lite Italian dressing (1 Tbsp.)	30	3	152
Lite Thousand Island dressing (1 Tbsp.)	40	3	143
Macaroni Salad (3.5 oz.)	160	7	216
Oil (1 Tbsp.)	130	14	<1
Pasta Salad (3.5 oz.)	80	1	322
Poppy Seed dressing (1 Tbsp.)	60	4	107
Potato Salad (1 cup)	260	17	127
Pudding, Butterscotch (3.5 oz.)	140	6	150
Pudding, Chocolate (3.5 oz.)	140	6	120
Pudding, Vanilla (3.5 oz.)	140	6	120
Ranch dressing (1 Tbsp.)	45	5	103
Mexican Bar			
Cheese Sauce, Regular (3.5 oz.)	420	17	365
Cheese Sauce, Nacho (3.5 oz.)	470	22	190
Refried Beans (3 oz.)	120	4	375
Sour Topping (3.5 oz.)	130	11	79
Spanish Rice (3.5 oz.)	90	<1	442
Spicy Meat Sauce (3.5 oz.)	80	4	751
Taco Sauce (3.5 oz.)	30	<1	806
Taco Shell	40	4	53
Tortilla	110	2	284
Tortilla Chips (1 oz.)	140	7	100
Pasta Bar			
Alfredo Sauce (3.5 oz.)	80	3	70
Chicken Noodle Soup (3.5 oz.)	40	<1	1,040
Cream of Broccoli Soup (3.5 oz.)	50	2	219
Parmesan Cheese Substitute (1 oz.)	80	4	1,000

Pasta Shells (3.5 oz.)	170	<4	2
Pasta/Vegetable Blend (3.5 oz.)	100	4	11
Rainbow Rotini (3.5 oz.)	180	4	9
Spaghetti (3.5 oz.)	140	4	1
Spaghetti Sauce (3.5 oz.)	80	<1	635
Spaghetti Sauce w/Meat (3.5 oz.)	150	8	419
Shakes and Desserts			
Chocolate Chip Cookies	130	6	65
Milkshake, Chocolate (without whip topping)	560	13	239
Milkshake, Strawberry (without whip topping)	560	13	226
Milkshake, Vanilla (without whip topping)	500	14	286
Whipped Topping, one dip	50	4	6

Taco Bell

	Calories	FAT g	Sodium g
Entrees			
Bean Burrito, Green Sauce	351	10	763
Bean Burrito, Red Sauce	357	10	888
Beef Burrito, Green Sauce	398	17	926
Beef Burrito, Red Sauce	403	17	1,051
Burrito Supreme, Green Sauce	407	18	796
Burrito Supreme, Red Sauce	413	18	921
Chicken Fajita	226	10	619
Cinnamon Crisps	259	15	127
Double Beef Burrito Supreme, Green Sauce	451	22	928
Double Beef Burrito, Red Sauce	457	22	1,053
Enchirito, Green Sauce	381	54	993
Enchirito, Red Sauce	382	20	1243
Guacamole	34	2	113
Hot Taco Sauce, packet	3	<1	82
Jalapeno Pepper	20	<1	1,370
Mexican Pizza	575	37	1,031
Meximelt	266	15	689
Nachos	346	18	399
Nachos Bell Grande	648	35	997
Pico De Gallo	8	<1	88
Pintos and Cheese, Green Sauce	184	9	518
Pintos and Cheese, Red Sauce	190	9	642
Ranch Dressing	236	25	571
Salsa	18	<1	376
Soft Taco	228	12	516
Soft Taco Supreme	275	16	516
Sour Cream	46	4	*
Steak Fajita	234	11	485
Super Combo Taco	286	16	462
Taco	183	11	276

Taco Bellgrande	355	23	472
Taco Light	410	29	594
Taco Salad without Shell	502	31	1,056
Taco Salad with Salsa	941	61	1,662
Taco Salad with Salsa, without Shell	520	31	1,431
Taco Sauce, Packet	2	<1	126
Tostado, Green Sauce	237	11	471
Tostado, Red Sauce	243	11	596

Wendy's

	Calories	FAT g	Sodium g
Breakfast Items			
Bacon, 2 strips	60	4	250
Breakfast Potatoes	360	22	745
Breakfast Sandwich	370	19	770
Buttermilk Biscuit	320	17	860
Danish, Cheese	430	21	500
Egg Fried, One	90	6	95
Eggs, Scrambled, 2 Eggs	190	12	160
French Toast, 2 slices	400	19	850
Omelet #1 - Ham & Cheese	290	21	570
Omelet #2 - Ham, Cheese & Mushrooms	250	17	405
Omelet #3 - Ham, Cheese, Onion & Green Pepper	280	19	485
Omelet #4 - Mushrooms, Onion & Green Pepper	210	15	200
Sausage, patty	200	18	405
White Toast with Margarine, 2 slices	250	9	410
Entrees			
Bacon Swiss Burger	710	44	1,390
Big Classic	580	34	1,015
Big Classic with Cheese	640	40	1,310
Chicken Breast Filet	430	19	705
Chili	230	9	960
Crispy Chicken Nuggets - 6 pieces cooked in animal/vegetable oil	290	21	615
Kid's Meal Cheeseburger	320	15	805
Kid's Meal Hamburger (2 oz. patty)	260	9	510
Philly Swiss Burger	510	24	975
Single Cheeseburger with Everything	490	28	1,100
Single Hamburger Patty (¼ lb.)	350	16	420
Single with Cheese	410	22	710
Single with Everything	430	22	805
Small Cheeseburger	320	15	805
Small Hamburger (2 oz. patty)	260	9	510
Taco Salad	660	37	1110

Take-Out Salads			
Chef Salad	180	9	140
Garden Salad	102	5	110
Side Dishes			
French Fries (cooked in animal/vegetable oil)	310	15	105
Bacon and Cheese Potato	570	30	1,180
Broccoli and Cheese Potato	500	25	430
Cheese Potato	590	34	450
Chili and Cheese Potato	510	20	610
Plain Potato	250	2	60
Sour Cream and Chives Potato	460	24	230
Shakes and Desserts			
"Frosty" Dairy Dessert	400	14	220
"Garden Spot" Salad Bar			
California Cole slaw (2 oz.)	60	6	140
Deluxe Three Bean Salad (¼ cup)	60	<1	15
Old Fashion Corn Relish (¼ cup)	35	<1	205
Pasta Deli Salad (¼ cup)	35	<1	120
Red Bliss Potato Salad	110	9	265
Butterscotch Pudding (¼ cup)	90	4	85
Chocolate Pudding (¼ cup)	90	4	70
Blue Cheese dressing (1 Tbsp.)	80	9	90
Celery Seed dressing (1 Tbsp.)	70	6	65
Creamy Peppercorn (1 Tbsp.)	80	8	135
French dressing (1 Tbsp.)	70	6	190
Golden Italian dressing (1 Tbsp.)	50	4	260
"Hidden Valley" Ranch dressing (1 Tbsp.)	50	6	115
Italian Caesar dressing (1 Tbsp.)	70	8	125
Oil (Tbsp.)	120	14	0
Reduced Calorie Bacon and Tomato (1 Tbsp.)	45	4	190
Reduced Calorie Creamy Cucumber (1 Tbsp.)	50	5	140
Reduced Calorie Italian (1 Tbsp.)	25	2	180
Reduced Calorie Thousand Island (1 Tbsp.)	45	4	125
Sweet Red French Dressing (1 Tbsp.)	70	6	130
Thousand Island Dressing (1 Tbsp.)	70	7	105
Wine Vinegar (1 Tbsp.)	2	<1	5

10

HINTS AND TIPS

Knowing and using the basic elements of food preparation are an important part of every meal. Meals are more than just eating food to keep our bodies going. Dining should be a pleasant experience. Meals do not need to be luxurious or fancy — a nicely done soup and salad luncheon can be a welcome break in a hectic day. Preparation and presentation are the keys to a memorable and enjoyable meal that you, your family and your friends will remember for a long time.

TEMPERATURE

This is the most basic element. Hot food should be served on hot plates. The food must be hot prior to plating and served immediately.

Cold food must be served on well-chilled plates and the food must be cold or kept on ice prior to serving.

REMEMBER: "Hot food served hot on hot plates."
"Cold food served cold on cold plates."

FLAVOR

All of the food on the plate is meant to be eaten. Therefore, all items must be well-seasoned and complement each other. Even though each individual food by itself might be well-prepared, if they do not complement each other, the meal will be undesirable.

COLOR

People eat with their eyes. In presenting food, you must keep in mind that multiple colors are much more appealing than foods that are similar in color. A plate with no contrasting colors looks dull and gives the impression that it tastes dull too. Use naturally bright-colored foods and prepare them properly.

TEXTURE

The key to texture is variety. Your plate should include foods with many different textures, not only for taste purposes, but also for eye appeal. Smooth, soft, crunchy, liquid, solid and firm textures should be used in a basic plate presentation. A well-balanced meal uses many textures to create a memorable experience.

SHAPES

Your presentation of food should utilize several different shapes. Use the natural shapes of food to highlight your presentation. Stay away from foods that have a similar shape. Also, wherever possible, add some height to your plate. This will create a completely different dimension.

GARNISH

This is the final touch to add before serving your meal. Use edible garnishes that complement your meal. Make them simple but creative. This will make a difference between having "dinner" or having a "dining experience."

MEASUREMENTS AND ABBREVIATIONS

tsp.	=	teaspoon
T	=	tablespoon
C	=	cup — 8 liquid ounces
oz.	=	ounce
g	=	gram
1 lb.	=	16 ounces
ea.	=	each
pt.	=	pint — 16 liquid ounces
qt.	=	quart — 32 liquid ounces
gal.	=	gallon — 128 liquid ounces

EQUIVALENTS

16 oz.	=	1 lb.
3 tsp.	=	1 T
16 T	=	1 C
2 C	=	1 pt.

2 pts.	=	1 qt.
4 qt.	=	1 gal.

THE BEST COOKING METHODS FOR LOW-FAT MEALS

POACHING: A method of gently cooking food completely covered in liquid (180-200 degrees).

For low-fat cooking, a defatted stock or bouillon is perfect. This should be seasoned with onions, celery, carrots and fresh herbs of your choice. Cook this liquid for 15-20 minutes to extract all of the flavors and strain. Use this liquid to poach your food items.

STEAMING: To cook food over a liquid that is boiling to create steam (212 degrees).

This is a terrific way to cook foods without adding fat. It preserves many nutrients and retains the natural flavor and color of many foods. There are many simple steaming units you can purchase for in-home use that are very easy to use.

BROILING: A transfer of heat through the air to brown and cook food.

This is an excellent method for cooking foods that have natural fat in them. Use a broiling rack to place food on to help eliminate excess fat. The major flavor given to food cooked with this method comes from the type of marinade you use on the food.

TIPS FOR LOW-FAT MEAL PREPARATION

1. Steam, poach or broil foods instead of sautéing, roasting or deep-fat frying.
2. If using any oils, think teaspoon instead of tablespoon.
3. Use skim milk instead of homogenized milk.
4. When cooking pastas, do not add oil to the water.
5. Use non-stick pans whenever possible to eliminate cooking with oils.
6. Use arrowroot or cornstarch for thickening instead of the animal or cooking fats used in rouxs.
7. Substitute fat-free food choices for high-fat foods.
8. Use fresh herbs in place of dried herbs if you can. They give a much better flavor.
9. Trim off all visual fat from any item that you are cooking.
10. Read all labels completely.
11. Choose meat labeled "very lean" or "extra lean."
12. Chill soups and stocks to make it easy to remove excess fat.
13. Use fat-free yogurts instead of low-fat yogurts.

14. Use flavored vinegars to season foods.
15. Purchase as many fresh products as possible.
16. Baste meats with defatted stocks instead of butter.
17. Make good use of stone-ground mustards, chutneys, lemon juice, garlic and onions.
18. Use a microwave to reheat leftover foods. This will eliminate adding fat to reheat.
19. If you use oils, try using infused oils. They add more flavor and you can get away with using less.
20. Purchase low-fat or fat-free salad dressings. These make great dips as well as dressings for use on salads and pastas.

QUALITY POTS AND PANS

Aside from using herbs and spices to supercharge foods with flavor, the next most important items are good pots and pans. Today's non-stick cookware is a far cry from what was available even only a few years ago.

Today you can pick from more than 40 different lines of non-stick cookware. And non-stick cookware is really the only type to consider, especially for low-fat cooking.

Non-stick pans offer the best in the way of low-fat, or even no-fat, cooking. Foods don't stick; you can use very small amounts of oil if you want to and the pans clean up ever so nicely.

All non-stick pans offer quick clean-up, but that's about as far as their similarities go. Different manufacturers make pans that differ in durability, price and performance. Some don't cook as well as others, and some are less durable than their competitors.

So which should you buy? It really depends on your cooking habits and the money that you want to spend. Do you really enjoy cooking? Is it an important part of your life? Or do you just want pans that let you cook quick and easy meals for your family and friends?

Good sets that will serve you well can be had for as little as $100, or you can spend up to $400 for high-end professional pans. You'll most likely find what you need in any good department store cooking department or at a specialty cooking shops.

At a minimum, here's what you'll need:

1. Two saucepans with lids — pick the size you use most often (somewhere in the 3-5 quart range).
2. One sauté pan, in the 10-12" size.
3. A one or two-burner griddle is very handy for vegetables, eggs, appetizers, small portions of meat and the ever-popular pancakes.
4. If you use them a lot, add specialty pieces such as an omelet pan or another

sauté pan.

TYPES OF PANS TO CONSIDER

Various types of pans are available. You can choose aluminum, cast or anodized aluminum, stainless steel and even glass.

I'd stay clear of the plain aluminum pans — they just aren't as durable. Coated cast or anodized aluminum is perhaps the very best heat conductor available. One warning: aluminum reacts with acidic foods like tomatoes, so be sure any aluminum pan is well coated with a non-aluminum, non-stick coating. Also make sure it covers the entire inside of the pan.

Stainless steel works well, but is not as good a heat conductor as aluminum. One way to solve this problem is to use stainless pans that have an aluminum or copper core to increase heat conductivity.

There are several non-stick coatings to choose from, and they all work well. Some companies spray on the coating, others dip the pan in the coating. Some manufacturers use one coat, others apply up to three coats of non-stick material. Obviously, the more the better.

Farberware sells non-stick pans made of stainless steel with an aluminum heat conductor on the bottom of the pan. These are good for browning and sautéing.

Millennium is popular with chefs, as is Excalibur and Castex. Excalibur is stainless steel, while Castex is anodized cast aluminum. Magnalite and Ultrex, both stainless steel with copper cores, are also popular.

Both Farberware and T-fal are popular for the home market due to their somewhat lower cost. T-fal's Resisteel, a stainless steel pan with a copper core, sells for about $170 for an eight-piece set.

Whichever brand you choose, it will all give you good service for years and the added benefit of low or no-fat cooking and spotlessly quick cleanup!

SELECTED SOURCES OF RELIABLE NUTRITION INFORMATION

American Dietetic Association
430 N. Michigan Ave.
Chicago, IL 60611

American Home Economics Association
Division of Public Affairs
2010 Massachusetts Ave. NW
Washington, DC 20036

American Institute of Baking
400 E. Ontario St.
Chicago, IL 60611

American Institute of Nutrition
9650 Rockville Pike
Bethesda, MD 20014

American Meat Institute
59 E. Van Buren St.
P.O. Box 3556
Washington, DC 20007

American Medical Association
Council on Foods and Nutrition
535 N. Dearborn St.
Chicago, IL 60610

American Public Health Association
1015 18th St. NW
Washington, DC 20036

American School Food Service
P.O. Box 10095
Denver, CO 80210

Children's Bureau
U.S. Department of Health, Education and Welfare
Washington, DC 20203

Food and Agriculture Organization (FAO) of the U.N.
c/o American Public Health Association
1740 Broadway
New York, NY 10019

Food and Drug Administration (FDA)
Parkland Building
5600 Fishers Lane
Rockville, MD 20852

Food and Nutrition Board
National Academy of Sciences
2101 Constitution Ave.
Washington, DC 20418

National Dietary Council
6300 N. River Rd.
Rosemont, IL 60018

National Foundation - March of Dimes
Health Information Department
P.O. Box 2000
White Plains, NY 10602

National Livestock and Meat Board
444 N. Michigan Ave.
Chicago, IL 60611

National Nutrition Consortium
24 Third St. NE Suite 200
Washington, DC 20002

Nutrition Foundation, Inc.
888 17th St. NW
Washington, DC 20016

Nutrition Information and Resource Center
Benedict House
Pennsylvania State University
University Park, PA 16802

Nutrition Today Society
101 Ridgly Ave.
P.O. Box 773
Annapolis, MD 21404

Society for Nutrition Education
1736 Franklin St.
Oakland, CA 94612

Superintendent of Documents
U.S. Government Printing Office
Washington, DC 20402

U.S. Department of Agriculture
Cooperative Extension Service
Home Economics
Washington, DC 20250

Nutrition Program Consumer and Food Economics Division
Agricultural Research Service
Hyattsville, MD 20782

Office of Communications
Washington, DC 20250

School Lunch Program
Information Division
Food and Nutrition Service
Washington, DC 20250

World Health Organization (WHO)
Distribution and Sales Service
1211 Geneva 27, Switzerland

Your local Cooperative Extension Service may also have free information available to give to you.

11

Biogenesis Basic Fundamentals Phase One

Biogenesis is many things because it can do so many things for you. It is a weight loss program, a fitness program, and physical therapy for your body. It is a good, healthy lifestyle. The original design concept was for weight loss, but when we put on our thinking caps, there were some obstacles to consider. Long-term weight loss and fitness are things that take time out of our schedules, and we decided if someone wanted to do this training it had to be quick and convenient to do. Spending 25% of your waking hours staying in shape to live an unguaranteed 10% longer life span really doesn't make sense. Trying to develop a habit that can be hard physical work has to be built upon. We believe in lifestyle change for the long haul!

The workout or training portion of Biogenesis is a multiphase resistance training program that builds on the fundamentals. There are a few fundamentals that you should know even before you start the program, and there are some you will pick up as you go through the phases. Some of them are basic fitness and human body knowledge fundamentals and there are also psychological fundamentals that, if developed, can transfer into your everyday life activities and conduct. Repetitions, sets, resistance styles, and body anatomy must be understood to get the most out your training. If these topics are not understood, Phase One should be repeated until the concepts are learned. The other fundamentals such as intensity, focus, desire and determination, to name a few, can be learned as you go. You will quickly learn that these fundamentals are the key difference between a good or mediocre program and a superior program that is Biogenesis. Master these fundamentals and make your mind control your body, willing it to change into what you imagine.

Let's take a closer look or each of these fundamentals. We can classify them into two categories, ones that are physical and ones that are psychological. The physical fundamentals of Biogenesis are ones that deal with how the workout is performed with your body and the environment around you. The psychological fundamentals are the ones that deal with our thoughts and state of mind before, during, and after working out. Remember, make the mind control the body. Not the other way around. This is why most people get out of shape in the first place.

RESISTANCE EXERCISE

Let's start with resistance exercise, what it is and why we use it. Whatever you want to call it, weight training, body building, strength training, or resistance training, it is pretty much the same in one aspect; oxygen, and the ability to use it, or not to use it, to burn fuel to provide energy for muscular contraction for work. This classifies exercise as aerobic (to use oxygen) or anaerobic,(without oxygen) to perform work. During resistance exercises we use stored energy to do the work. This does not last long and it is how difficult the work is that determines how long we will do the exercise.

Think of an electrical battery that has a given amount of charge in it to be exhausted. You can make it put out all of its power in short bursts or in a long, slow stream like aerobics. It will take some time to recharge, like your muscles; but the interesting thing with resistance training is that every time the battery recharges, the battery gets stronger, and that's what your muscles do. So what does this mean? A stronger battery, or muscle, means the ability to do more work and burn up more energy.

If one person lifts 100 lbs. straight up for a total of 5 feet and the task takes him five seconds to do, he has done a certain amount of work, right? Now, let's take that same 100 lbs. and put it on a cart with wheels and pull it up an incline that is 5 feet high but is 500 feet long and it takes someone five minutes to pull the cart the same distance and height. This is relatively the same amount of work the same amount of energy expenditure. The difference is in the time it took to perform the work. Now look at all the free time you have if you decided to lift the weight straight up compared to the other way.

This leads us to the time factor of why this program starts out as only 10 minutes. The average person does not have a long power output at high levels of work load and their energy can be spent in a few moments. What is important is how much work is performed, not how long the work is performed. Take the same scenario with the weight. Let's say someone was paying you to do it by the pound and they gave you 10 minutes to do it. How would you perform the work? If you chose to lift the weight straight up you have the right frame of mind to do Biogenesis. For those of you who picked the other method, you might want to stick to walking if you can find the time.

Now let's look at workout jargon, like repetitions and sets. If you lifted that 100 lbs. one time that would be one repetition. If you lift it several times and then stop to rest, that would be called a set, or a set of repetitions. In ten minute workouts we divide the work into different exercises that require a given number of sets of repetitions. This is the basic structure and design of many successful resistance exercise programs.

This brings us to execution of exercises. In the first phase of Biogenesis we want to eliminate as much confusion as possible. Many of you have never been exposed to resistance training or its fundamentals. Equipment like weights and different types of exercise machines can be very intimidating. The Biogenesis exercises are designed to provide resistance, or force, to make the body work to expend energy. Some exercises use gravity and our body weight to provide the resistance; some exercises pit one body part against another, and others are a combination of gravity and opposite body parts that are isometric. Isometric is a term used to describe force, or work, that does not require motion. This is perfect for beginners because no investments in equipment are required. This also helps you understand how your body works and moves while you work out and the focus is on the body instead of equipment.

Knowing what your body does during an exercise and how it does a certain exercise are very important and will be useful for the rest of the phases. How your body moves from muscular contractions can be confusing at first, but when you start Phase One you will observe that when you do a certain motion several times with resistance, you feel it in a certain area of your body. Take note of this infor-

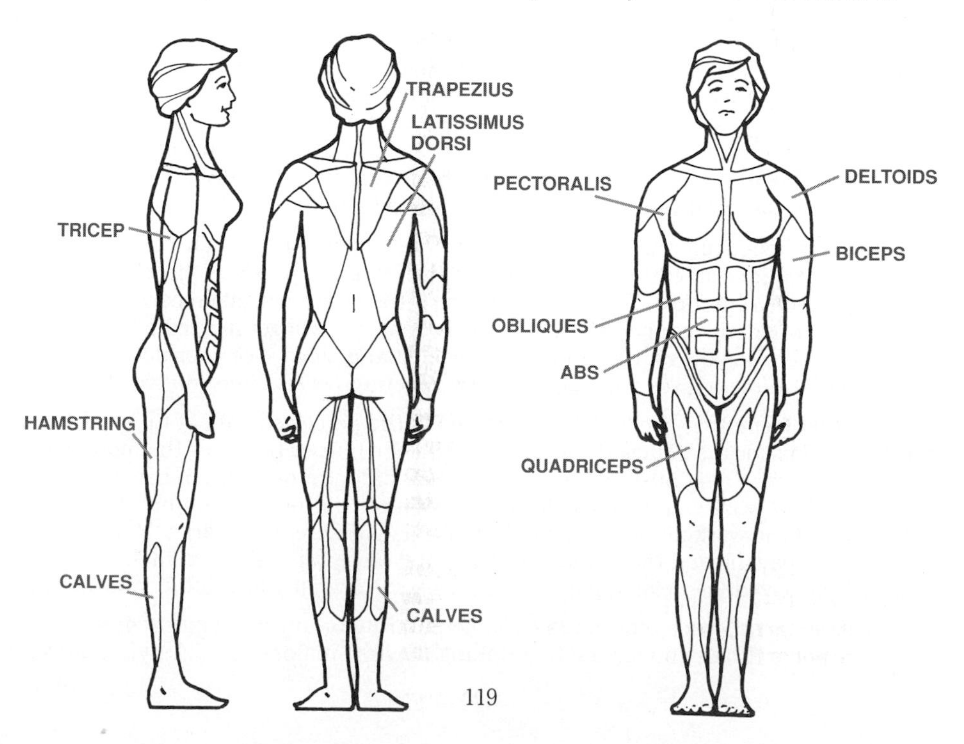

mation and remember the cause and effect relationship of movement and the muscular contraction feel. This way you can work on the muscles that are the focus of that particular day of working out. Doing sloppy execution of exercises just to get through the workout is not as effective as feeling each contraction from every repetition that you perform during the workout.

The diagram of the muscular anatomy can be an important tool in shaping your body. Once you get to the last phase of Biogenesis you will be able to identify what body parts need more or less work.

How you shape your body is dependent upon what exercises you perform. What it comes down to is you can't change something as complex as the human body unless you learn how it is put together and how it works. Once you understand some of the basics you will see how easy it is to control your physique.

When performing your workout it is important to understand that there will be perceived pain and discomfort. The only pain that you may encounter is lactic acid accumulation from repetitive muscular contractions and delayed muscle soreness. Lactic acid build up is a temporary condition and can be severe depending on a person's pain threshold and is a direct result of muscular contractions that are being performed at that given time. Push this limit as far as you can stand; after awhile you will look forward to the challenge of lactic acid. This pain builds up with every repetition and eases as soon as you stop.

Another so-called pain that we get is from delayed muscle soreness. What causes the discomfort is the damage that the muscle sustains as a result of the workout. It can last a couple days if the muscles that you are working are not used to getting much activity. After a while you will actually start measuring your workout intensity by how sore you got and be proud of the physical work you did to make this happen. You may think we are crazy when we tell you this, but it is true. These feelings make you aware of your body and that it is alive. However, don't get this confused with being injured or having a muscle tear.

If you do feel pain, and it happens on the first repetition, first check your form and see if you are executing the movement right. If it still persists, the likely culprits can be past injuries. They can resurface if they were not taken care of when the injuries originally happened. It is unlikely that you will get injured from Biogenesis because the movements are controlled and slow. See your doctor if a particular movement gives you pain on every repetition every time you try it.

Another issue that needs to be addressed is the perceived pain of the workout. Most people associate pain with hard work, and the harder the work the more pain received from it. Don't misunderstand these two different qualities of resistance training. Hard work can be uncomfortable, but it should not be painful. If pain is received and the workout is not hard, then that is a different scenario. Hard work has positive payoffs and the harder the work, the more it pays out results. So don't let perceived, associated pain get in your way of what you want in your body.

Before starting your Biogenesis exercise program or any workout program there are some things you should be thinking of when making this lifestyle change.

Is this a temporary change or is it going to be permanent? If you think it will be temporary, just to get some weight off or to get in shape for some event in the near future, remember, being in shape and improving your health can be addicting and it can influence others to do the same. This is a good thing. If you use this program and follow it as close as you can, you will get awesome results and it will become a permanent thing. A little health never seems to be enough.

Visualization is an important aspect of training with Biogenesis. If you can't imagine or dream of what you can look like before you start, you never will get to where you want to look like. There should be a plan for your exercises and what they are going to do for you. When you get up in the morning to go to work, you don't just get in your car and drive around and end up at work. You plan out a route which you will execute and arrive at work in an allotted amount of time. This sounds simple and makes sense, and it is no different with a fitness program. Biogenesis plans out the route and gives you the vehicle to get there, but it is up to you as to where you are going with your body. If you have never been in shape, you must visualize this. If you have been in shape at one point in time, you know a little about where you would like to go, but you must still visualize the goal.

Focus is a fundamental that is overlooked often when engaging in an exercise and diet program. When you are working on your body don't detach yourself from the workout, get into it as much as possible, almost a Zen-like state. Watching television or trying to do something else while working out does not seem to be beneficial to making progress. Biogenesis is an intense style of working out and requires mental and physical focus. This refers to the mind-body link. Make the "mind power the body" and you will see changes that you never thought you could attain. Master this link with quality focus and visualization techniques. For example, you see a picture in a magazine of a celebrity or model with tremendous legs. Look at it for a few moments and store it in your long term memory. Now, when it is time to work on your legs, visualize the image and focus your mind on the movements that will forge your legs to look like the photograph. This technique is used by the best built physiques in the world and is a training tool considered to be one of the best motivational techniques to change your appearance.

On the Biogenesis program you must ask yourself some questions concerning desire, determination, dedication and discipline. Everyone has some level of these qualities. Constantly review these qualities in yourself to influence your work ethic. Staying in shape, losing weight, getting fit or shaping your body the way you want it takes a good work ethic. If these qualities are high and you have a good work ethic, there should no stopping you from attaining your goals set for your body.

Biogenesis Phase One is an entry level resistance training program that is made up of fifteen progressive workouts. It is set into 10 minute workouts that train two to three body parts without weights or equipment. Resistance is applied from body weight, isometrics and opposite body parts. Without the use of equipment, the workout intensity is up to you. Therefore, the more you put into your workout the more you get out of it. Remember, if an exercise seems easy it probably won't do much for you, so apply more intensity. Here are some training tips and hints to make these 10 minute workouts more effective and productive.

- At least 10 minutes are recommended if you are a beginner; do additional repetitions and put more time in if you are more advanced.

- Do the workouts in the order they are presented; don't fall into the trap of doing the workouts you like and avoiding the ones you dislike.

- Doing more than two workouts in one day is okay; doing more than four consecutive workouts in one day can cause overtraining symptoms. There are fifteen progressive workouts; pace yourself daily. Consistency is a critical factor in your success.

- When doing gravity movements like squats, lunges, calf raises, crunches, push-ups and hyperextensions, going deep as possible with as much range of motion will increase the exercise's intensity.

- Isometric and opposite body part exercises like palm presses, curls, rows and extensions are done with as much tension as one can apply for the given repetitions or time.

-Don't get disappointed if you cannot do a certain exercise for a specific number of reps. With resistance training it is not what you can do, but what you attempt to do that makes your body change.

- Breathing deeply while working out is a good thing. Never hold your breath while exercising.

- Your heart rate should not elevate that high during your ten minute workouts. If you feel it is high, count your heartbeat for six seconds; it should not exceed 15 beats during that time. If it is less than 8 you need to apply more intensity or speed up the movements.

- A towel is sometimes used to link opposite body parts so they can be worked against each other. When using a towel to link body parts keep the tension of the towel to a maximum between the body parts; never let slack form in the towel.

One more concept before you start; resistance training is a little different from other exercise programs. Failures in most areas of life are deemed negative because we strive to succeed. But, in resistance training, success is made by efforts to exhaust you to failure from the intensity of resistance. For example, if the workout calls for ten repetitions and you do them fairly easily with little effort, do you think that did you as much good as putting out 100% effort and only being able to do seven or eight repetitions? Most people would think that achieving the ten reps are more productive than the failure of only doing seven or eight.

If we forget all about the numbers of reps, which scenario was the more intense set? Of course, the one in which you were not able to complete all ten repetitions. Why? Because you put an all-out effort to get to ten, failed, but gave 100% intensity. You did not exhaust yourself with the easy set. Our bodies adapt to stress. Once we adapt we stop changing. The higher the levels of stress, the more we adapt and change. Remember, intensity of the exercise is more important than completing all the exercises with ease when striving for long term success. Short term failures of the exercise program add up to long term results. This idea is one of the most important aspects of your training and getting the results you desire.

This phase is called Bio Speed Shape and has a workout tape that is the same as the workout out program that is pictured. There is a tremendous amount of information in these workout tapes in ability that is difficult to put into writing because they are better learned through visual instruction. These videotapes are available for men or women. Refer to the Biogenesis order line located in the last chapter of the book.

STRETCHING

Flexibility is an often overlooked component of fitness. Everyone is so concerned with form that they seem to neglect the function of their bodies. It is useless to have a great looking shape that you can't do anything with. But many people overlook the reason and applications of being fit and healthy. It is a fact that a healthy, fit individual can do everything better than someone of equal talent but of a lesser fitness level. Being flexible provides many unseen advantages that most may never pay any attention to. Tying your shoes, putting on your coat and scratching an itch on your back are simple activities that are easier if you are flexible, and a chore if you are not. Being flexible can also prevent many injuries like low back pain, upper neck tension headaches, and sprains and strains from day-to-day activities.

Stretching is not part of the workouts; it is a supplement to the workouts, so make extra time to perform your stretching routine. There isn't a perfect time to do stretching activities and that is exactly why they are often not performed. Stretching should be done before and after workouts, but it can be done anytime or anyplace. It can be done as much as you feel like stretching. There isn't a bad time to stretch. If you know what stretches go with what muscles it is convenient to stretch between exercises. Here are some general guidelines for stretching with the biogenesis program phases.

- Stretching is recommended before and after every workout. Flexibility is an important part of fitness that is often overlooked, so stretch often throughout the day.

- Stretches are usually held for 20 seconds in each position, longer if time is permitted. Stretches should not be painful but should have good tension that is slightly uncomfortable.

- Do not bounce or rock with motion when stretching.

- Discomfort when stretching correctly should be felt in the muscular area, not in joints of the body.

- Ease yourself into the stretch slowly.

- Stretches to be performed:

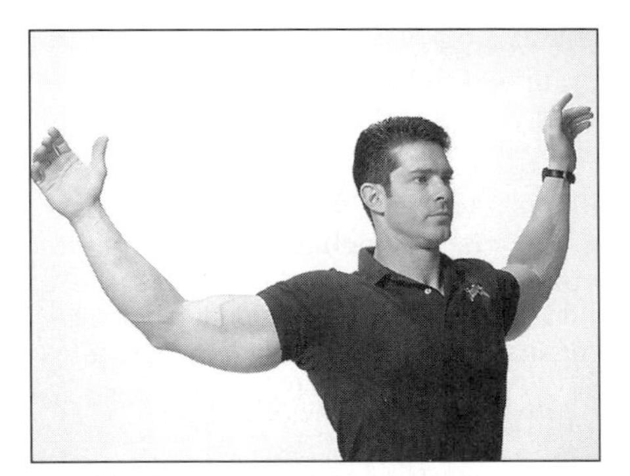

Double biceps stretch

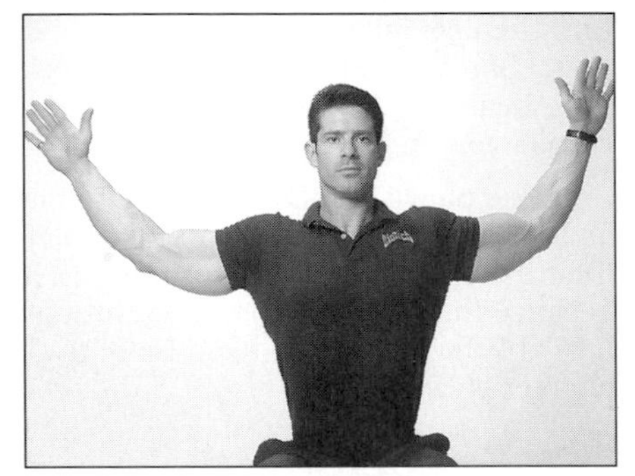

Pectoral stretch (both arms out and back)

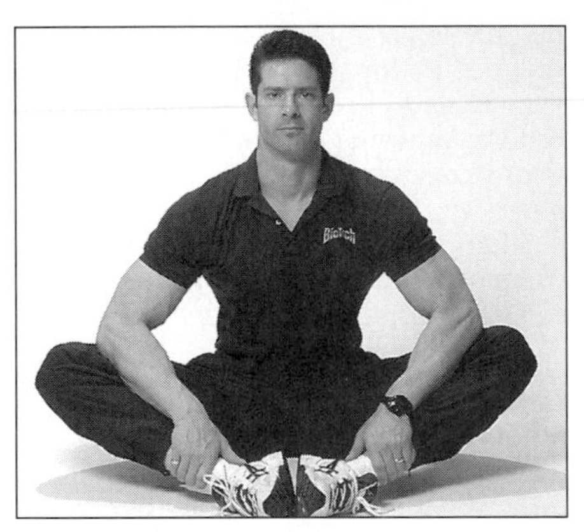

Seated groin

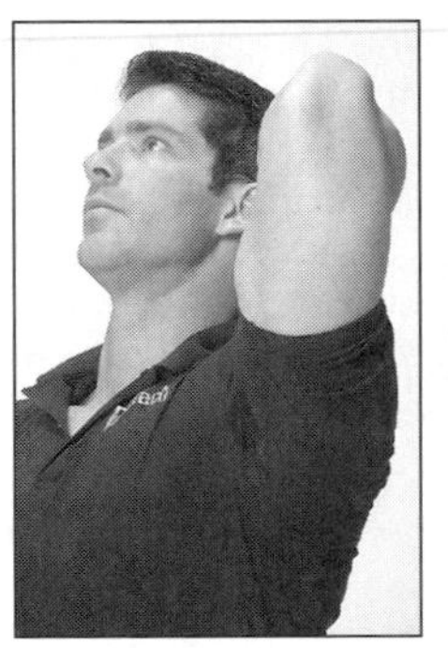

Triceps hand behind head R/L

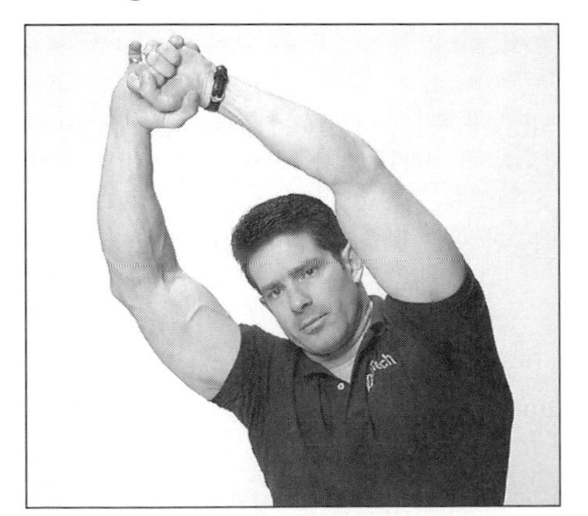

Overhead back stretch R/L

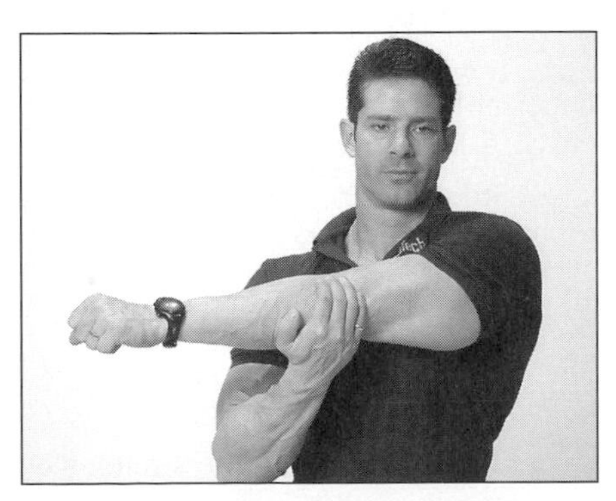

Rear lateral delt stretch R/L

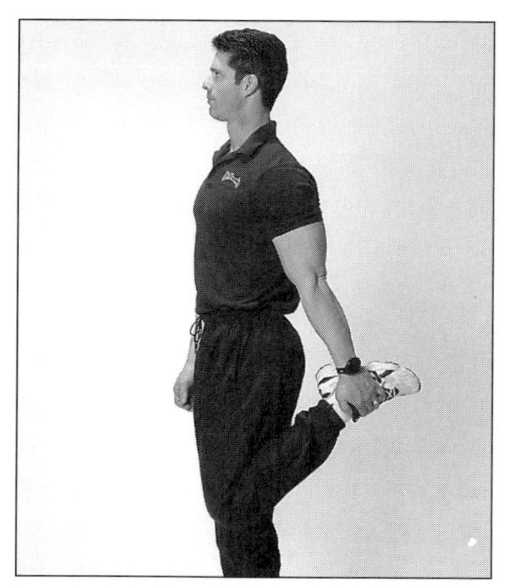

Quad stretch R/L

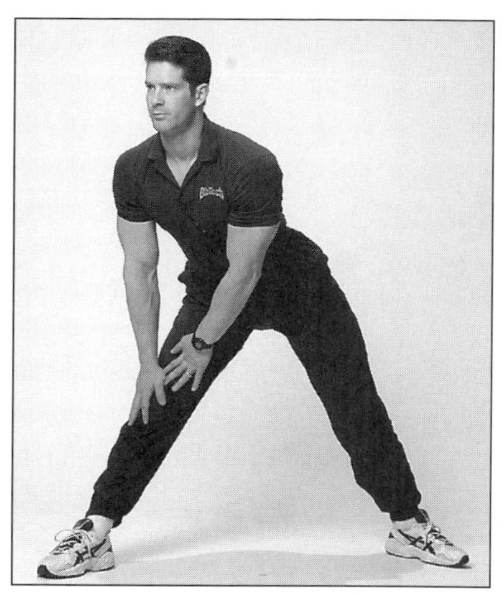

Standing low back and hamstring R/L

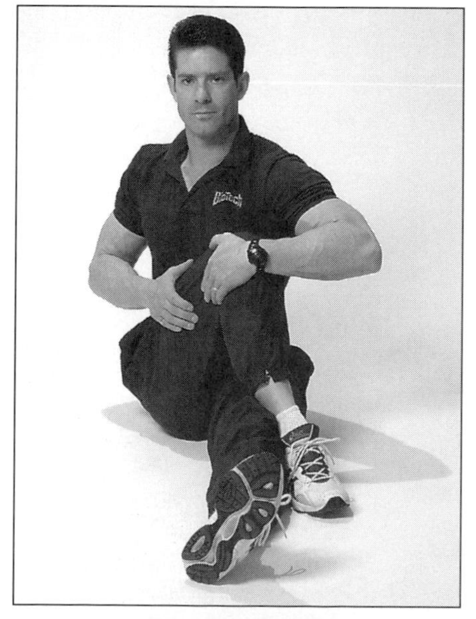

Glute-low back leg cross R/L

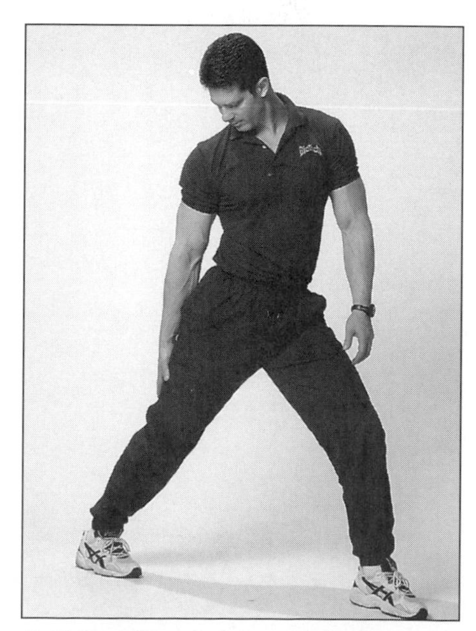

Calf stretch

12

Introduction to Biogenesis Phase Two

The second phase of Biogenesis is very basic in design and has the same movements and time involved as Phase One. The basic change from Phase One to Phase Two is that now we introduce equipment to the resistance program. We introduce weights and a bench to the workout to increase the intensity of the workout. You should be getting fitter from the first phase and be ready for a new challenge. Depending on your ability, going to the next phase is up to you.

Each phase increases in difficulty and intensity, and each phase prepares you for the next. If you are having difficulty on one particular phase, don't go to the next if you are not physically or mentally prepared. Go through that phase again until it is mastered and all of the concepts and techniques are understood. The ideas for this program to build your knowledge of exercise and nutrition and how it interacts with your body. You are only cutting yourself short if you don't use all of the tools that are in the Biogenesis program.

Exercise intensity can be elevated for maximum results in many different ways. Intensity can be increased by adding equipment, adding time, different training techniques and even subtracting time, such as rest between exercises. All of these techniques should be used at one point or another to change the intensity and monotony of resistance training. This is why many people are not successful with resistance training and some people are. There are many ways to make your workout effective by being creative. If you have an arsenal of exercises and several techniqucs to cnhance them, you will see constant progress toward your goals.

EQUIPMENT

The weights used in this program are dumbbells and a bench, which is used to incorporate more movements to the workout. There are several reasons for the introduction of dumbbells to this program rather than some expensive weight machine. One reason for the use of dumbbells is to learn basic free form movements that require coordination and balance of the arms and legs. Machines can't give this same free movement. There will be a time in the later phases of Biogenesis for machines. We don't condemn them, but we just want you to concentrate on your body and not equipment. Another reason to use dumbbells is that the best physiques in the world are built with dumbbells, so they ought to be good enough for you. Finally, dumbbells are very inexpensive and are very versatile as far as home gyms are concerned.

We also use a bench in this phase of Biogenesis. This is used for a couple reasons. A workout bench will give you greater range of motion and a variety of angles in which to put your body. You have to change the angle and position of your body to work different muscles and since dumbbells only have resistance in an up and down motion, position must be altered to change your range of motion to accommodate this fact. Another reason is the bench will be a place to sit and exercise because some movements require a seated position. We also use the bench in a variety of ways for support for certain exercises.

If you do not have a firm grasp of the concepts in Phase One, go back and repeat Bio Speed Shape until you understand the concepts of the first training phase. Biogenesis was put together with the basics in mind. However, some novices to body shaping may take a longer period of time to adjust to the mental and physical demands. Some professionals in the fitness industry may think the basics are made up of a simple routine that anyone can follow. This presents the problem of the word "routine" in the ever-changing world of fitness exercise programs. If your workouts do not change, you will not change, period. One particular workout may be effective for a while but it will not work for long. The returns will diminish and your progress will come to a halt and then your workout program fails. We understand that fundamental skills are important, but there are other skills that need to be learned before any equipment is even used.

At Biotech Research we have analyzed why people don't get results from resistance training programs. Dave and Frank have more than 50,000 hours in personal training with clients and have unique insights as to why people often fail in various fitness and diet programs. Dave and Frank also spend a great amount of time in the gym developing new techniques and setting higher standards in the fitness and nutrition industry.

In the first phase of Biogenesis you learned differences in exercises that involve the same body parts. For example, squats, leg extensions and curls for your thighs. You should have learned that all of the exercises just mentioned work parts of the thigh, but they are different exercises. Another important topic is learning muscle groups and how they move the body or body parts. This is critical because you have to know what the contraction of that muscle feels like in order to work it effectively with other movements or exercises. After the completion of Phase One, if shoulders are mentioned, you should be thinking of which exercises work that body part and what these exercise movements looks like.

In Phase One, techniques that make training with resistance different from other programs are the sequence of exercises. In some of the workouts you train only certain muscles on a particular day. The idea behind this is to give maximum stimulation to that area and then allow the area or muscle to rest and recover for a few days. The workout intensity creates a stimulus that tells your body to change. Then the rest and recovery period provides the nutrition that will repair and rebuild the muscles you have stimulated. If you train too often without the proper recovery, you will overtrain and become sore and tired all the time. This aspect is often overlooked with beginners who run themselves into the ground receive poor results and then quit the program.

SUPER SETS

An additional technique you may have noticed in Phase One is two exercises done back to back for the same body part. This is called super setting. You do two different exercises, the hard one first and then finish that body part off with whatever strength you have left. This is usually considered an advanced style of training and is for experts only, but we feel that if these techniques are learned from the beginning your training program will be accelerated, which will produce results much faster. Phase Two has many super set workouts and these really create a physical challenge. For example, if we are training the chest, or the pectoral muscles, we will execute ten repetitions of push-ups and then move to a bench and do dumbbell bench presses. Both exercises work on the chest, but in one exercise you are on the floor facing down and in the other you are on a bench facing up. Just remember the second set is going to be harder because you are already fatigued from the first.

GIANT SETS

Another technique for Phase Two is called giant sets. This is similar to super sets in that we are focusing on one body part and adding one or two more exercises to the set. This is just one more step above super sets. Let's look at the previous example of the chest super set and make it a giant set. First you perform the ten push-ups and then do the dumbbell bench presses. Now, instead of taking a break, you do one or two more different exercises for your chest with no rest. This is really demanding on your system and makes your body adapt to the high levels of stress this type of technique can provide. When you perform these giant sets, you will notice that you become more and more fatigued with each exercise. The weights you would normally use if you were fresh are now so heavy that you must use a lighter than normal weight. This is okay and you will take some time to adapt your muscular endurance to this training technique. Also, you will learn your limits of training intensity without thinking.

STRIP SETS

Strip sets are another technique you will encounter during Phase Two. This intensity generating method is really simple and effective. This is done with one exercise for two to four sets with a reduction in weight after each set has been completed. For example, let's use dumbbell curls and a strip set for three sets of ten reps. You start off doing ten reps with a heavy weight. After ten reps, you reduce the weight of the dumbbells and do another ten repetitions. When those ten repetitions are done, you reduce the weight again and try to do ten more repetitions. There is very little rest between these sets. Reductions in weight should be about twenty-five percent each time you reduce the weight.

These three techniques are simple ways to get the most out of your body workout in the shortest amount of time. These techniques can even be combined for more creative workouts. The more effort you put into your body, the greater the reward; it is that simple. So if your workout is easy and you can sail through it without any problem, you might want to reevaluate the program and see where you can make it more difficult.

Not only do these techniques raise the intensity of the workout, but they also eliminate the downtime between sets. If you are doing a standard resistance training program that requires six to eight sets per body part and you have to train two body parts, it can consume thirty to forty minutes of your time. With these methods you can train them in roughly ten minutes. What we are trying to do is put more work into the workout and take out the rest periods in between the exercises.

Phase Two of Biogenesis is a ten minute workout program. Try to keep within the time limits. The Phase Three program will add some volume to your training program and will consume more time. Phase Two also has more workouts in it and more techniques throughout, so don't be afraid to repeat this phase a couple of times. We have had clients stay at this phase for years, get great results, and not progress to the third phase. It is up to you how far you want to go with your fitness level and you can always go back to a lower phase if conditions require this to happen. For example, if you go on vacation and you don't want to take your weights and bench with you, you can still work out with Phase One.

One other tip before you start your workout, read through the entire workout for each body part so you can adjust your dumbbells at the start. This will help in keeping within the ten minute time frame and keep the workout intensity high.

Do the same stretching routine that you did during Phase One. Get your bench and weights set up correctly and get ready do some work.

13

Biogenesis Phase Three

(STAR MODEL)

Biogenesis Phase Three is similar to Phase Two in that it requires only dumbbells and a bench for equipment. The difference in intensity level comes from more volume and greater resistance. What this means is that instead of doing three to six sets per muscle group, we are now going to slow the pace down, add some more sets to each body part and train with more weight. In Phase One we concentrated on how resistance training is done, the feel of it, and some of the psychological fundamentals that make this type of training effective. Phase Two concentrated on working with minimal equipment and some of the techniques, like super sets, giant sets, and strip sets that make workouts creative and challenging.

In this phase we are going to concentrate on one body part at a time during your workout. In the previous two phases we put several body parts together for ten minutes and rotated the use of each body part during the workout. Now we are going to work one body part straight until it is done, then move to the next. This raises the intensity because the one body part you are working on gets all the focus and intensity for that time period with little rest.

This phase of the program is referred to as the "Star Model" program because it was a program Dave designed for some of the celebrities with whom he has worked. Keeping in mind that most people don't know how to get started with a custom resistance program, we put a two-body part workout program together that is 25 minutes a day, five days a week. This is roughly twice the amount of time of the Phase Two program, so allotting the time to exercise is crucial in planning your workout times.

Doing the stretches and workout, you should have approximately 35 minutes of time invested. Actually, there are two workouts that come with the Star Model Program. The workouts are basically the same format on paper, but you will alternate from a low weight/high repetition workout one week to a heavy weight/low repetition workout the next week.

Making a change in weights and repetitions can change a workout dramatically and this experience is something you will want to take note of. The reason for doing this is so you can feel the difference between fatigue from lactic acid and fatigue from muscular failure.

These two different training styles for the same workout have different effects on the body. Low weight/high rep training provides high energy expenditure with high lactic acid production and causes little muscle soreness the next couple of days. As you contract muscles in the body lactic acid builds up causing a hot or burning sensation if enough repetitions are performed. Usually, this takes at least 15 plus repetitions for this condition to occur. It probably occurred in some of the other previous phase workouts, but possibly you did not pay attention to the fact that it was from high repetition exercises. This type of work makes your heart rate more elevated than the heavy weight/low repetition format. It also makes you burn more energy during the workout than the heavy weight/low reps workout.

On the other hand, heavy weight/low rep training does not cause lactic acid burn but will give some delayed onset of muscle soreness, which activates post workout energy expenditure. This style seems more difficult for several reasons. Obviously, we are working with more weight and this can have some negative psychological responses. Don't worry about getting all the reps during this phase. It is not what you can accomplish in the workout, it is what you attempt to do. This is one of the biggest points that has to be made over and over to make resistance training work its magic!

If you can perform all the reps in every workout every time, it is definitely time to increase the amount of weight. Not properly increasing the amount of weight used in the workout is one of the biggest fundamentals that keep people from reaching their goals. These two styles have their pros and cons but both should be utilized for a synergistic effect to reduce body fat and increase your metabolic potential.

This is the last phase of the Biogenesis workouts designed for a small budget home gym. But, this phase can also be done at a gym and be as effective. When you reach this phase, you should be well on your way to fully understanding the different types of training movements and why they are applied. Phase Three is a short phase and only six to eight weeks should be spent doing this workout program. No question about it, it is very effective. It is a program that will bridge the gap to the Fourth Phase, Ultragenesis.

PHASE THREE STAR MODEL PROGRAM
REFER TO PHOTOS IN PHASE TWO
WOMEN'S WORKOUT (Alternate between heavy and light weights weekly)

WORKOUT #1 SHOULDERS AND CALVES

SHOULDERS
Light weight / high reps workout
Side lateral raise with dumbbells
Set of 15 reps
Rear lateral raise with dumbbells
Set of 15 reps
Frontal raise with dumbbells
Set of 15 reps
Dumbbell press
Set of 15 reps
Upright row
Set of 15 reps
Repeat three times each arm.

CALVES
Calves raised together 150 reps

SHOULDERS
Heavy weight / low reps workout
Side lateral raise with dumbbells
8 reps
Rear lateral raise with dumbbells
8 reps
Frontal raise with dumbbells
8 reps
Upright row to side
8 reps
Dumbbell press
8 reps
Repeat four times each arm.

CALVES
One foot calf raise on bench right/left/both 30/30/30
Repeat 2x

WORKOUT #2 BICEPS AND TRICEPS

Light weight / high reps workout

Bench dip 20 reps feet in close
Overhead dumbbell tricep extensions 15 reps
Dumbbell kick back, right-left 15 reps both arms
Repeat tricep exercises three times
Supinated curls 20 reps
Hammer curls 15 reps
Concentration curls 15 reps
Repeat bicep exercises three times each arm

Heavy weight / low reps workout

Overhead dumbbell tricep extension 10 reps
Bench dip 10 reps feet in close
Dumbbell kick back, right-left 10 reps both arms
Repeat tricep exercises four times
Supinated curls 10 reps
Hammer curls 10 reps
Concentration curls 10 reps
Repeat circuit four times each arm
Repeat bicep exercises

WORKOUT #3 LEGS AND GLUTES

Light weight / high reps workout

Step up with dumbbell right/left 25 reps
Lunge with dumbbell right/left 25 reps
Dumbbell squat 25 reps
Repeat three times
Dumbbell dead lift 25 reps
Hip extension right/left 25 reps
Leg curl 20 reps on incline bench
Repeat three times

Heavy weight / low reps workout

Step up with dumbbell right/left 12 reps
Lunge with dumbbell right/left 12 reps
Dumbbell squat 10 reps
Repeat four times
Dumbbell dead lift 10 reps
Hip extension right/left 25 reps
Leg curl 10 reps on incline bench
Repeat four times

WORKOUT #4 BACK AND OBLIQUES

Light weight / high reps workout

One arm dumbbell row-right/left 20 reps each
Dumbbell pullover 20 reps
Dumbbell row both arms 15 reps
Two arm dumbbell row elbows out 15 reps
Repeat two times
Dumbbell shrugs 20 reps
Hyperextensions 30 reps
Repeat two times
Side bends with dumbbells 25 reps each side
Side floor crunch 25 reps each side
Repeat two times.

Heavy weight / low reps workout

One arm dumbbell row right/left 10 reps each
Dumbbell pullover 10 reps
Dumbbell row both arms 10 reps
Two arm dumbbell row elbows out 10 reps
Repeat two times
Dumbbell shrugs 10 reps
Repeat circuit three times
Hyperextensions 20 reps with dumbbell
Repeat two times
Side bends with dumbbell 15 reps each side
Side floor crunch with dumbbell 15 reps each side
Repeat two times

WORKOUT #5 CHEST AND ABS

Light weight / high reps workout

Incline fly 10 reps
Incline dumbbell press 10 reps
Dumbbell fly 10 reps
Knee push-up 10 reps
Repeat four times
Tucks 100 reps
Crunches 100 reps

Heavy weight / high reps workout

Incline dumbbell fly 10 reps
Incline dumbbell press 10 reps
Dumbbell fly 10 reps

Knee push-up 10 reps
Repeat five times
Tucks with dumbbell 50 reps
Crunches with dumbbell 50 reps

PHASE THREE STAR MODEL PROGRAM
REFER TO PHOTOS IN PHASE TWO
MEN'S WORKOUT (Alternate between heavy and light weights weekly)

WORKOUT #1 SHOULDERS AND CALVES

SHOULDERS
Light weight / high reps workout
Rear lateral raises super set with rear upright rows
3 sets of 15 reps
Front raises super set with shoulder press
3 sets of 15 reps
Lateral raise super set with upright rows
3 sets of 15 reps
Heavy weight / low reps workout
Rear lateral raise super set with rear upright row
3 sets of 8 reps
Front raise super set with shoulder press
3 sets of 8 reps
Lateral raise super set with upright rows
3 sets of 8 reps

CALVES
Light weight / high reps workout
Alternating one leg calf raises
Calf raise together
200 reps total any combination of reps

Heavy weight / high reps workout
6 sets of 30 reps each leg

WORKOUT #2 BICEPS AND TRICEPS

BICEPS
Light weight / high reps workout
Hammer curl super set with regular dumbbell curl
3 sets of 15 reps
Alternating hammer curl

3 sets of 15 reps
Alternating regular curl
3 sets of 15 reps

Heavy weight / low reps workout
Hammer curl super set with regular dumbbell curl
3 sets of 8 reps
Alternating hammer curl
3 sets of 8 reps
Alternating regular curl
3 sets of 8 reps

TRICEPS
Light weight / high reps workout
Tricep bench dip two sets of maximum repetitions
Overhead dumbbell extension
3 sets of 15 reps
Lying tricep extension both arms
3 sets of 15 reps

Heavy weight / low reps workout
Tricep push-up two sets of maximum repetitions
Tricep double kick back
3 sets of 8 reps
Overhead tricep extension
3 sets of 8 reps

WORKOUT # 3 LEGS AND GLUTES

Light weight / high reps workout
Dumbbell lunge 15 reps
Dumbbell squat close stance 15 reps
Dumbbell squat wide stance 15 reps
Dumbbell dead lift 15 reps
This is a giant set that will repeat 4x
Leg kick 50 reps each leg 3 sets alternating

Heavy weight / low reps workout
Dumbbell lunge with rear foot up alternating legs 3 sets of 10 reps
Dumbbell step up alternating legs 3 sets of 10 reps
Dumbbell squat 3 sets of 10 reps
Dumbbell dead lift 3 sets of 10 reps
Dumbbell leg bench curl 3 sets of 10 reps

WORKOUT #4 BACK AND OBLIQUES

Light weight / high reps workout

Seated dumbbell row elbows out
3 sets of 15 reps stripping weight each set approximately 20 %
Seated dumbbell row elbows close
3 sets of 15 reps stripping weight each set approximately 20%
Seated straight arm row
3 sets of 15 reps stripping weight each set approximately 20%
Dumbbell shrugs
20 reps super set with dumbbell pullovers 15 reps
3 sets
Dumbbell side bend
2 sets of 25 reps for each side

Heavy weight / low reps workout

One arm dumbbell row wide
3 sets of 10 reps each side
One arm dumbbell row close
3 sets of 10 reps each side
Straight arm row super set with pullover
3 sets of 10 reps each
Dumbbell side crunch
2 sets of 20 reps each side

WORKOUT #5 CHEST AND ABS

Light weight / high reps workout

Incline fly super set with incline press
3 sets of 10 reps each movement
Flat fly super set with flat dumbbell press
3 sets of 10 reps each movement
Push-ups on bench
Feet up on bench for 10 reps then hands on bench for 10 reps
3 sets
V-crunch 20 reps
Tucks 20 reps
Crunches 20 reps
3 sets

Heavy weight / low reps workout

Feet on bench push-up
3 sets of max reps
Incline fly
3 sets 10 reps

Flat fly
3 sets 10 reps
Hands on bench push-ups
3 sets of max reps
Dumbbell V-crunch 10 reps
Dumbbell tuck 10 reps
Dumbbell crunch 10 reps
3 sets

TIPS AND HINTS

- Stated repetitions are only targets, shoot for them and do more if you can.
- If overshooting target reps often, it is time to increase your weights.
- Never go easy on yourself, if you think you can do more, do it.
- During resting phases do not take more than 2 minutes to start next set.
- Super setting, strip setting and giant setting require only 10 to 20 seconds of rest between the exercises.
- Stretch before and after each workout.
- Do all the workouts and exercises, don't play favorites with ones you like so your physique won't become unbalanced.
- Remember the fundamentals from the previous phases.

14

PHASE FOUR ULTRAGENESIS

If you have reached Phase Four you are on your way to being in control of what your body can do and knowing your body's capabilities. Many people that practice this type of a training and diet program never make it this far. They are normally stuck somewhere between Phase Two and Three.

At this point you will notice a significant difference in your appearance. If there isn't a noticeable difference in your appearance, you have not mastered the first three phases and need to apply more intensity to those phases. Everything that you have been exposed to in the preceding phases prepared you to start making changes to your workout and to tailor your workout to match your goals. This is a crucial point. You now should know what exercises work the different muscle groups and how to apply different training techniques to increase the level of difficulty in your workout. If you are not at the level to start Ultragenesis training, you can still benefit and increase your overall knowledge by reading this chapter. What you will learn in Phase Four is invaluable to the long-term success of your workout program.

Developing your own workouts seems to be complicated. Most people prefer to be shown what to do and then just execute the workout. This will eventually slow their progress or they will just lose interest in the workout. They may end up finding something else to do to that won't be as effective as resistance training. When you complete Phase Four, you will be the creator of your workouts and your body will reflect your ability to be creative in designing your workouts. Eventually, you will enjoy the confidence that you can go into any workout environment and make it effective.

There are so many things that can pull you off track when it comes to an exercise program. You need to learn how to get around problems like making time to workout, injuries, vacations, training with other people, different equipment, crowded gyms, and the combinations of all of these problems. Refer to Chapter Two on the mental aspect of discipline and fitness if you need a refresher. You need to learn how to prioritize your time for fitness and the other aspects of your life. We both have families who are important in our lives, yet we still have the mental discipline to maintain our training schedule. During Phase Four you will continue to develop these fitness and diet skills. Those who have the discipline to deal with various issues and still make progress or maintain progress will excel at Phase Four. Remember that you never stop learning in life. Ultragenesis can increase your mental and physical capabilities. Your potential is unlimited.

TRAINING PARTNER

What is a training partner and what beneficial role could one have for you? A training partner is someone with whom you workout. There are many roles a training partner should play if they are to be an asset toward helping you to achieve your goals. In the first three phases of the Biogenesis program a training partner would be used more to keep you company as opposed to actually being able to increase the productivity of your workout. Since Phase Four requires the absolute maximum effort, there may be times when you may need a little nudge from your partner to keep you going.

We will explain some of the reasons you may want to get a training partner. If you are not a member of the financially secure minority that can afford an adequate home gym, then you will need to join a gym or health club. If you are already a member of a gym or club then the hardest part about Phase Four is the actual workout. But, if you have never been a member of a gym or it has been awhile since you have been, the hardest part may be actually walking in the front door of your local gym or health club and saying, "I want to sign up." Believe me, you are not alone. Walking into the front door of a gym can be so overwhelming that you may want to go back home and say, "I think I'll stick to Phase Three." This is a great reason to have a training partner. It's much easier to handle a new challenge or strange atmosphere with a friend by your side.

If you have worked very hard through your first three phases, you are fully prepared to walk into any gym and not embarrass yourself. Chances are very good that you have already acquired more knowledge through the first three phases of Biogenesis than 90% of the people you will meet in the gym.

Now let's discuss the "real" roles of a training partner. When choosing a training partner, you should choose someone whose personality does not clash with your own. For example, if you are nervous or timid about being in the gym, then you may not want a training partner who is loud or does things to draw unwanted attention to you while you're working out.

In your situation it may be a poor choice for you to pick a partner that has already been working out for a while. Many times this type of person will try to instill their training methods on you because of their training experience. Just because a person has been in the gym for a long time does not mean that they are working out properly. We have seen and talked to people in gyms who have been using incorrect training techniques for years!

There is a funny story we would like to tell you. We were giving a seminar at a very exclusive health club where the clientele consisted of mostly millionaire members. We noticed a gentleman doing some unusual exercise that was actually very strenuous and dangerous for his knees. The man was about eighty pounds overweight, which made the exercise all the more dangerous. We watched the man for about fifteen minutes only to discover that all of his exercises were bizarre!

"You have to be careful when you give somebody pointers or tips," Frank said. "If you don't word it correctly, he may think you are making fun of him because we are in better shape then he is."

Frank approached the man and suggested some alternate exercises he could utilize for training his legs that would be less dangerous to his knees. This gentleman, not knowing who we were proceeded to tell us to mind our own business. The man said, "I pay one hundred dollars a day with a personal trainer from this club who put me on this program. I have been doing this program for three years now and it works great."

Frank asked the gentleman how much weight he had lost over the three years. "I lost 40 pounds but gained some of it back when I hurt my knee and had to take some time off," replied the man. As ridiculous as this sounds, and to make this story more strange, the man was a cardiologist.

The point to this story is that you have two of the best trainers on the planet instructing you. You can be very confident the exercises you do on the Biogenesis program are both safe and effective. The cardiologist we spoke of was eighty pounds overweight and continued to do the same exercise routine year after year. He thought that since it was getting easier to do that he was making progress. You can do the wrong thing over and over and, no matter how many times you do it or how easy it gets, it's still wrong. So please don't make the mistake of choosing a training partner just for the amount of time that they have spent in the gym.

You want to pick a person who is motivated and has similar goals to yourself. An example of a bad choice is to pick a partner whose objective is to get as huge as humanly possible if your goal is to merely continue the Biogenesis process. It would also not be in your best interest to pick someone who would rather be socializing instead of concentrating on the workout. This can be a very uncomfortable situation for you especially if that person is your friend. How do you tell a friend that you no longer want to work out with them because they bring enough positives to the partnership?

Not having a training partner isn't the end of the world. In fact, when David is training for a show he prefers to not have a partner. He states that one of the drawbacks to having a partner is that you can't do whatever you want while you're in the gym; and when you are getting ready for a show you have to be selfish.

"The nice thing about having a training partner," says David, "is that when you are training in a very intense manner you often get burnt out. You don't feel like going to the gym. But when you have a partner, you have to go. You have a responsibility to show up and push each other. When you find the right person, it makes working out that much sweeter."

It makes the training partnership much easier when the two of you have an understanding from the beginning. Both of you are going to the gym to train. To sum it up, when looking for a training partner you should look for a person who shares your goals and motivation. You may not be able to find someone to fit that criteria right away. That's all right. It is better to train alone then with a person who makes working out an uncomfortable and frustrating experience. You can keep an eye out while you are training for another person who trains the same time that you do and seems to have an understanding of how to workout correctly. Talk to them. Show them your Biogenesis program and perhaps you'll hit it off and find a great training partner.

FINDING A GYM

Finding a gym should be easier than choosing your workout partner. What we recommend is that, if at all possible, you go to whichever gym or health club you are considering at the "slow times." The slow times at most gyms are usually between ten in the morning and four in the afternoon. By going during these hours you will be able to comfortably look at the facility and ask the manager any questions you may have. When inspecting the gym look for things like cleanliness, condition of the equipment and friendliness of the staff. Just because you train at a gym doesn't mean it has to smell like one.

Phase Four was developed for people who are ready to take it to the extreme. This is hard to do in one of those fancy clubs where people spend more time sitting on the equipment reading the newspaper than actually using the machines to exercise. Neon lights and a rubber-coated jogging floor are nice, but clean, up to date equipment and a serious atmosphere are more likely to help you achieve what you are looking for. Your lean, muscular body is obviously something you take seriously, so make sure your gym atmosphere is serious too.

There are a few final things for you to keep in mind when going to the gym for your first couple of times. If you feel intimidated by people, try and go during off peak hours. Ask the manager when the busiest times are and avoid them. Don't be afraid to ask for help.

When David first started to work out in the gym, he had an embarrassing and potentially dangerous situation. David was on the bench press and was unable to complete the last repetition. The weights came about halfway up and his strength just left. The bar was stuck across his chest and getting heavier by the second. There were lots of people in the gym at the time but he was too embarrassed to ask anyone to help pick the bar off his chest. He started to push up on just one side so the weights would slide off. Well, the weights did slide off but the weights on the other side made the bar flip over and hit a man in the back of the head, knocking him nearly unconscious. What do you think is more embarrassing, asking for help or hitting a man twice David's size in the head? David never went back to that gym again.

CHOOSING THE PROPER CLOTHING AND EQUIPMENT

You need to wear comfortable clothing. Be as comfortable as possible. Well, let's rephrase that. Be as comfortable as possible without showing everyone in the gym parts of you that only a select few people should be seeing.

Today there are many companies that produce sportswear for workouts and fitness clubs. You can be fashionable and comfortable, or you can wear the old and comfortable grey sweat pants and T-shirt.

The equipment that you use to work out with in the gym needs to be kept in good condition in order to protect and support your body. Personal equipment that could play a part in your progress includes workout belts, knee wraps, wrist straps, cross training shoes and workout gloves.

Workout belts should be worn for protection of the lower back on only your heaviest sets. Some people wear their belts during their entire workout. This is not good for two reasons. By wearing your belt all of the time you never allow that part of your back to develop as much as the surrounding areas. If you had to have a weaker link in your body, the lower back would probably be the last place you would want it to be. Your lower back connects your upper body to your lower body and is involved to some extent in nearly every exercise you do.

Another reason you do not want to wear your workout belt all the time is it will make your waist bigger. You're wondering how this could be possible? If you look at all of the movements in Phase One Bio Speed Shape you're are not using any weights or equipment. Your muscle development comes from isometric movements. What do you think is happening to your stomach muscles if they are pushing against your tight belt for thirty or forty minutes? Your stomach is being isometrically trained for thirty or forty minutes, therefore the stomach muscles are increasing in size. A belt can definitely provide some protection against back injuries but should only be worn when needed.

Knee wraps are not recommended unless you already have some sort of knee injury. Some people like to use them while doing heavy squats or leg presses. We'll leave that up to you.

Wrist straps are used mostly when training back muscles. They are used to help hold on to extremely heavy weights. As you get stronger you will probably need to invest in some wrist straps. Your back is a bigger and stronger muscle then your biceps and forearms, so to stimulate your back into growth you are going to be using weights that you may not be able to handle. When you reach the point where your grip gives out before your back does then it is time to invest in some straps. They will cost you anywhere from five to ten dollars.

The shoes you wear should give your arches strong support. When leg training you want to wear shoes that are as flat and comfortable as possible. In most cases regular gym shoes are good enough.

Workout gloves are always a good option. They not only add support to your grip but also prevent calluses from developing on your hands. They also keep you from coming in direct contact with the equipment with your hands.

IMPORTANT TIPS

Don't expect to master all of the equipment right away. No one can. Take notes and ask the staff for help. It is far less embarrassing to ask the staff for help than to end up doing a triceps push down on a chest pull over machine. Take your Biogenesis book with you for reference or ask a staff member for help. If you follow the Ultragenesis Campitelli and Dearth training methods you will be fine.

Remember, Phase Four is designed to be a push to the limit workout. Don't overdo it right off the bat. If you push yourself too hard, you will be so sore you'll never want to work out again. Almost everyone is sore after their first couple of workouts. The soreness usually is maximized or "maxed out" around the forty eight-hour mark. This is called Delayed Onset Muscle Soreness. Don't freak out. Your muscles aren't used to this new work.

Briefly, here is what is happening to your body. When you are training a certain body part, you are forcing a large amount of blood to that area. This is referred to as "getting a pump." You may feel a burning sensation while doing exercises that create a pump. This is because the large amount of blood flow into the muscle is pushing the lactic acid out. With all of the blood pumping into the muscle cell microscopic rips will occur. These microscopic rips cause a little pain. You've all heard the old saying "no pain no gain." This is the kind of pain referred to. The good news is that after the muscles recover and repair themselves they become stronger and harder to rip. So after working out for a couple of weeks you will not be as sore, unless you have an extra great workout.

Next, we say don't be embarrassed. Don't feel embarrassed at not lifting very much weight. Don't think other people are staring at you or talking about you. The more you focus on other people the less you are concentrating on yourself. The weight will eventually improve. When we train, sometimes we go for high repetitions at lower weights; sometimes as high as 100 reps in a row. Dave weighs 230 pounds. To the untrained eye it may appear very funny if you were to walk into the gym toward the end of one of our high repetition sets and see us screaming in pain using the twenty pound dumbbells.

RULES

Once you have joined a gym or health club, there are several things you want to keep in mind. Besides the rules the gym has posted, there are also some unwritten rules. These are not so much rules as they are common courtesy. For example, if someone is using a machine or a piece of equipment you want to use, politely ask them if you can work in. When you work in with someone you take turns with them. It is recommended that you only work in when there are not a lot of additional adjustments for you to make, such as adding or subtracting weights or readjusting the seat position. It's quite common for you to work in with another person, so don't be apprehensive about asking. It's also a common courtesy for you to allow others to work in with you as well. On the other hand, it is very impolite for you to stand near and watch someone working out on a machine wait for them to finish. The best thing for you to do in that situation is either ask the person if you can work in or ask them how much longer they will be.

If you need help adjusting one of the machines or forget how to use a piece of equipment, it's best to ask someone on staff. Usually they are more than happy to lend a hand.

If you are working out alone and aren't sure whether or not you will be able to complete your set, it is common to ask someone on staff or someone who is in between sets to give you a spot. When you get a spot from someone, this means that another person stands over you to assist you in case you are unable to complete the exercise on your own. When using heavy weights it is always best to have someone spot you.

There are several other things to remember as far as gym courtesy. Don't spit in the drinking fountain. This needs no explanation.

Don't drop your dumbbells or throw your weights around. Besides looking foolish, this also damages the equipment and is very distracting to others. Always put your weights back where you got them.

Always wipe off your equipment. Some people perspire more then others. Even if you don't sweat on the equipment always wipe it off when you complete your set. Wouldn't you rather use a machine that someone had just wiped off as opposed to one someone hadn't?

The unwritten rule for cardio equipment is thirty minutes. Most gyms have limited cardio equipment. Treadmills, stair steppers and exercise bikes are considered cardio equipment and should be used with consideration. If there is no one waiting for the equipment then obviously it is okay to go longer then thirty minutes. Treat the gym the way you would a guest in your home and you should have no problems.

ULTRAGENESIS

Now that we have the basics done, we need to get into an area that very few advanced exercise programs elaborate. There definitely has to be a different physiological approach to phase four than your previous three phases. The Ultragenesis program requires you to put forth the maximum effort your body is capable of. You must constantly strive to do one of two things, either increase the weights you are using or the amount of repetitions you are doing.

Here is one example. Let's say that one week you are bench pressing one hundred and twenty pounds for eight repetitions. It would not be beneficial for you to continue to do this week after week. Your body would adjust to the stress on the muscle and you would no longer get the results that one hundred and twenty pounds had previously given you. This is where you need to push yourself. Remember, it is impossible for you to get stronger without creating more muscle.

MENTAL FOCUS

Intensity 1: the quality or state of being intense; esp: extreme degree of strength, force, or energy. 2. the magnitude of force or energy.

To tell you that you need to be intense without teaching you how to increase your intensity would be nothing more then a pep talk. There are certain ways to create intensity and these are what we will discuss now.

Intensity is the high level of strength, force or energy that you put into your workout. Here is a formula to follow. The amount of intensity that you put into your workout is directly related to the amount of results that you will see, as well as the period of time in which you will see results. The less intense your workout, the longer it will take you to see results.

How does one go about creating intensity? By using extreme concentration or focusing on every repetition of every set. This means that prior to actually picking up your dumbbells, or even getting on the machine, you clear your mind of anything that may distract your total attention on the set at hand. While in the gym you will most likely see some of the local "muscle heads" yelling and screaming at each other in feeble attempts to psyche each other up. All they are doing is wasting energy ranting and raving while they could be using that energy toward their set. Do not fall into this trap. If you yell louder, that does not mean you are stronger. You want to visualize yourself from the beginning of the movement all the way through to the end. Picture how heavy the weight will be and see yourself driving through the movement with extreme force. Once you have visualized this several times in your mind, all that is left is for you to actually do it. You have already imagined how heavy and hard the set will be so you won't be overwhelmed when you attempt the first repetition. By focusing on each repetition and set before you actually do the movement, you eliminate any outside distractions.

David takes these visualization techniques to an even further extreme prior to contests. Dave says, "The night before I would go to the gym, I would lay in my bed and picture the next day's workout in its entirety. I would think of every little detail, even what workout outfit I was going to wear. I would see every machine and exercise I was going to use and picture the intensity I was going to apply toward each set. I would play the workout in my mind so many times that by the time I got to the gym the next day, all I had to do was switch my brain to automatic pilot and I was off. I would not have to waste any time or energy thinking about what I had to do once I got there."

Now this may be a little extreme for most of us who are not professional bodybuilders, but you can see where visualization can play an important role in developing intensity. As you progress in your training you will begin to develop techniques that will be tailored toward your style of training. But until you do, we suggest you try our form of visualizing your set before you do it. We are a firm believer that if you are going to do something, do it correctly and to the best of your ability. With consistent, intense training your body has absolutely no choice but to respond in a very positive manor. It's the most awesome feeling in the world when you are able to sculpt your body to look the way you want it. It's a feeling of confidence and power, but mostly a feeling of satisfaction. Nothing seems impossible once you make this kind of training a part of your daily regimen.

WORKOUT

Now comes the fun part, the actual workout. Unlike the first three phases where we gave you an actual workout routine to follow, Phase Four allows you some freedom to develop your own program. We are going to give you the information that is pertinent in constructing your program as well as information that is more general and flexible. As in Phase Three there is more emphasis on each individual body part and you split your body into four to five different days.

Here is an example of how a Four Day split should look.

Monday: chest and shoulders
Tuesday: back and abs
Thursday: biceps and triceps
Friday: quads, hams and calves (legs)
Wednesday: off
Saturday and Sunday would be off days.

If you wanted to split your body over a Five Day period it may look like this.

Day one: chest
Day two: back
Day four: shoulders abs, and calves
Day five: biceps and triceps
Day six: quads and hams (legs)
Day three: off
Day seven: off

Let's say we are training chest, the workout should start like this. You would start by stretching out your pecs, followed with a couple of light sets on the bench press doing around fifteen to twenty repetitions. Once you are fully warmed up it is time to begin with your first real set. Hopefully, you have found an adequate training partner or a reliable person to spot you. It's always best to be safe and use a spotter when training with heavy weights.

You should use a weight with which you can complete eight to ten repetitions. The next set you will add weights to the bar and try to do six to eight reps. For your third set you will again add weights and shoot for three to six reps. Finally on the fourth set, if you are feeling strong, add a little more weight and go for three reps. Keep track of your workout in your logbook. This is how your four sets on the bench press would look in your logbook.

The first column is for the number of sets. Follow this with an "X." The next space is for the amount of repetitions and follow that with another "X." Finally, in the last space put the weight that you used. Your log would look like this:

Bench Press
1 x 8 x 150 (One set of eight repetitions at 150 pounds)
1 x 6 x 165
1 x 4 x 170
1 x 3 x 175

After completing your bench pressing you should move onto the next exercise. We'll use dumbbell fly's. Again you would use the same sort of descending sets that you did on the bench press, but instead of doing four sets you may want to do only three.

Dumbbell Fly's This is how 3 sets of Dumbbell Fly's will look in your log.
1 x 8 x 40 (One set of eight repetitions at 40 pounds)
1 x 8 x 45
1 x 6 x 50

For the third chest exercise we'll choose the incline dumbbell press.

Dumbbell Press
1 x 8 x 60 (One set of eight repetitions at 60 pounds)
1 x 6 x 60
1 x 4 x 65

And finally we will finish the chest off with standing cable crossovers. Instead of changing the weights here, we will just do three sets of eight to ten reps.

Standing Cable Crossovers
3 x 10 x 50 (Three sets of ten repetitions at 50 pounds)

Your chest should be "pretty fried" at this point. Make sure with every workout that you take five to ten minutes to stretch out the body part you just trained. This is just one example of a possible chest workout you might do to add some quality muscle to your upper body. One key to remember is that the number of reps you do is not as important as pushing yourself until failure. Actually, the best thing that can happen to you is that you do not get in all of the reps that you had planned on. This means you are pushing yourself to complete failure. This is one time where failure is a good thing.

The more you tear those muscles down the bigger the muscle cell becomes when it repairs itself. So train hard, but train smart. Always use perfect form and make sure you keep good track of your workouts in your training log. This will help you keep track of your progress and serve as a motivational tool for you to continue to try to beat your previous workout.

If you are trying to gain muscle but at the same time lean your body fat down then you will probably want to do a program using higher repetitions. Try to keep your reps between ten and twenty. Using the chest work out we just showed you, your training log may look like this.

Bench Press
1x15x120
1x15x130
1x12x140
1x10x150

Dumbbell Fly's
1x15x40
1x15x40
1x10x45

Incline Dumbbell Presses
1x15x50
1x12x50
1x10x55

Standing Cable Crossovers
3x20x40

For the ultimate results we suggest that you cycle your training, going with heavy weight and low repetitions for several weeks then switching over to lighter weights, with higher reps for the next few weeks. By doing this you will never allow your body to adapt to any one particular way of training. This will ensure you constant results with very few periods where your progress slows down. Although training consistently and maintaining a high level of intensity is important, your diet and nutritional supplementation will still account for about seventy five percent of your results.

It does not matter how hard you train if you are not consuming the proper amounts of protein and other nutrients needed to rebuild your muscle. By keeping your protein very high and your carbohydrates and fats low, you will ensure optimum muscle gains while at the same time lowering your body fat. We hesitate calling any of the first three phases "bodybuilding" phases, but in all actuality any form of resistance training is bodybuilding.

Your objective with resistance training is to build your body's muscles so that you require more calories to sustain your structure. By cutting back on your calories or cutting out foods that will impede your fat loss you are able to obtain a lean and toned physique. Phase Four is designed to take it to a higher level than just looking firm. Ultragenesis is designed to give you a body that stands out from everybody else's. Many times we hear people say they don't want to look big and "freaky." Please don't come to the conclusion that by following this program you will go to bed on Wednesday looking like you do now and follow the Phase Four program for a couple of days and wake up on Saturday looking like the authors of this book. The awesome thing about the Biogenesis program is that you can go to any level you desire. And if taking your physique to the highest level you have ever done is what you are looking to do, well then Phase Four is definitely for you.

Getting back to the nutritional aspect of Phase Four, if you want to get big then you can't be afraid to eat. We suggest that you eat four to six times per day. If you are looking to get more muscular while at the same time achieving and maintaining a lower body weight, you need only to be eating three to five times per day. You can do one of three things: 1) alter the Fat-Flush Diet to fit your Phase Four training program; 2) contact Frank or Dave at www.biogenesis.net and get yourself a personalized diet; or 3) consult with your family physician. We have included a page from David Dearth's actual contest diet journal. Remember this is his diet, so you can imagine how many calories he consumed in the off season when he competed.

Meal one:
- 6 egg whites
- 3 whole eggs
- 100 grams of oatmeal
- 1 slice toast
- 1 tsp. peanut butter

Meal two:
- 100 grams of chicken
- 5 grams red meat
- 100 grams of rice
- 50 grams green beans

Meal three:
- 100 grams chicken breast
- 100 grams red meat
- 50 grams broccoli

Meal four:
- 75 grams chicken
- 75 grams fish
- 3 whole eggs
- 50 grams rice

Meal five:
- 15 egg whites

Meal six:
- 100 grams red meat
- 100 grams chicken
- 75 grams potato
- 2 whole eggs

These are the meals he would eat. Notice that protein shakes are not included here. Along with these six meals per day he would consume three to four protein shakes which consisted of about 50 grams of protein each. Keep in mind that this diet was being used while he was doing three hours a day on the treadmill and training with weights twice a day. This kind of diet and training routine is far too extreme for 99.9% of the people in the world, and David does not train and eat like this today. However, when David was a professional, his motivation was financial. You have to find what motivates you to complete Biogenesis.

Phase Four is about challenging yourself, pushing yourself to the limit in the gym. You have the rest of the twenty-three hours in the day to go to work, clean the house, take care of the kids, mow the yard or whatever it is that you do for everyone else all day long. Make the time you spend in the gym personal quality time. You will be amazed at how little time it actually takes out of the week to get and maintain a great body. All it takes is a strong desire and knowing what to do and when to do it. No matter what your goals are, Phase Four is where you ultimately want to be. The first three phases of Biogenesis follow set routines. And if you are like most people, set routines become boring. When working out becomes boring chances are very good that you will not stick with it. Phase Four gives you more freedom to be creative. You are living a fitness lifestyle rather then following a fitness routine.

The next few pages include a sample workout for each body part. If you are still not completely comfortable putting together your own workout routine, feel free to follow this one until you are settled into the gym. We have split your body up so that you are training each body part once a week. You may want to follow this workout until you stop seeing progress. At this point, substitute a different exercise for one pictured in this book or use similar or new equipment in your own gym.

This workout is on a four day per week training schedule. Each workout should last no longer then forty-five minutes. If it is taking you longer then forty-five minutes to do this workout, you are taking too much time in between sets. Good Luck.

ULTRAGENESIS WORKOUT

This is the four day workout plan. We guarantee great results if you follow this plan along with the Biogenesis nutritional program.

DAY ONE WORKOUT. CHEST AND DELTOIDS

Start by stretching out your chest and shoulders. Since the chest is a bigger muscle, we will start here.

Chest

Bench Press
1x15 reps
1X12 reps
1X10 reps
1X 8 reps

Incline Bench Press
1X10
1X10
1X 8

Dumbbell Fly's
1X10
1X10
1X 8

Peck Deck
1X15
1X15

Deltoids

Straight bar shoulder press (to the front)
1X15

1X10
1X 8
1X 6

Lateral dumbbell raises
1X10
1X10
1X 8

Rear dumbbell raises
1X10
1X10
1X10

Cable upright rows
1X15
1X15

With each set the final repetition should be extremely hard or even impossible to achieve. This will ensure that you are pushing yourself to failure.

DAY TWO WORKOUT. BACK AND ABDOMINALS.

Back

Lat pull downs to the front
1X15
1X15
1X10
1X10

Low cable rows
1X10
1X10
1X8

One arm dumbbell rows
1X8
1X8
1X8

Dumbbell pull over
1X15
1X15

Abdominals

Crunches

1X100
1X100

Tucks
1X50
1X50

Hanging leg lifts
1X50
1X50

DAY THREE WORKOUT. BICEPS AND TRICEPS.

Biceps

Standing straight bar curls
1X15
1X10
1X10
1X8

Alternate dumbbell curls
1X12
1X10
1X8

Hammer curls
1X20
1X20

Bicep curl machine
1X15
1X15

Triceps

Tricep cable push downs
1X20
1X15
1X15
1X10

Seated one arm dumbbell extensions
1X15
1X15
1X15

One arm dumbbell kick backs
1X15
1X15
1X15

Lying barbell extensions
1X25

DAY FOUR WORKOUT. QUADRICEPS, HAMSTRINGS, AND CALVES.

Quadriceps

Leg press
1X25
1X20
1X15
1X10
1X6

Hack squats
1X15
1X15
1X10

Leg extensions
1X25
1X25
1X10

Hamstrings

Stiff leg dead lifts
1X20
1X15
1X10

Lying leg curls
1X20
1X15
1X10
1X8

Calves

Standing calf raises
1X20
1X15
1X10

Seated calf raises
1x50
1x25
1x25

This would conclude your entire week's workout program. One key thing to remember is with each set, try to add a little weight so that every set is heavier than the last. Obviously if you are really pushing yourself, by adding weight to each set you shouldn't be able to do as many repetitions. By adding weight to each set and dropping the amount of reps you do, you have created a type of training called pyramiding. Pyramiding can also be done in the reverse. In the reverse situation you would start with the heaviest weight first when you were at your strongest. Then as your energy depletes you decrease the weight. If you train this way, you would want to keep your rep scheme all the same. In other words, instead of going ten, then eight, then six, you would just shoot for three sets of ten. Decrease your weight with each set to ensure you get as close to ten reps as possible. Remember that proper form is always important. It is much easier to learn the correct way right from the start then learning it after you blow out a shoulder or a knee.

15

Biogenesis Phase One Photographs

women's workout

week 1

day 1 – back and chest

a.

Towel Row Elbows Out

Hold towel with overhand position, towel should be long enough to go around arch of the foot with legs and arms straight. Keep back straight with chest out during all phases of movement. Push with foot for resistance during all phases of rowing movement.

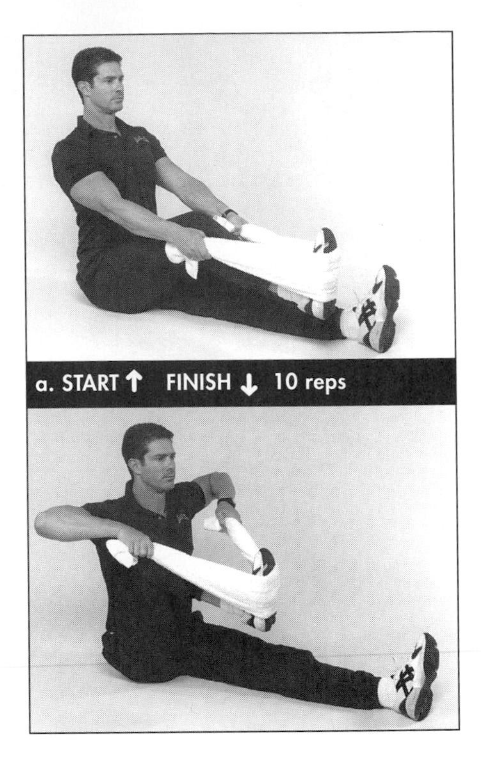

a. START ↑ FINISH ↓ 10 reps

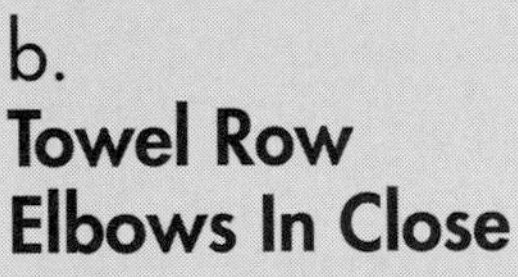

b.

Towel Row Elbows In Close

Hold towel with overhand position, towel should be long enough to go around arch of the foot with legs and arms straight. Keep back straight with chest out during all phases of movement. Push with foot for resistance during all phases of rowing movement.

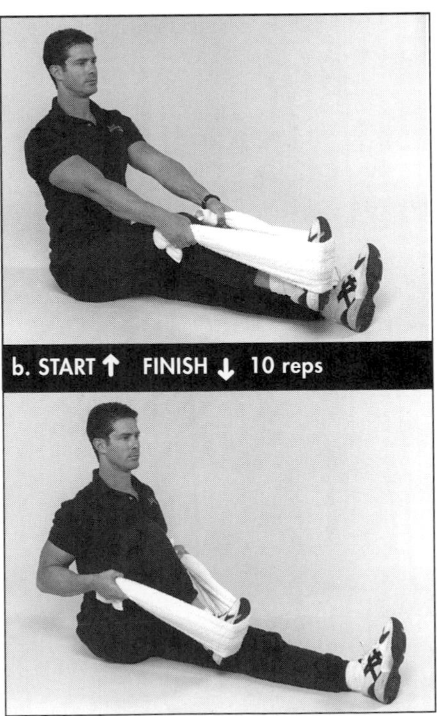

b. START ↑ FINISH ↓ 10 reps

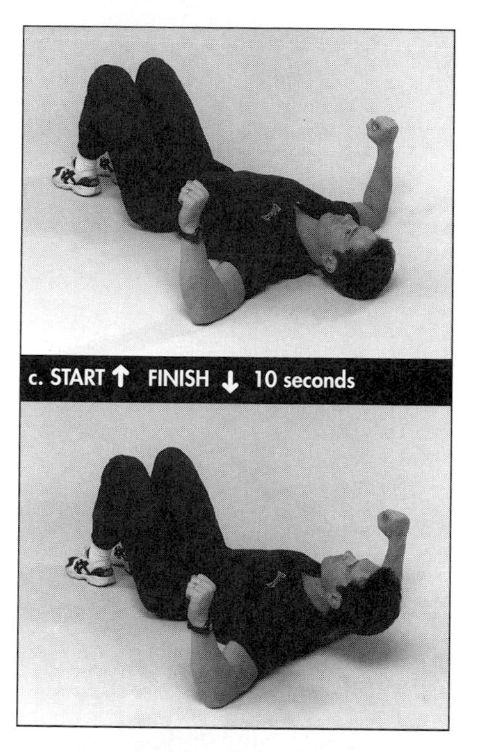

c. START ↑ FINISH ↓ 10 seconds

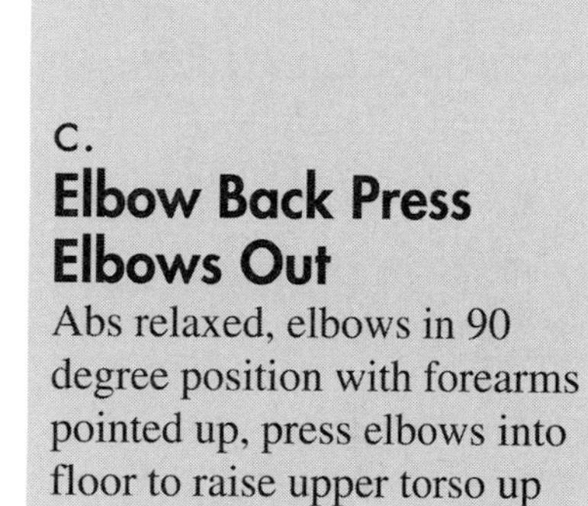

c.

Elbow Back Press Elbows Out

Abs relaxed, elbows in 90 degree position with forearms pointed up, press elbows into floor to raise upper torso up for duration of exercise, head in alignment with body.

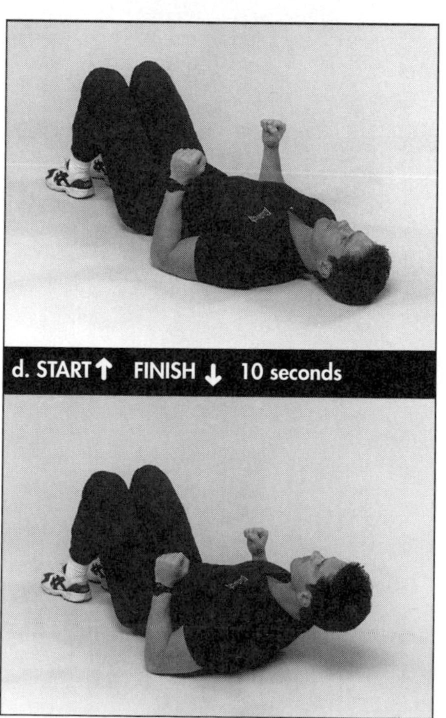

d. START ↑ FINISH ↓ 10 seconds

d.

Elbow Back Press Elbows In Close

Abs relaxed, elbows in 90 degree position with forearms pointed up, press elbows into floor to raise upper torso up for duration of exercise, head in alignment with body.

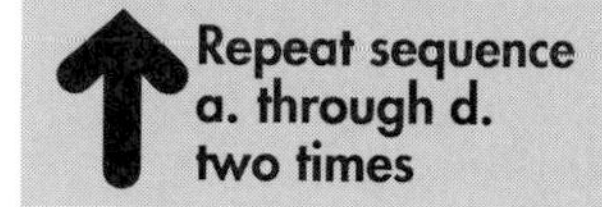

e.
Isometric Chest Fly

Hips and back straight, hands much wider than shoulder width, fingers pointed out, lower upper torso as close to floor as possible.

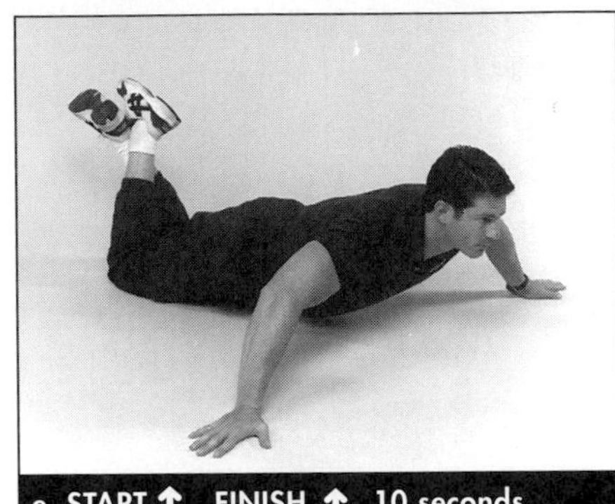

e. START ↑ FINISH ↑ 10 seconds

f.
Isometric Palm Press

Press palms together with elbows out, hands positioned 12 inches away from chest.

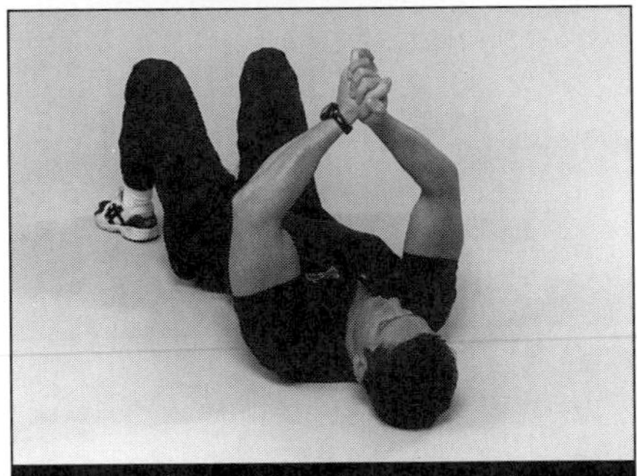

f. START ↑ FINISH ↑ 10 seconds

g.
Push-Up From Knees

Back straight, head up, shoulder width hand position, lower body as far as you can and return.

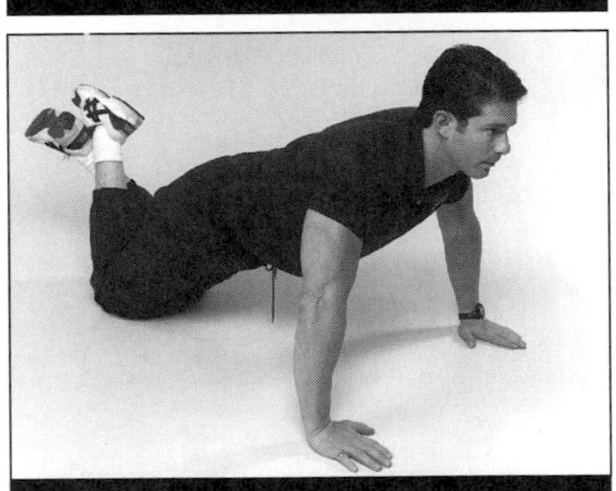

g. START ↑ FINISH ↓ 10 reps

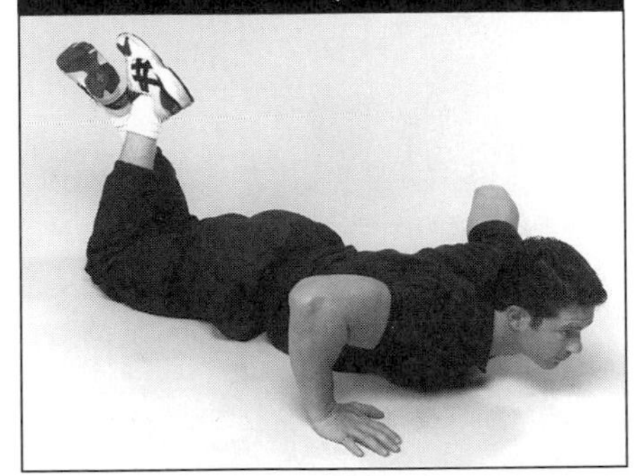

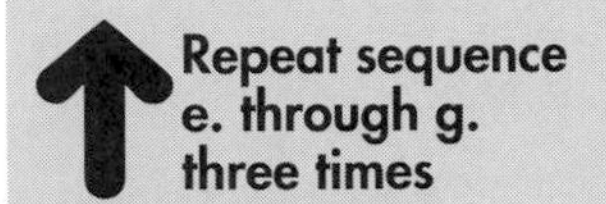

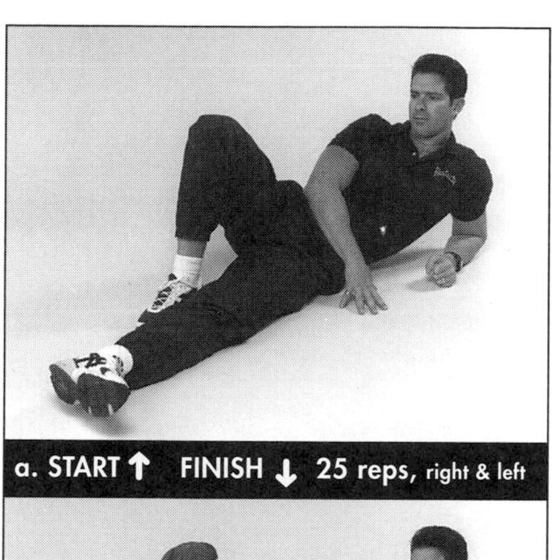

a. START ↑ FINISH ↓ 25 reps, right & left

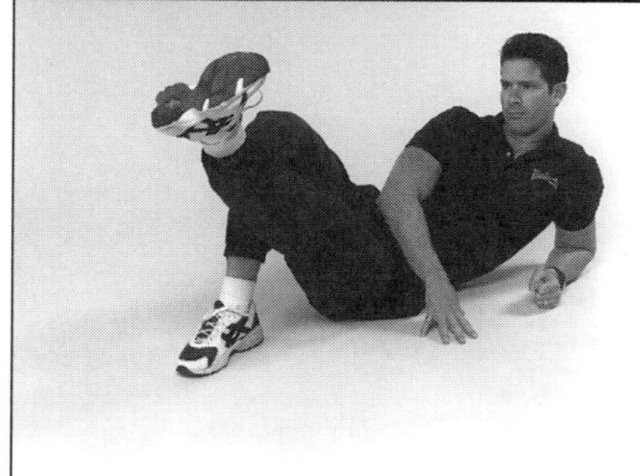

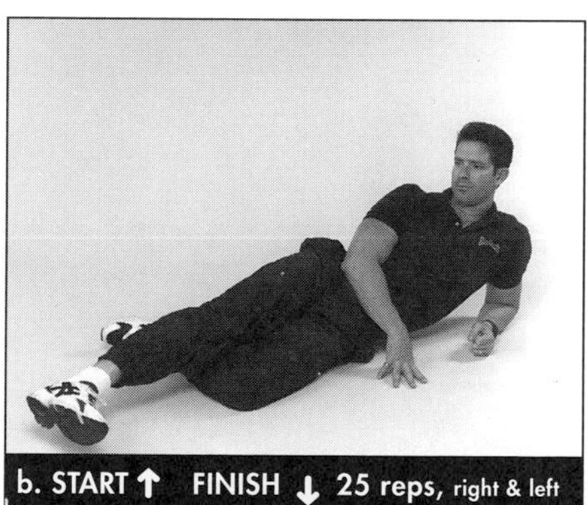

b. START ↑ FINISH ↓ 25 reps, right & left

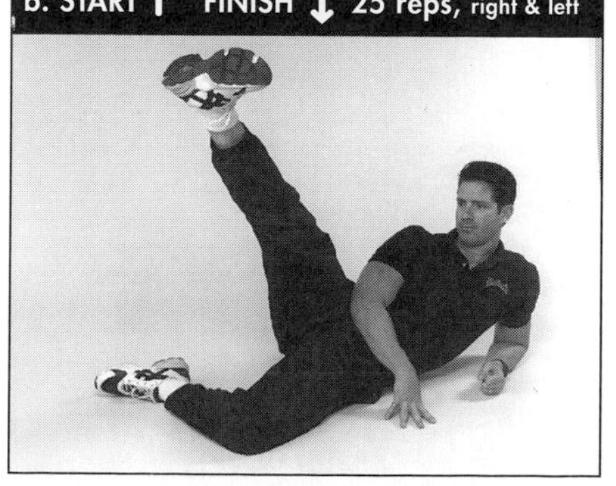

women's workout week 1

day 2 – abs, thighs, glutes

a.

Inner Thigh Adduction

Lay on side with bottom leg straight and other leg bent with foot on floor, raise the lower leg 2 feet from the ground with toes pointed out so that it is parallel to the floor. Lower foot 2 inches from the floor and return.

b.

Outer Thigh Abduction

Lay on side with bottom leg bent and top leg straight, rotate foot parallel to floor and raise three feet from floor and return.

c.
Hip Extension Out

On hands and knees kick heel of one leg out by extending the hip, bend hip to return, back straight, head up.

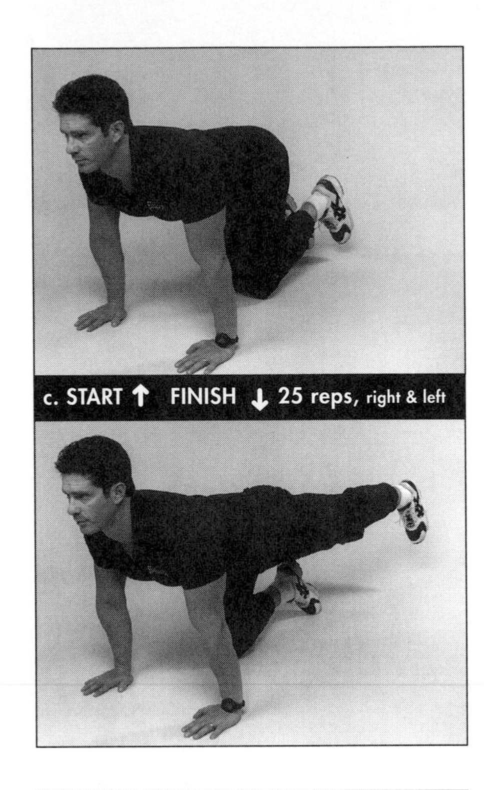

c. START ↑ FINISH ↓ 25 reps, right & left

d.
Crunches

Lay on back, eyes up, head back, hands on chest or on back of neck, breathe out and raise shoulder blades from floor, inhale on return motion.

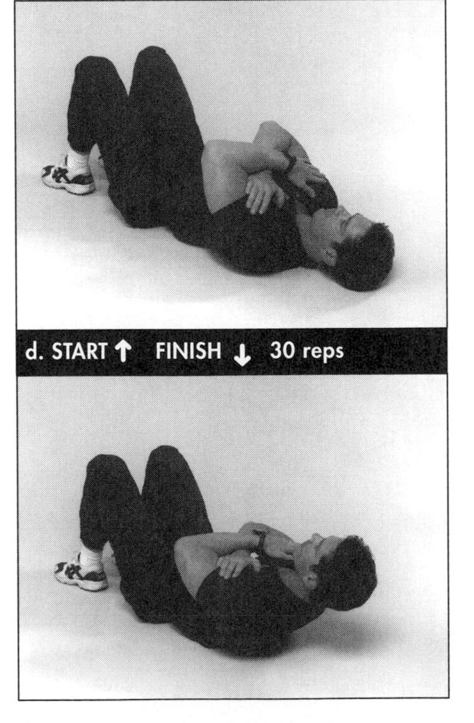

d. START ↑ FINISH ↓ 30 reps

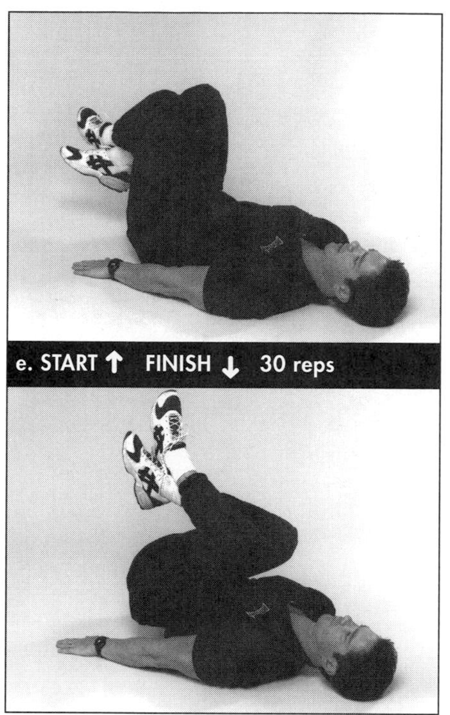

e. START ↑ FINISH ↓ 30 reps

e.
Tucks

Lay on back, ankles crossed, knees bent, hands by sides. Raise feet off floor pulling knees to face, exhaling at same time, inhale when lowering feet back to floor.

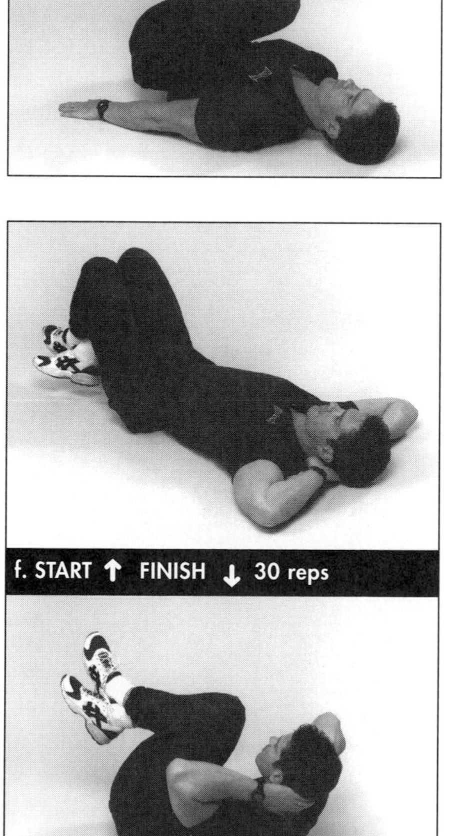

f. START ↑ FINISH ↓ 30 reps

f.
V-Crunches

Lay on back with knees bent, hands behind neck. Breathe out and raise feet and shoulders off floor simultaneously, inhale when lowering shoulders and feet.

women's workout
week 1

day 3 – legs

a.
Lunge
Feet should be twice the width of shoulders, toes of both feet point in same direction, keep back leg as straight as possible, bend front knee and hip to lower into lunge position and push to return, head up, back straight, chest out.

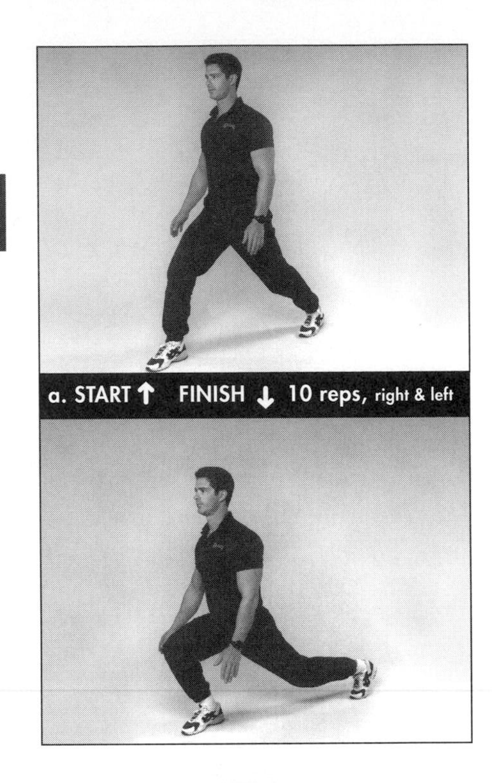
a. START ↑ FINISH ↓ 10 reps, right & left

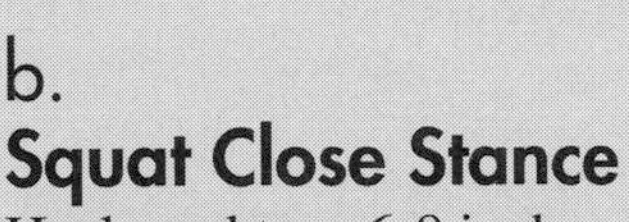

b.
Squat Close Stance
Heels and toes 6-8 inches apart, heels stay on floor during all ranges of exercise, head up, back straight, chest out. Bend knees and hips to lower upper body into squat position and return.

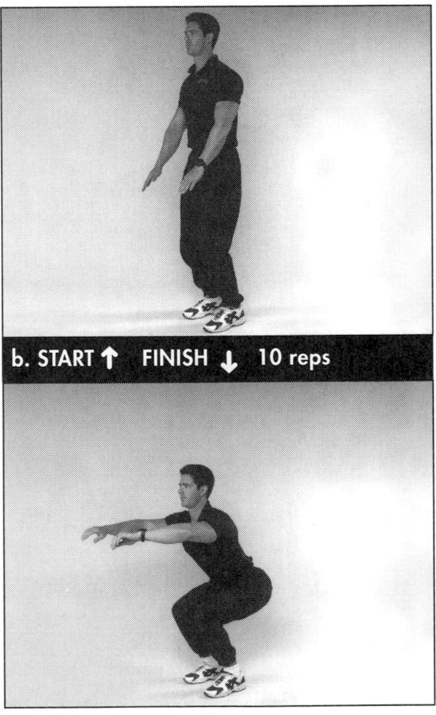
b. START ↑ FINISH ↓ 10 reps

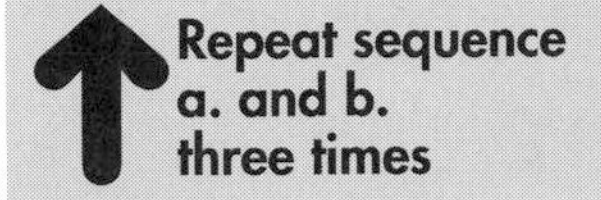
Repeat sequence a. and b. three times

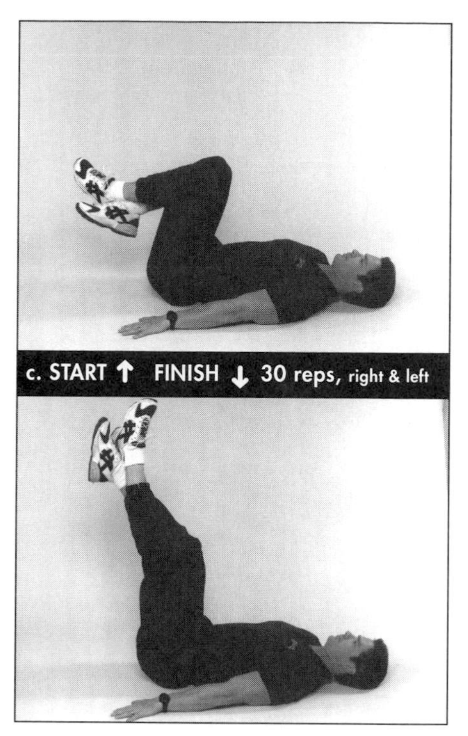
c. START ↑ FINISH ↓ 30 reps, right & left

c.

Leg Extension/Curl

Lay on back with knees up and ankles crossed, push lower shin area and back of ankle together for resistance, straighten and bend knees while applying pressure through all ranges of motion, switch ankle position to put resistance on the opposite muscles.

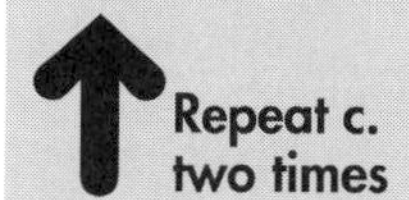

women's workout week 1

day 4 – bicep, tricep, shoulder

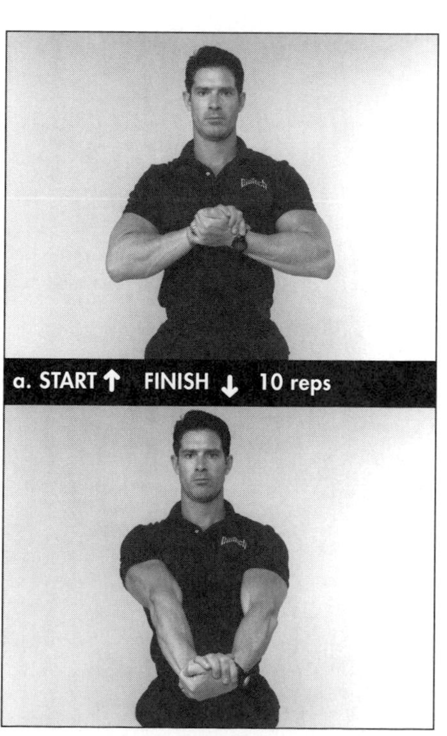
a. START ↑ FINISH ↓ 10 reps

a.

Bicep/Tricep Press

Place palms together for resistance, rotate wrist positions until back of one hand is facing you and the other is facing away, press arms straight then return to chest.

b.

Bicep/Tricep Pull

Place one hand on back of other grasping with fingers and pull for resistance, flex and extend hands away from body by bending elbows, resistance through all ranges of motion.

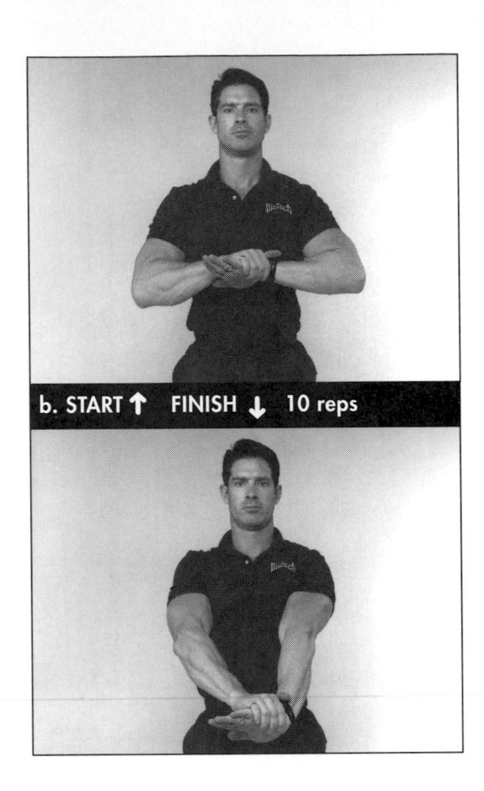

b. START ↑ FINISH ↓ 10 reps

c.

Front Raise

Working arm straight, place other hand on working arm wrist area, press down on working arm as far as it will go down, return with as much pressure from top hand as working shoulder and arm can withstand.

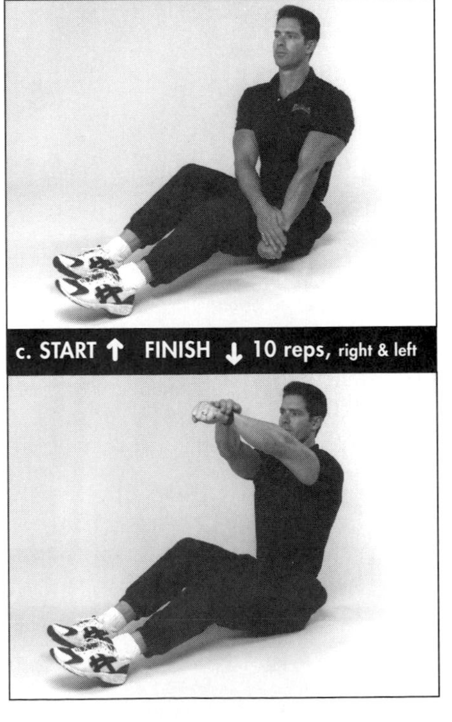

c. START ↑ FINISH ↓ 10 reps, right & left

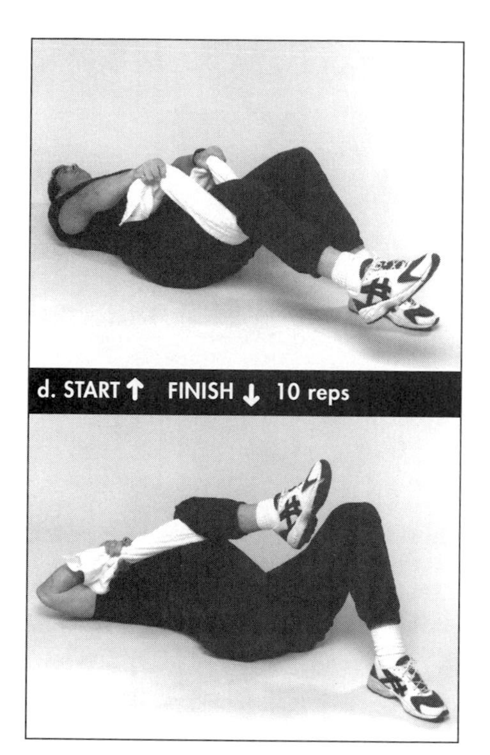

d. START ↑ FINISH ↓ 10 reps

d.

Upright Row

Towel around the back of knee with overhand position, draw elbows up toward ears while pulling leg with towel, return keeping elbows out, use leg pressure on towel for added resistance.

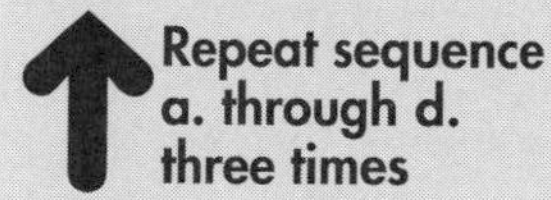

women's workout week 1

day 5 – abs, calves, lower back

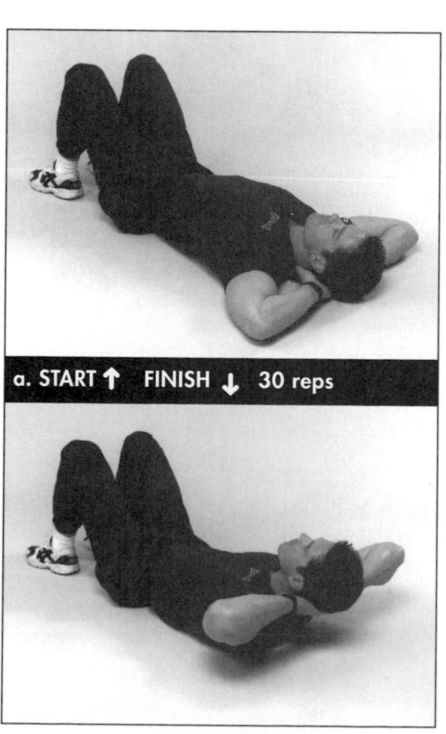

a. START ↑ FINISH ↓ 30 reps

a.

Crunches

Lay on back, eyes up, head back, hands on chest or on back of neck, breathe out and raise shoulder blades from floor, inhale on return motion.

b. Tucks

Lay on back, ankles crossed, knees bent, hands by sides. Raise feet off floor pulling knees to face, exhaling at same time, inhale when lowering feet back to floor.

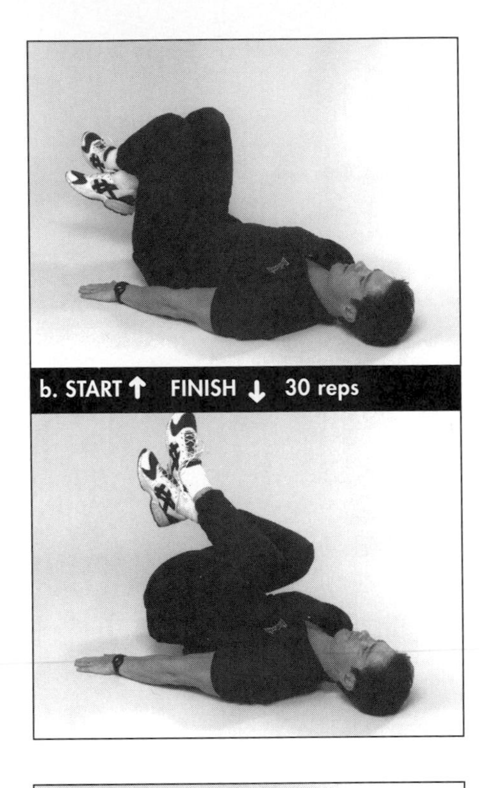

b. START ↑ FINISH ↓ 30 reps

c. V-Crunches

Lay on back with knees bent, hands behind neck. Breathe out and raise feet and shoulders off floor simultaneously, inhale when lowering shoulders and feet.

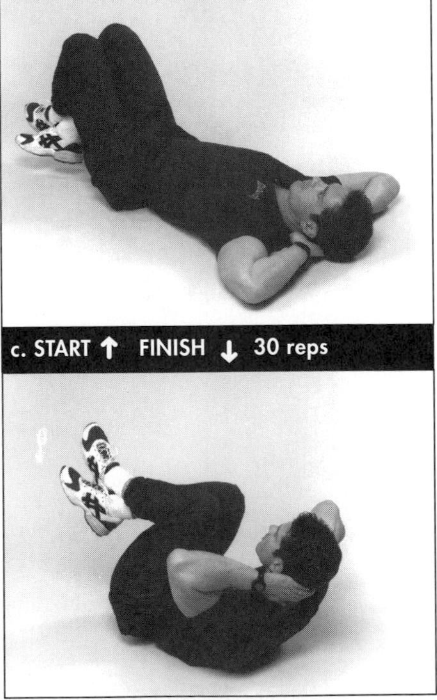

c. START ↑ FINISH ↓ 30 reps

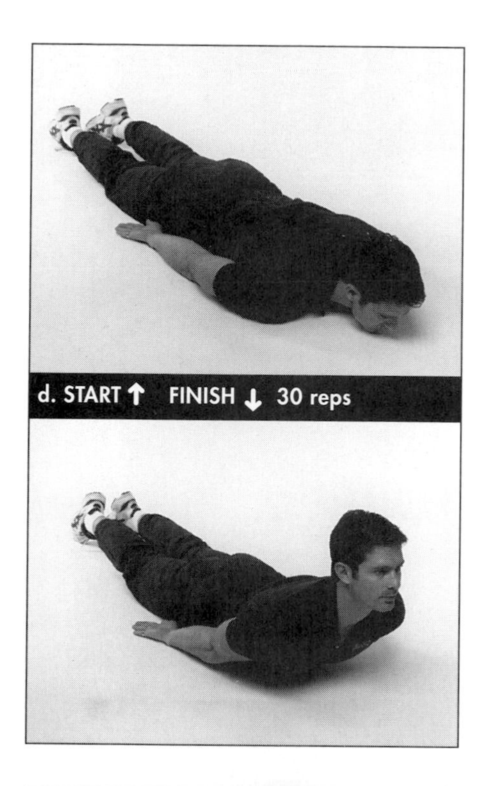

d. START ↑ FINISH ↓ 30 reps

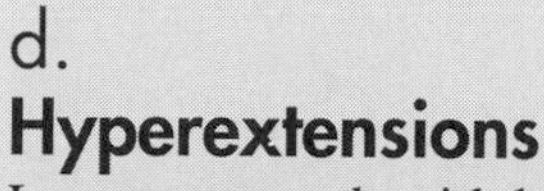

d. Hyperextensions

Lay on stomach with hands by sides for easy resistance, behind head for moderate resistance, straight out in front for maximum resistance, raise head, shoulders and chest from floor and return.

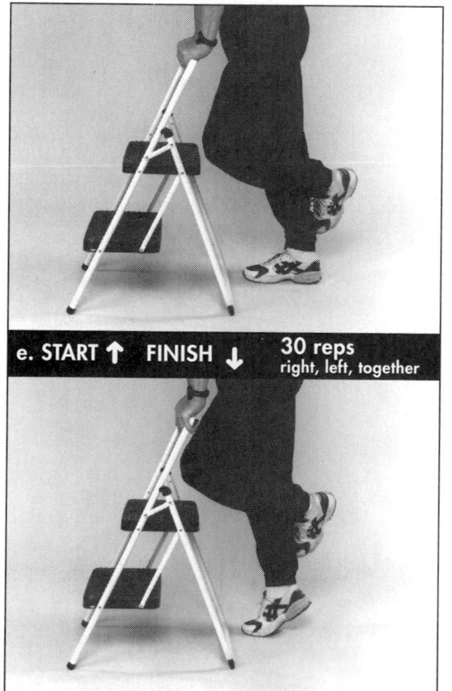

e. START ↑ FINISH ↓ 30 reps right, left, together

e. Calf Raise

Standing on one foot, raise heel from floor 2-3 inches and return. For double calf raise, stand on both feet, raise heels from floor 2-3 inches and return.

women's workout

week 2

day 1 – back and chest

a.

Elbow Back Press Elbows Out

Abs relaxed, elbows in 90 degree position with forearms pointed up, press elbows into floor to raise upper torso up for duration of exercise, head in alignment with body.

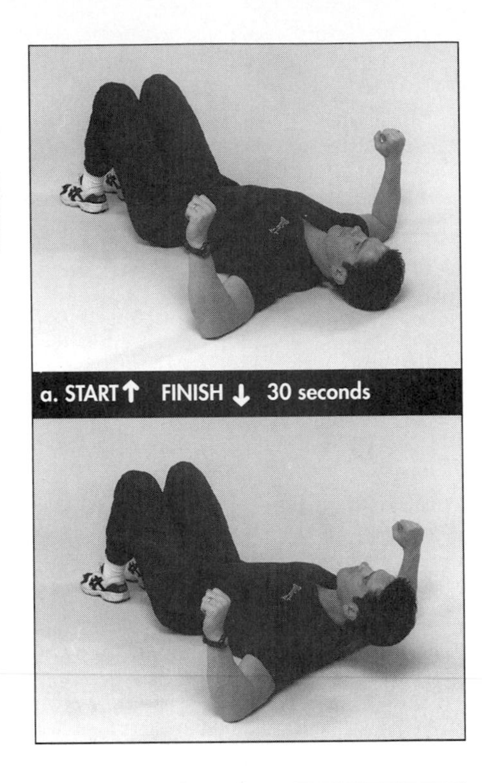
a. START ↑ FINISH ↓ 30 seconds

b.

Elbow Back Press Elbows In Close

Abs relaxed, elbows in 90 degree position with forearms pointed up, press elbows into floor to raise upper torso up for duration of exercise, head in alignment with body.

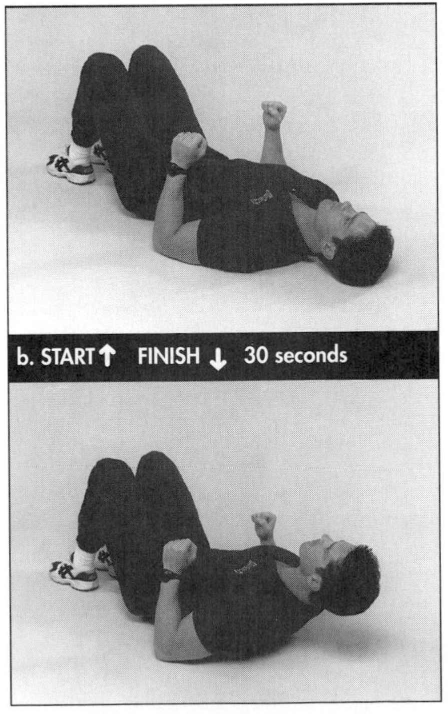
b. START ↑ FINISH ↓ 30 seconds

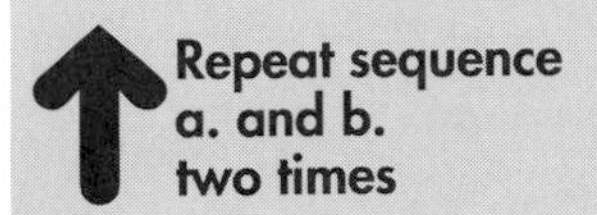

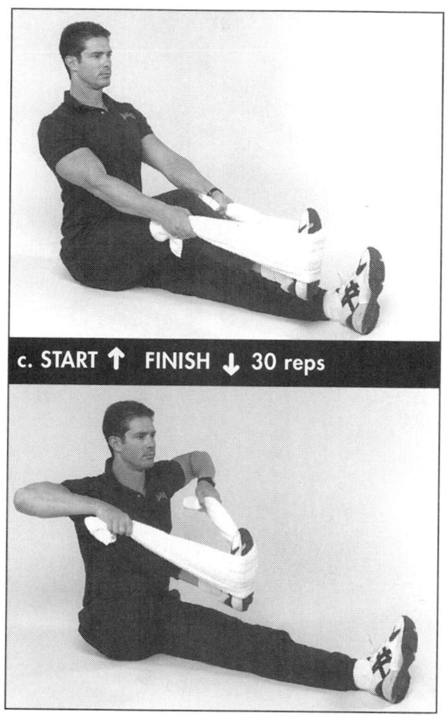

c. START ↑ FINISH ↓ 30 reps

c.
Towel Row Elbows Out

Hold towel with overhand position, towel should be long enough to go around arch of the foot with legs and arms straight. Keep back straight with chest out during all phases of movement. Push with foot for resistance during all phases of rowing movement.

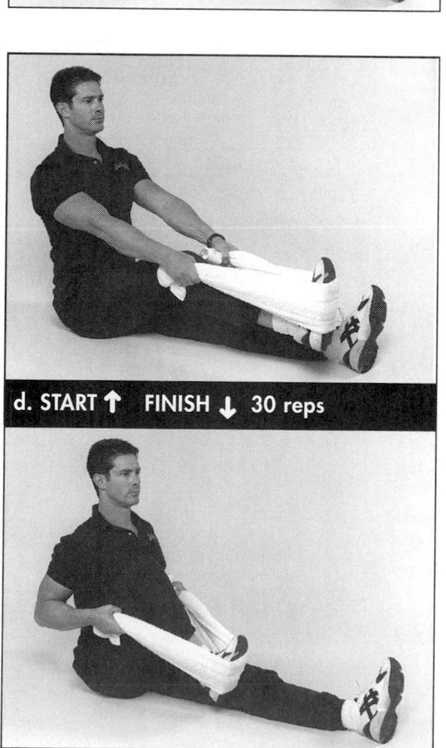

d. START ↑ FINISH ↓ 30 reps

d.
Towel Row Elbows In Close

Hold towel with overhand position, towel should be long enough to go around arch of the foot with legs and arms straight. Keep back straight with chest out during all phases of movement. Push with foot for resistance during all phases of rowing movement.

e.
Isometric Palm Press
Press palms together with elbows out, hands positioned 12 inches away from chest

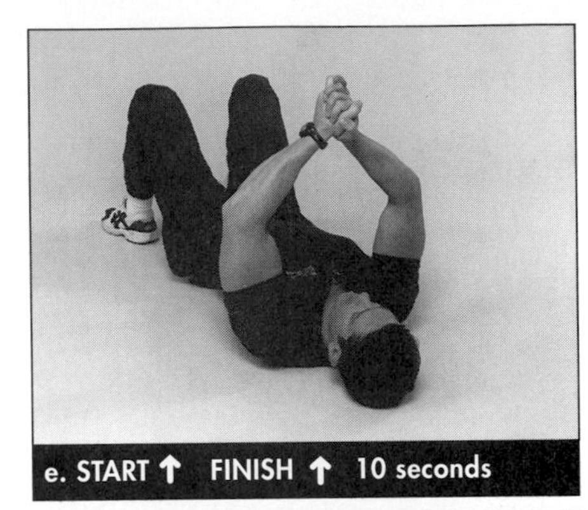

e. START ↑ FINISH ↑ 10 seconds

f.
Isometric Chest Fly
Hips and back straight, hands much wider than shoulder width, fingers pointed out, lower upper torso as close to floor as possible.

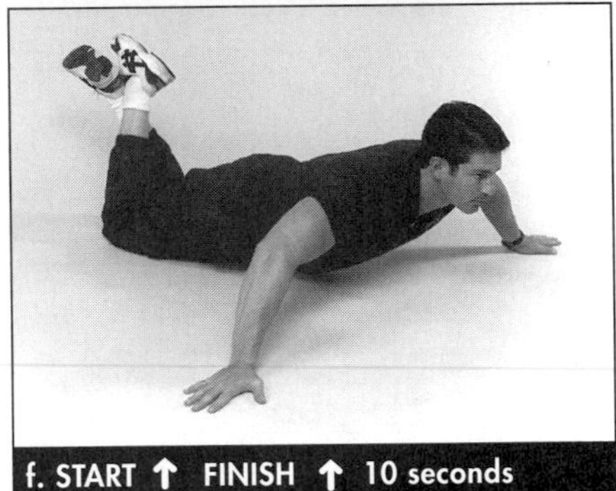

f. START ↑ FINISH ↑ 10 seconds

↑ Repeat sequence e. and f. two times

g.
Push Up From Knees
Back straight, head up, shoulder width hand position, lower body as far as you can and return.

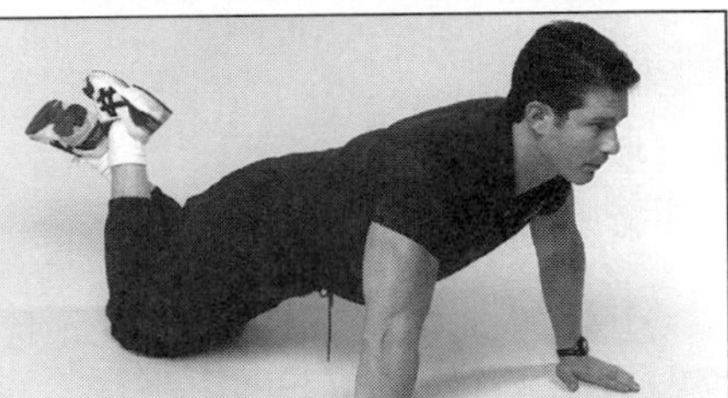

g. START ↑ FINISH ↓ 30 reps

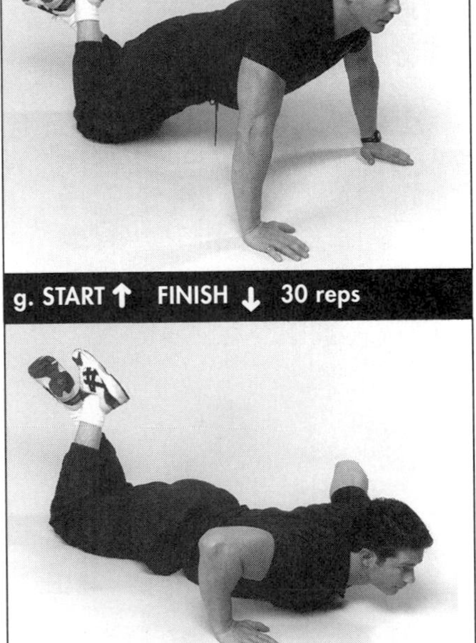

women's workout week 2

day 2 – abs, thighs, glutes

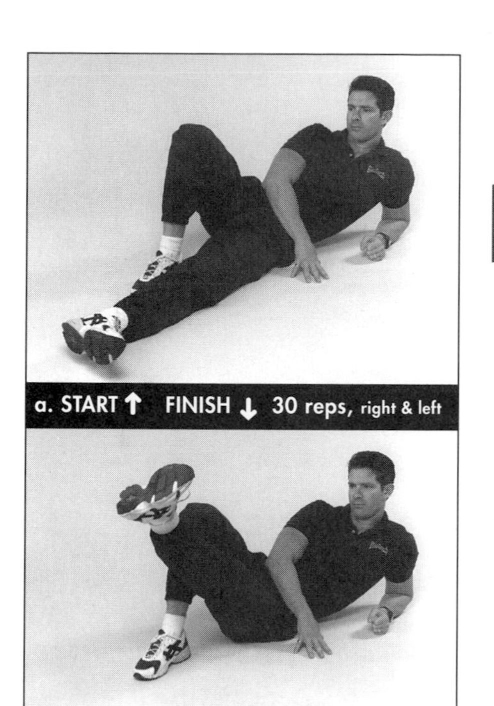

a. START ↑ FINISH ↓ 30 reps, right & left

a. Inner Thigh Adduction

Lay on side with bottom leg straight and other leg bent with foot on floor, raise the lower leg 2 feet from the ground with toes pointed out so that it is parallel to the floor. Lower foot 2 inches from the floor and return.

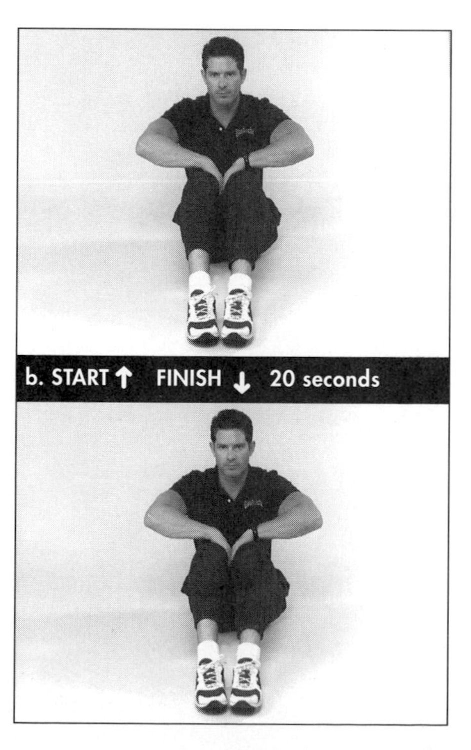

b. START ↑ FINISH ↓ 20 seconds

b. Isometric Thigh Adduction

Sit with knees in 90 degree position. Place hands between knees and pull knees apart while squeezing together with knees.

c.
Outer Thigh Abduction

Lay on side with bottom leg bent and top leg straight, rotate foot parallel to floor and raise three feet from floor and return.

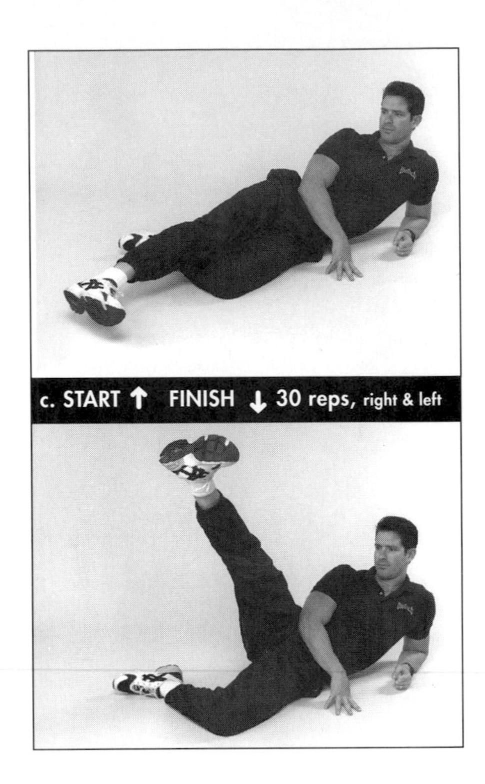
c. START ↑ FINISH ↓ 30 reps, right & left

d.
Isometric Thigh Abduction

Sit with knees in 90 degree position. Place hands on outside of knees pushing in with hands while pushing out with knees.

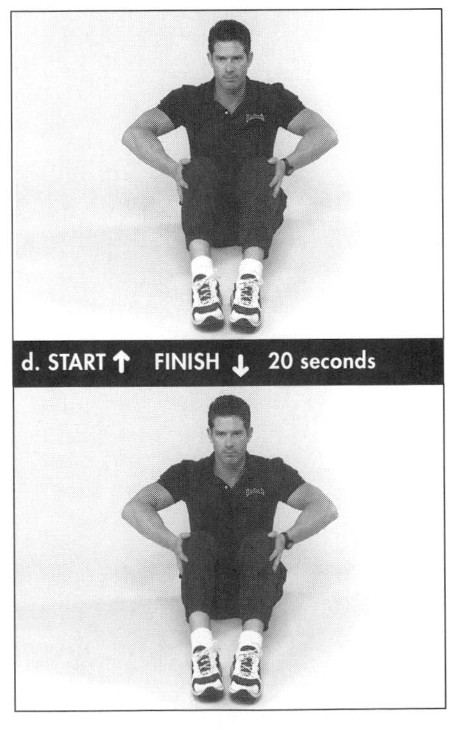
d. START ↑ FINISH ↓ 20 seconds

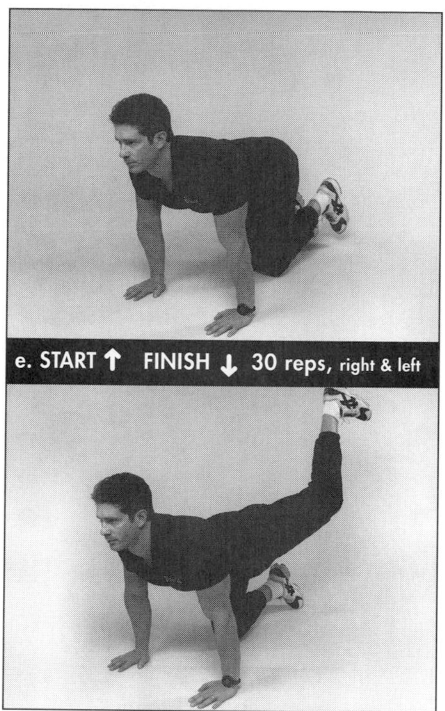

e.
Kneeling Heel Push Straight Up

On hands and knees, lift one knee and extend foot back and up and return.

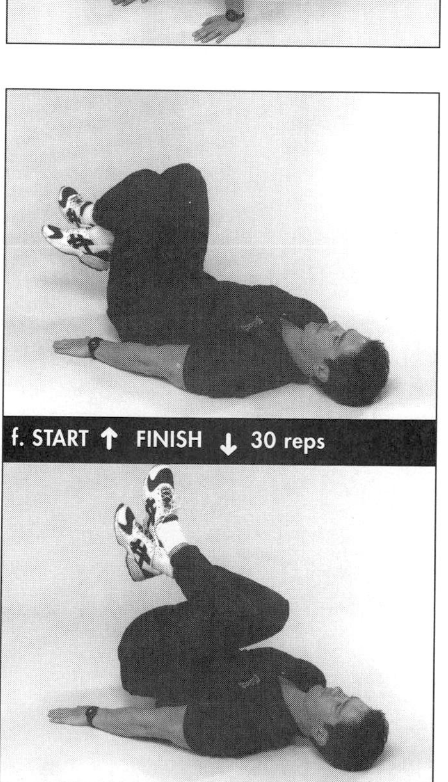

f.
Tucks

Lay on back, ankles crossed, knees bent, hands by sides. Raise feet off floor pulling knees to face, exhaling at same time, inhale when lowering feet back to floor.

g.
Crunches

Lay on back, eyes up, head back, hands on chest or on back of neck, breathe out and raise shoulder blades from floor, inhale on return motion.

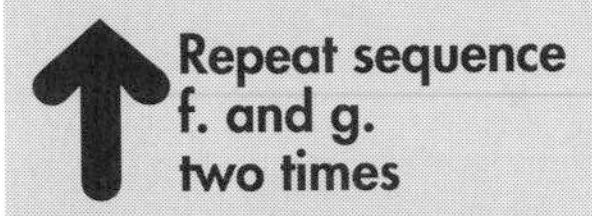
Repeat sequence f. and g. two times

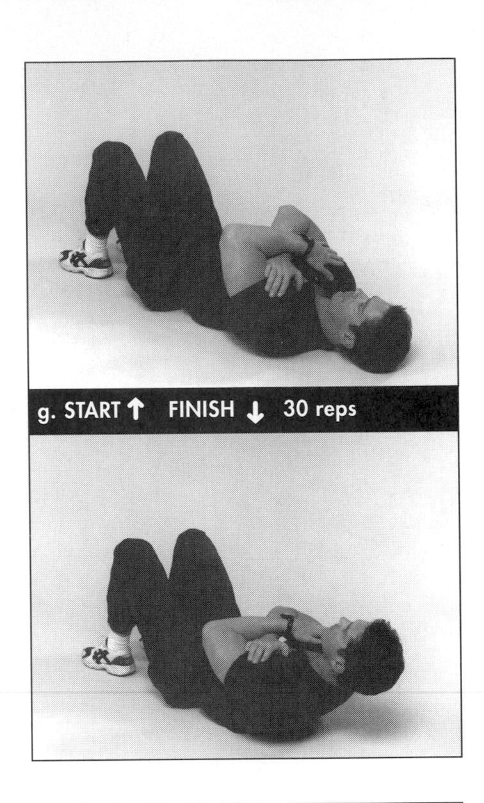
g. START ↑ FINISH ↓ 30 reps

women's workout
week 2
day 3 – legs

a.
Isometric Squat Close Stance

Heels and toes 6-8 inches apart, bend knees and hips to lower body into squat position and hold for recommended time, heels stay down, chest out, head up, back straight.

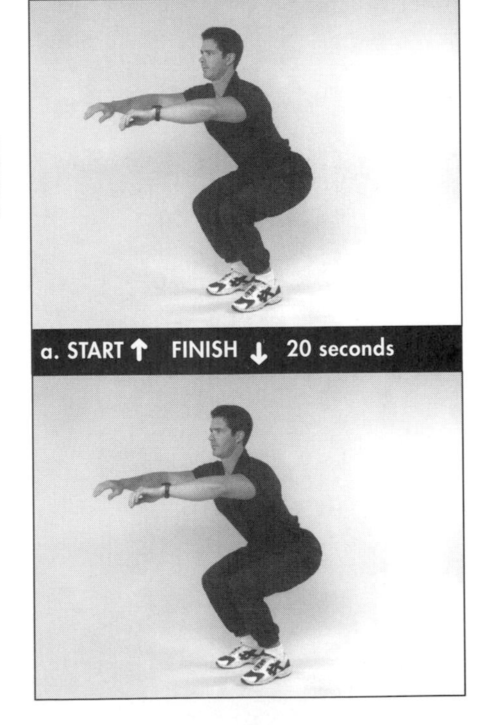
a. START ↑ FINISH ↓ 20 seconds

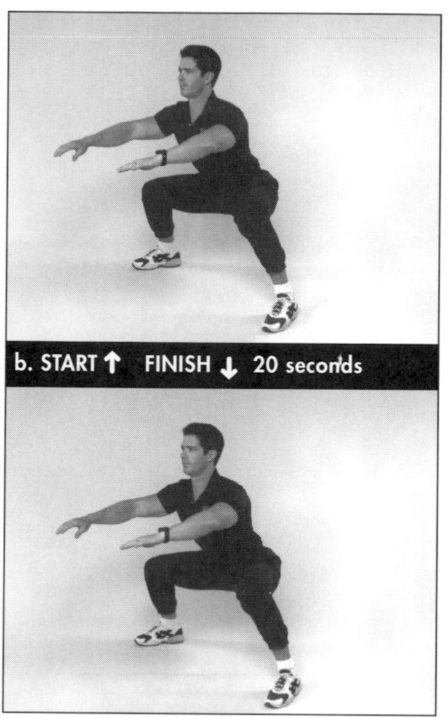

b.

Isometric Squat Wide Stance

Heels twice as wide as shoulder width with toes pointing out slightly, bend knees and hips to lower body into squat position and hold for recommended time, back straight, head up, heels down.

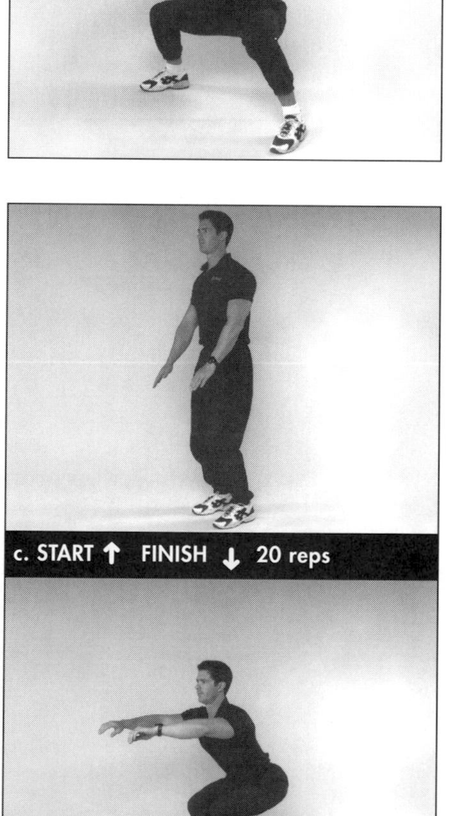

c.

Squat Close Stance

Heels and toes 6-8 inches apart, heels stay on floor during all ranges of exercise, head up, back straight, chest out, bend knees and hips to lower upper body into squat position and return.

d.

Squat Wide Stance

Heels twice as wide as shoulder width with toes pointing out slightly, heels stay down, head up, back straight, chest out, bend knees and hips to lower upper body into squat position and return.

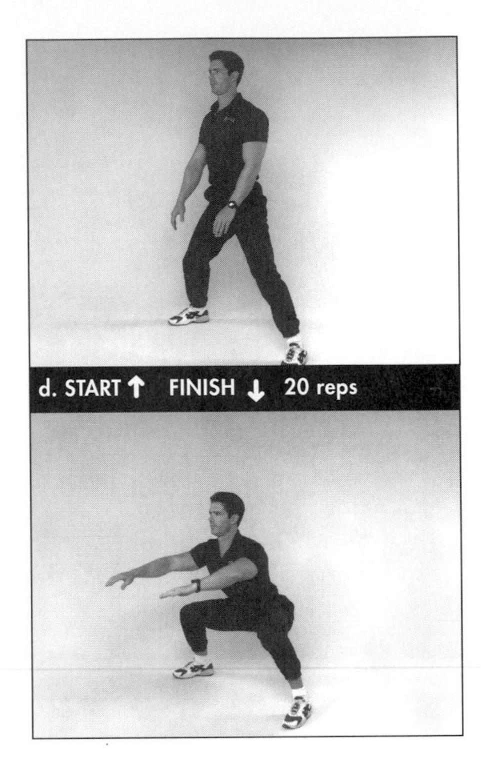

d. START ↑ FINISH ↓ 20 reps

↑ Repeat sequence a. through d. three times

e.

Ankle Cross Extension/Curl

Lay on back with knees up and ankles crossed, push lower shin area and back of ankle together for resistance, straighten and bend knees while applying pressure through all ranges of motion, switch ankle position to put resistance on the opposite muscles.

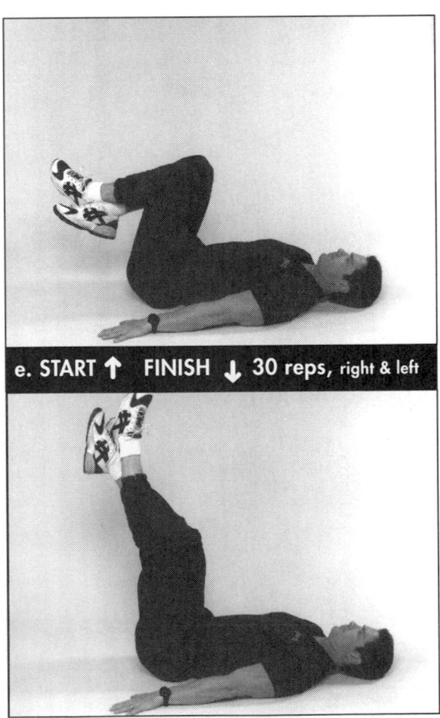

e. START ↑ FINISH ↓ 30 reps, right & left

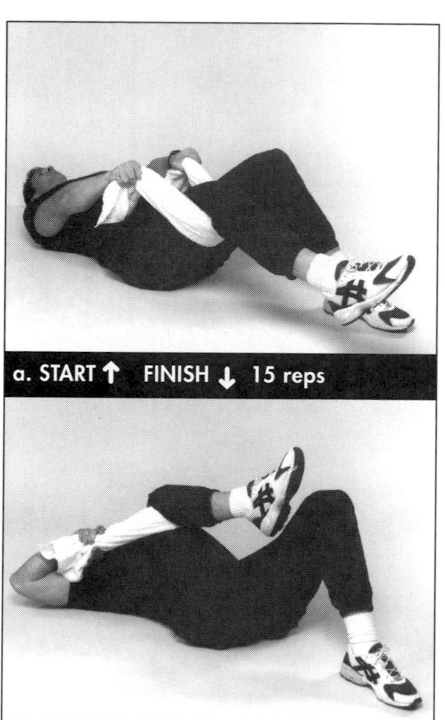

a. START ↑ FINISH ↓ 15 reps

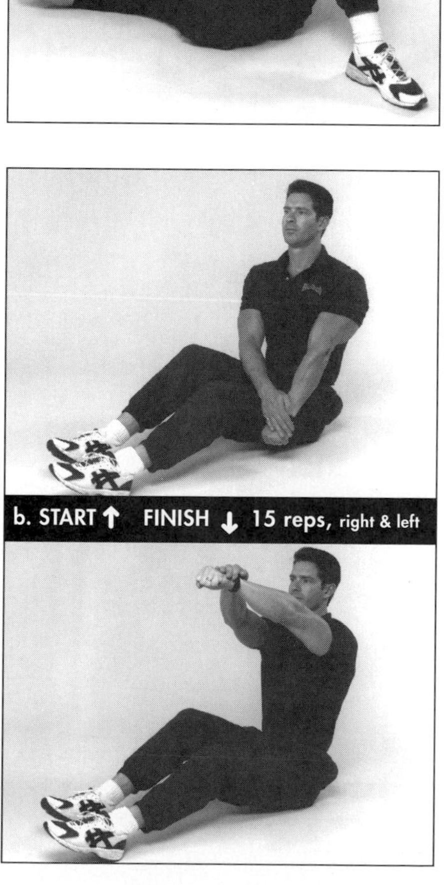

b. START ↑ FINISH ↓ 15 reps, right & left

women's workout week 2

day 4 – bicep, tricep, shoulder

a.
Upright Row With Towel

Towel around the back of knee with overhand position, draw elbows up toward ears while pulling leg with towel, return keeping elbows out, use leg pressure on towel for added resistance.

b.
Frontal Raise

Working arm straight, place other hand on working arm wrist area, press down on working arm as far as it will go down, return with as much pressure from top hand as working shoulder and arm can withstand.

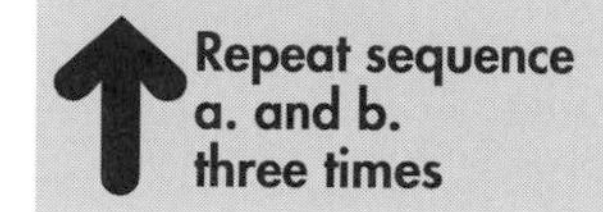

Repeat sequence a. and b. three times

c.
Bicep Towel Curl

Use underhand position with towel under back of knee, apply pressure with leg for resistance, bend elbows to pull knee to upper body and return.

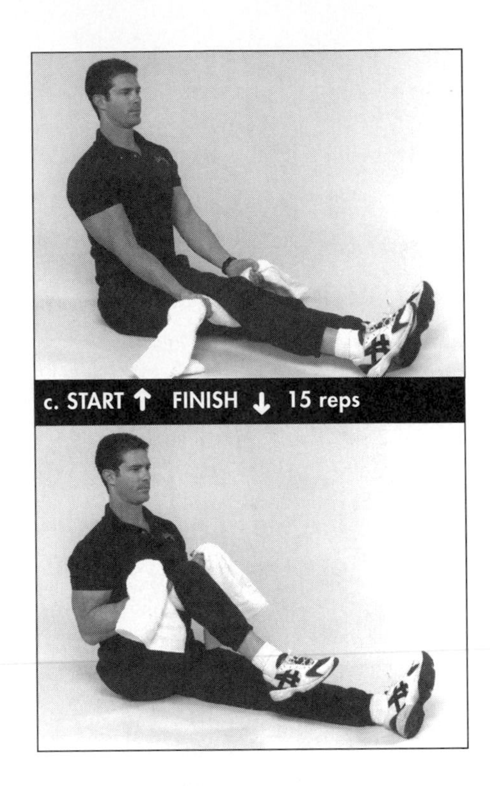

c. START ↑ FINISH ↓ 15 reps

d.
Double Tricep Extension

Laying on back with towel in overhand position, elbows out with 90 degree bend, forearms pointed straight up, pull towel with both hands to apply resistance to opposing triceps, apply resistance through full range of motion when flexing and straightening each arm.

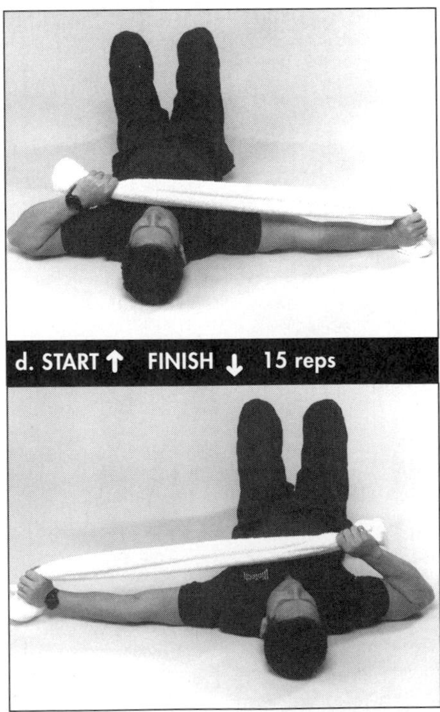

d. START ↑ FINISH ↓ 15 reps

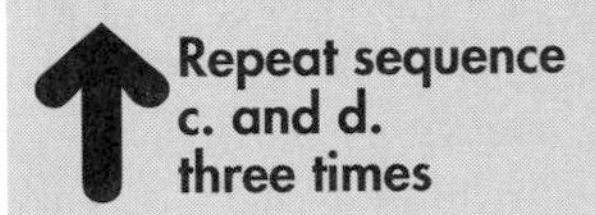

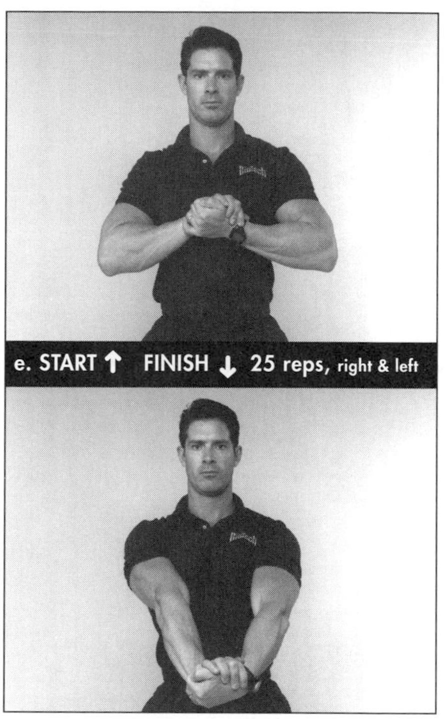

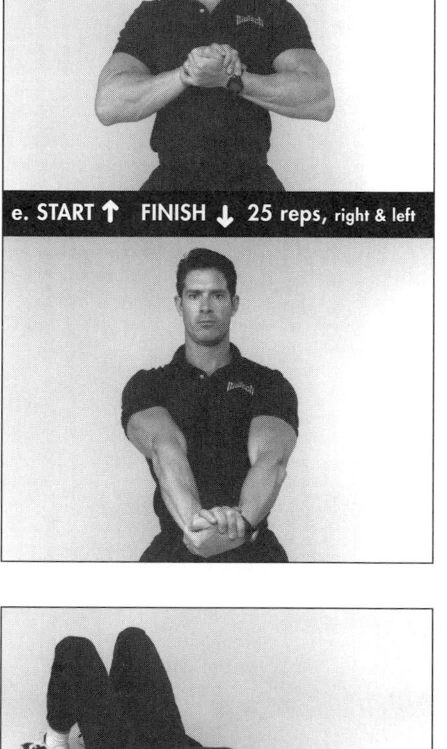

e. START ↑ FINISH ↓ 25 reps, right & left

e.

Bicep/Tricep Curl Press

Place palms together for resistance, rotate wrist positions until back of one hand is facing you and the other is facing away, press arms straight then return to chest.

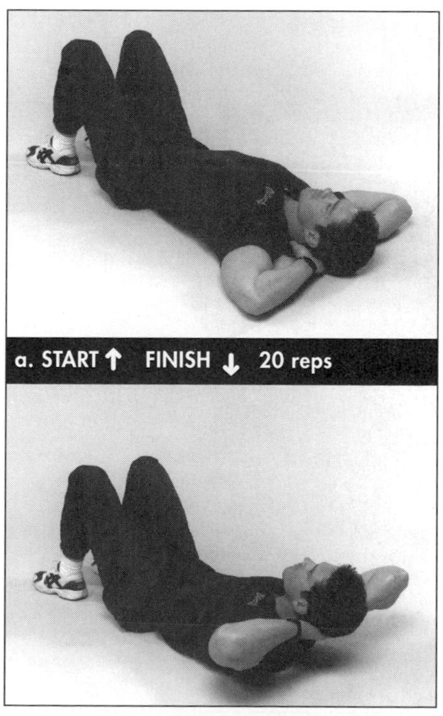

a. START ↑ FINISH ↓ 20 reps

women's workout week 2

day 5 – obliques, abs, lower back, calves

a.

Crunches

Lay on back, eyes up, head back, hands on chest or on back of neck, breathe out and raise shoulder blades from floor, inhale on return motion.

b.
Tucks

Lay on back, ankles crossed, knees bent, hands by sides. Raise feet off floor pulling knees to face, exhaling at same time, inhale when lowering feet back to floor.

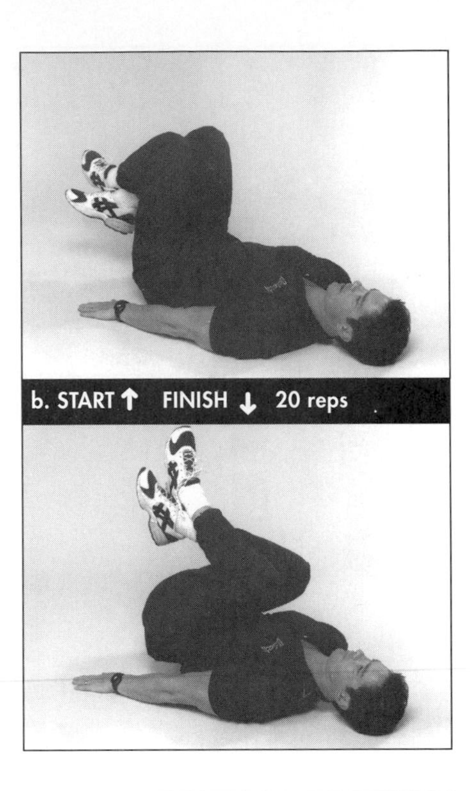

b. START ↑ FINISH ↓ 20 reps

c.
Side Crunch

Lay on side with hips flexed and knees bent, bottom arm supporting head with elbow off the floor, top arm straight, exhale while reaching for ankle, inhale and return.

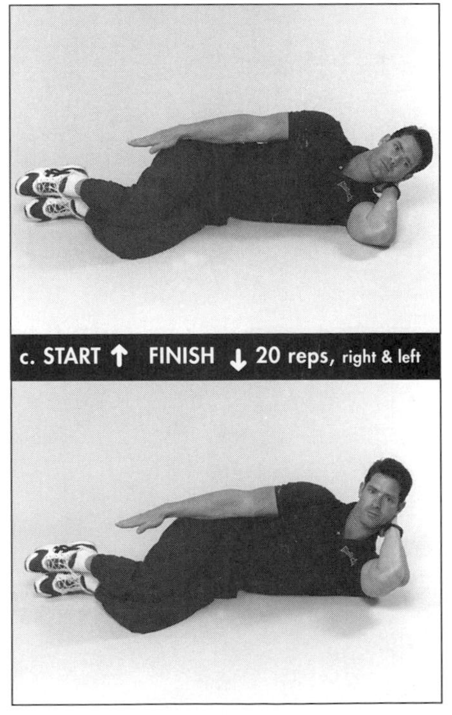

c. START ↑ FINISH ↓ 20 reps, right & left

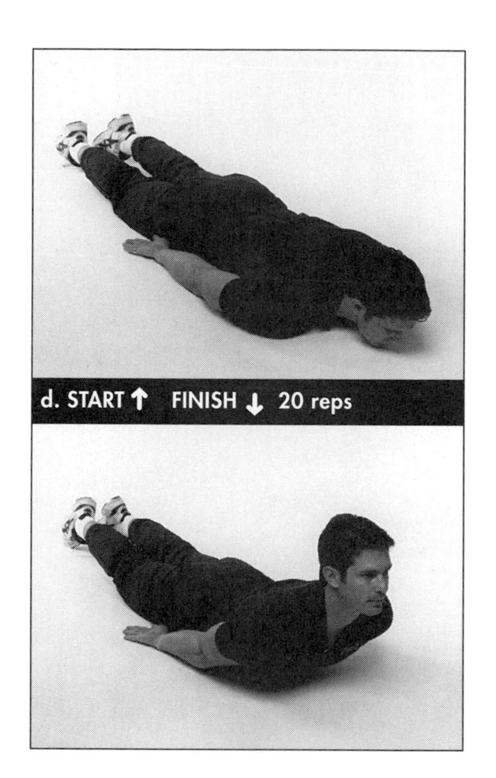
d. START ↑ FINISH ↓ 20 reps

d.

Hyperextensions

Lay on stomach with hands by sides for easy resistance, behind head for moderate resistance, straight out in front for maximum resistance, raise head, shoulders and chest from floor and return.

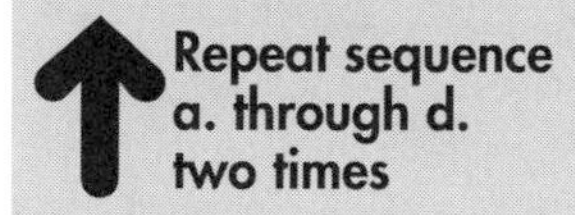

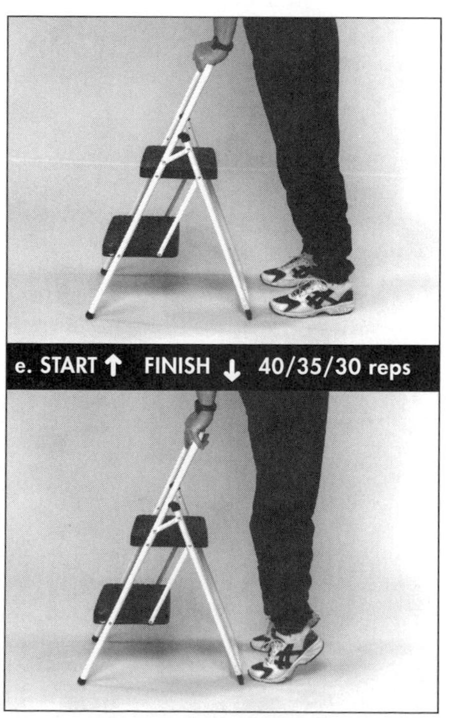
e. START ↑ FINISH ↓ 40/35/30 reps

e.

Calf Raise Together

Standing on both feet, raise heels from floor 2-3 inches and return.

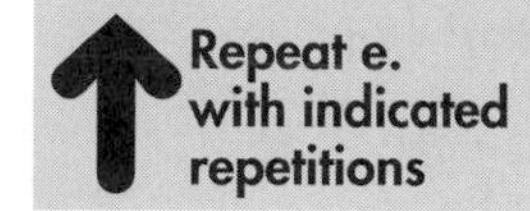

women's workout
week 3

day 1 – back and chest

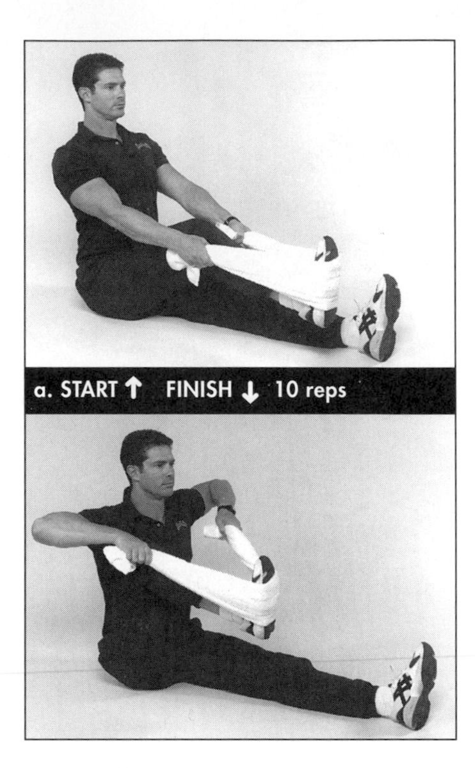

a. START ↑ FINISH ↓ 10 reps

a.

Towel Row Elbows Out

Hold towel with overhand position, towel should be long enough to go around arch of the foot with legs and arms straight. Keep back straight with chest out during all phases of movement. Push with foot for resistance during all phases of rowing movement.

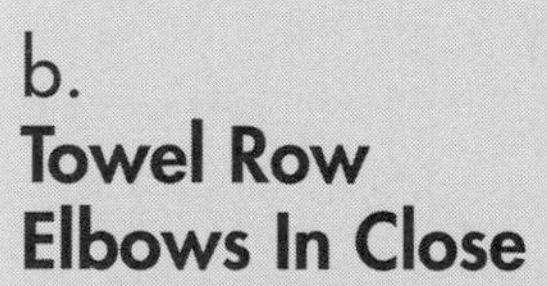

b.

Towel Row Elbows In Close

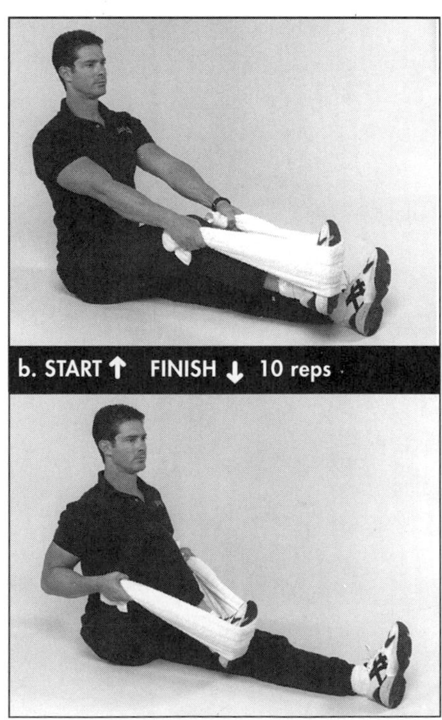

b. START ↑ FINISH ↓ 10 reps

Hold towel with overhand position, towel should be long enough to go around arch of the foot with legs and arms straight. Keep back straight with chest out during all phases of movement. Push with foot for resistance during all phases of rowing movement.

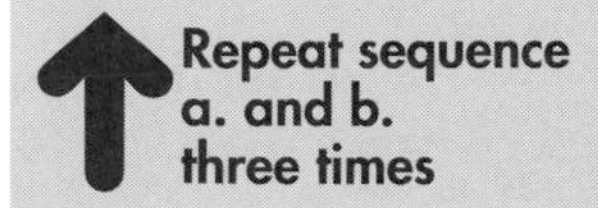

Repeat sequence a. and b. three times

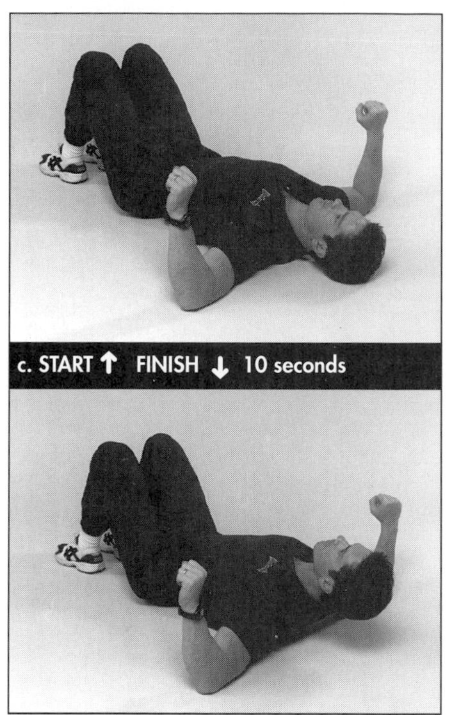

c. START ↑ FINISH ↓ 10 seconds

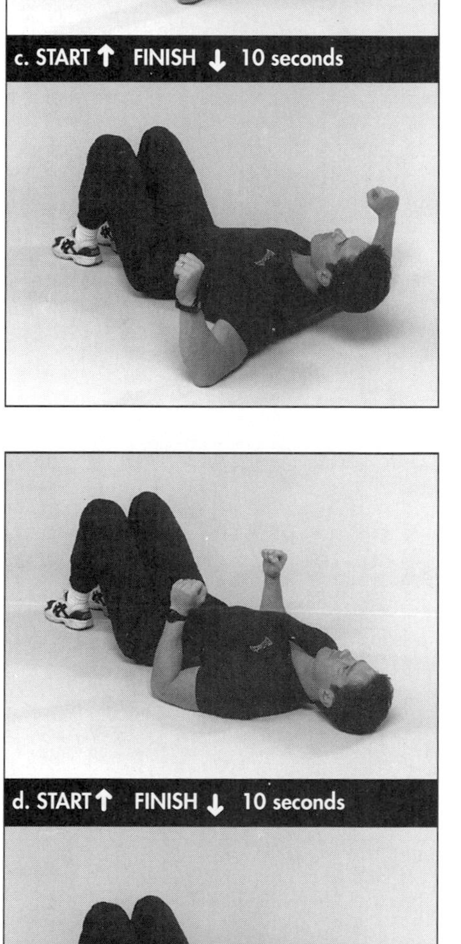

c.
Elbow Back Press Elbows Out

Abs relaxed, elbows in 90 degree position with forearms pointed up, press elbows into floor to raise upper torso up for duration of exercise, head in alignment with body.

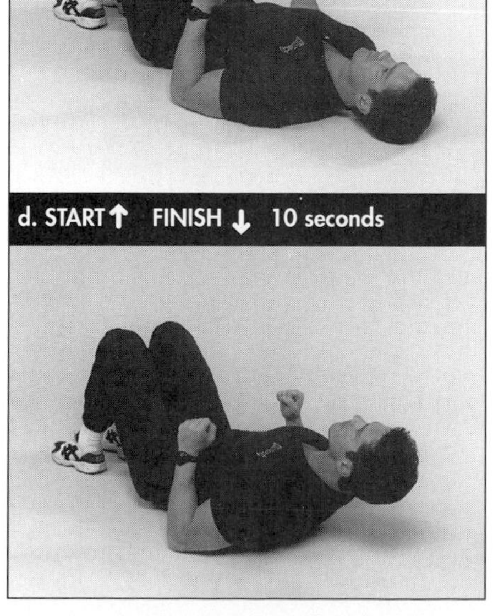

d. START ↑ FINISH ↓ 10 seconds

d.
Elbow Back Press Elbows In Close

Abs relaxed, elbows in 90 degree position with forearms pointed up, press elbows into floor to raise upper torso up for duration of exercise, head in alignment with body.

↑ Repeat sequence c. and d. three times

e.
High Palm Press
Press palms together with elbows out, hands positioned 12 inches away from nose.

f.
Medium Palm Press
Press palms together with elbows out, hands positioned 18 inches away from chest.

g.
Low Palm Press
Press palms together with elbows out, hands positioned 12 inches away from navel.

Repeat sequence e. through g. two times

h.
Chest Fly
Hips and back straight, hands much wider than shoulder width, fingers pointed out, lower upper torso as close to floor as possible.

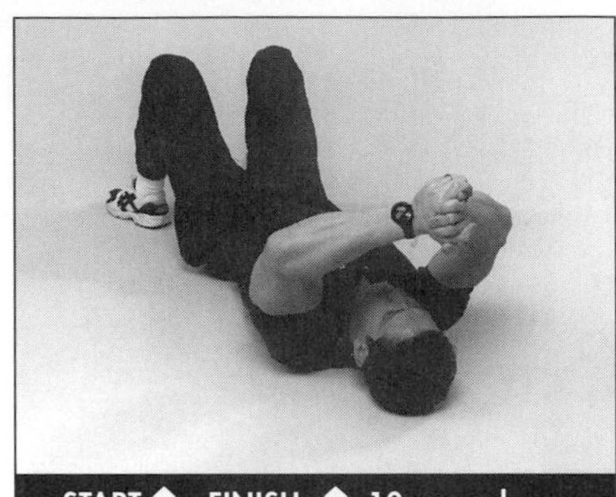
e. START ↑ FINISH ↑ 10 seconds

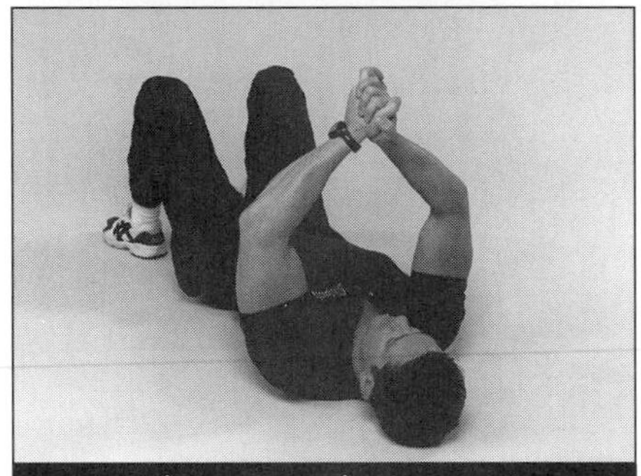
f. START ↑ FINISH ↑ 10 seconds

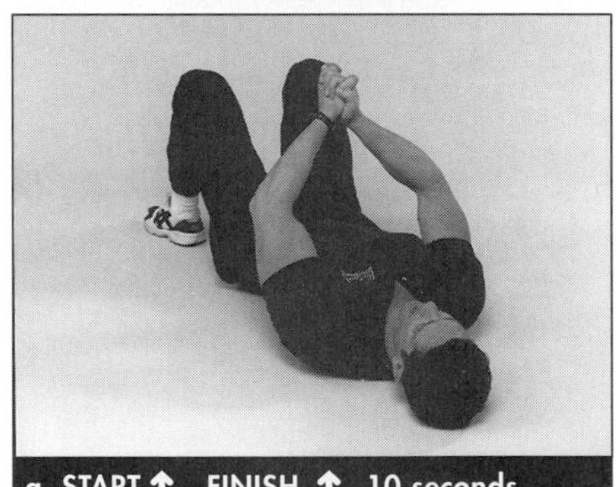
g. START ↑ FINISH ↑ 10 seconds

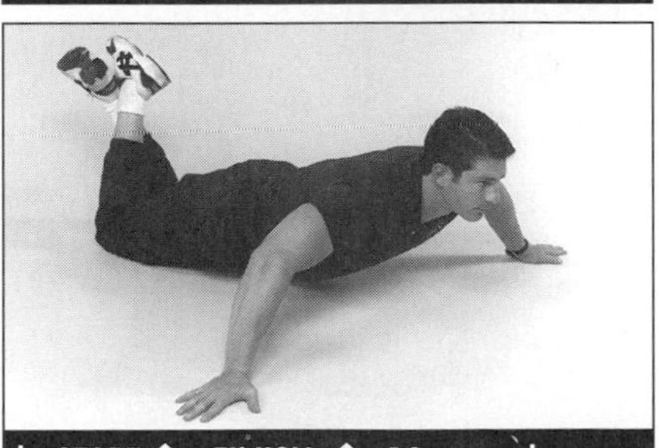
h. START ↑ FINISH ↑ 10 seconds

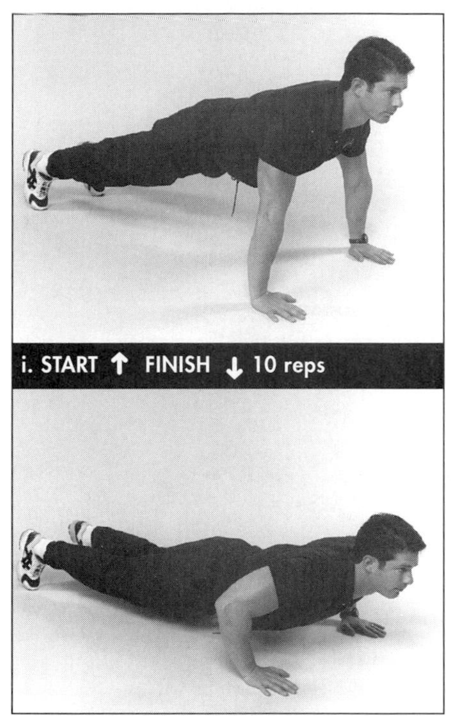

i. START ↑ FINISH ↓ 10 reps

i.

Push Up

Back straight, head up, shoulder width hand position, lower body as far as you can and return.

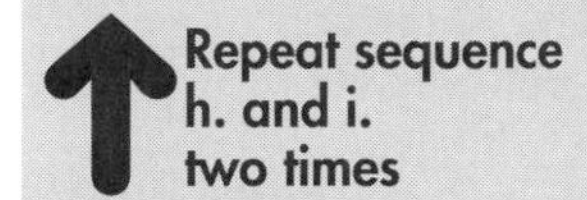

women's workout week 3

day 2 – abs, thighs, glutes

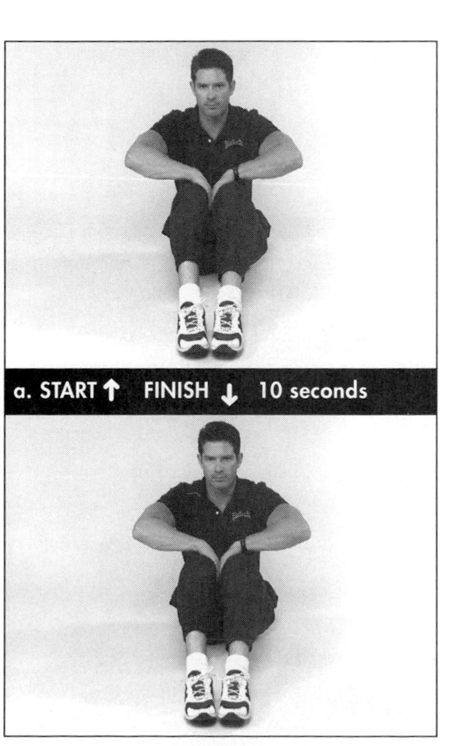

a. START ↑ FINISH ↓ 10 seconds

a.

Isometric Thigh Adduction

Sit with knees in 90 degree position. Place hands between knees and pull knees apart while squeezing together with knees.

b.

Isometric Thigh Abduction

Sit with knees in 90 degree position. Place hands on outside of knees pushing in with hands while pushing out with knees.

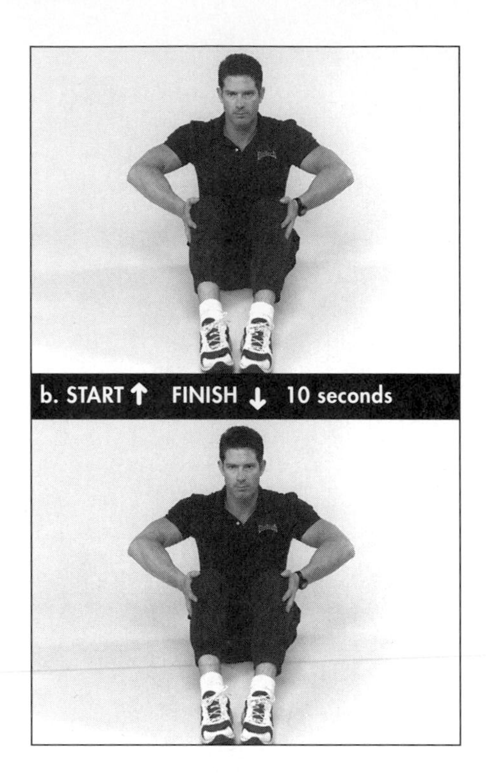

b. START ↑ FINISH ↓ 10 seconds

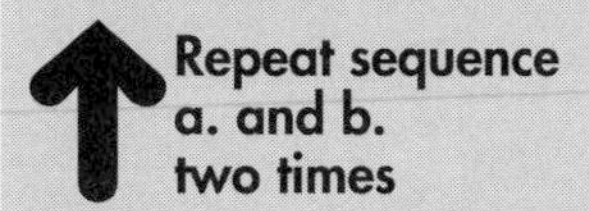

c.

Supine Heel Press Into Floor

Lay on back with one leg straight up, other leg down with knee bent no more than 90 degrees. Push heel into floor to raise lower body off floor.

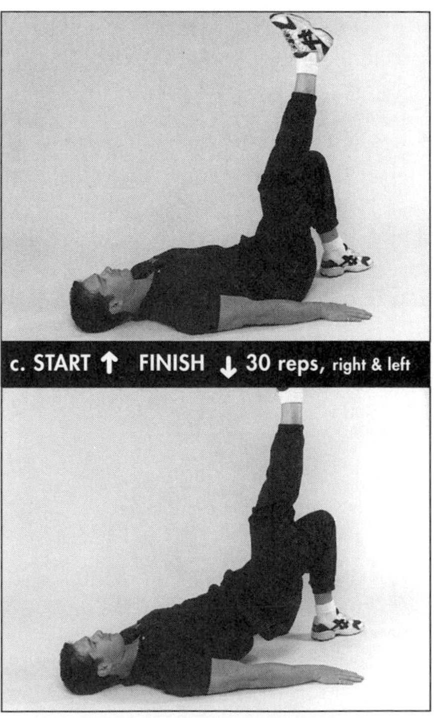

c. START ↑ FINISH ↓ 30 reps, right & left

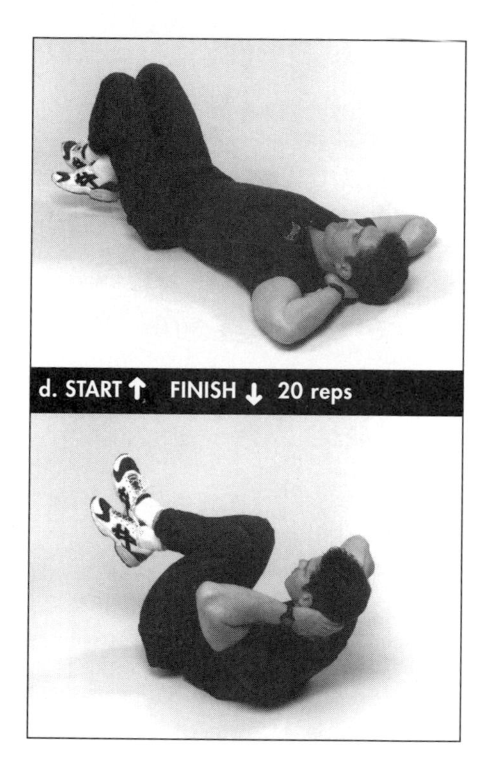

d.
V-Crunch

Lay on back with knees bent, hands behind neck, breathe out and raise feet and shoulders off floor simultaneously, inhale when lowering shoulders and feet.

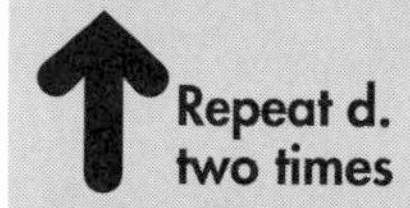

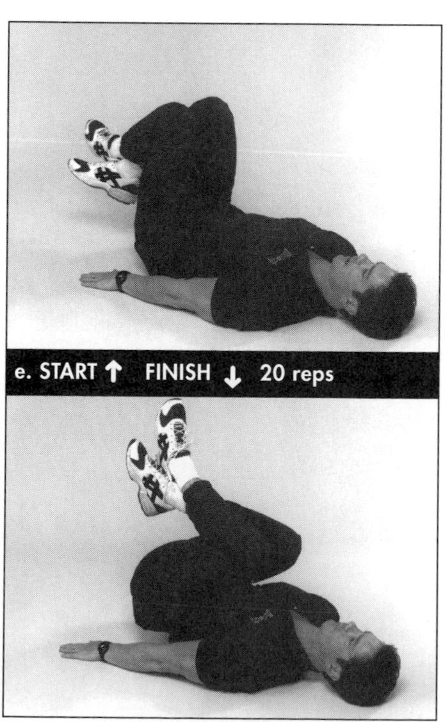

e.
Tucks

Lay on back, ankles crossed, knees bent, hands by sides, raise feet off floor pulling knees to face exhaling at same time, inhale when lowering feet back to floor.

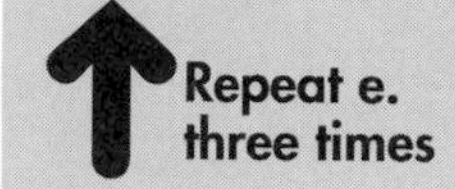

women's workout

week 3

day 3 – legs

a.

Ankle Cross Extension/Curl

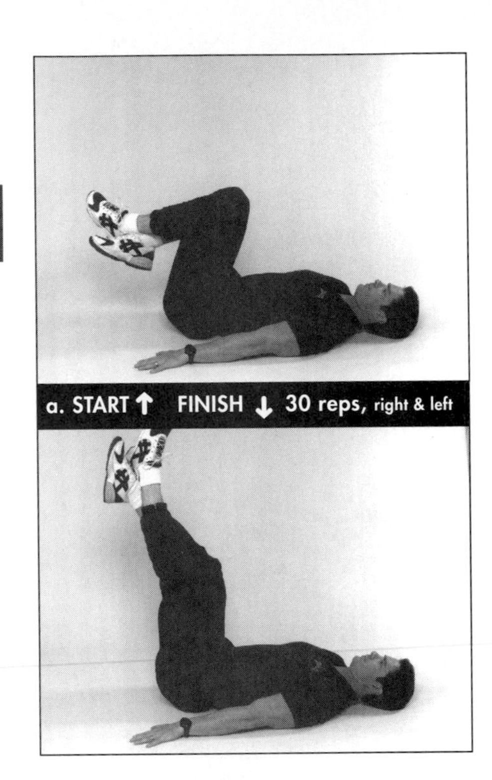
a. START ↑ FINISH ↓ 30 reps, right & left

Lay on back with knees up and ankles crossed, push lower shin area and back of ankle together for resistance, straighten and bend knees while applying pressure through all ranges of motion, switch ankle position to put resistance on the opposite muscles.

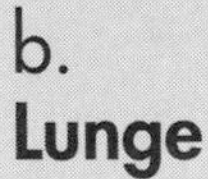
b.

Lunge

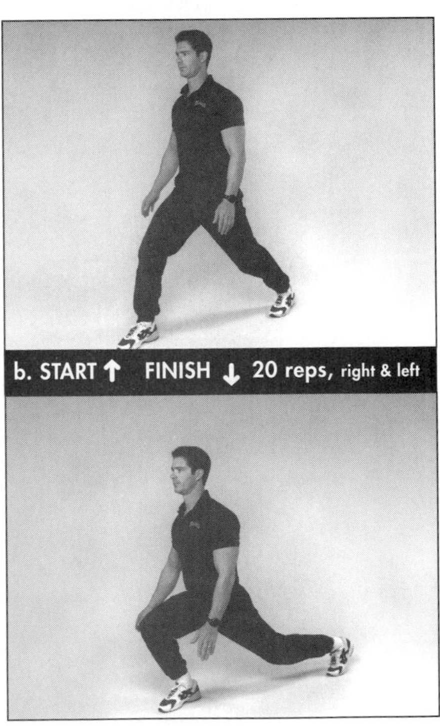
b. START ↑ FINISH ↓ 20 reps, right & left

Feet should be twice the width of shoulders, toes of both feet point in same direction, keep back leg as straight as possible, bend from front knee and hip to lower into lunge position and push to return, head up, back straight, chest out.

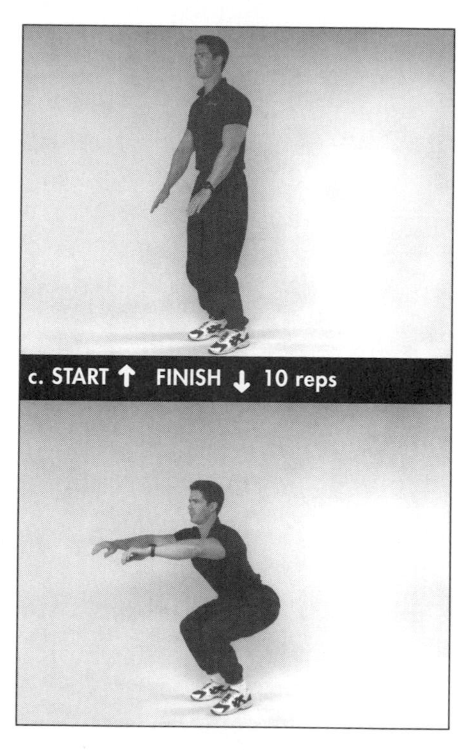

c.

Squats Close Stance

Heels and toes 6-8 inches apart, heels stay on floor during all ranges of exercise, head up, back straight, chest out. Bend knees and hips to lower upper body into squat position and return.

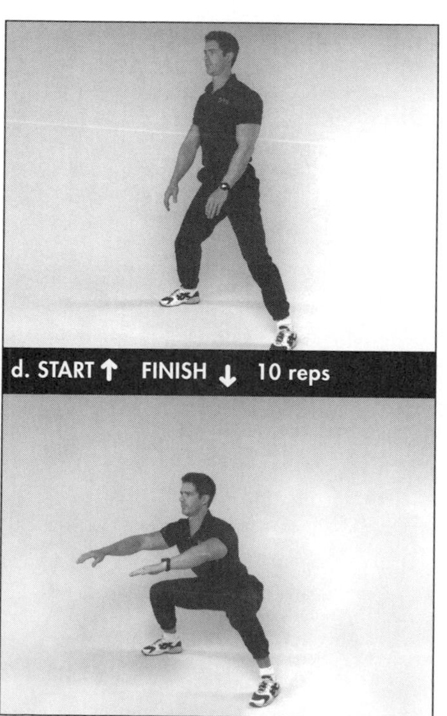

d.

Squats Wide Stance

Heels twice as wide as shoulder width with toes pointing out slightly, heels stay down, head up, back straight, chest out, bend knees and hips to lower upper body into squat position and return.

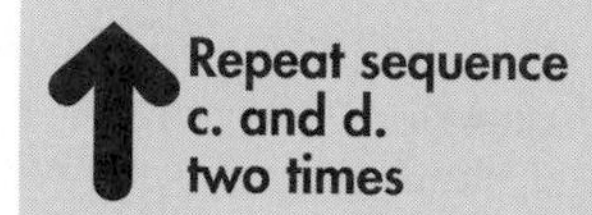

e.

Isometric Squat Close Stance

Heels and toes 6-8 inches apart, bend knees and hips to lower body into squat position and hold for recommended time, heels stay down, chest out, head up, back straight.

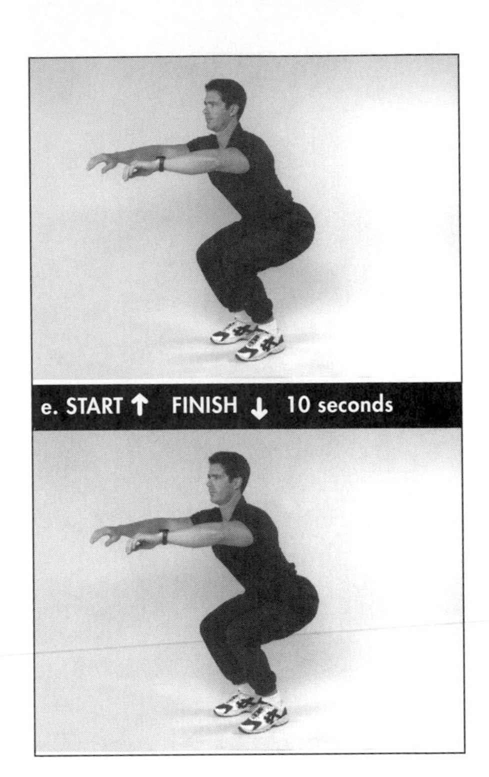

e. START ↑ FINISH ↓ 10 seconds

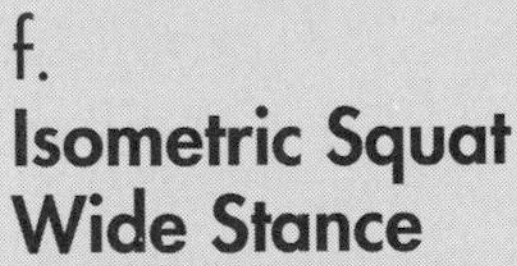

f.

Isometric Squat Wide Stance

Heels twice as wide as shoulder width with toes pointing out slightly, bend knees and hips to lower body into squat position and hold for recommended time, back straight, head up, heels down.

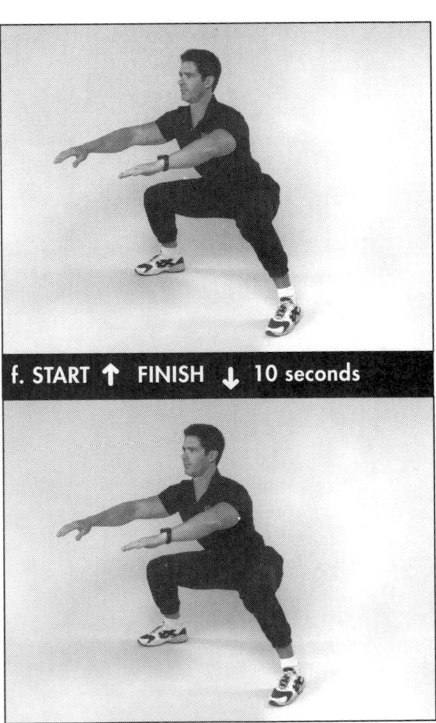

f. START ↑ FINISH ↓ 10 seconds

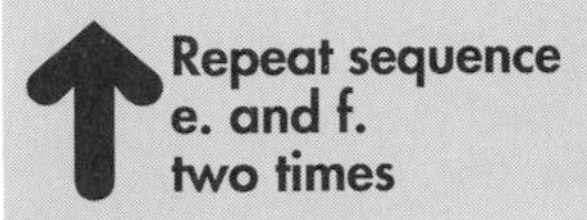

Repeat sequence e. and f. two times

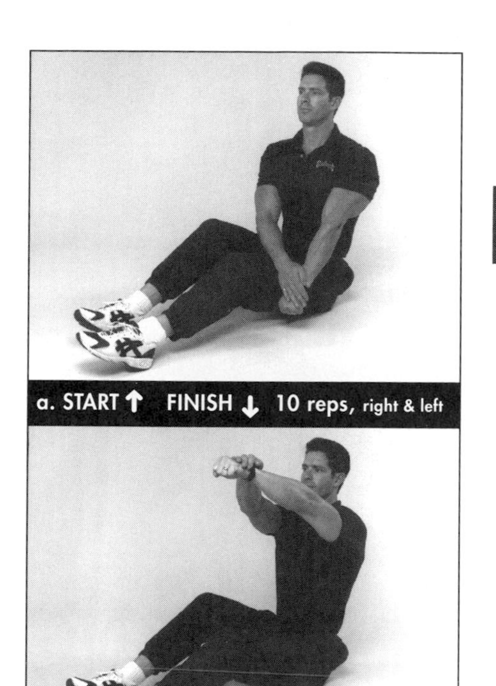

a. START ↑ FINISH ↓ 10 reps, right & left

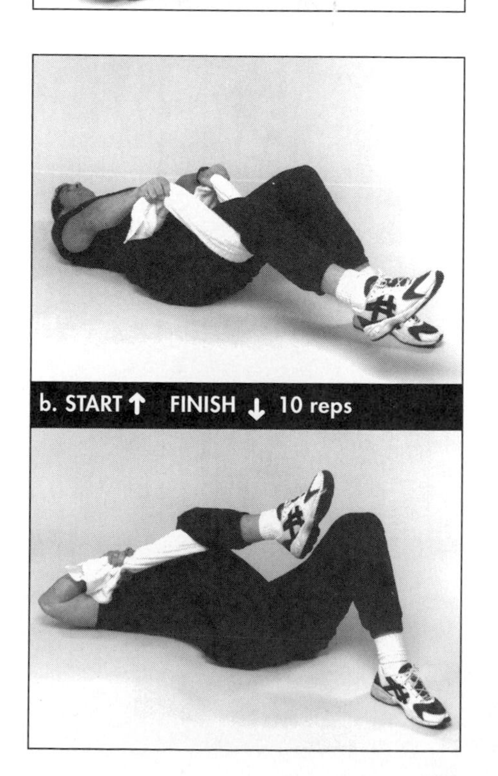

b. START ↑ FINISH ↓ 10 reps

women's workout week 3

day 4 – bicep, tricep, shoulder

a.
Front Raise

Working arm straight, place other hand on working arm wrist area, press down on working arm as far as it will go down, return with as much pressure from top hand as working shoulder and arm can withstand.

b.
Towel Upright Row

Towel around the back of knee, with overhand position draw elbows up toward ears while pulling leg with towel, return keeping elbows out, use leg pressure on towel for added resistance.

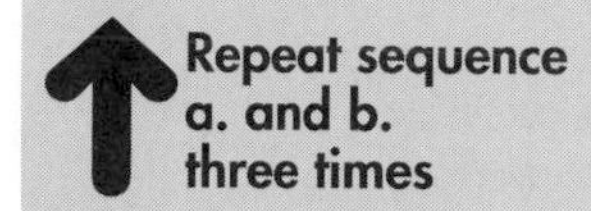

Repeat sequence a. and b. three times

c.
Bicep/Tricep Palm Press

Place palms together for resistance, rotate wrist positions until back of one hand is facing you and the other is facing away, press arms straight then return to chest.

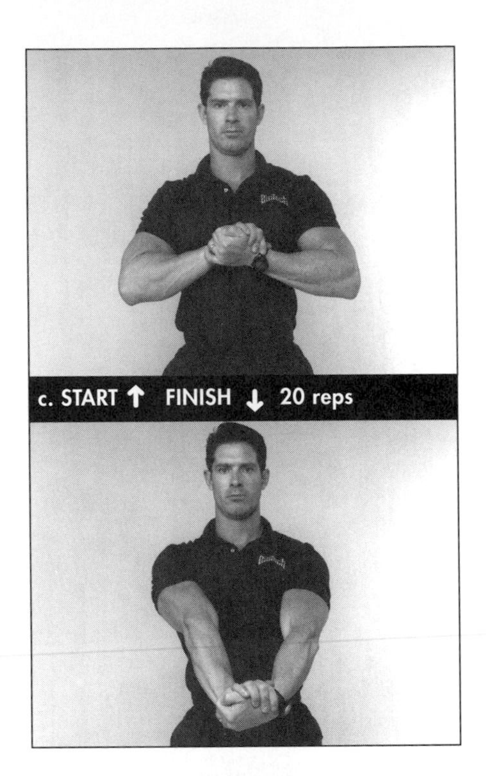

c. START ↑ FINISH ↓ 20 reps

d.
Bicep/Tricep Palm Pull

Place one hand on back of other grasping with fingers and pull for resistance, flex and extend hands away from body by bending elbows, resistance through all ranges of motion.

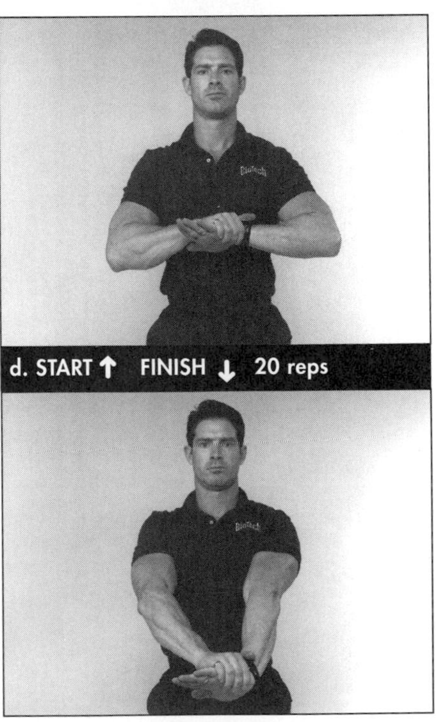

d. START ↑ FINISH ↓ 20 reps

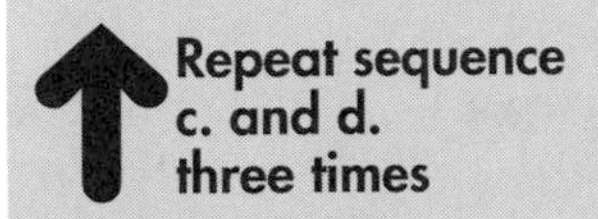

Repeat sequence c. and d. three times

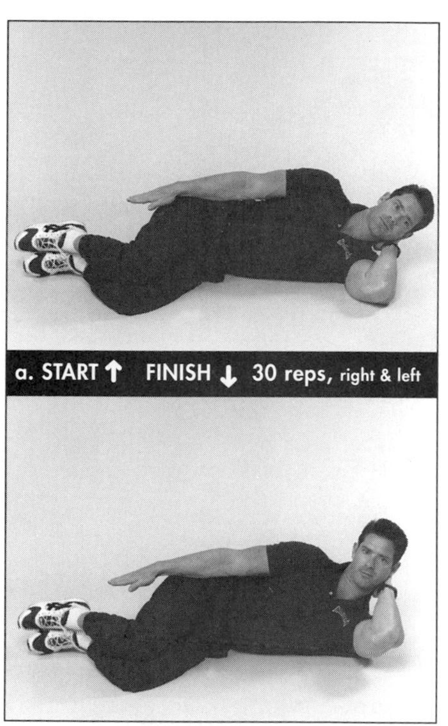

a. START ↑ FINISH ↓ 30 reps, right & left

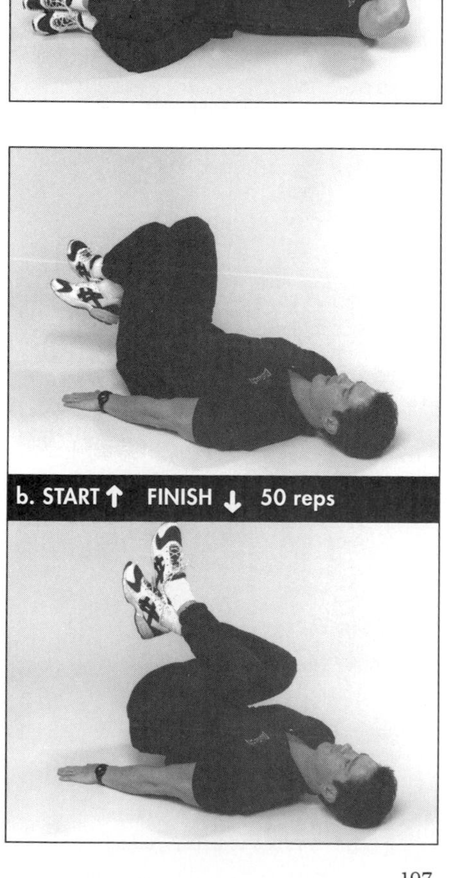

b. START ↑ FINISH ↓ 50 reps

women's workout week 3

day 5 – obliques, abs, lower back, calves

a. Side Crunch

Lay on side with hips flexed and knees bent, bottom arm supporting head with elbow off the floor, top arm straight, exhale while reaching for ankle, inhale and return.

b. Tucks

Lay on back, ankles crossed, knees bent, hands by sides. Raise feet off floor pulling knees to face exhaling at same time, inhale when lowering feet back to floor.

c.
Hyperextension Superman

Lay on stomach with hands out in front of head. Raise head, shoulders, chest, and toes from floor and return.

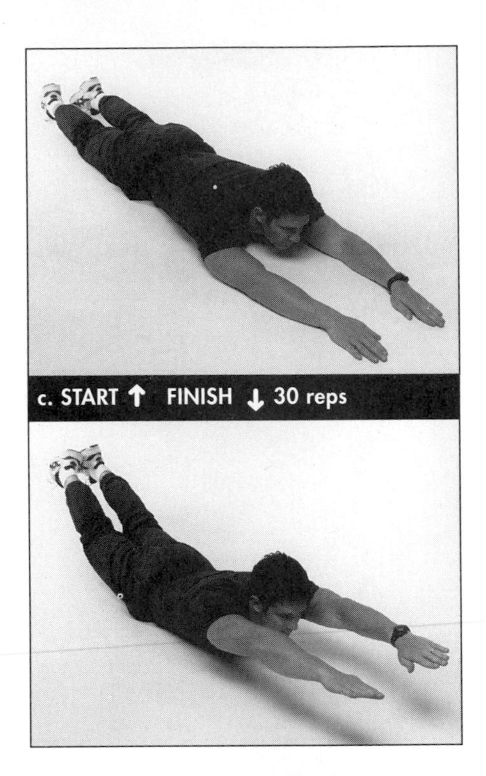

d.
Calf Raise

Standing on one foot, raise heel from floor 2-3 inches and return.

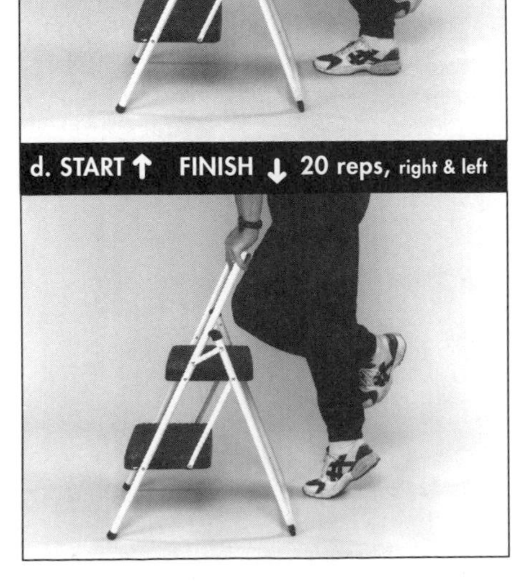

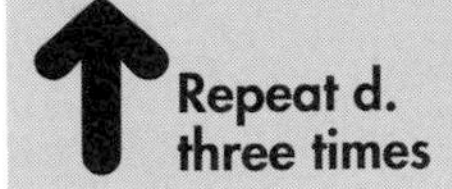

Repeat d. three times

men's workout

week 1

day 1 – back and chest

a.

Isometric Palm Press

Press palms together with elbows out, hands positioned 18 inches away from chest.

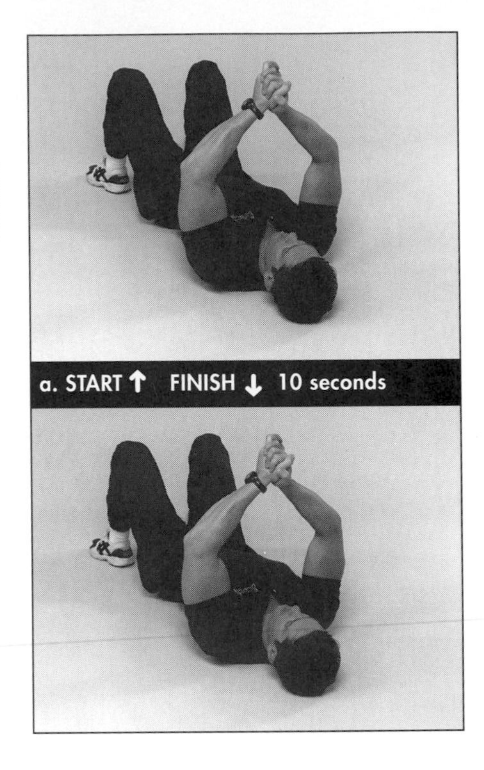

a. START ↑ FINISH ↓ 10 seconds

b.

Push-Up

Back straight, head up, shoulder width hand position, lower body as far as you can and return.

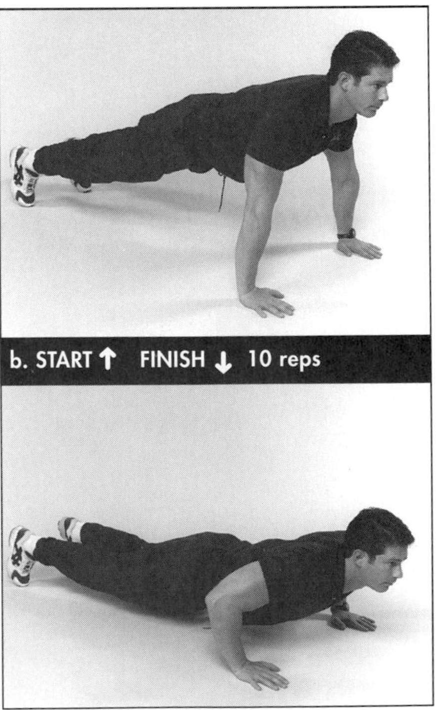

b. START ↑ FINISH ↓ 10 reps

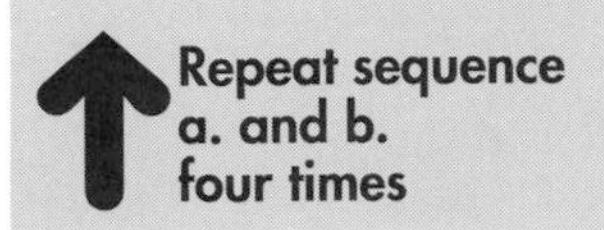

Repeat sequence a. and b. four times

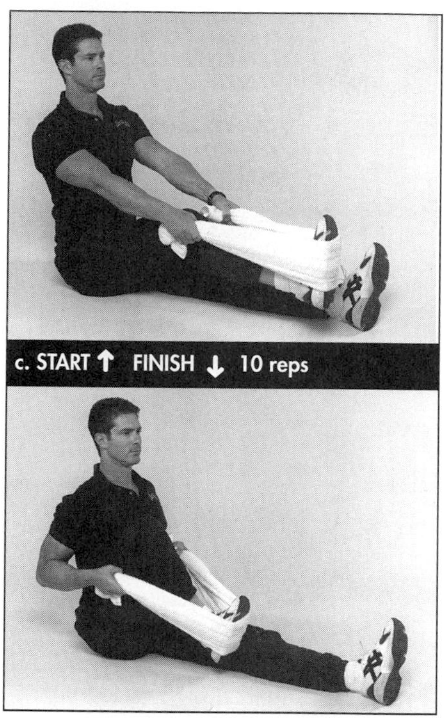

c.

Towel Row Elbows In Close

Hold towel with overhand position, towel should be long enough to go around arch of the foot with legs and arms straight. Keep back straight with chest out during all phases of movement. Push with foot for resistance during all phases of rowing movement.

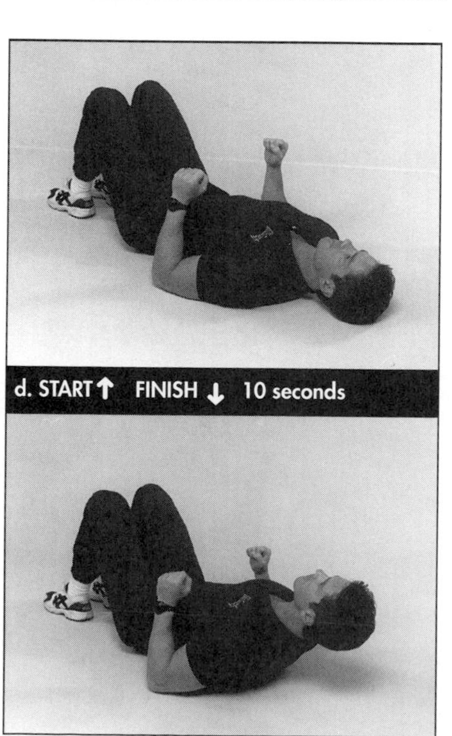

d.

Elbow Back Press Elbows In Close

Abs relaxed, elbows in 90 degree position with forearm pointed up, press elbows into floor to raise upper torso up for duration of exercise, head in alignment with body.

↑ Repeat sequence c. and d. four times

men's workout

week 1

day 2 – abs, obliques, glutes

a.
Crunches
Lay on back, eyes up, head back, hands on chest or on back of neck, breathe out and raise shoulder blades from floor, inhale on return motion.

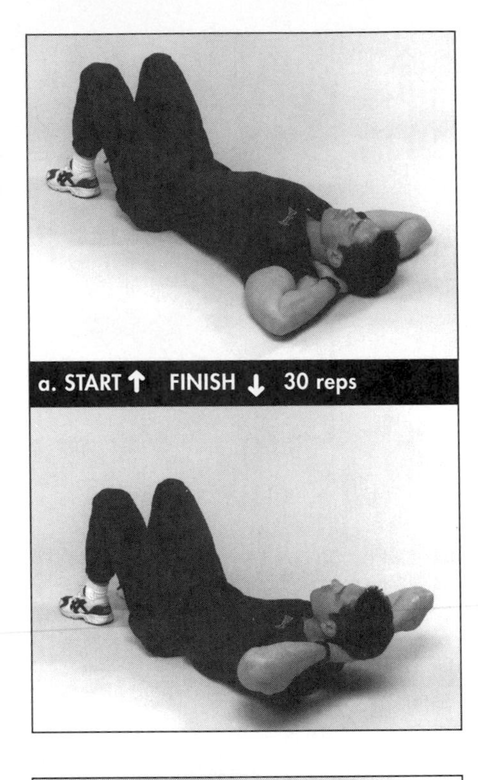

a. START ↑ FINISH ↓ 30 reps

b.
Tucks
Lay on back, ankles crossed, knees bent, hands by sides. Raise feet off floor pulling knees to face, exhaling at same time, inhale when lowering feet back to floor.

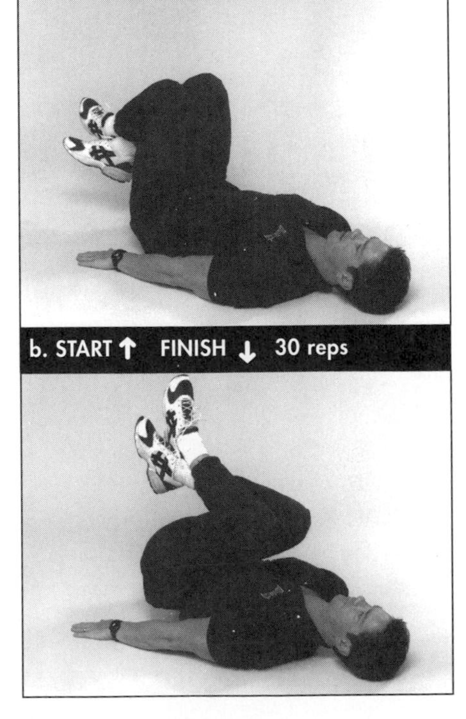

b. START ↑ FINISH ↓ 30 reps

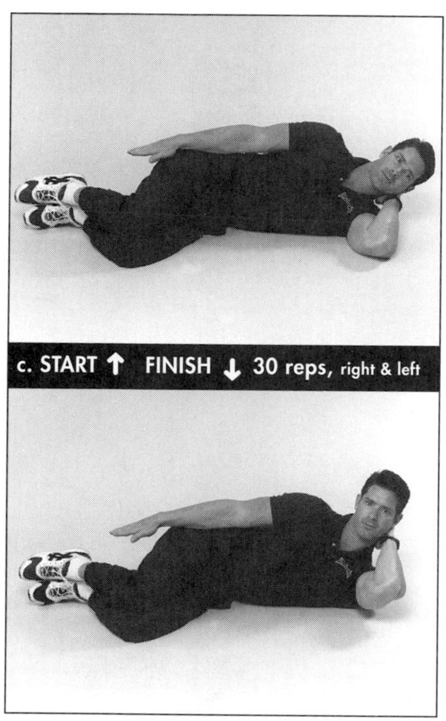

c. START ↑ FINISH ↓ 30 reps, right & left

c.
Side Crunch

Lay on side with hips flexed and knees bent, bottom arm supporting head with elbow off the floor, top arm straight, exhale while reaching for ankle, inhale and return.

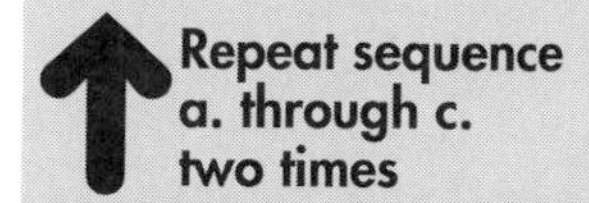

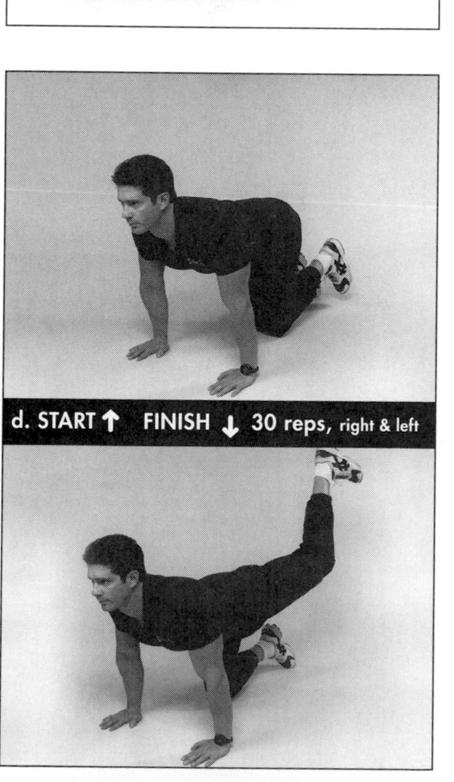

d. START ↑ FINISH ↓ 30 reps, right & left

d.
Hip Extension

On hands and knees kick heel of one leg out by extending the hip, bend hip to return, back straight, head up.

men's workout

week 1

day 3 – legs

a.

Isometric Squat Close Stance

Heels and toes 6-8 inches apart, bend knees and hips to lower body into squat position and hold for recommended time, heels stay down, chest out, head up, back straight.

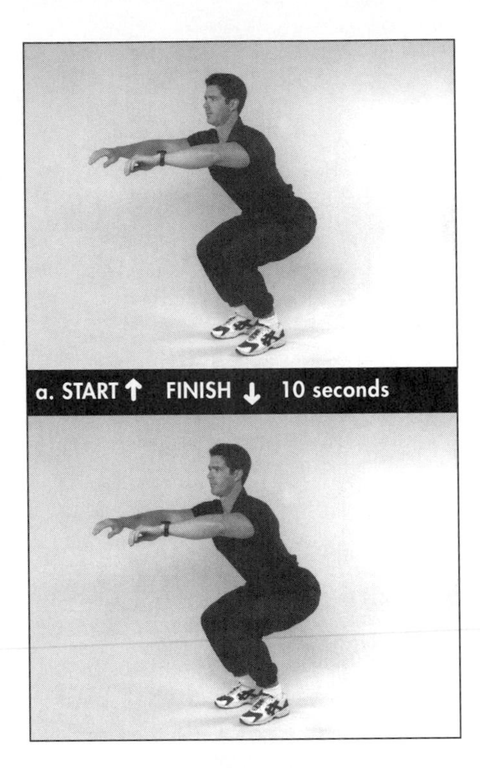

a. START ↑ FINISH ↓ 10 seconds

b.

Squat Close Stance

Heels and toes 6-8 inches apart, heels stay on floor during all ranges of exercise, head up, back straight, chest out, bend knees and hips to lower upper body into squat position and return.

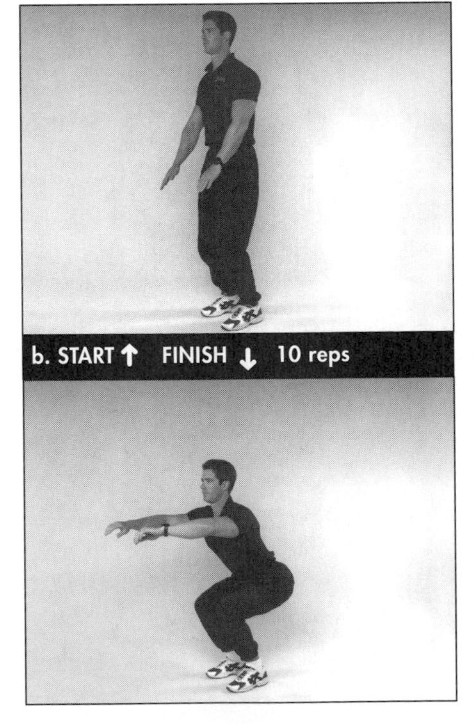

b. START ↑ FINISH ↓ 10 reps

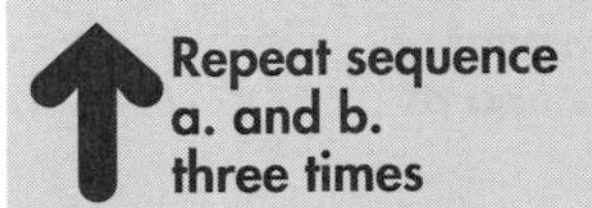

Repeat sequence a. and b. three times

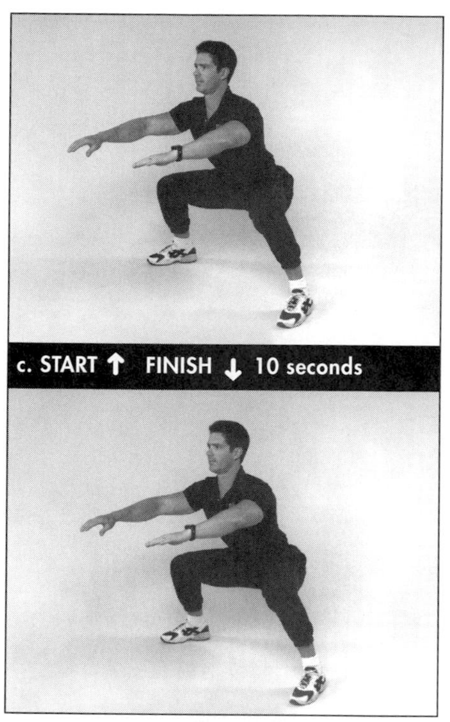
c. START ↑ FINISH ↓ 10 seconds

c.
Isometric Squat Wide Stance

Heels twice as wide as shoulder width with toes pointing out slightly, bend knees and hips to lower body into squat position and hold for recommended time, back straight, head up, heels down.

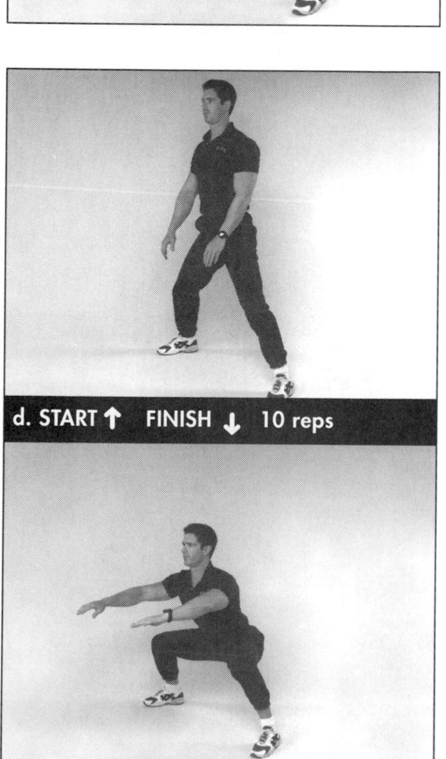
d. START ↑ FINISH ↓ 10 reps

d.
Squat Wide Stance

Heels twice as wide as shoulder width with toes pointing out slightly, heels stay down, head up, back straight, chest out, bend knees and hips to lower upper body into squat position and return.

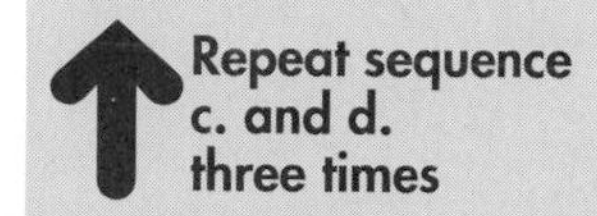

men's workout

week 1

day 4 – bicep, tricep, shoulder

a.

Upright Row

Towel around the back of knee with overhand position, draw elbows up toward ears while pulling leg with towel, return keeping elbows out, use leg pressure on towel for added resistance.

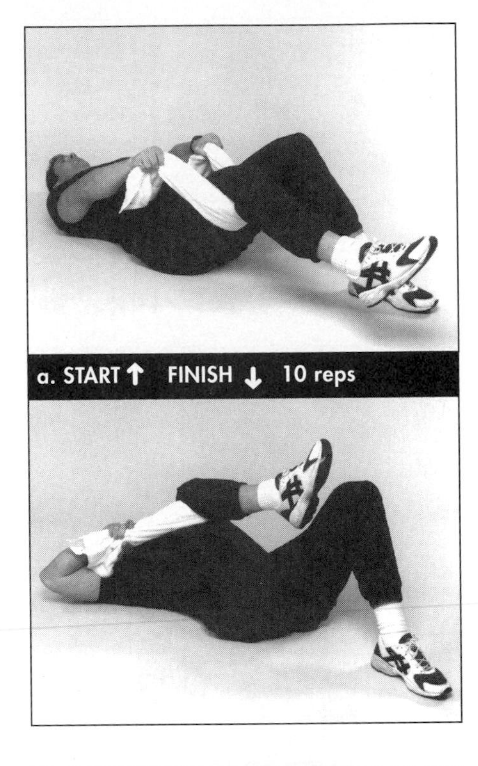

a. START ↑ FINISH ↓ 10 reps

b.

Front Raise

Working arm straight, place other hand on working arm wrist area, press down on working arm as far as it will go down, return with as much pressure from top hand as working shoulder and arm can withstand.

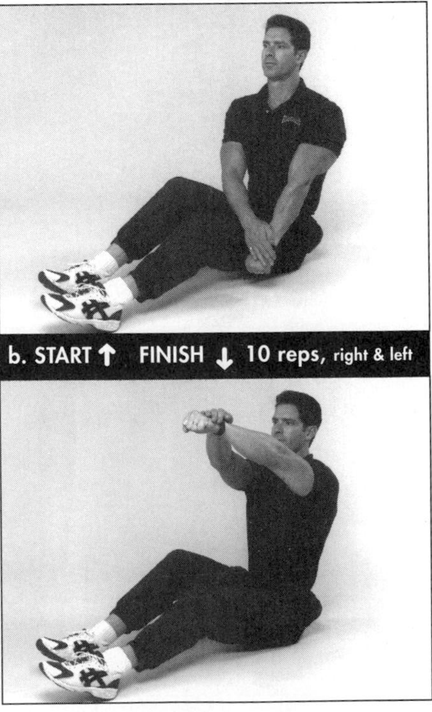

b. START ↑ FINISH ↓ 10 reps, right & left

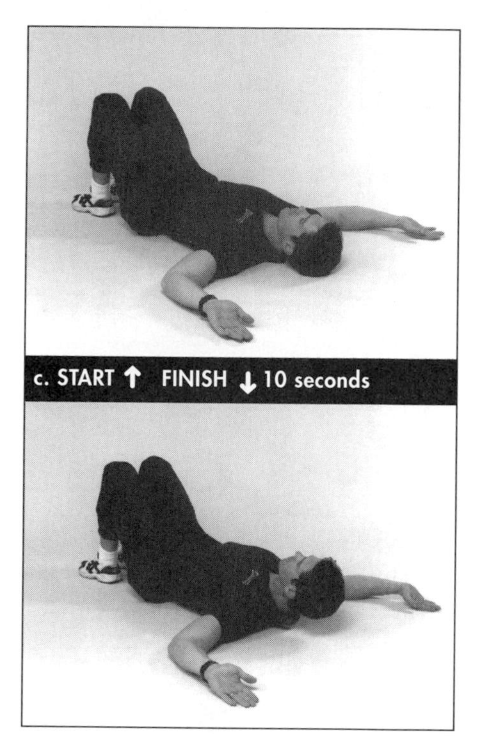

c. START ↑ FINISH ↓ 10 seconds

c.

Rear Deltoid Press

Lay on back, knees bent, elbows bent 90 degrees. Press back of wrist into floor for desired time.

Repeat sequence a. through c. two times

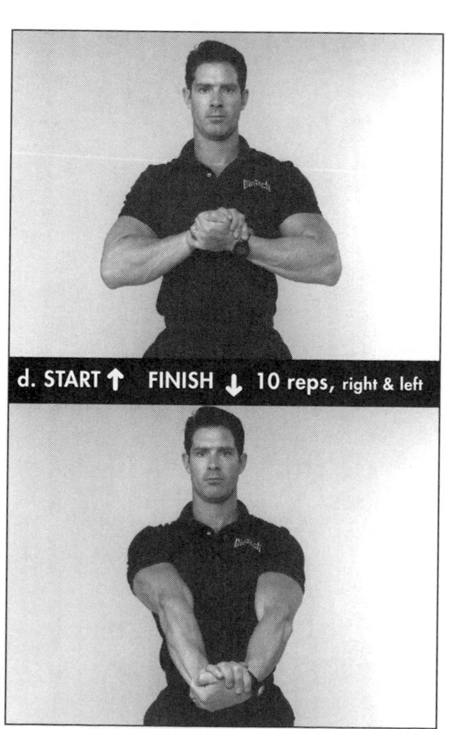

d. START ↑ FINISH ↓ 10 reps, right & left

d.

Bicep/Tricep Press

Place palms together for resistance, rotate wrist positions until back of one hand is facing you and the other is facing away, press arms straight then return to chest.

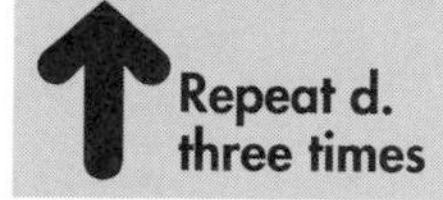

men's workout

week 1

day 5 – abs, calves, lower back

a.

Crunches

Lay on back, eyes up, head back, hands on chest or on back of neck, breathe out and raise shoulder blades from floor, inhale on return motion.

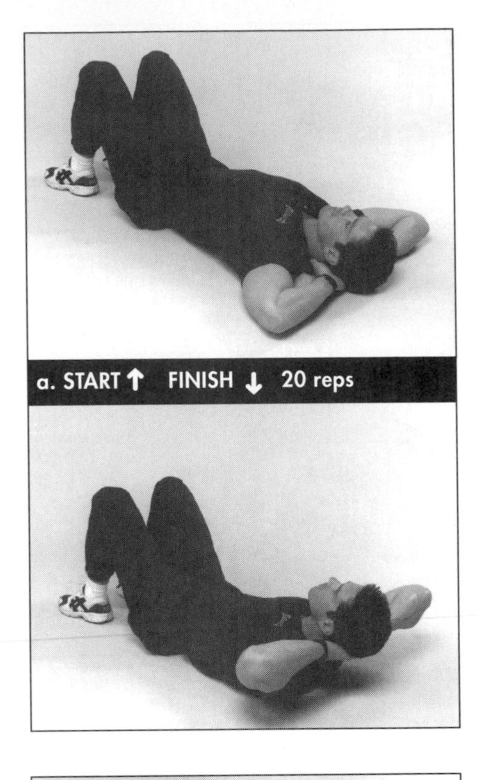

a. START ↑ FINISH ↓ 20 reps

b.

Tucks

Lay on back, ankles crossed, knees bent, hands by sides. Raise feet off floor pulling knees to face, exhaling at same time, inhale when lowering feet back to floor.

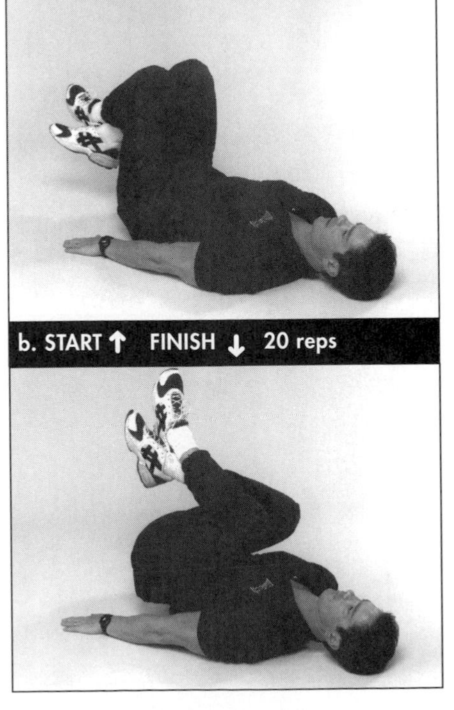

b. START ↑ FINISH ↓ 20 reps

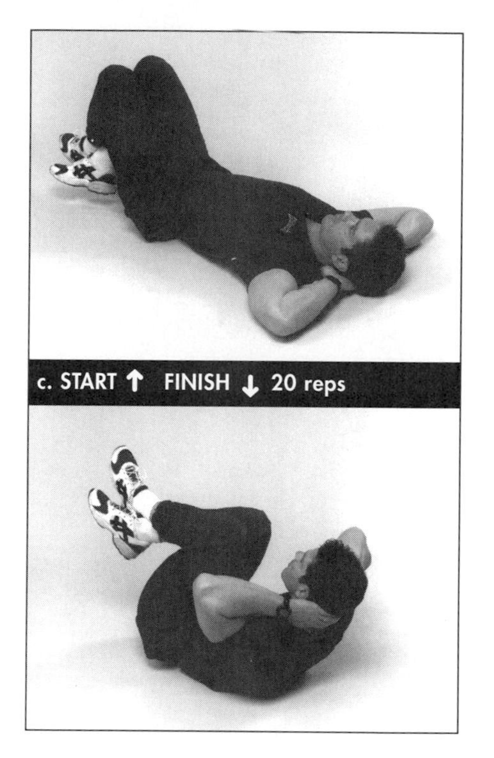

c. START ↑ FINISH ↓ 20 reps

c.

V-Crunch

Lay on back with knees bent, hands behind neck, breathe out and raise feet and shoulders off floor simultaneously, inhale when lowering shoulders and feet.

↑ Repeat sequence a. through c. two times

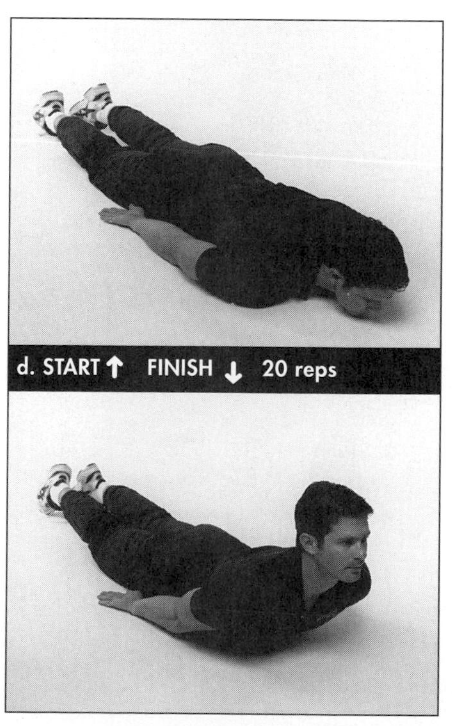

d. START ↑ FINISH ↓ 20 reps

d.

Hyperextensions

Lay on stomach with hands by sides for easy resistance, behind head for moderate resistance, straight out in front for maximum resistance, raise head, shoulders and chest from floor and return.

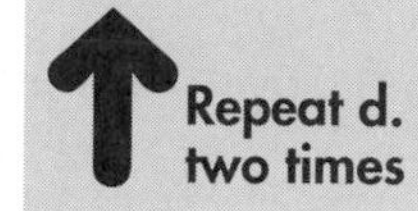

e.
Calf Raises

Standing on one foot, raise heel from floor 2-3 inches and return. For double calf raise, stand on both feet, raise heels from floor 2-3 inches and return.

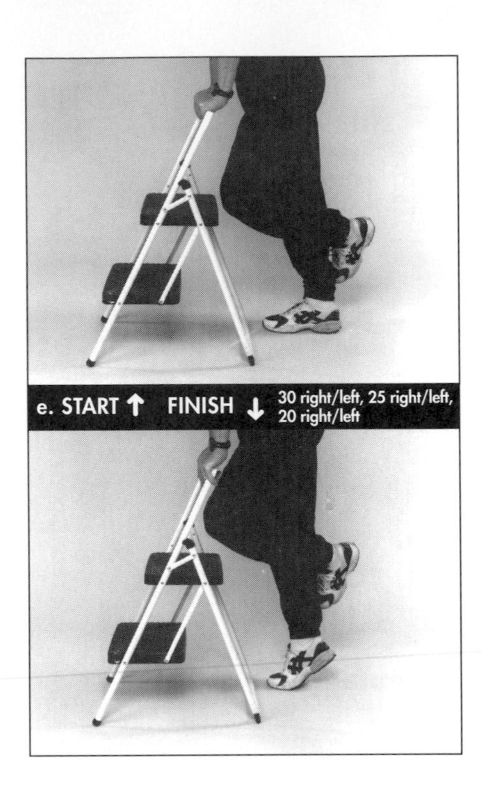

e. START ↑ FINISH ↓ 30 right/left, 25 right/left, 20 right/left

men's workout week 2

day 1 – back and chest

a.
Isometric Palm Press

Press palms together with elbows out, hands positioned 12 inches away from chest

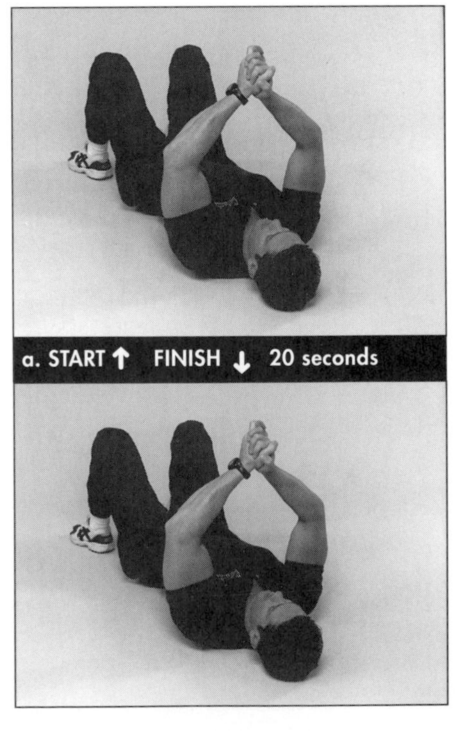

a. START ↑ FINISH ↓ 20 seconds

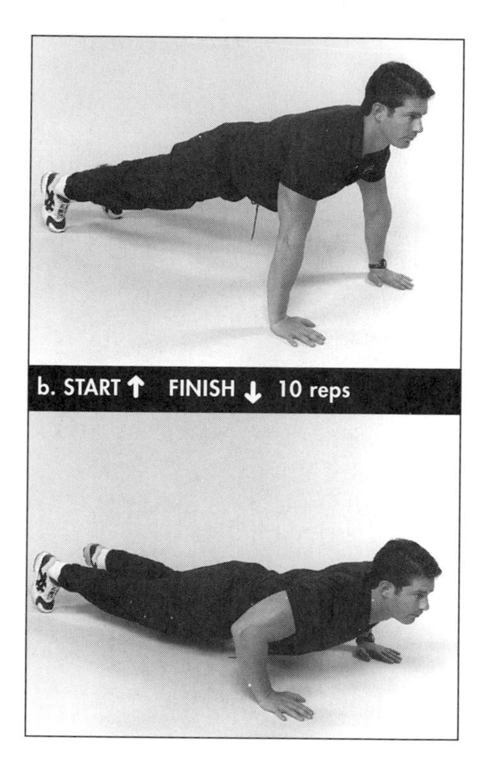

b. START ↑ FINISH ↓ 10 reps

b.

Push-Up

Back straight, head up, shoulder width hand position, lower body as far as you can and return.

↑ **Repeat sequence a. and b. four times**

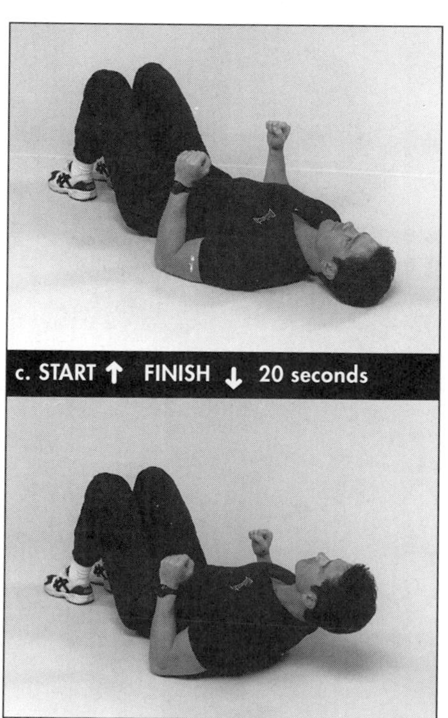

c. START ↑ FINISH ↓ 20 seconds

c.

Elbow Back Press Elbows In Close

Abs relaxed, elbows in 90 degree position with forearm pointed up, press elbows into floor to raise upper torso up for duration of exercise, head in alignment with body.

d.

Towel Row Elbows Out

Hold towel with overhand position, towel should be long enough to go around arch of the foot with legs and arms straight. Keep back straight with chest out during all phases of movement. Push with foot for resistance during all phases of rowing movement.

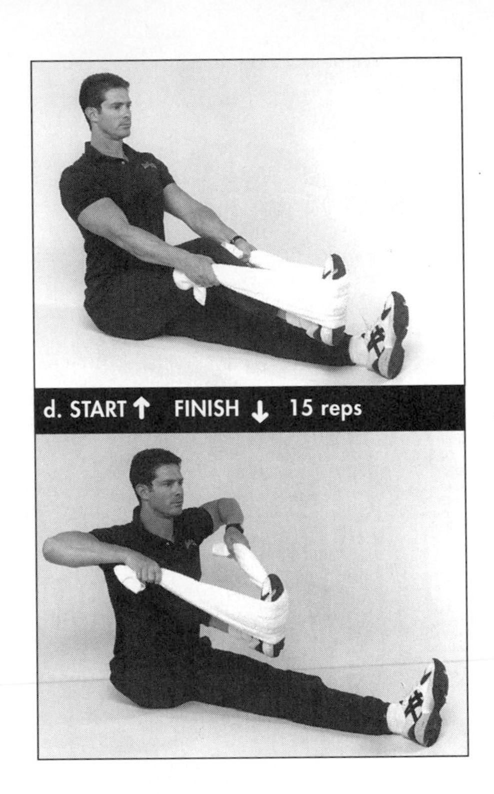

d. START ↑ FINISH ↓ 15 reps

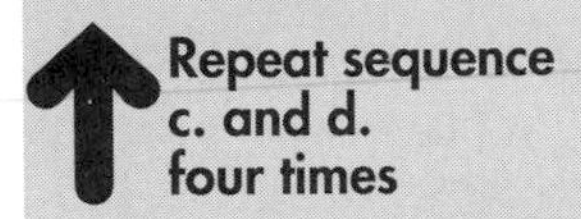

Repeat sequence c. and d. four times

men's workout week 2

day 2 – abs, obliques, glutes

a.

V-Crunch

Lay on back with knees bent, hands behind neck, breathe out and raise feet and shoulders off floor simultaneously, inhale when lowering shoulders and feet.

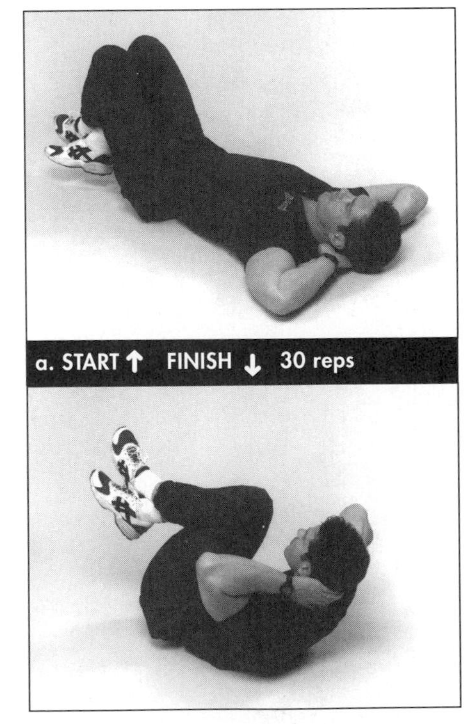

a. START ↑ FINISH ↓ 30 reps

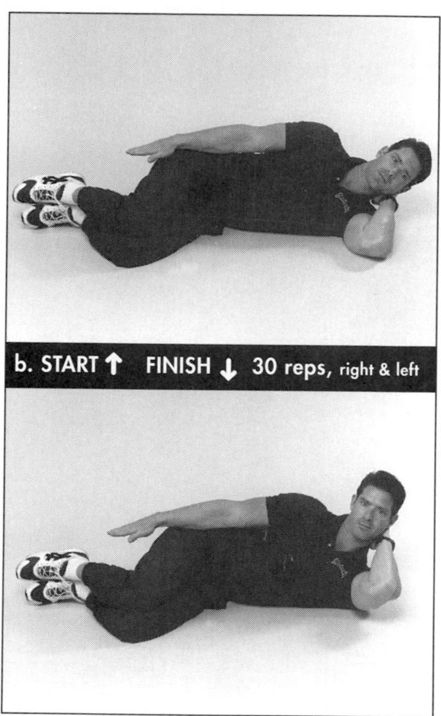

b. START ↑ FINISH ↓ 30 reps, right & left

b.
Side Crunch

Lay on side with hips flexed and knees bent, bottom arm supporting head with elbow off the floor, top arm straight, exhale while reaching for ankle, inhale and return.

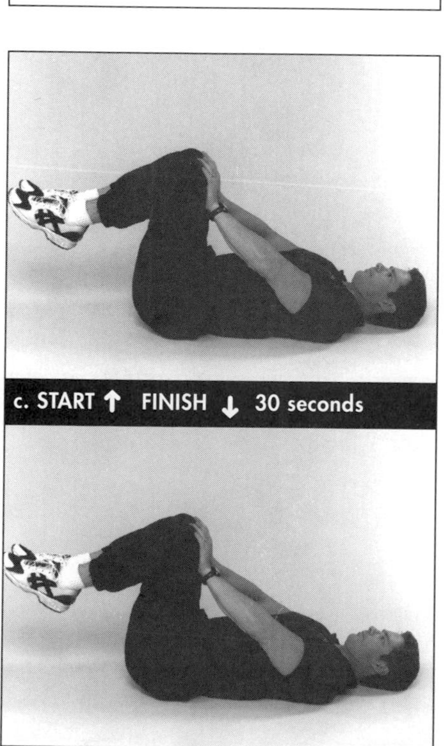

c. START ↑ FINISH ↓ 30 seconds

c.
Thigh Press

Lay on back with knees bent. Breathe out slowly while pushing your thighs down, don't let feet touch the floor, hold for recommended time.

↑ **Repeat sequence a. through c. two times**

d.

Hip Extension

On hands and knees kick heel of one leg out by extending the hip, bend hip to return, back straight, head up.

Repeat d. two times

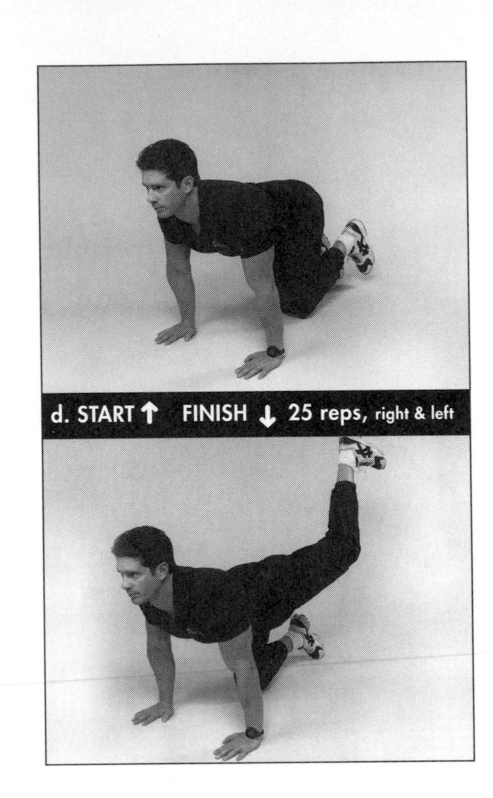

d. START ↑ FINISH ↓ 25 reps, right & left

men's workout

week 2

day 3 – legs

a.

Ankle Cross Extension/Curl

Lay on back with knees up and ankles crossed, push lower shin area and back of ankle together for resistance, straighten and bend knees while applying pressure through all ranges of motion, switch ankle position to put resistance on the opposite muscles.

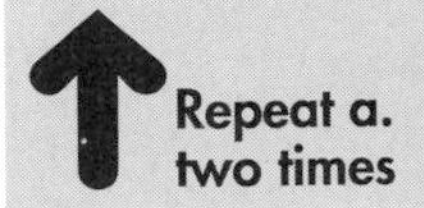

Repeat a. two times

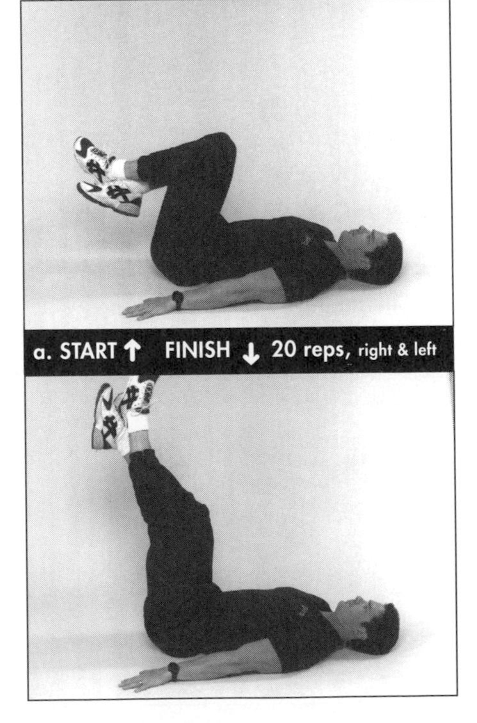

a. START ↑ FINISH ↓ 20 reps, right & left

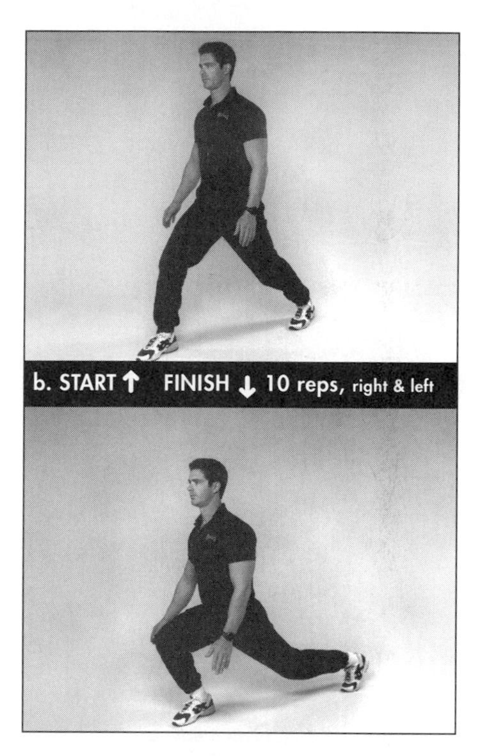

b.
Lunge
Feet should be twice the width of shoulders, toes of both feet point in same direction, keep back leg as straight as possible, bend from front knee and hip to lower into lunge position and push to return, head up, back straight, chest out.

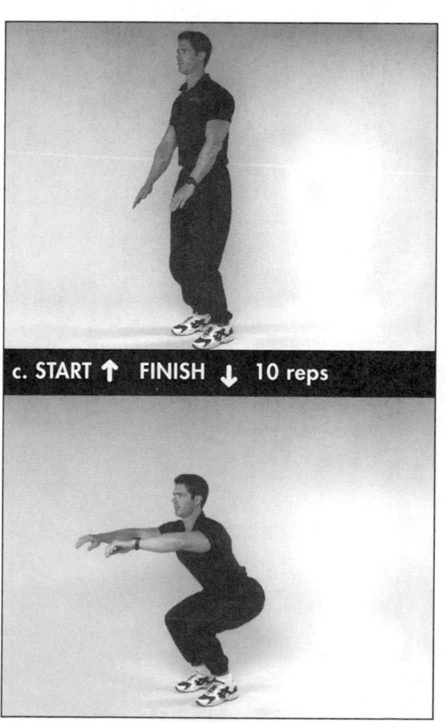

c.
Squats Close Stance
Heels and toes 6-8 inches apart, heels stay on floor during all ranges of exercise, head up, back straight, chest out. Bend knees and hips to lower upper body into squat position and return.

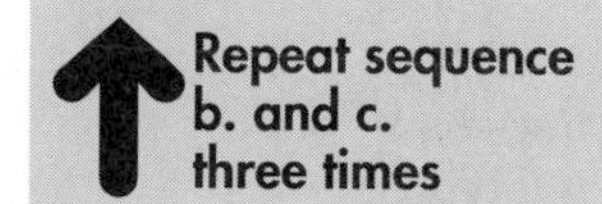

men's workout

week 2

day 4 – bicep, tricep, shoulder

a.

Bicep/Tricep Curl Press

Place palms together for resistance, rotate wrist positions until back of one hand is facing you and the other is facing away, press arms straight then return to chest.

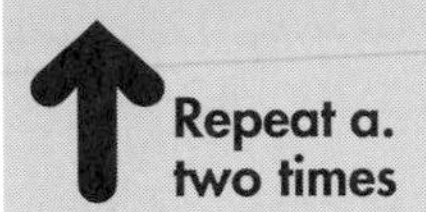

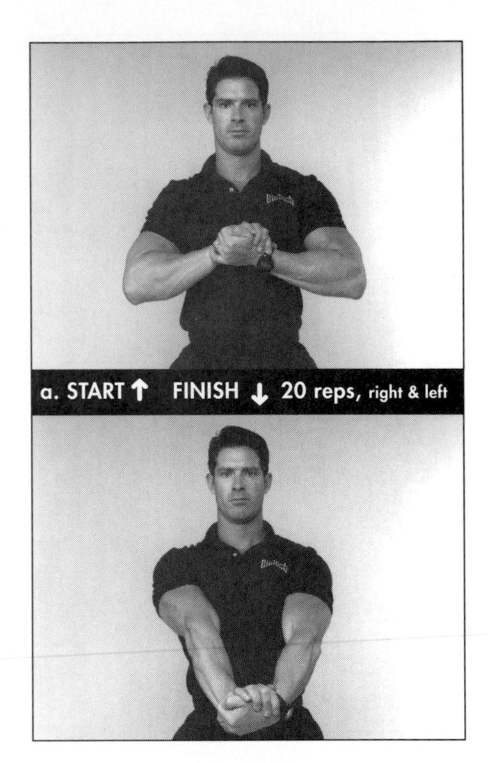

a. START ↑ FINISH ↓ 20 reps, right & left

b.

Bicep/Tricep Pull

Place one hand on back of other grasping with fingers and pull for resistance, flex and extend hands away from body by bending elbows, resistance through all ranges of motion.

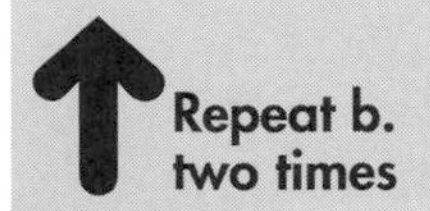

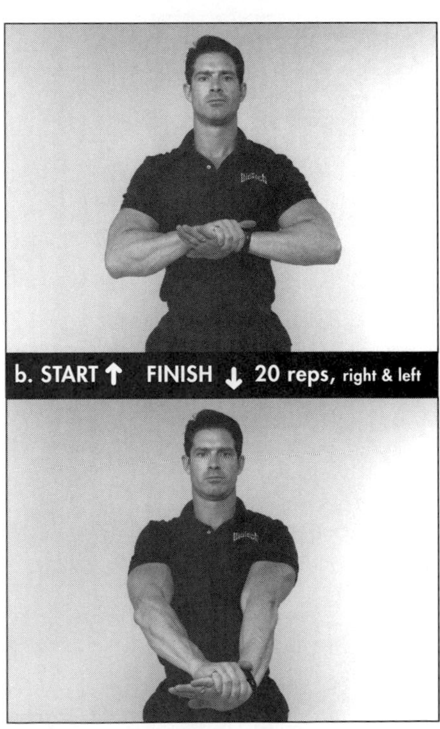

b. START ↑ FINISH ↓ 20 reps, right & left

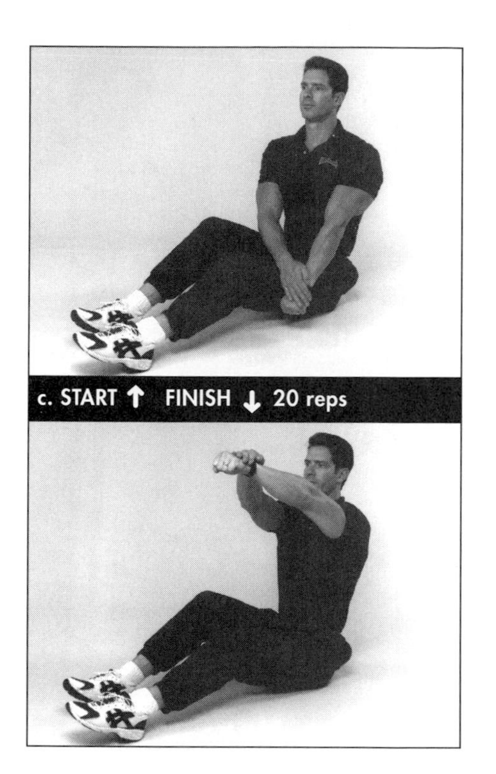

c. START ↑ FINISH ↓ 20 reps

c.
Frontal Raise

Working arm straight, place other hand on working arm wrist area, press down on working arm as far as it will go down, return with as much pressure from top hand as working shoulder and arm can withstand.

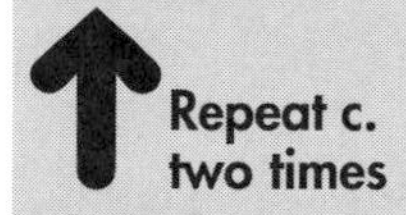

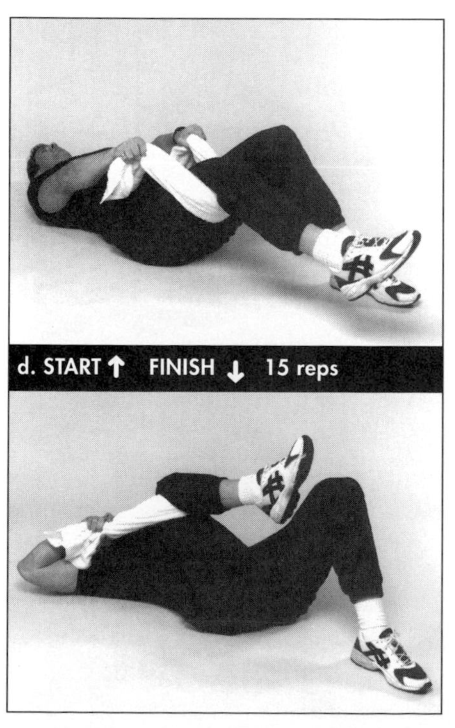

d. START ↑ FINISH ↓ 15 reps

d.
Upright Row

Towel around the back of knee with overhand position, draw elbows up toward ears while pulling leg with towel, return keeping elbows out, use leg pressure on towel for added resistance.

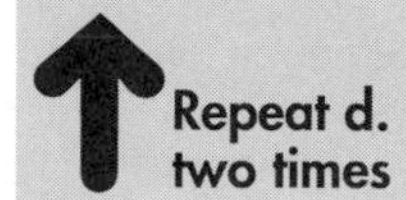

men's workout

week 2

day 5 – abs, calves, lower back

a.

Crunches

Lay on back, eyes up, head back, hands on chest or on back of neck, breathe out and raise shoulder blades from floor, inhale on return motion.

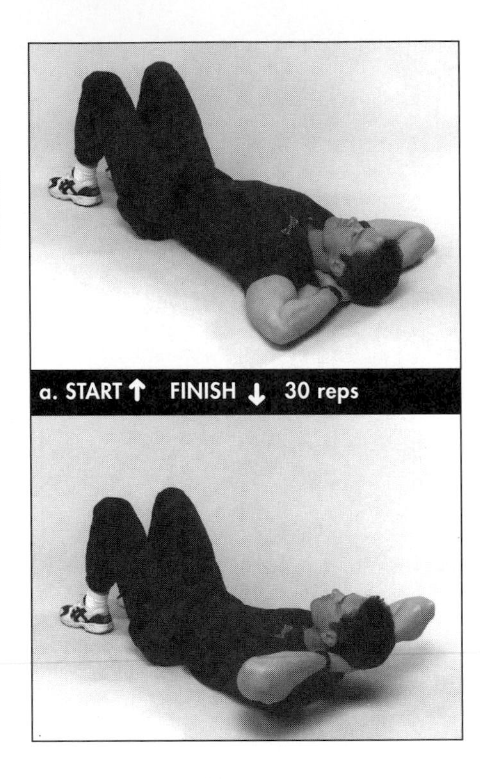

a. START ↑ FINISH ↓ 30 reps

b.

Tucks

Lay on back, ankles crossed, knees bent, hands by sides. Raise feet off floor pulling knees to face, exhaling at same time, inhale when lowering feet back to floor.

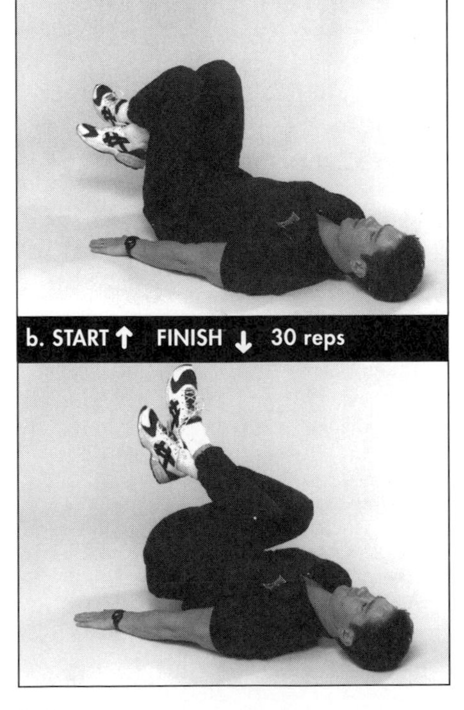

b. START ↑ FINISH ↓ 30 reps

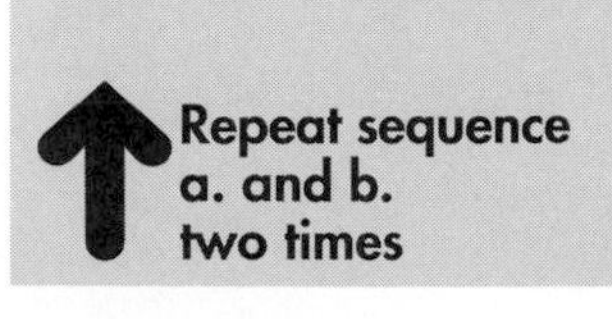

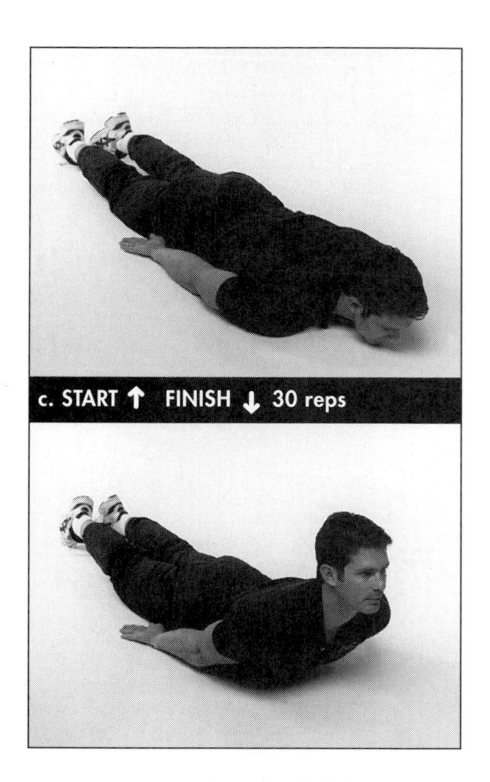

c. START ↑ FINISH ↓ 30 reps

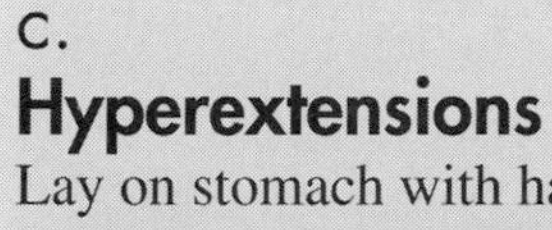

c.

Hyperextensions

Lay on stomach with hands by sides for easy resistance, behind head for moderate resistance, straight out in front for maximum resistance, raise head, shoulders and chest from floor and return.

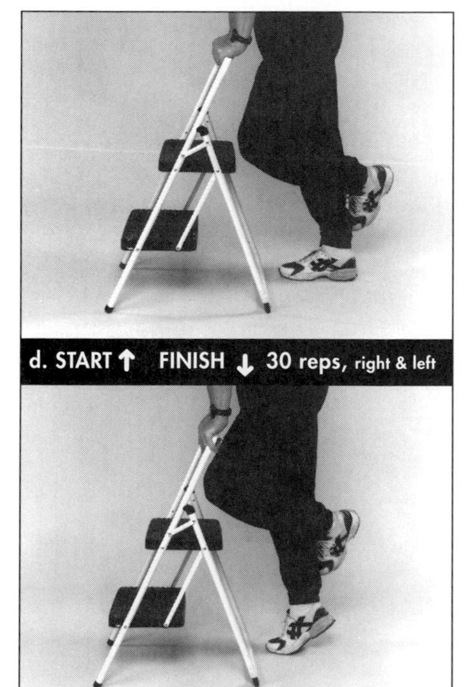

d. START ↑ FINISH ↓ 30 reps, right & left

d.

Calf Raise

Standing on one foot, raise heel from floor 2-3 inches and return.

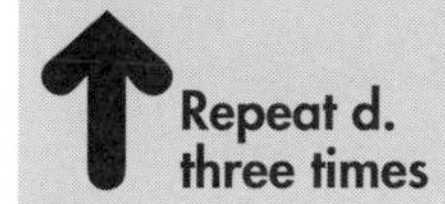

men's workout

week 3

day 1 – back and chest

a.

Isometric Chest Fly

Hips and back straight, hands much wider than shoulder width, fingers pointed out, lower upper torso as close to floor as possible.

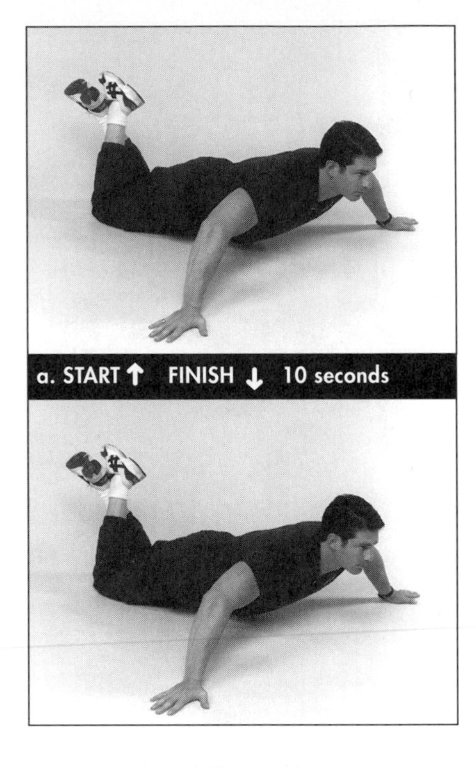

a. START ↑ FINISH ↓ 10 seconds

b.

Push-Up Wide Hand Position

Back straight, head up, hands much wider than shoulder position, lower body as far as you can and return.

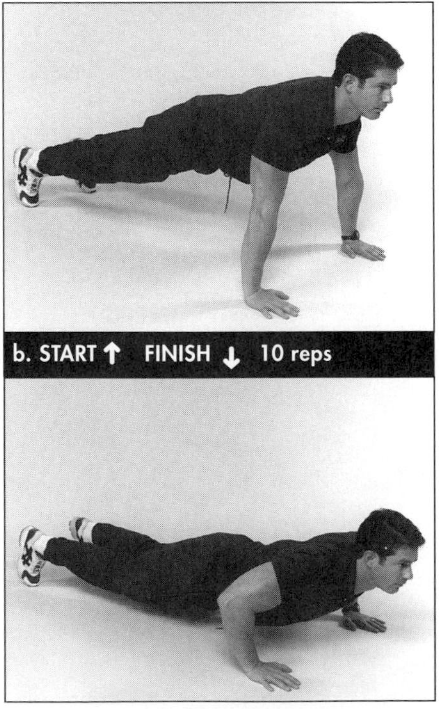

b. START ↑ FINISH ↓ 10 reps

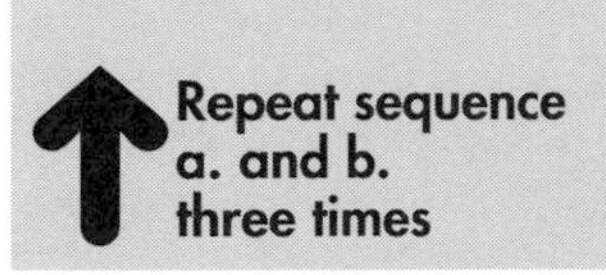

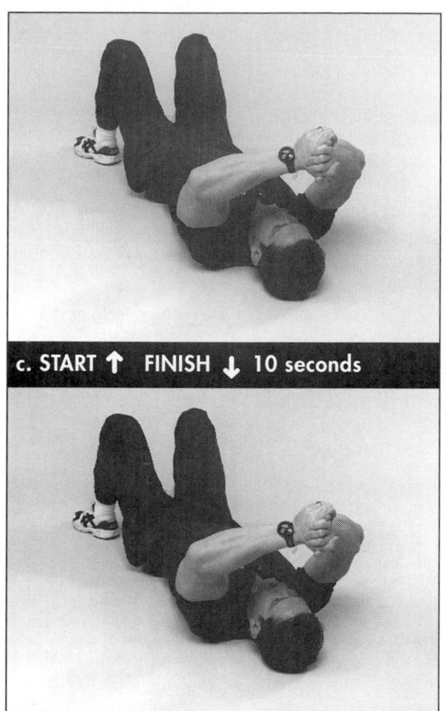

c. START ↑ FINISH ↓ 10 seconds

c.

High Palm Press

Press palms together with elbows out, hands positioned 12 inches away from nose.

↑ Repeat c. three times

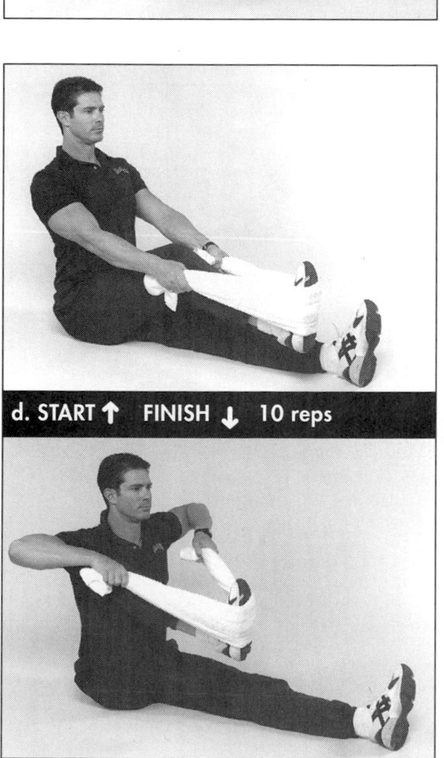

d. START ↑ FINISH ↓ 10 reps

d.

Towel Row Elbows Out

Hold towel with overhand position, towel should be long enough to go around arch of the foot with legs and arms straight. Keep back straight with chest out during all phases of movement. Push with foot for resistance during all phases of rowing movement.

e.
Towel Row
Elbows In Close

Hold towel with overhand position, towel should be long enough to go around arch of the foot with legs and arms straight. Keep back straight with chest out during all phases of movement. Push with foot for resistance during all phases of rowing movement.

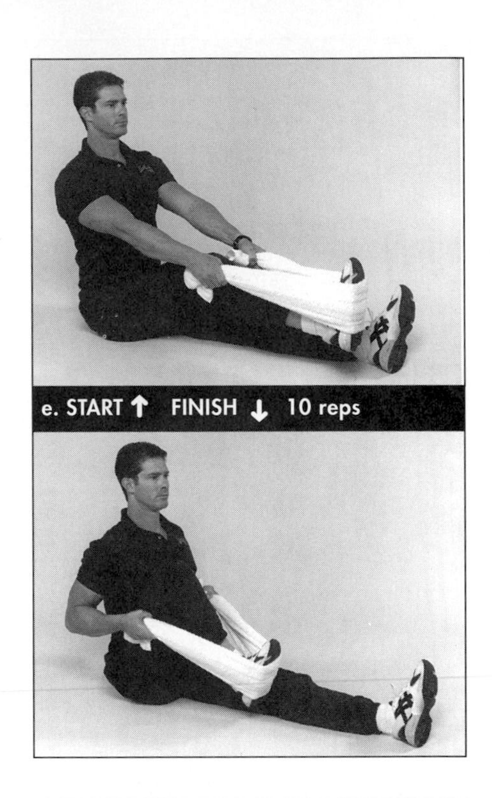

e. START ↑ FINISH ↓ 10 reps

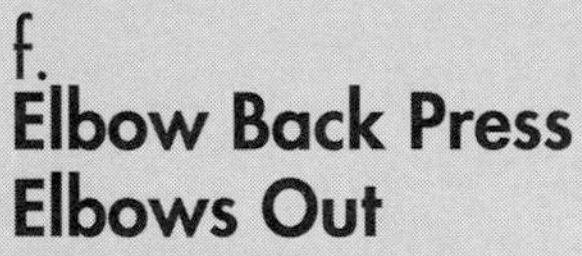

f.
Elbow Back Press
Elbows Out

Abs relaxed, elbows in 90 degree position with forearm pointed up, press elbows into floor to raise upper torso up for duration of exercise, head in alignment with body.

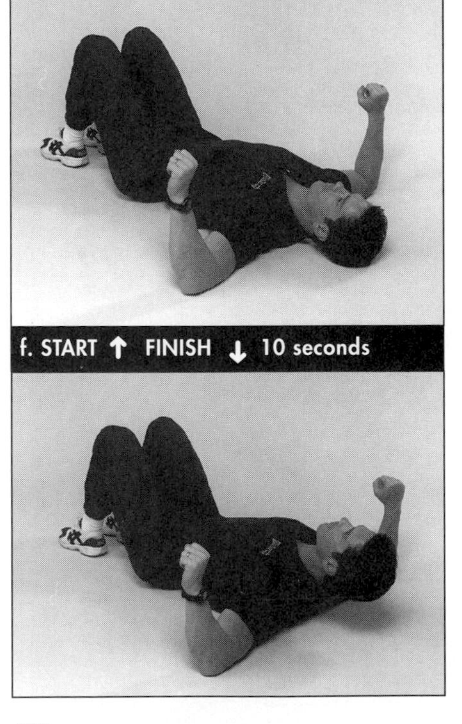

f. START ↑ FINISH ↓ 10 seconds

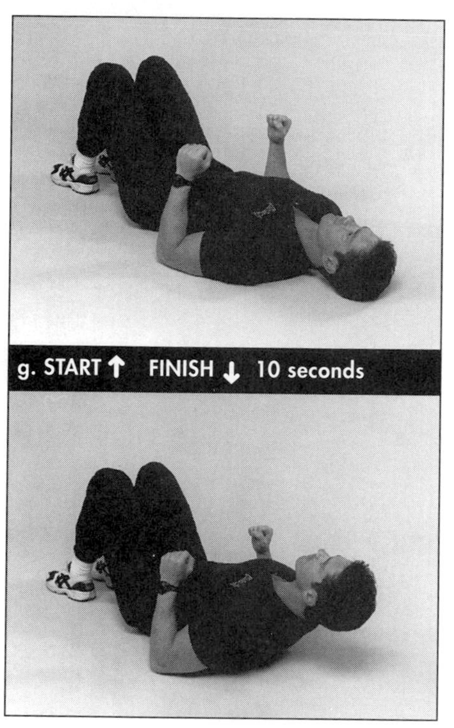

g. START ↑ FINISH ↓ 10 seconds

g.

Elbow Back Press Elbows In Close

Abs relaxed, elbows in 90 degree position with forearm pointed up, press elbows into floor to raise upper torso up for duration of exercise, head in alignment with body.

↑ **Repeat sequence d. through g. two times**

men's workout week 3

day 2 – abs, obliques, glutes

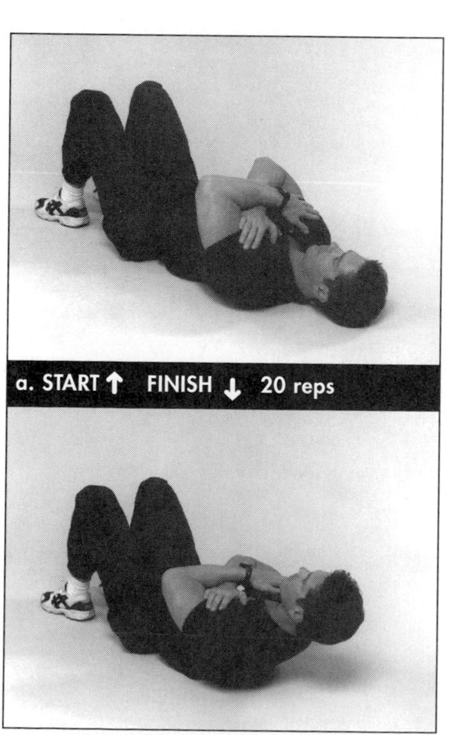

a. START ↑ FINISH ↓ 20 reps

a.

Crunches

Lay on back, eyes up, head back, hands on chest or on back of neck, breathe out and raise shoulder blades from floor, inhale on return motion.

b.
Thigh Press

Lay on back with knees bent. Breathe out slowly while pushing your thighs down, don't let feet touch the floor, hold for recommended time.

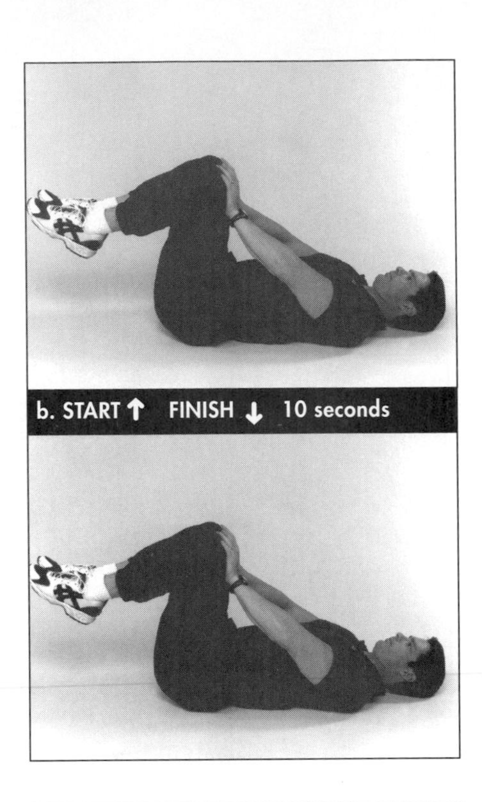

b. START ↑ FINISH ↓ 10 seconds

↑ Repeat sequence a. and b. two times

c.
Tucks

Lay on back, ankles crossed, knees bent, hands by sides. Raise feet off floor pulling knees to face, exhaling at same time, inhale when lowering feet back to floor.

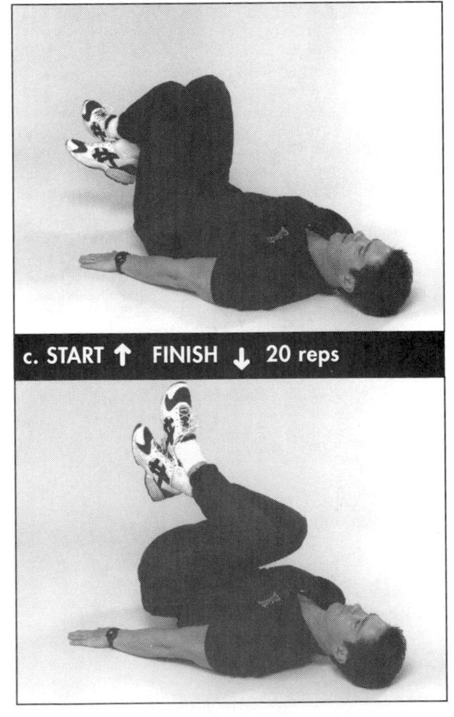

c. START ↑ FINISH ↓ 20 reps

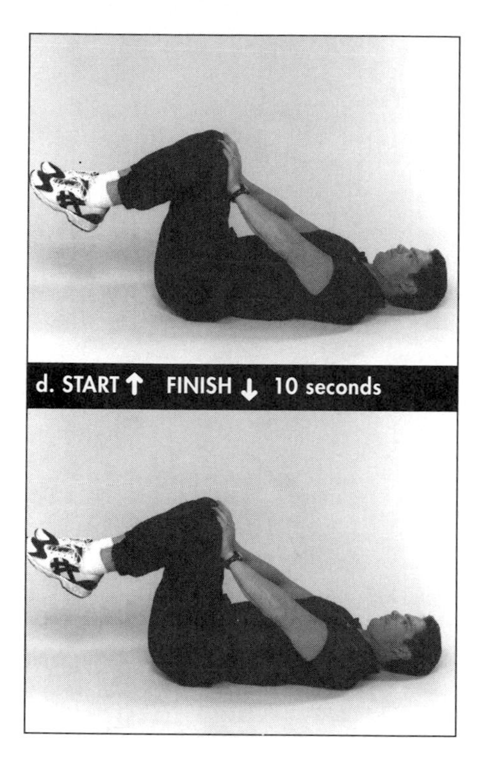

d. START ↑ FINISH ↓ 10 seconds

d.

Thigh Press

Lay on back with knees bent. Breathe out slowly while pushing your thighs down, don’t let feet touch the floor, hold for recommended time.

↑ **Repeat sequence c. and d. two times**

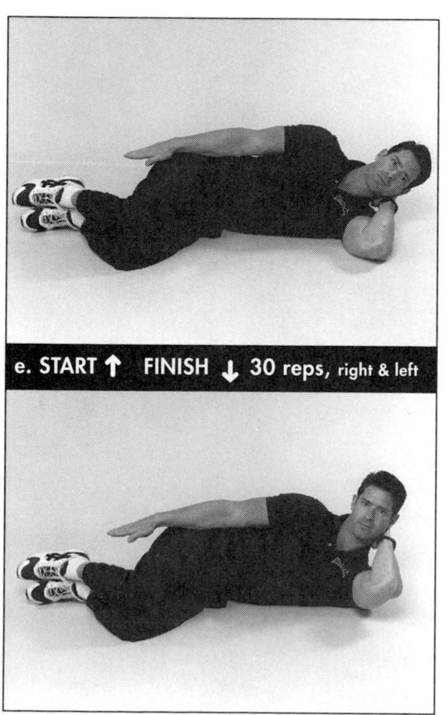

e. START ↑ FINISH ↓ 30 reps, right & left

e.

Side Crunch

Lay on side with hips flexed and knees bent, bottom arm supporting head with elbow off the floor, top arm straight, exhale while reaching for ankle, inhale and return.

f.
Heel Press

Lay on back with one leg straight up, other leg down with knee bent no more than 90 degrees. Push heel into floor to raise lower body off floor.

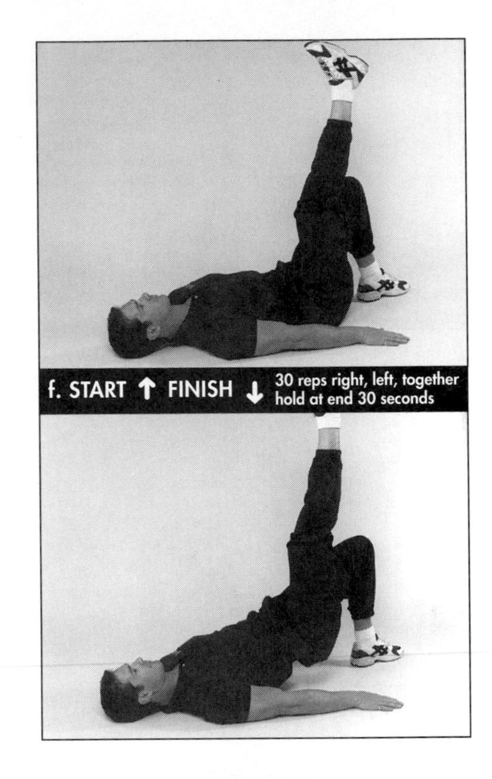
f. START ↑ FINISH ↓ 30 reps right, left, together hold at end 30 seconds

men's workout
week 3

day 3 – legs

a.
Lunge

Feet should be twice the width of shoulders, toes of both feet point in same direction, keep back leg as straight as possible, bend from front knee and hip to lower into lunge position and push to return, head up, back straight, chest out.

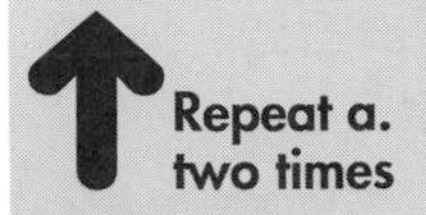
Repeat a. two times

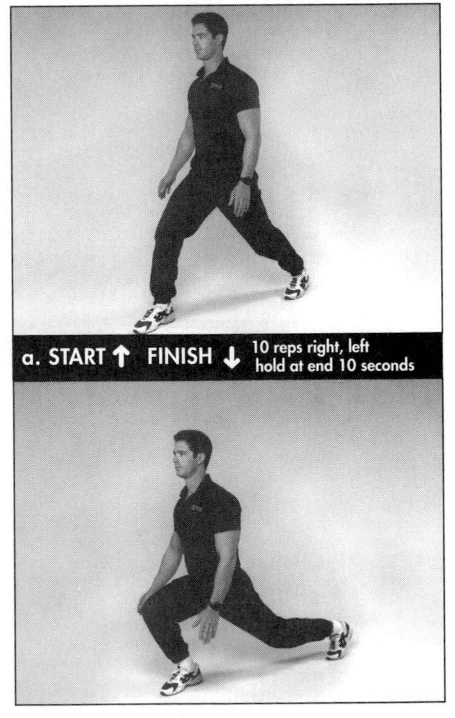
a. START ↑ FINISH ↓ 10 reps right, left hold at end 10 seconds

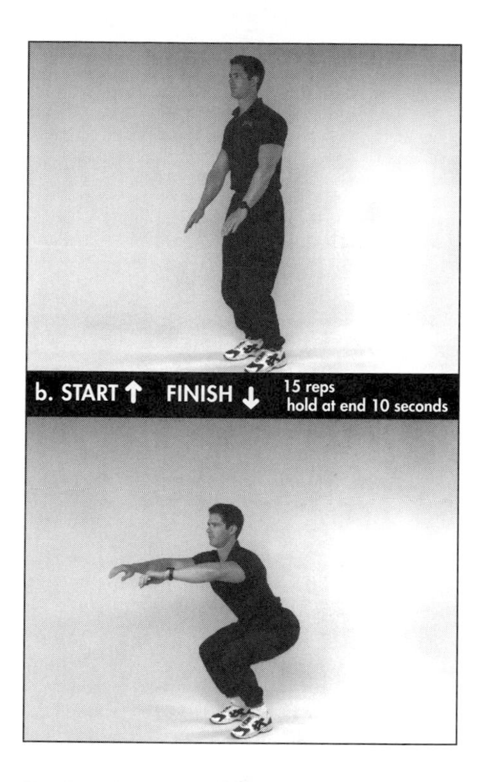

b.
Squats Close Stance

Heels and toes 6-8 inches apart, heels stay on floor during all ranges of exercise, head up, back straight, chest out. Bend knees and hips to lower upper body into squat position and return.

Repeat b. two times

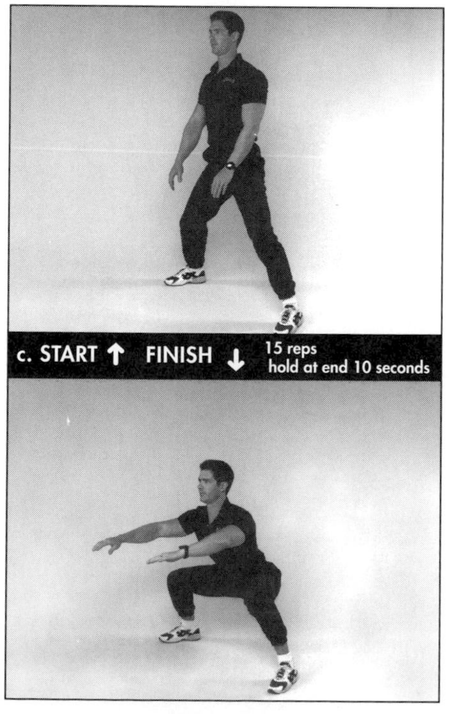

c.
Squats Wide Stance

Heels twice as wide as shoulder width with toes pointing out slightly, heels stay down, head up, back straight, chest out, bend knees and hips to lower upper body into squat position and return.

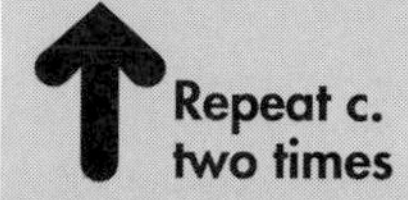

d.
Ankle Cross Extension/Curl

Lay on back with knees up and ankles crossed, push lower shin area and back of ankle together for resistance, straighten and bend knees while applying pressure through all ranges of motion, switch ankle position to put resistance on the opposite muscles.

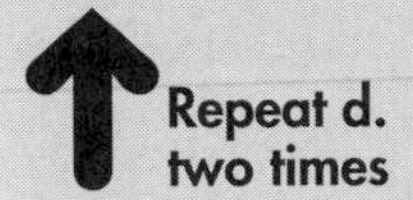
Repeat d.
two times

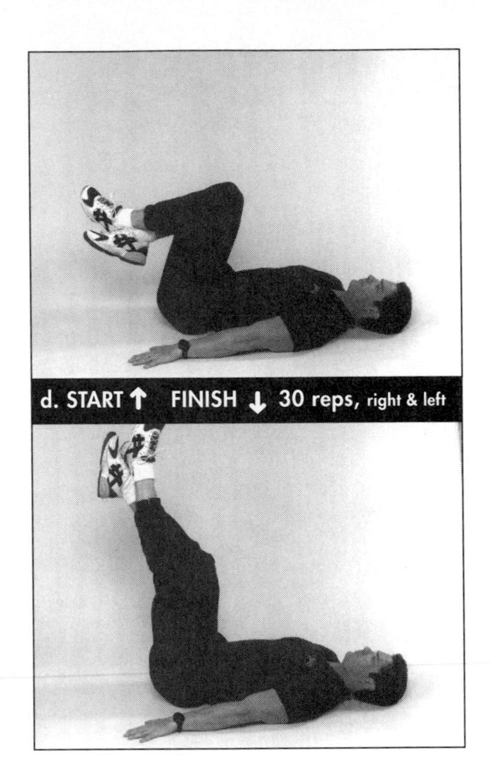
d. START ↑ FINISH ↓ 30 reps, right & left

men's workout week 3

day 4 – bicep, tricep, shoulder

a.
Supinated Bicep Curl With Towel

Sit with towel under back of knee. Hold towel with underhand grip, pull leg to chest and return.

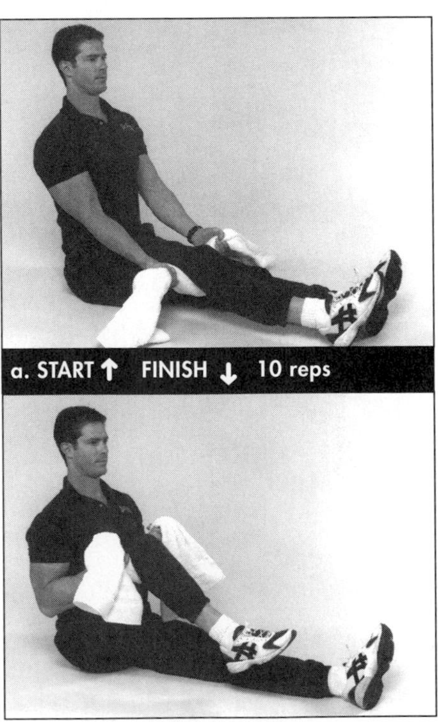
a. START ↑ FINISH ↓ 10 reps

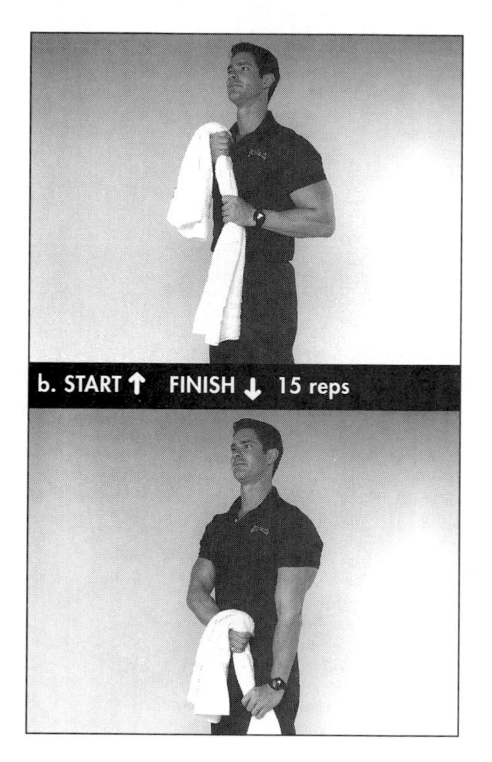

b.
Hammer Curl With Towel

Stand holding towel in overhand position with 4 to 6 inches between hands, pull towel with both hands.

↑ **Repeat sequence a. and b. two times**

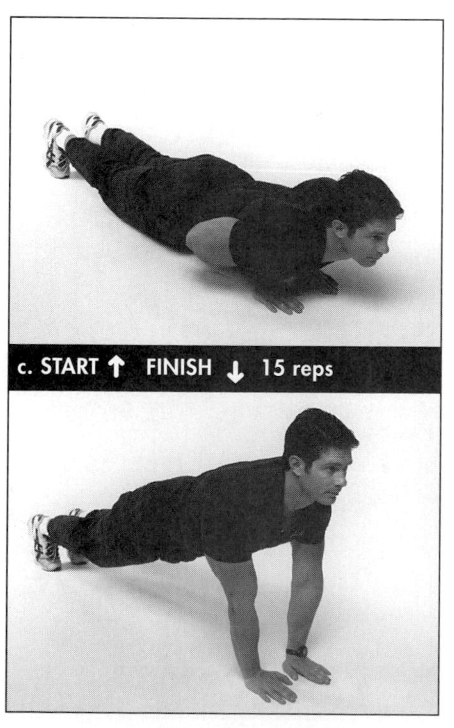

c.
Tricep Push-Up

Start with push up position from toes or from knees. Place hands together, lower body 6 to 8 inches from floor and return.

d.
Double Tricep Extension

Laying on back with towel in overhand position, elbows out with 90 degree bend, forearms pointed straight up, pull towel with both hands to apply resistance to opposing triceps, apply resistance through full range of motion when flexing and straightening of each arm.

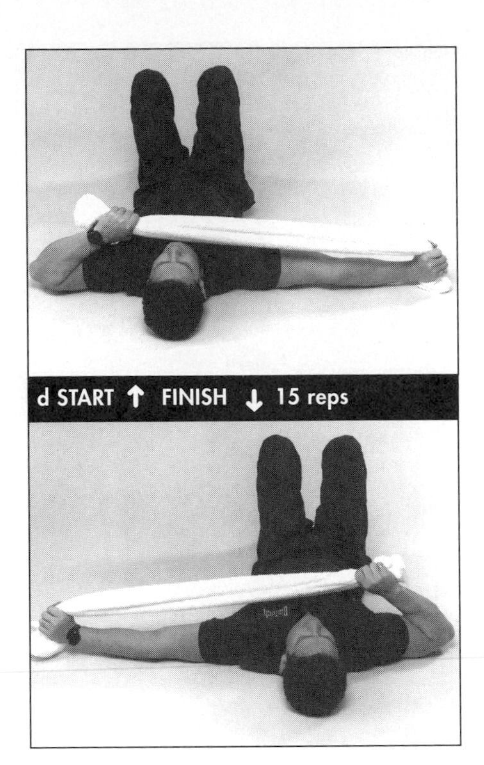

d START ↑ FINISH ↓ 15 reps

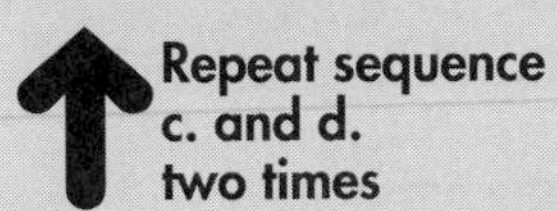

Repeat sequence c. and d. two times

e.
Bicep/Tricep Curl Press

Place palms together for resistance, rotate wrist positions until back of one hand is facing you and the other is facing away, press arms straight then return to chest.

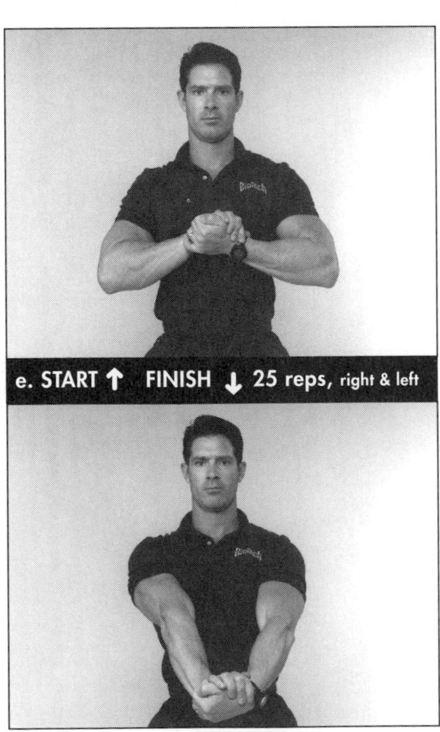

e. START ↑ FINISH ↓ 25 reps, right & left

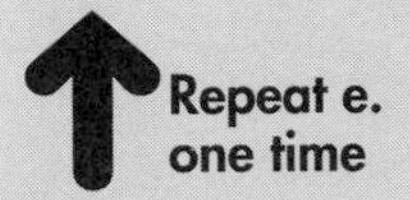

Repeat e. one time

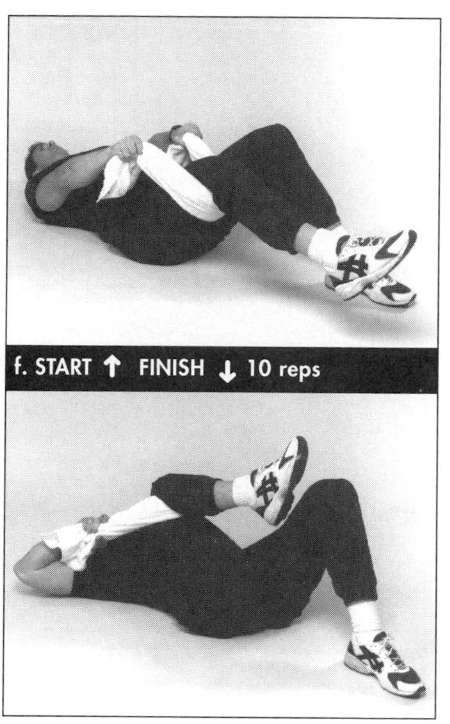

f. START ↑ FINISH ↓ 10 reps

f.
Upright Row

Towel around the back of knee with overhand position, draw elbows up toward ears while pulling leg with towel, return keeping elbows out, use leg pressure on towel for added resistance.

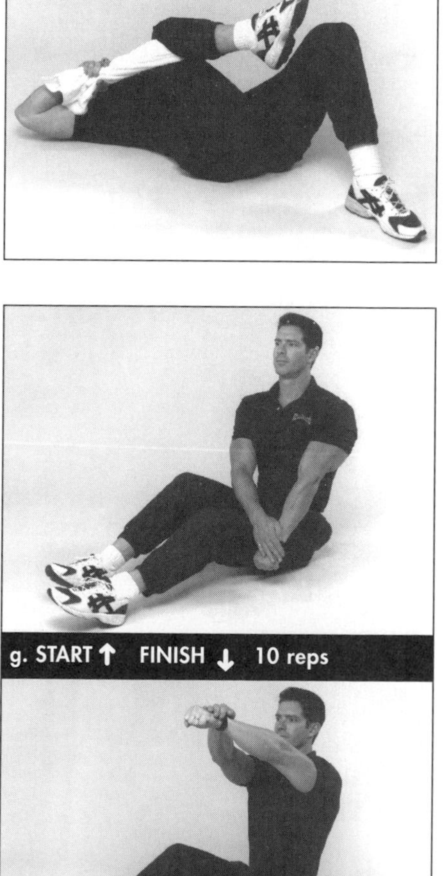

g. START ↑ FINISH ↓ 10 reps

g.
Front Raise

Working arm straight, place other hand on working arm wrist area, press down on working arm as far as it will go down, return with as much pressure from top hand as working shoulder and arm can withstand.

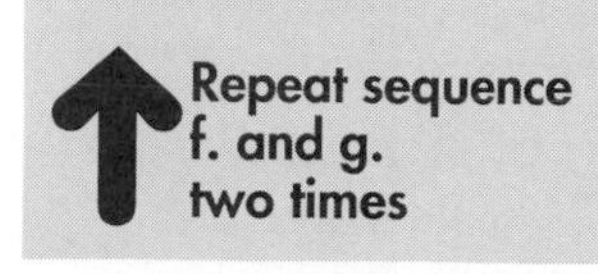

men's workout

week 3

day 5 – abs, lower back, calves

a.

Thigh Press

Lay on back with knees bent. Breathe out slowly while pushing your thighs down, don't let feet touch the floor, hold for recommended time.

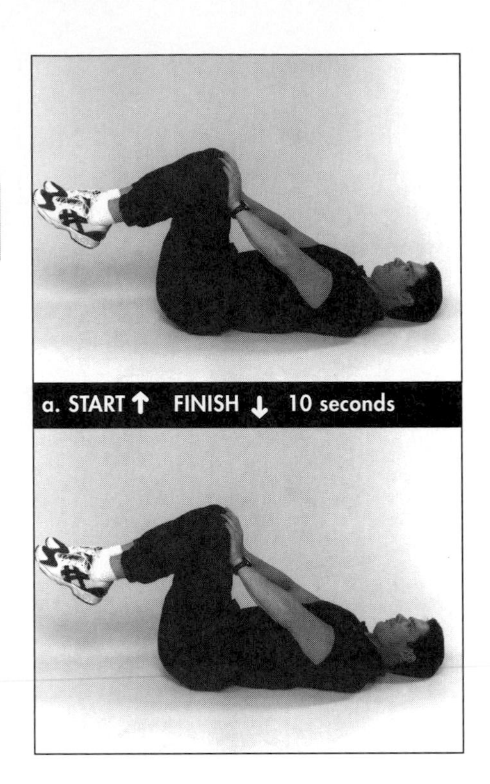

a. START ↑ FINISH ↓ 10 seconds

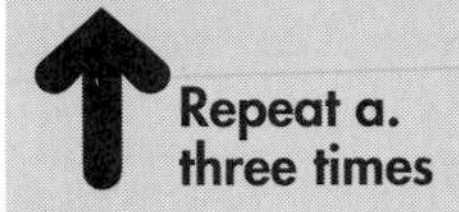

b.

Tucks

Lay on back, ankles crossed, knees bent, hands by sides. Raise feet off floor pulling knees to face, exhaling at same time, inhale when lowering feet back to floor.

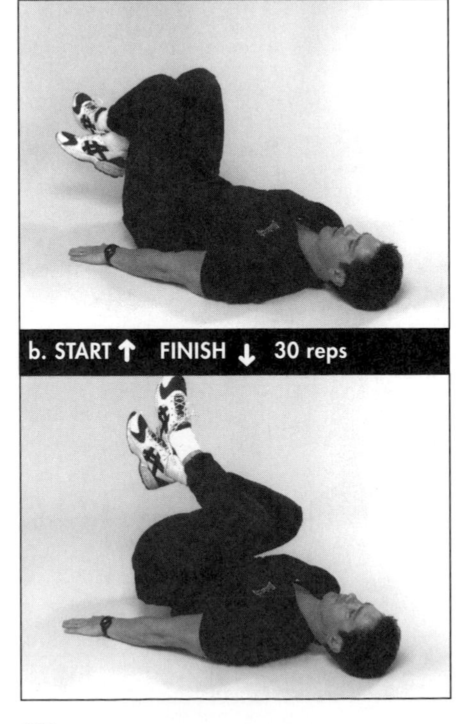

b. START ↑ FINISH ↓ 30 reps

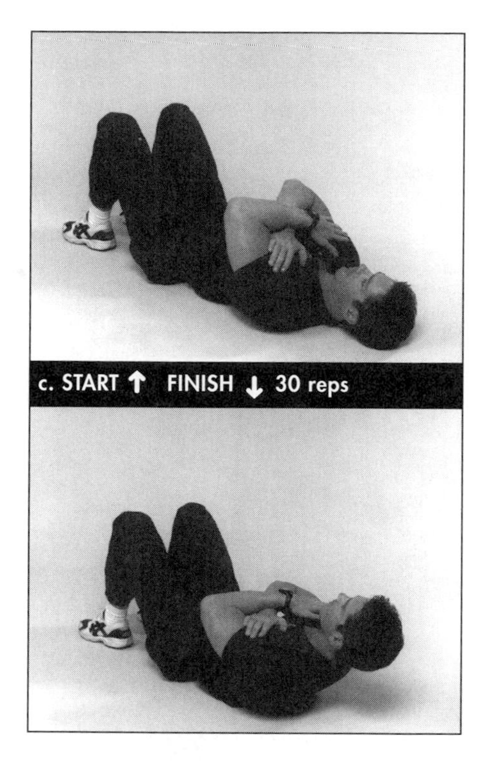

c. START ↑ FINISH ↓ 30 reps

c.
Crunches

Lay on back, eyes up, head back, hands on chest or on back of neck, breathe out and raise shoulder blades from floor, inhale on return motion.

↑ **Repeat sequence b. and c. two times**

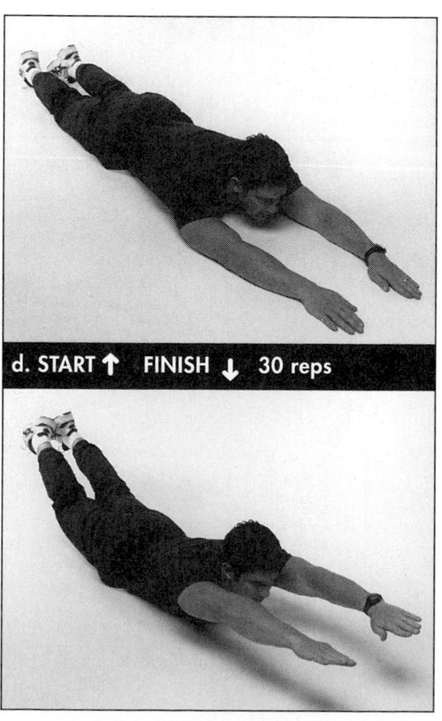

d. START ↑ FINISH ↓ 30 reps

d.
Hyperextension Superman

Lay on stomach with hands out in front of head. Raise head, shoulders, chest, and toes from floor and return.

e.

Calf Raises

Standing on one foot, raise heel from floor 2-3 inches and return. For double calf raise, stand on both feet, raise heels from floor 2-3 inches and return.

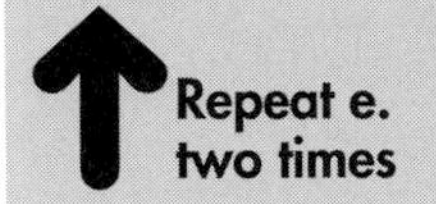

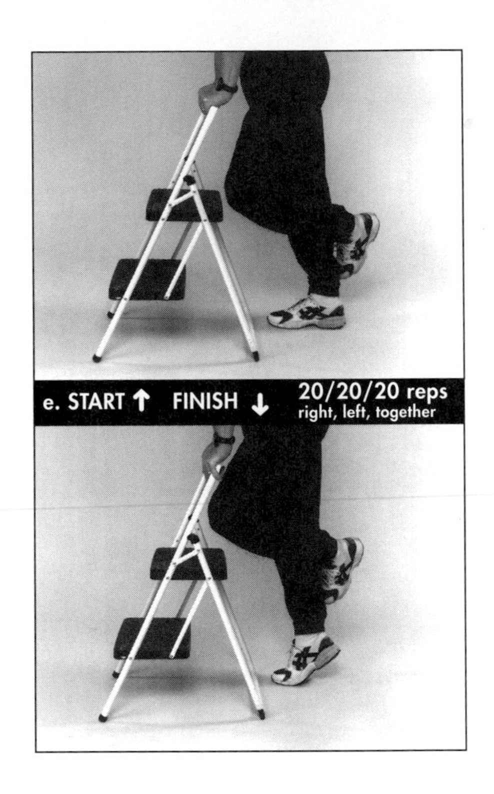

16

Biogenesis Phase Two and Three Photographs

THE CAMPITELLI ADVANCED 10 MINUTE EXERCISE METHOD

WOMEN'S WORKOUT #1 • PAGE 1

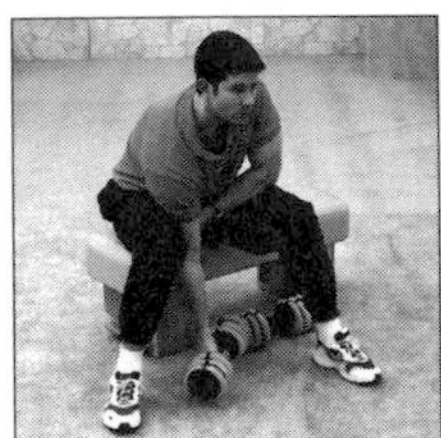

START FINISH

1. Concentration Curl
15 reps Right/Left

- Brace curling arm inside thigh for support.
- Use other hand for additional support.

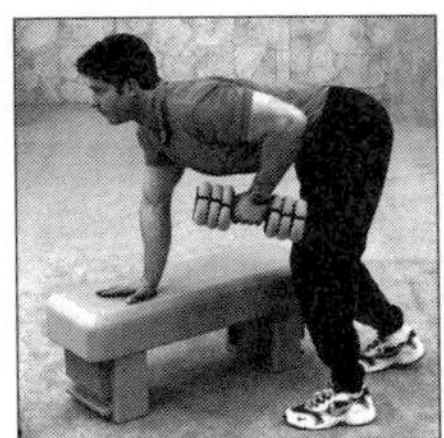
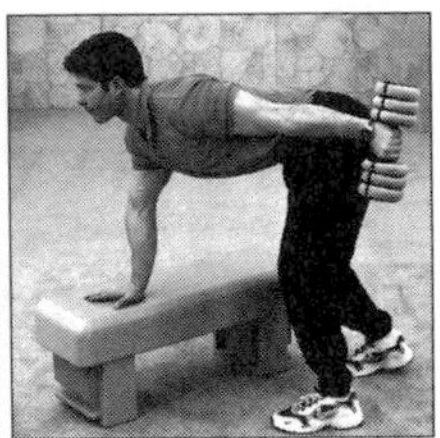

START FINISH

2. Tricep Kick Back
15 reps Right/Left

- Support upper body with non-working arm.
- Extend arm until parallel to floor and hold.
- Don't swing weight at bottom.

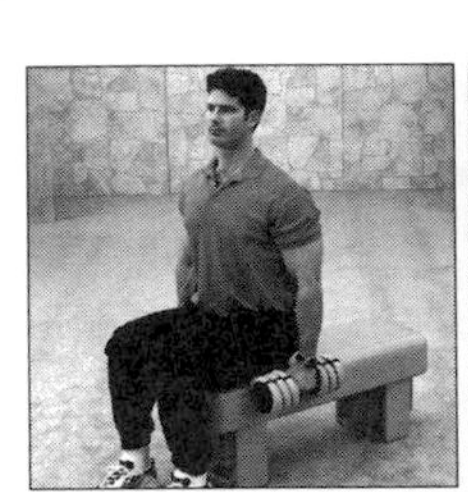
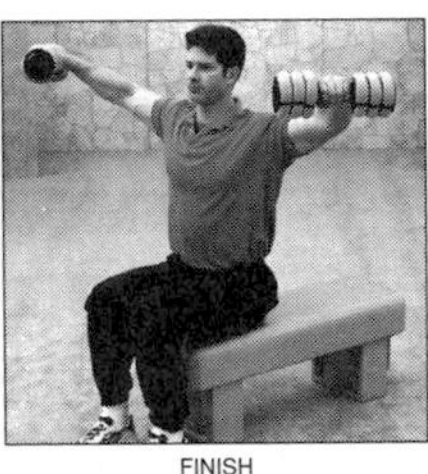

START FINISH

3. Lateral Raise
15 reps

- Raise DBs out to the side keeping palms down.
- Concentrate on raising your elbows, not the DBs.

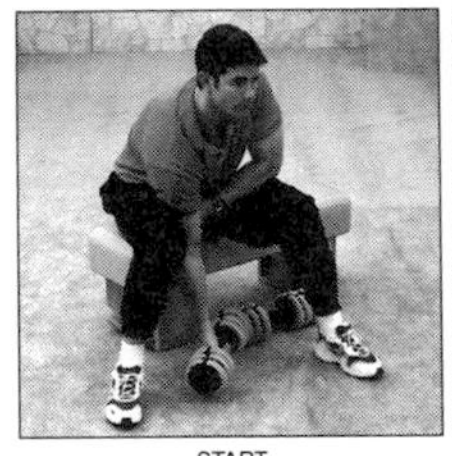
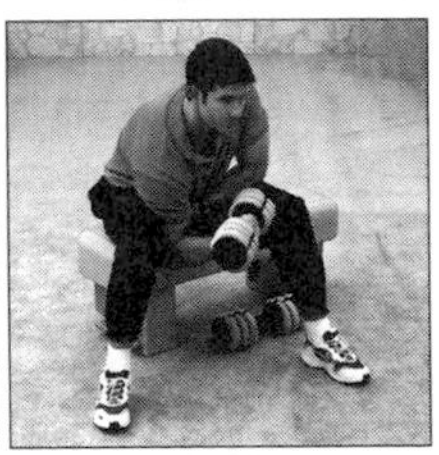

START FINISH

4. Concentration Curl
15 reps Right/Left

- Brace curling arm inside thigh for support.
- Use other hand for additional support.

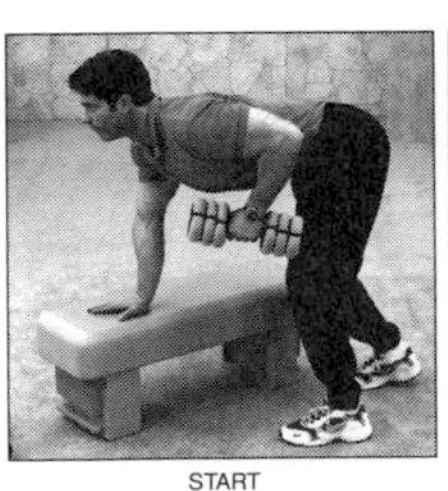
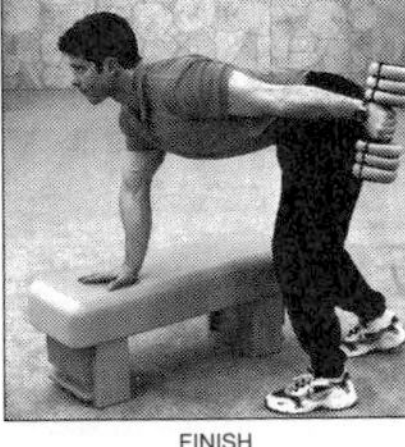

START FINISH

5. Tricep Kickback
15 reps Right/Left

- Support upper body with non working arm.
- Extend arm until parallel to floor and hold.
- Don't swing weight at bottom.

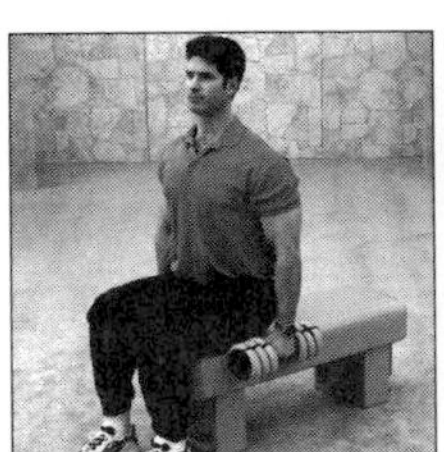
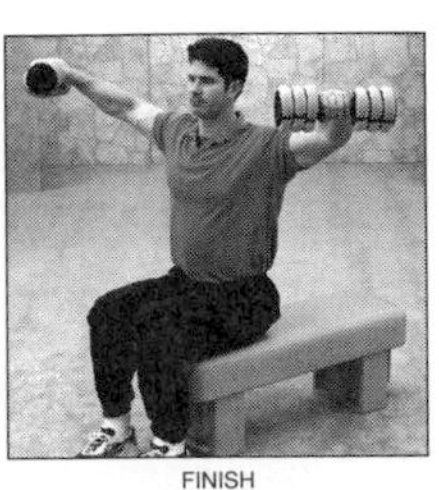

START FINISH

6. Lateral Raise
15 reps

- Raise DBs out to the side keeping palms down.
- Concentrate on raising your elbows, not the DBs.

END OF ROUTINE. NO PAGE 2.

THE CAMPITELLI ADVANCED 10 MINUTE EXERCISE METHOD

WOMEN'S WORKOUT #2 • PAGE 1

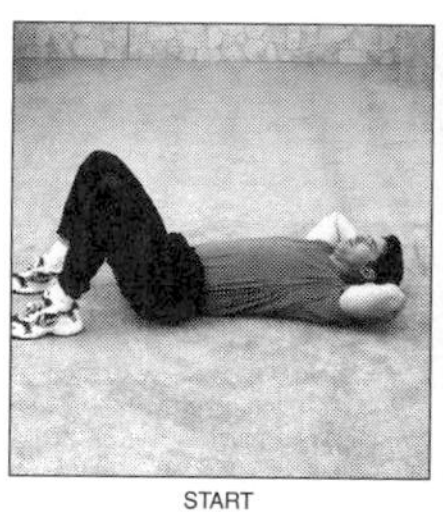

START FINISH

1. Crunch
30 reps

- Push lower back into floor.
- Focus on ceiling, not knees.
- Breathe out as you go up.

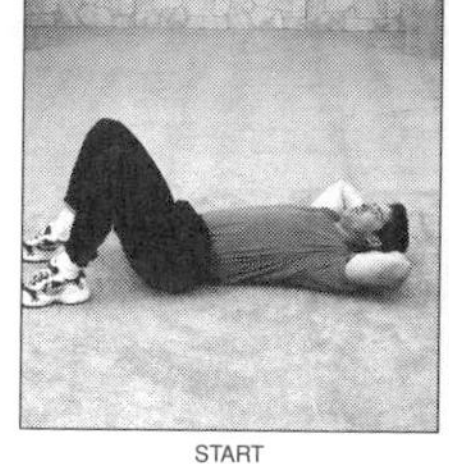

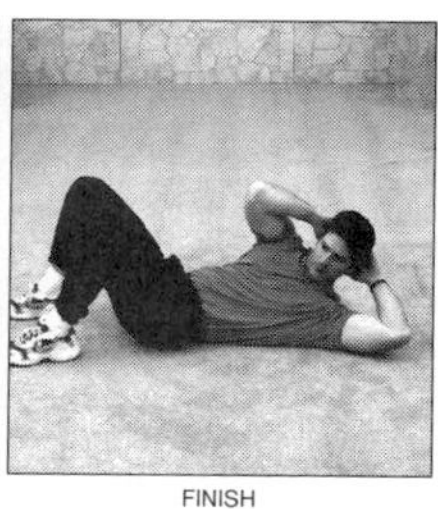

START FINISH

2. Twisting Crunch
30 reps Left

- Start same as Crunch. Right elbow to left knee
- Exhale on the way up.
- Inhale going down.

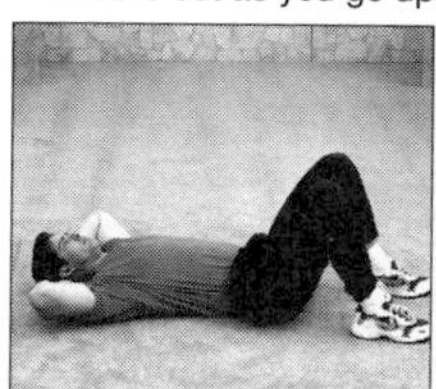

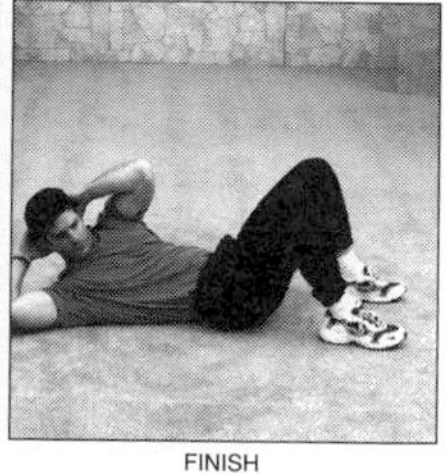

START FINISH

3. Twisting Crunch
30 reps Right

- Start same as Crunch. Left elbow to right knee
- Exhale on the way up.
- Inhale going down.

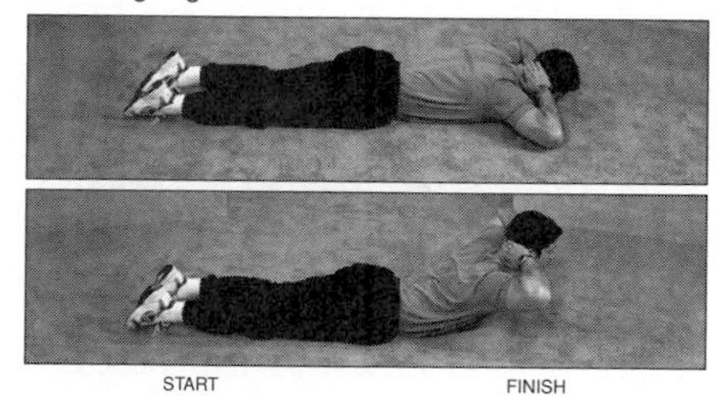

START FINISH

4. Hyper Extension
30 reps Right/Left

- Raise upper body off floor feeling contraction in mid to low back.

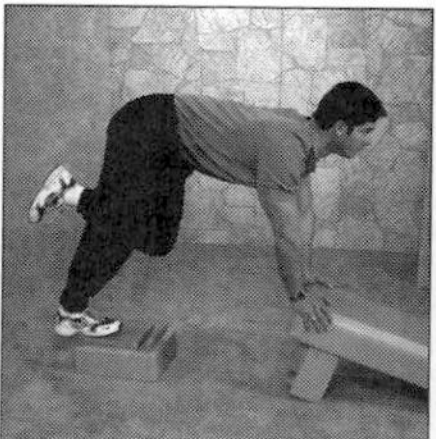

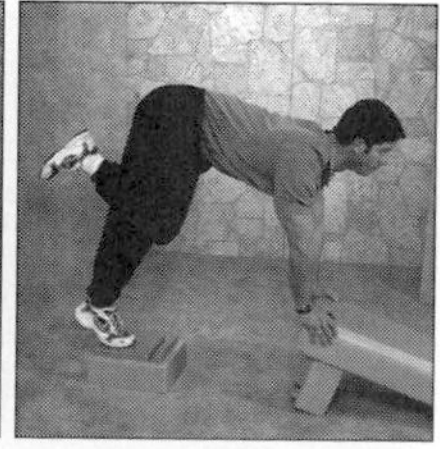

START FINISH

5. Donkey Calf Raise
30 reps Right/Left

- Place ball of foot on step or book and raise heal.
- Keep knee straight.

THE CAMPITELLI ADVANCED 10 MINUTE EXERCISE METHOD

WOMEN'S WORKOUT #2 • PAGE 2

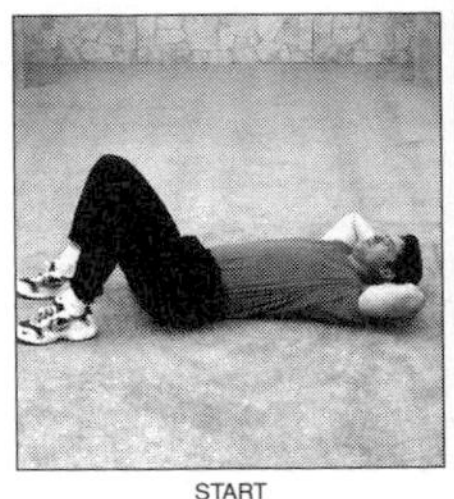

START FINISH

6. Crunch
20 reps

- Push lower back into floor.
- Focus on ceiling, not knees.
- Breathe out as you go up.

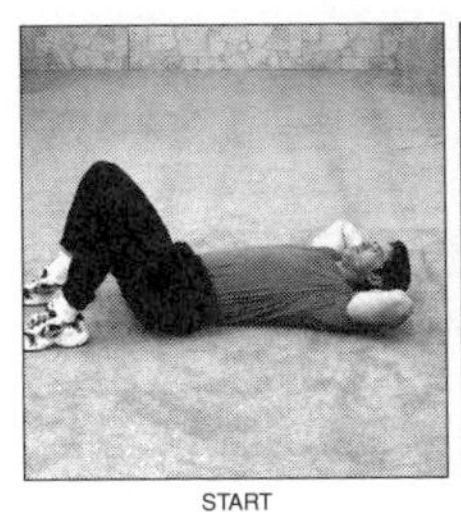

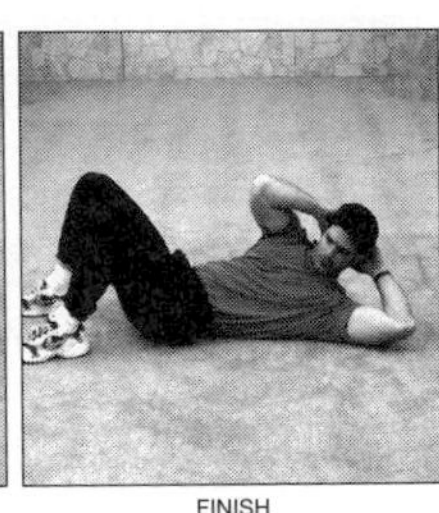

START FINISH

7. Twisting Crunch
20 reps Left

- Start same as Crunch. Right elbow to left knee
- Exhale on the way up.
- Inhale going down.

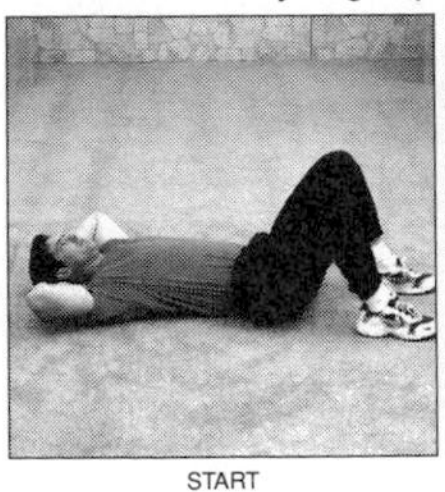

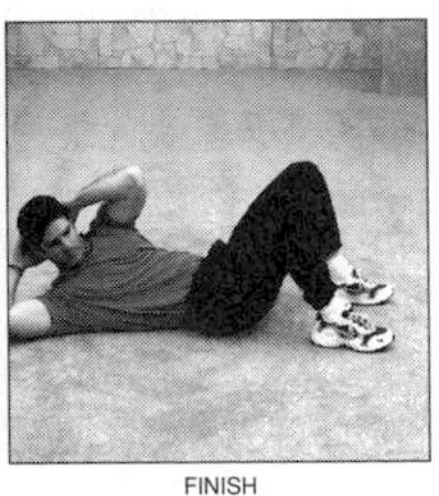

START FINISH

8. Twisting Crunch
20 reps Right

- Start same as Crunch. Left elbow to right knee
- Exhale on the way up.
- Inhale going down.

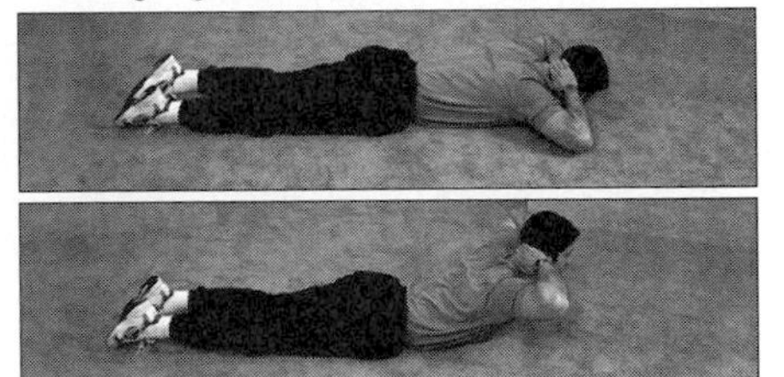

START FINISH

9. Hyper Extension
20 reps Right/Left

- Raise upper body off floor feeling contraction in mid to low back.

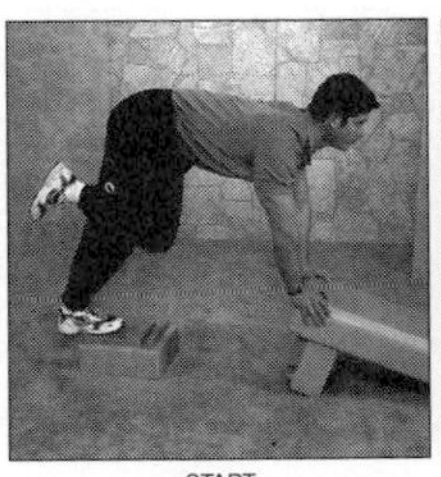

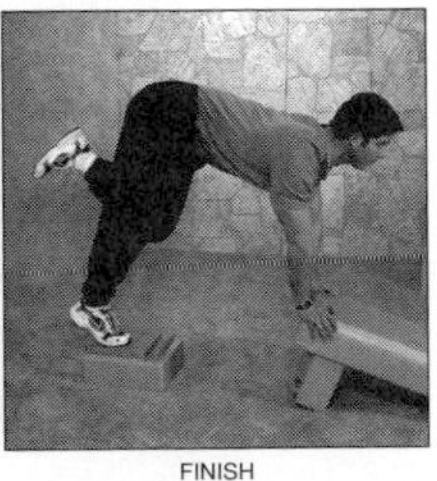

START FINISH

10. Donkey Calf Raise
20 reps Right/Left

- Place ball of foot on step or book and raise heal.
- Keep knee straight.

THE CAMPITELLI ADVANCED 10 MINUTE EXERCISE METHOD

WOMEN'S WORKOUT #3 • PAGE 1

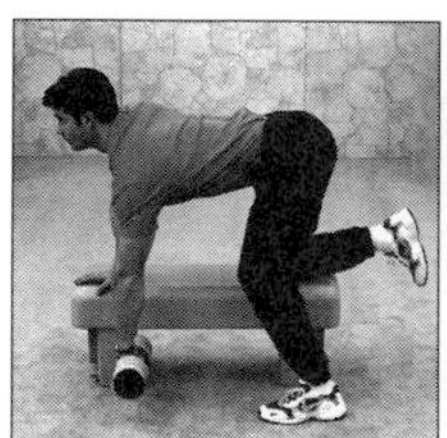

START FINISH

1. Single Arm Dumbbell Row Wide Grip
15 reps Right/Left

- Back flat, use hand to support body.
- Pull elbow up and away from body.
- Head up.

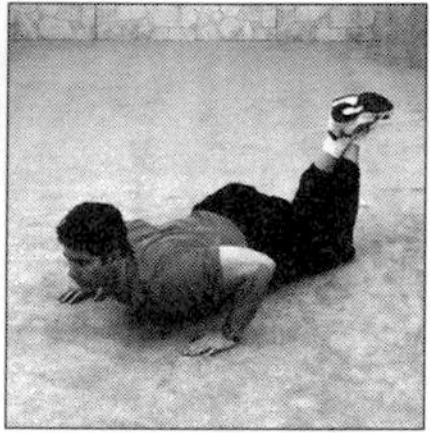

START FINISH

2. Modified Pushup
15 reps

- Start from knees.
- Hands shoulder width.
- Head up.

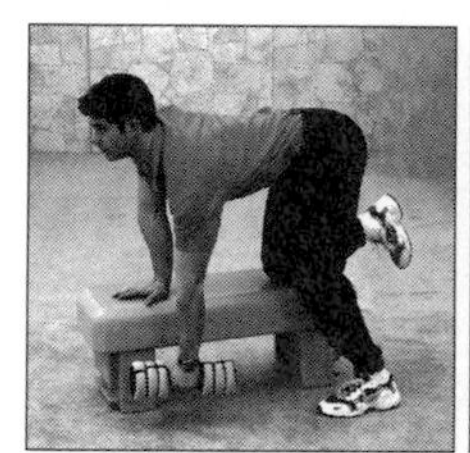

START FINISH

3. Single Arm Dumbbell Row Close Grip
15 reps Right/Left

- Back flat, use hand to support body.
- Pull DB close to side.
- Head up.

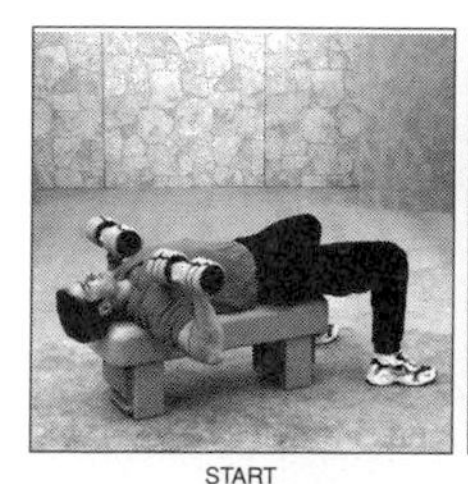

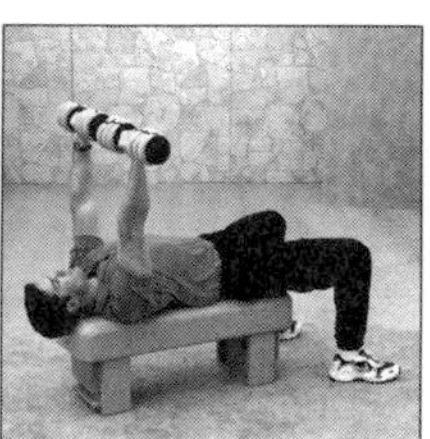

START FINISH

4. Dumbbell Press
15 reps

- Hold weights palms toward knees.
- Relax abdomen.
- Lower weights until even with chest.

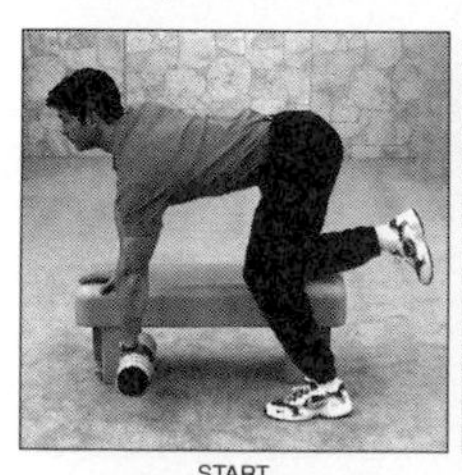

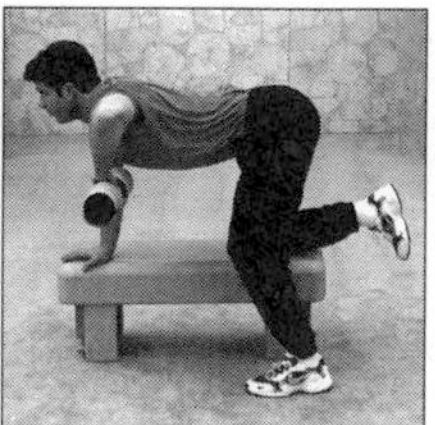

START FINISH

5. Single Arm Dumbbell Row Wide Grip
15 reps Right/Left

- Back flat, use hand to support body.
- Pull elbow up and away from body.
- Head up.

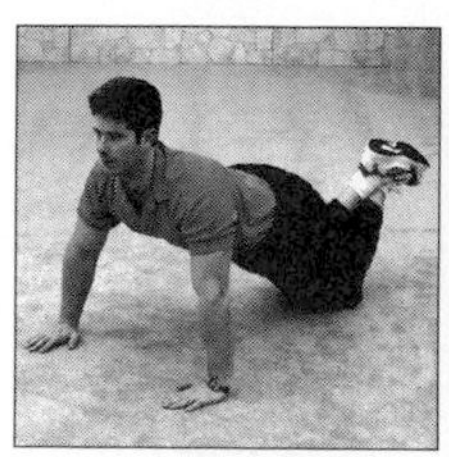

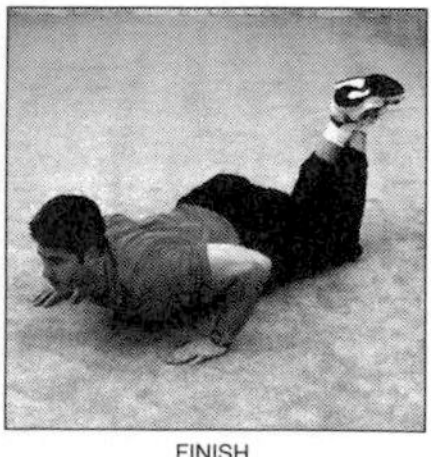

START FINISH

6. Modified Pushup
15 reps

- Start from knees.
- Hands shoulder width.
- Head up.

THE CAMPITELLI ADVANCED 10 MINUTE EXERCISE METHOD

WOMEN'S WORKOUT #3 • PAGE 2

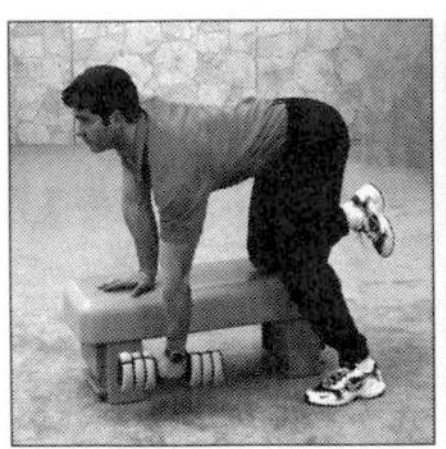

START FINISH

7. Single Arm Dumbbell Row Close Grip
15 reps Right/Left

- Back flat, use hand to support body.
- Pull DB close to side.
- Head up.

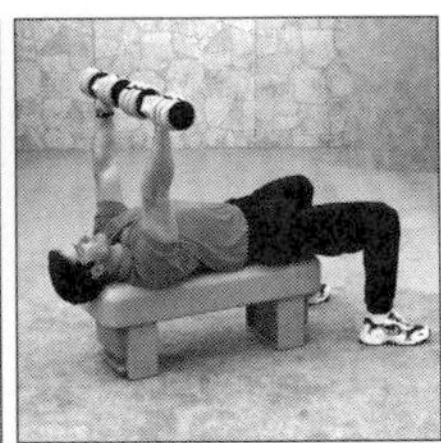

START FINISH

8. Dumbbell Press
15 reps

- Hold weights palms toward knees.
- Relax abdomen.
- Lower weights until even with chest.

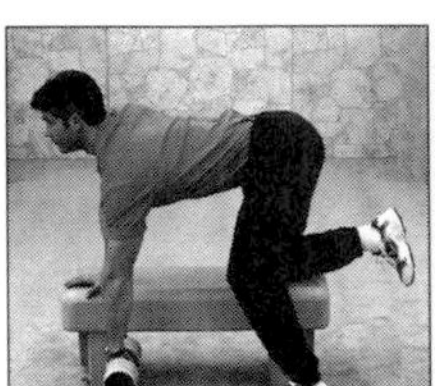

START

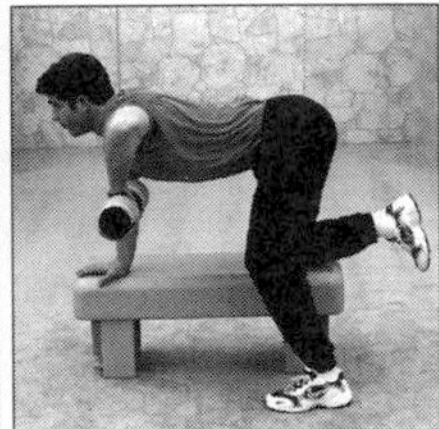

FINISH

9. Single Arm Dumbbell Row Wide Grip
15 reps Right/Left

- Back flat, use hand to support body.
- Pull elbow up and away from body.
- Head up.

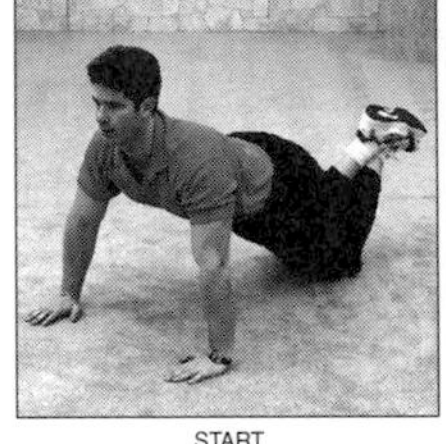

START

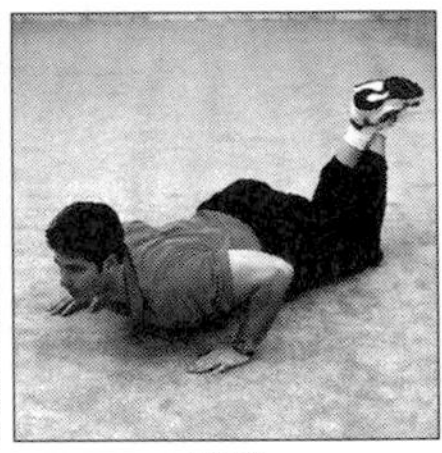

FINISH

10. Modified Pushup
15 reps

- Start from knees.
- Hands shoulder width.
- Head up.

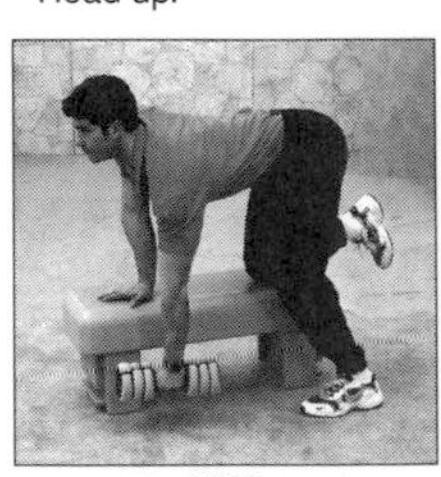

START

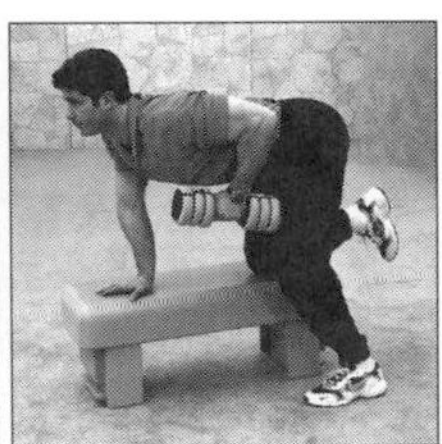

FINISH

11. Single Arm Dumbbell Row Close Grip
15 reps Right/Left

- Back flat, use hand to support body.
- Pull DB close to side.
- Head up.

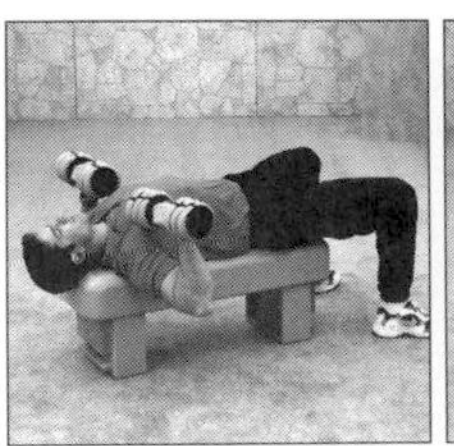

START

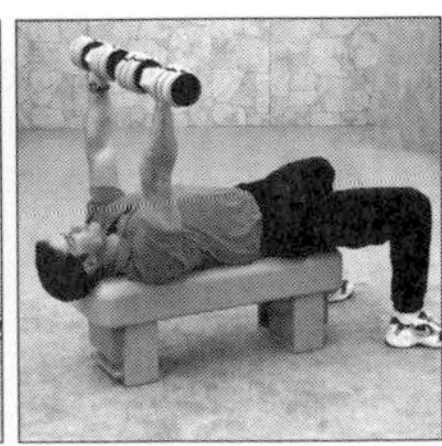

FINISH

12. Dumbbell Press
15 reps

- Hold weights palms toward knees.
- Relax abdomen.
- Lower weights until even with chest.

THE CAMPITELLI ADVANCED 10 MINUTE EXERCISE METHOD

WOMEN'S WORKOUT #4 • PAGE 1

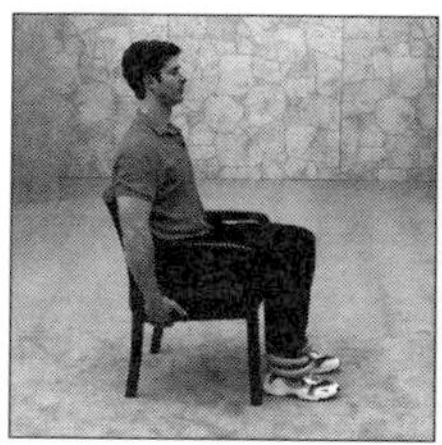

START

FINISH

1. Leg Extension with Ankle Weights
15 reps Right/Left

- Extend foot out with weights, hold leg straight for a brief pause and then return.

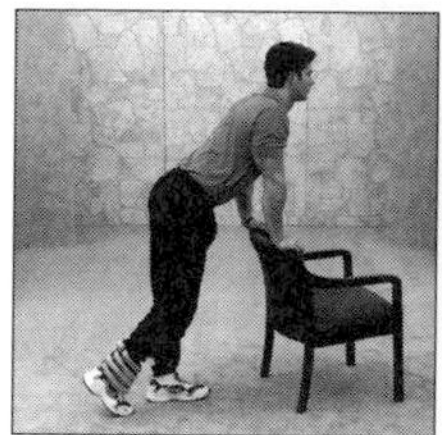

START

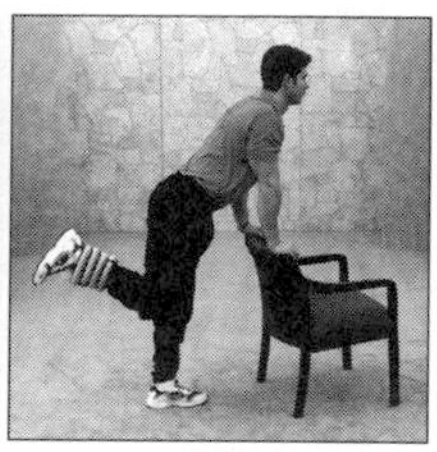

FINISH

2. Standing Leg Curl with Ankle Weights
15 reps Right/Left

- Raise leg bending knee.
- Use chair for balance. Keep toe pointed down.
- Hold briefly at top position.

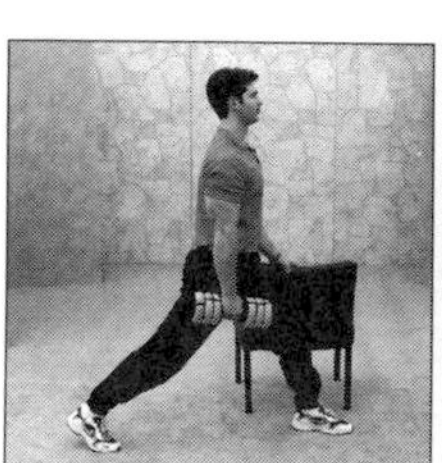

START

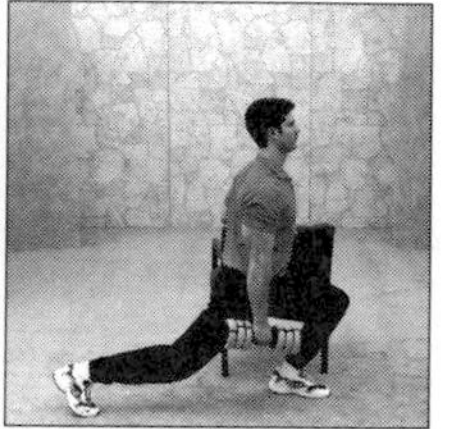

FINISH

3. Dumbbell Lunge
20 reps Right/Left

- Use chair for balance.
- Heel to toe. Stance to 4 feet apart.
- Back straight. Chest out.

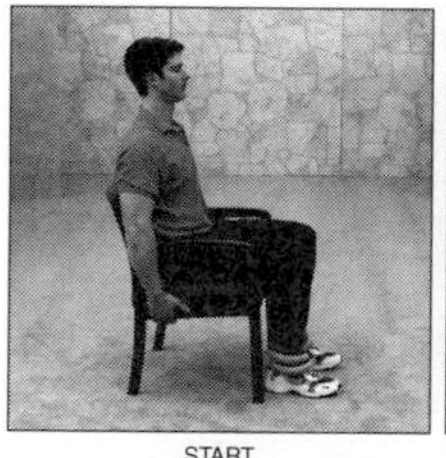

START

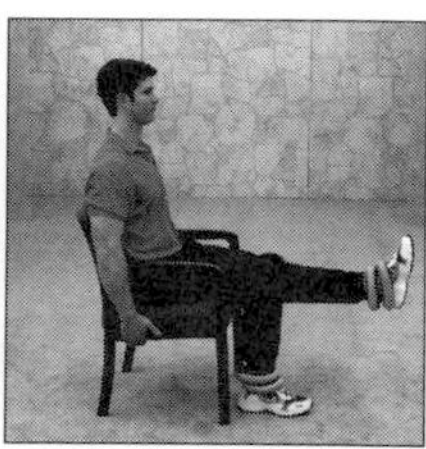

FINISH

4. Leg Extension with Ankle Weights
15 reps Right/Left

- Extend foot out with weights, hold leg straight for a brief pause and then return.

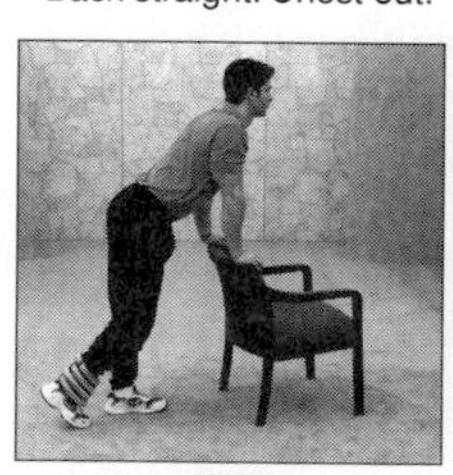

START

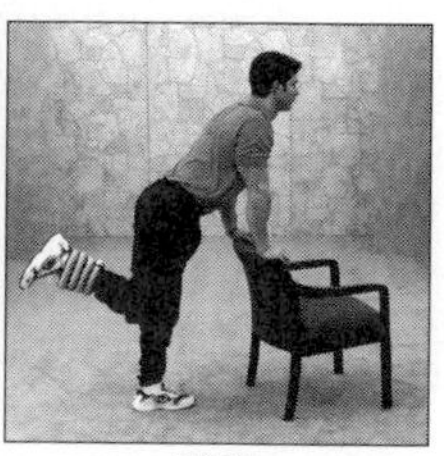

FINISH

5. Standing Leg Curl with Ankle Weights
15 reps Right/Left

- Raise leg bending knee.
- Use chair for balance. Keep toe pointed down.
- Hold briefly at top position.

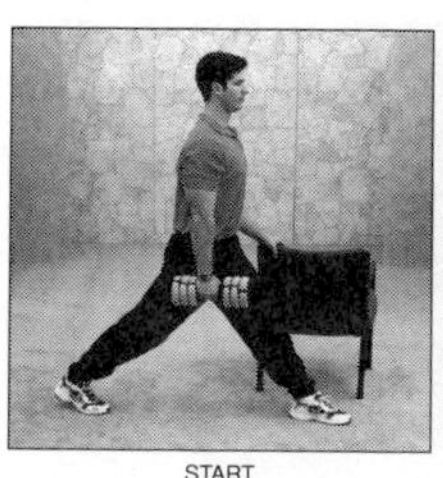

START

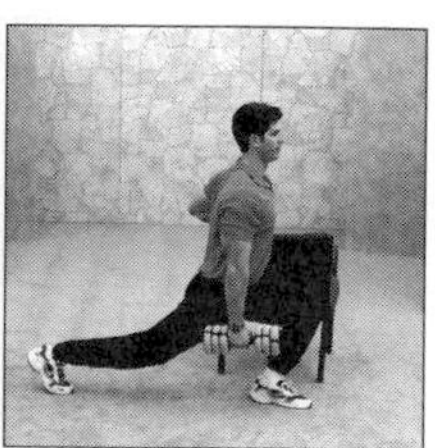

FINISH

6. Dumbbell Lunge
20 reps Right/Left

- Use chair for balance. Heel to toe. Stance to 4 feet apart.
- Back straight. Chest out.

END OF ROUTINE. NO PAGE 2.

THE CAMPITELLI ADVANCED 10 MINUTE EXERCISE METHOD

WOMEN'S WORKOUT #5 • PAGE 1

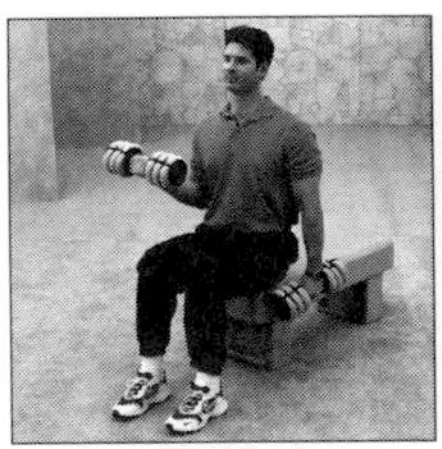
START

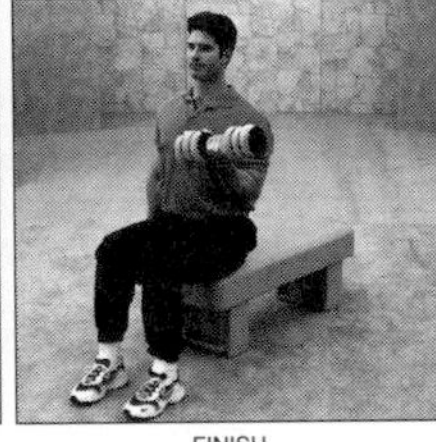
FINISH

1. Alternating Seated Dumbbell Curl
10 reps each arm

- Chest out and shoulders back.
- Keep elbows to your side.
- Palms up at top. • Don't swing weights.

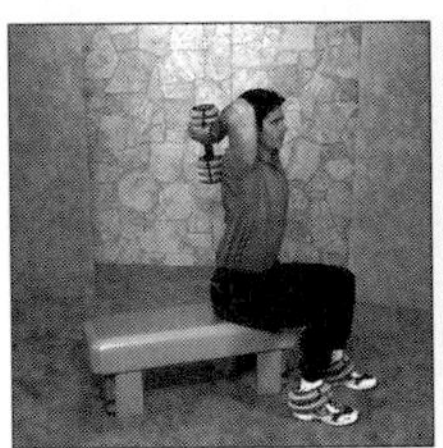
START

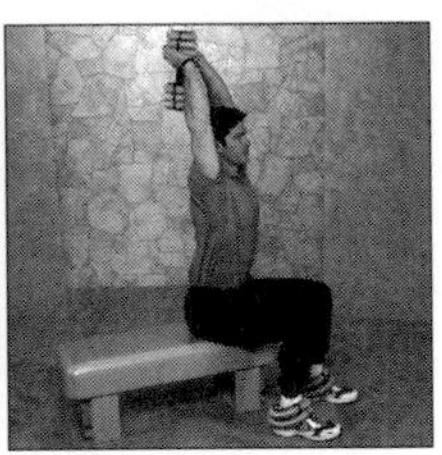
FINISH

2. Overhead Tricep Extension
10 reps

- Extend weight over head.
- Keep elbows up and close to head.

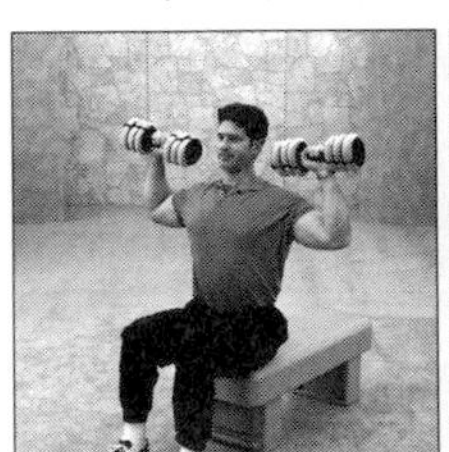
START

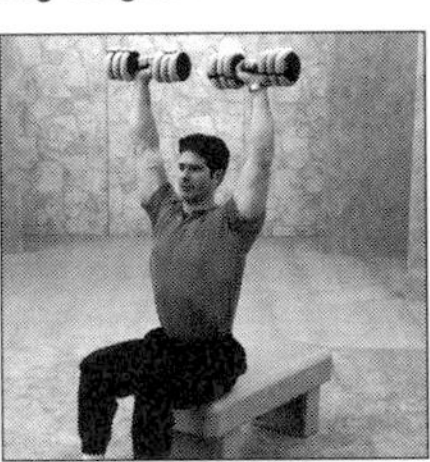
FINISH

3. Shoulder Press
15 reps

- Press weights with elbows out from sides.
- Palms facing forward.

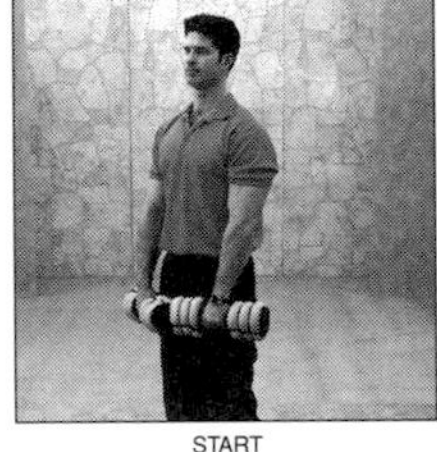
START

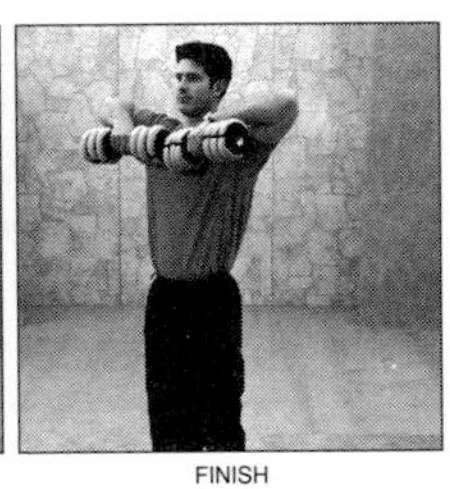
FINISH

4. Upright Rows
15 reps

- Pull weights to chin.
- Elbows should be higher than weights at finish.

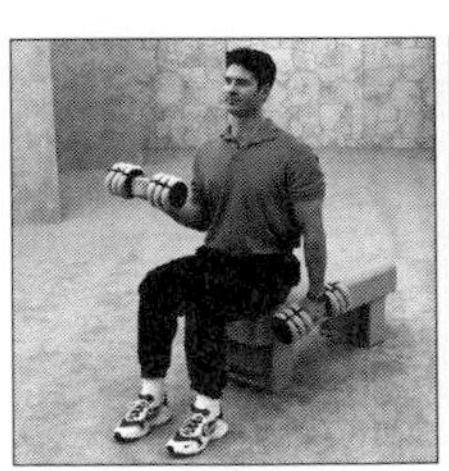
START

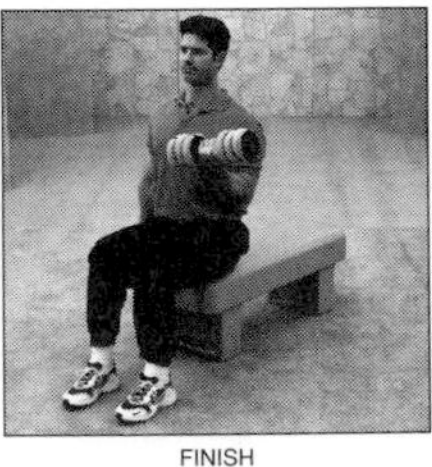
FINISH

5. Alternating Seated Dumbbell Curl
10 reps each arm

- Chest out and shoulders back.
- Keep elbows to your side.
- Palms up at top. • Don't swing weights.

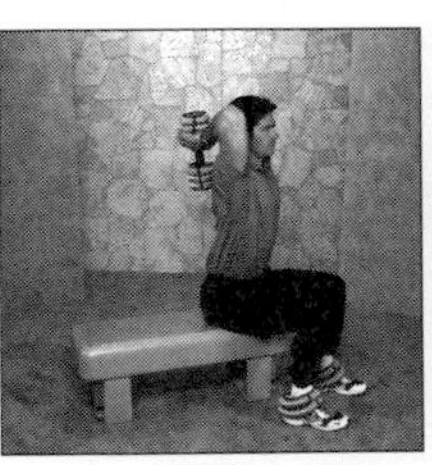
START

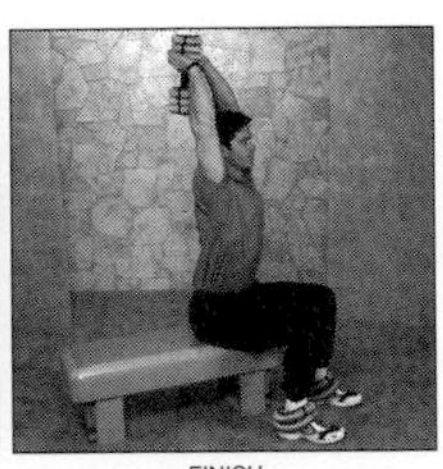
FINISH

6. Overhead Tricep Extension
10 reps

- Extend weight over head.
- Keep elbows up and close to head.

THE CAMPITELLI ADVANCED 10 MINUTE EXERCISE METHOD

WOMEN'S WORKOUT #5 • PAGE 2

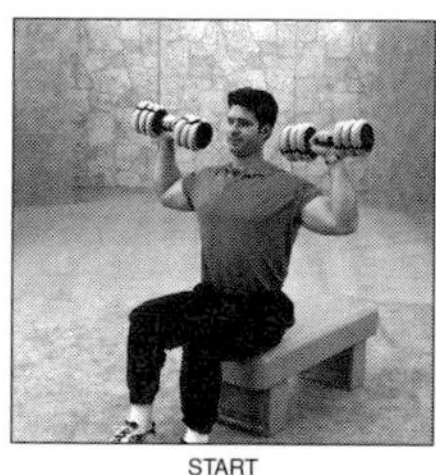

START

FINISH

7. Shoulder Press
15 reps

- Press weights with elbows out from sides.
- Palms facing forward.

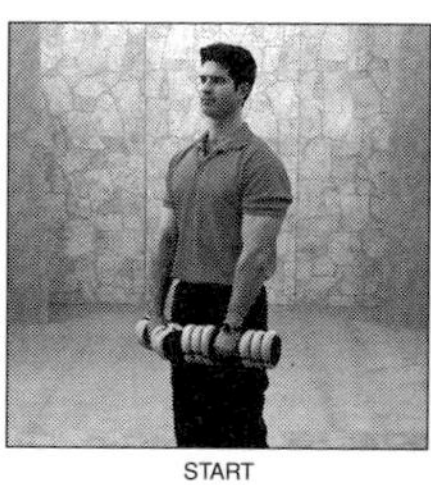

START

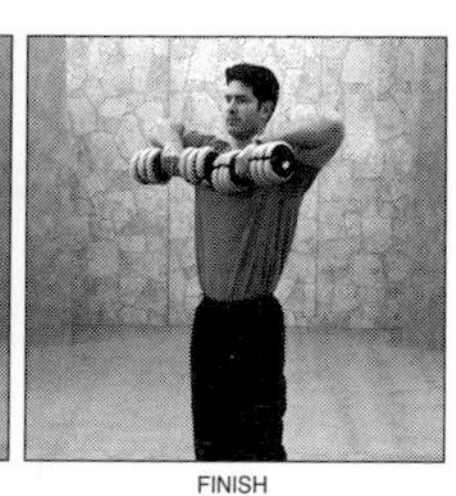

FINISH

8. Upright Rows
15 reps

- Pull weights to chin.
- Elbows should be higher than weights at finish.

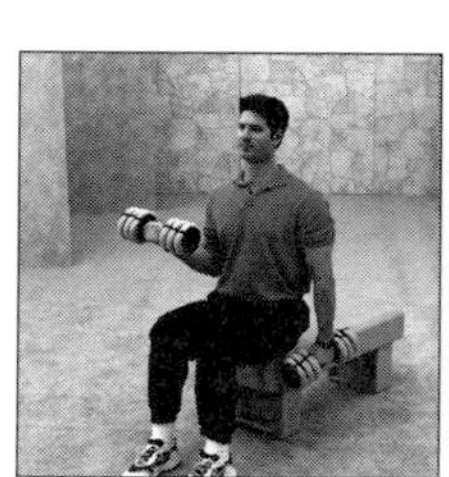

START

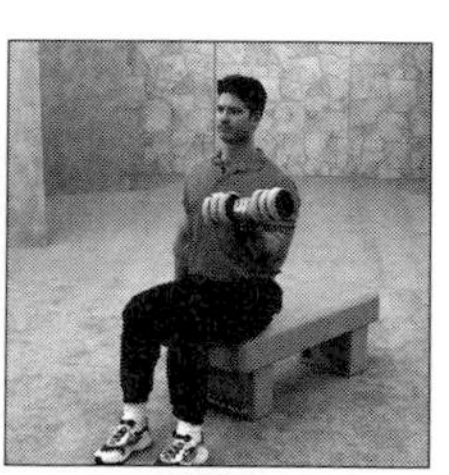

FINISH

9. Alternating Seated Dumbbell Curl
10 reps each arm

- Chest out and shoulders back.
- Keep elbows to your side.
- Palms up at top. • Don't swing weights.

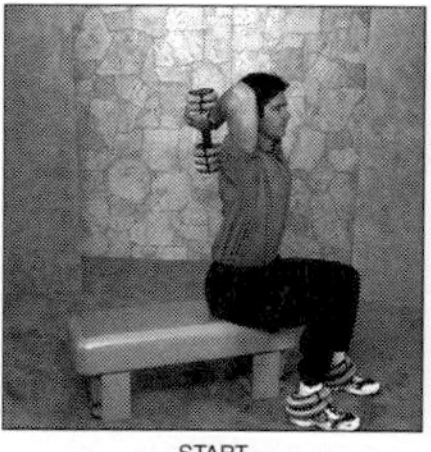

START

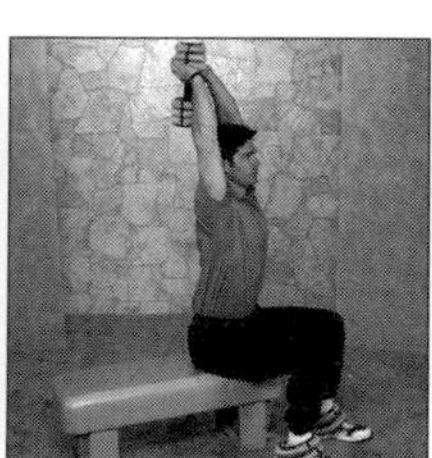

FINISH

10. Overhead Tricep Extension
10 reps

- Extend weight over head.
- Keep elbows up and close to head.

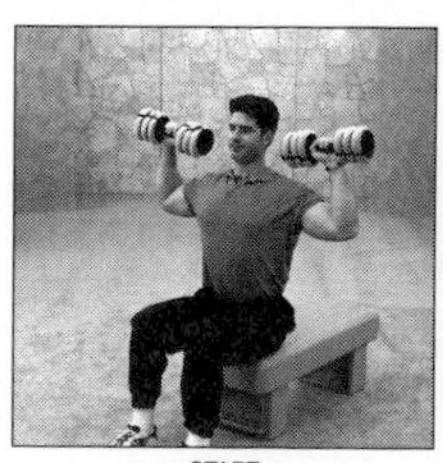

START

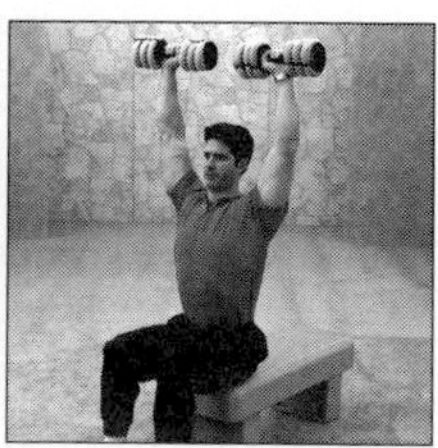

FINISH

11. Shoulder Press
15 reps

- Press weights with elbows out from sides.
- Palms facing forward.

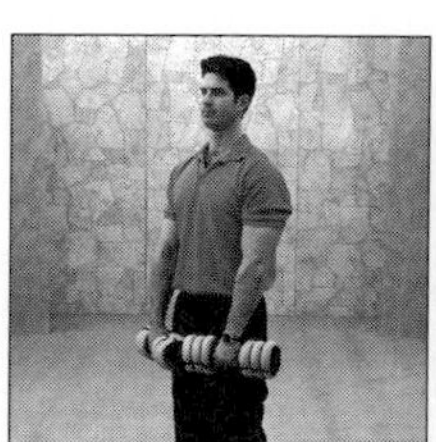

START

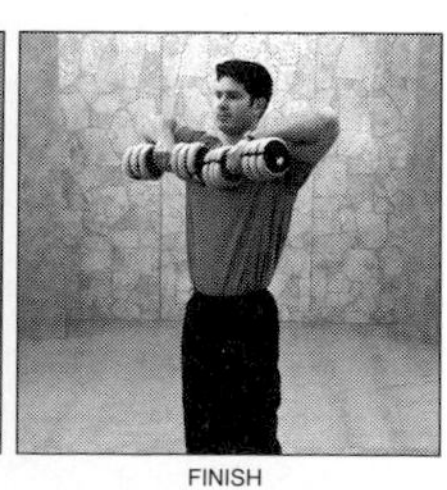

FINISH

12. Upright Rows
15 reps

- Pull weights to chin.
- Elbows should be higher than weights at finish.

THE CAMPITELLI ADVANCED 10 MINUTE EXERCISE METHOD

WOMEN'S WORKOUT #6 • PAGE 1

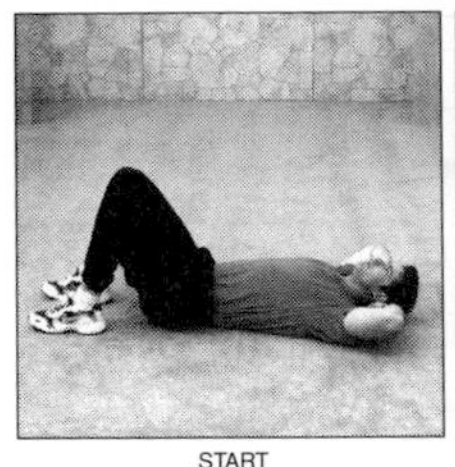
START

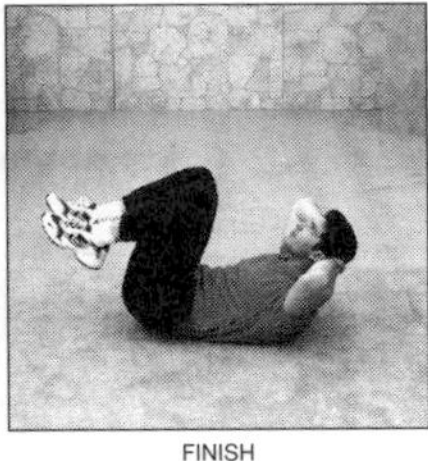
FINISH

1. V-Crunch
20 reps

- Draw knees to chest as you lift shoulder from the floor.
- Exhale as knees and shoulders come up.

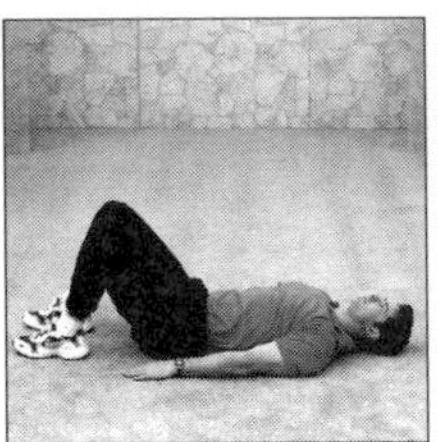
START

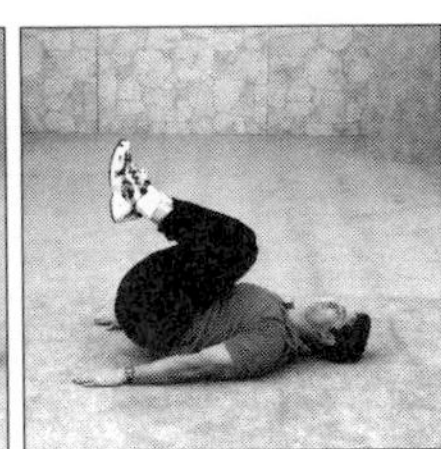
FINISH

2. Tucks
20 reps

- Knees stay bent.
- Curl up until glutes come off floor.
- Exhale as knees come toward head.

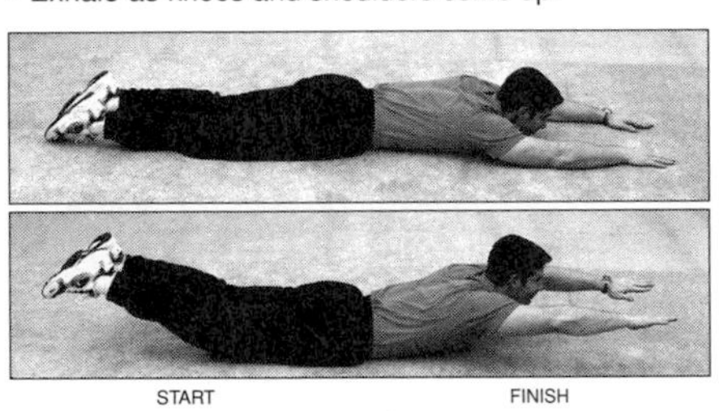
START FINISH

3. Supermans
20 reps

- Raise both hands and legs at the same time.
- Hold briefly at top.

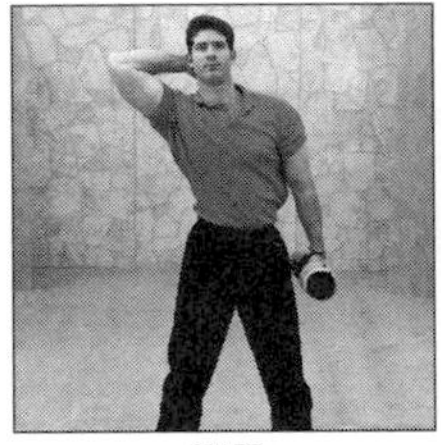
START

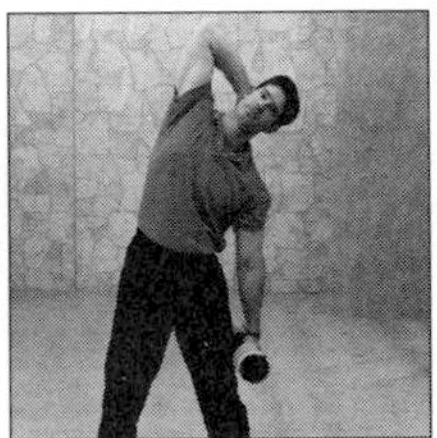
FINISH

4. Side Bends with Dumbbell
20 reps Right/Left

- Feet shoulder width apart.
- Pull DB up the side of leg.
- Keep shoulders, back and chest out.

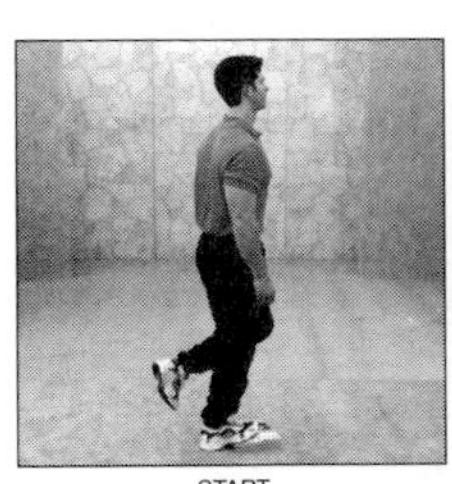
START

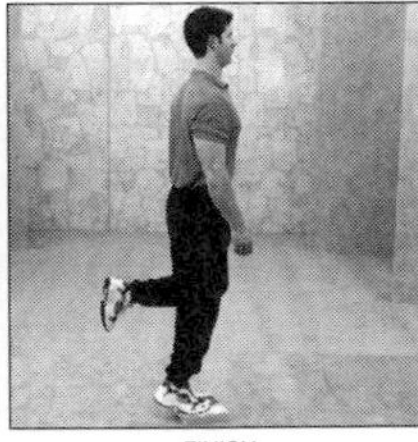
FINISH

5. Standing Calf Raise
20 reps Right/Left

- Place ball of foot on step or book and raise heal.
- Keep knee straight.

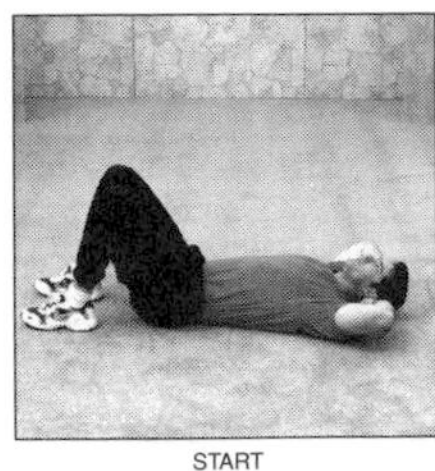
START

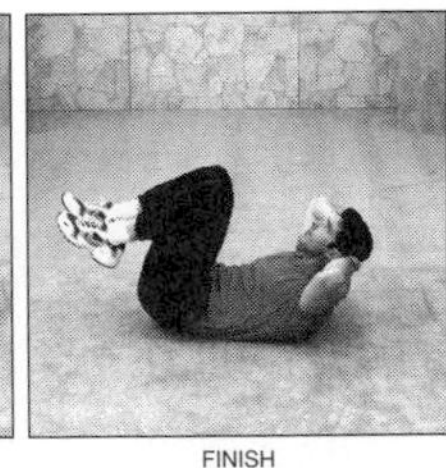
FINISH

6. V-Crunch
20 reps

- Draw knees to chest as you lift shoulder from the floor.
- Exhale as knees and shoulders come up.

THE CAMPITELLI ADVANCED 10 MINUTE EXERCISE METHOD

WOMEN'S WORKOUT #6 • PAGE 2

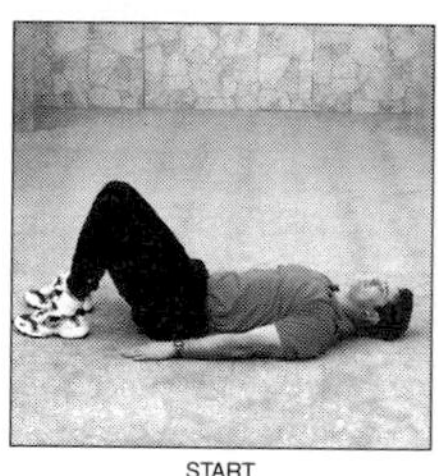

START FINISH

7. Tucks
20 reps

- Knees stay bent.
- Curl up until glutes come off floor.
- Exhale as knees come toward head.

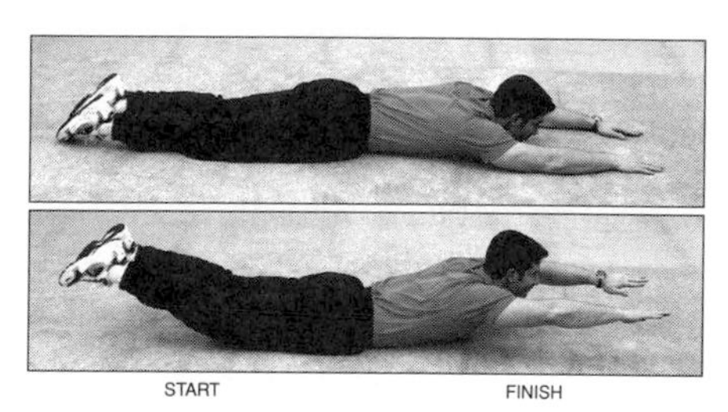

START FINISH

8. Superman's
20 reps

- Raise both hands and legs at the same time.
- Hold breifly at top.

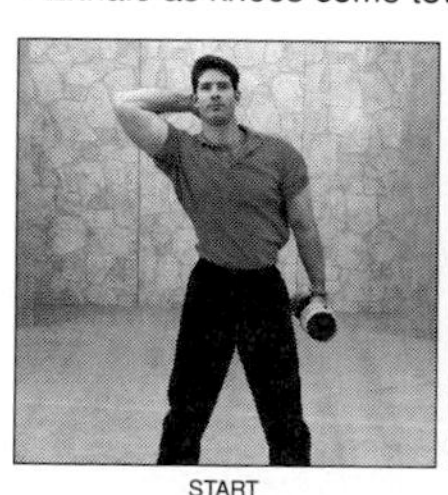

START

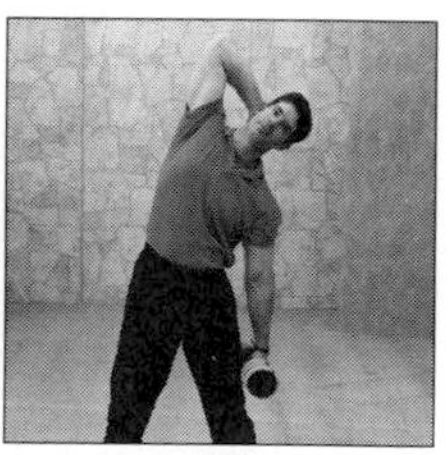

FINISH

9. Side Bends with Dumbbell
20 reps Right/Left

- Feet shoulder width apart.
- Pull DB up the side of leg.
- Keep shoulders, back and chest out.

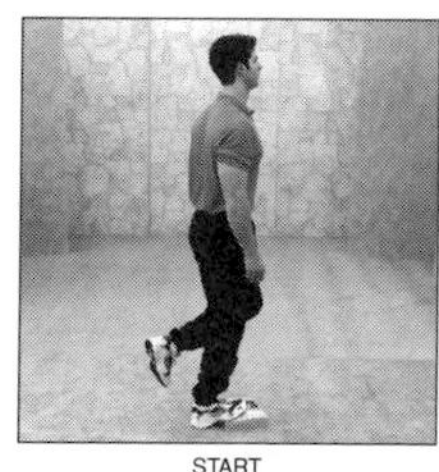

START

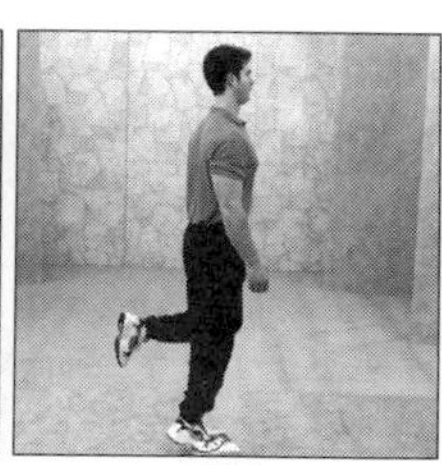

FINISH

10. Standing Calf Raise
20 reps Right/Left

- Use step or book for elevation.
- Raise heel up.
- Keep knees straight during movement.

THE CAMPITELLI ADVANCED 10 MINUTE EXERCISE METHOD

WOMEN'S WORKOUT #7 • PAGE 1

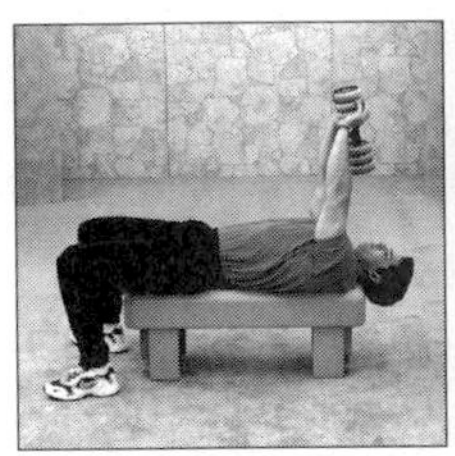

START

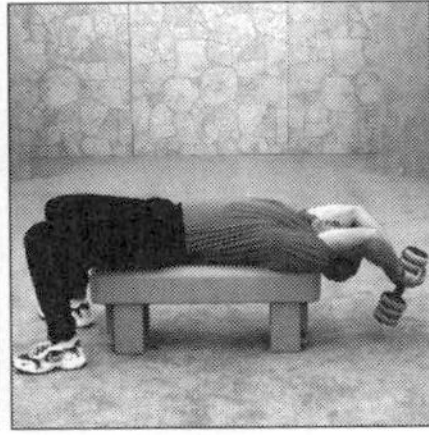

FINISH

1. Dumbbell Pullover
20 reps

- Relax abdomen. Keep elbows in toward body.
- Inhale as weight goes over head.
- Exhale as weight is pulled up.

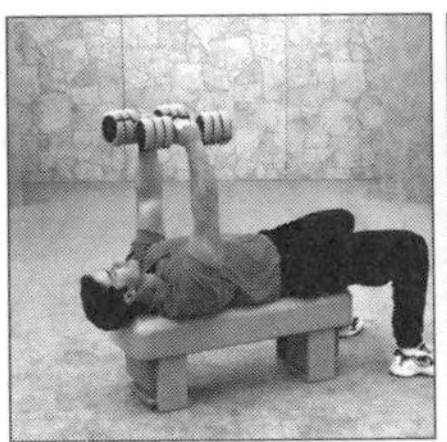

START

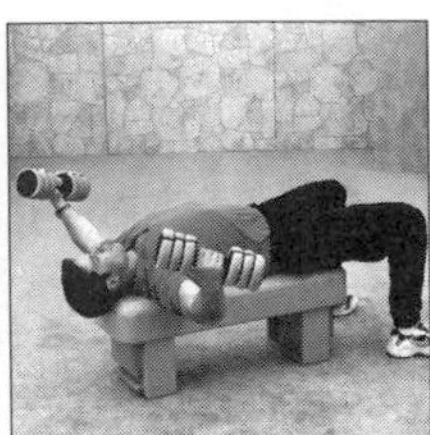

FINISH

2. Dumbbell Fly
20 reps

- Elbows slightly bent with palms facing each other.
- Lower weights out to the side of body until weight is parallel to body. Keep elbow slightly bent.

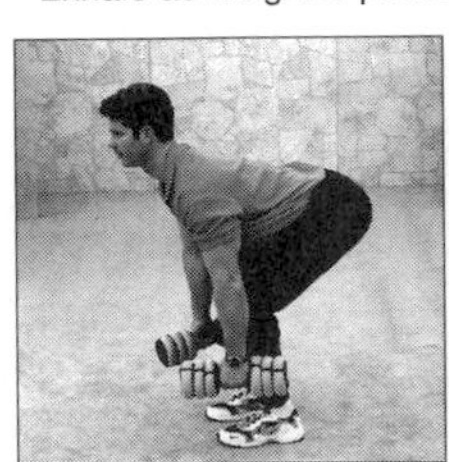

START

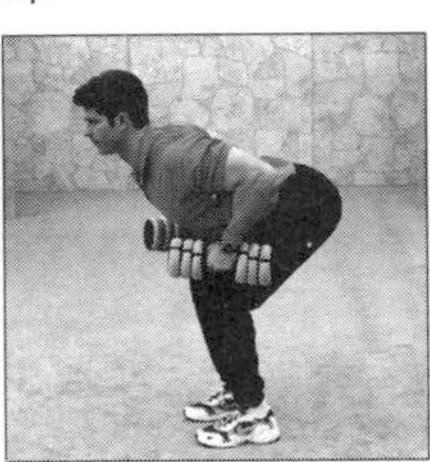

FINISH

3. Dumbbell Row Close Grip
20 reps

- Feet together. Bend at hips, not at waist.
- Back straight. Chest out.
- Head up. Pull weights with elbows close to body.

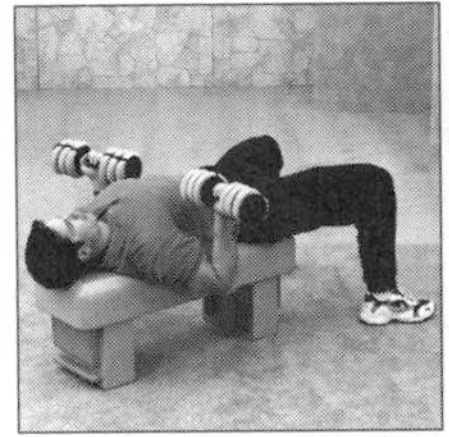

START

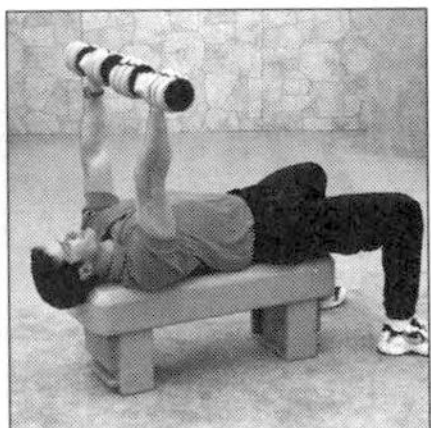

FINISH

4. Lying Dumbbell Press
20 reps

- Hold weights palms toward knees.
- Relax abdomen.
- Lower weights until even with chest.

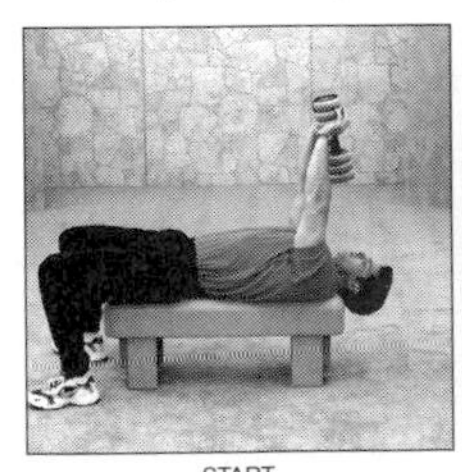

START

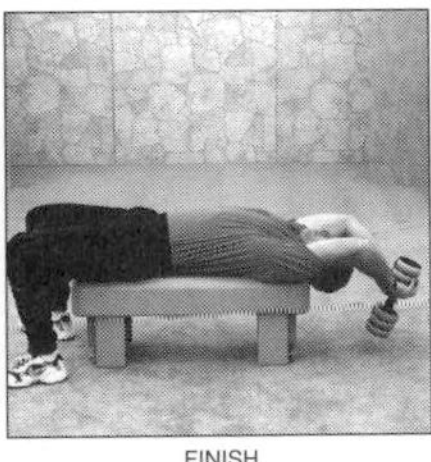

FINISH

5. Dumbbell Pullover
20 reps

- Relax abdomen. Keep elbows in toward body.
- Inhale as weight goes over head.
- Exhale as weight is pulled up.

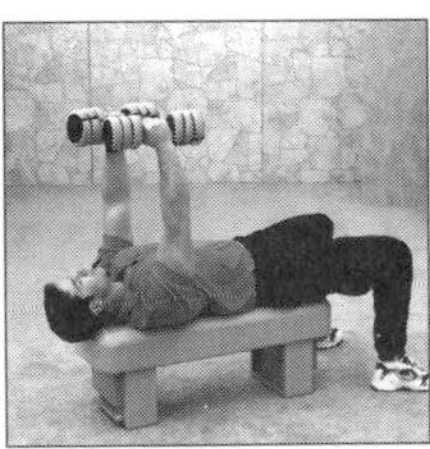

START

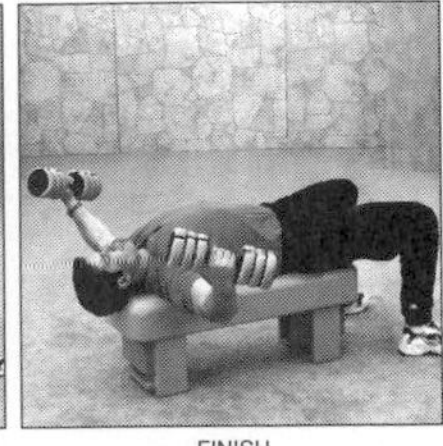

FINISH

6. Dumbbell Fly
20 reps

- Elbows slightly bent with palms facing each other.
- Lower weights out to the side of body until weight is parallel to body. Keep elbow slightly bent.

THE CAMPITELLI ADVANCED 10 MINUTE EXERCISE METHOD

WOMEN'S WORKOUT #7 • PAGE 2

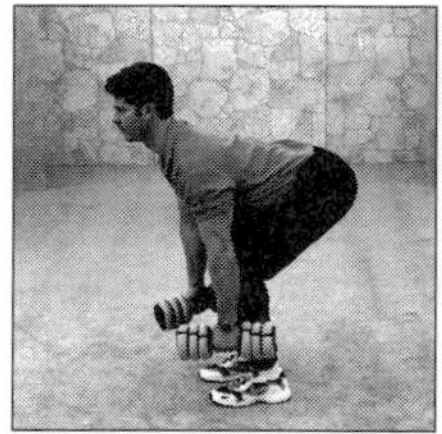

START FINISH

7. Dumbbell Row Close Grip
20 reps

- Feet together. Bend at hips, not at waist.
- Back straight. Chest out.
- Head up. Pull weights with elbows close to body.

START FINISH

8. Lying Dumbbell Press
20 reps

- Hold weights palms toward knees.
- Relax abdomen.
- Lower weights until even with chest.

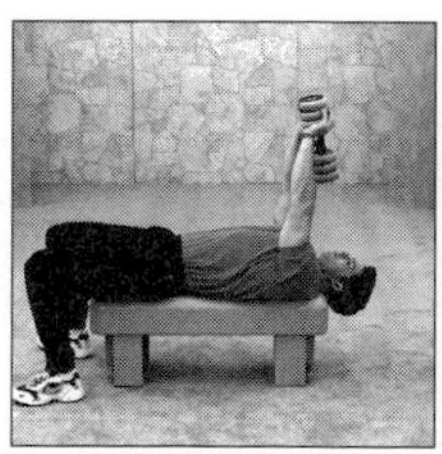

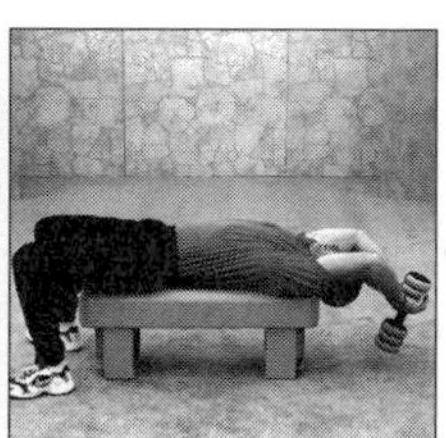

START FINISH

9. Dumbbell Pullover
20 reps

- Relax abdomen. Keep elbows in toward body.
- Inhale as weight goes over head.
- Exhale as weight goes up.

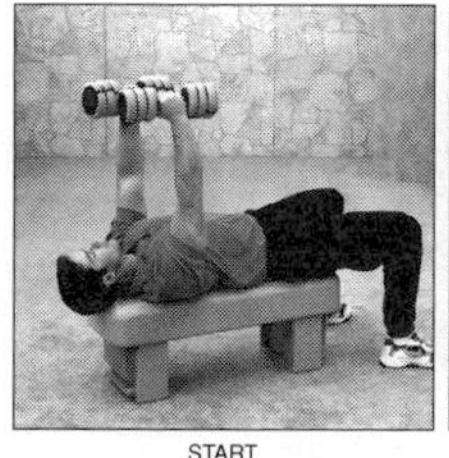

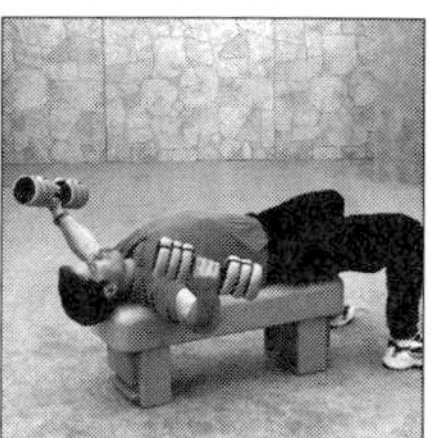

START FINISH

10. Dumbbell Fly
20 reps

- Elbows slightly bent with palms facing each other.
- Lower weights out to the side of body until weight is parallel to body. Keep elbow slightly bent.

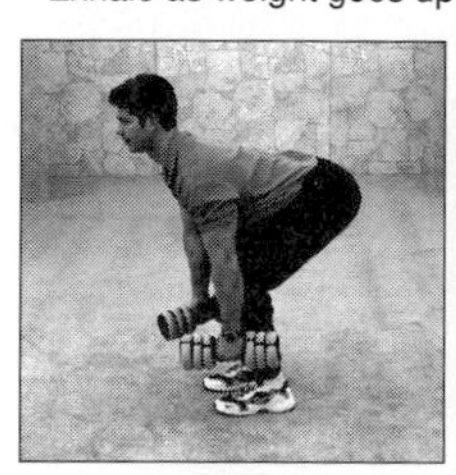

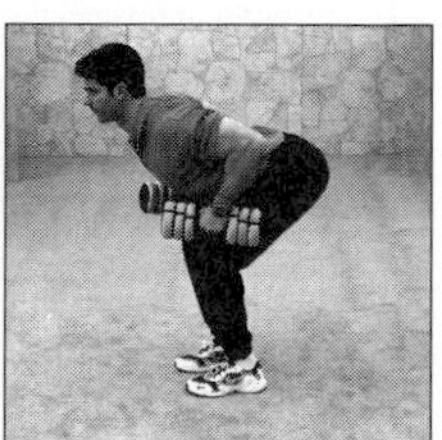

START FINISH

11. Dumbbell Row Close Grip
20 reps both arms

- Feet together. Bend at hips, not at waist.
- Back straight. Chest out.
- Head up. Pull weights with elbows close to body.

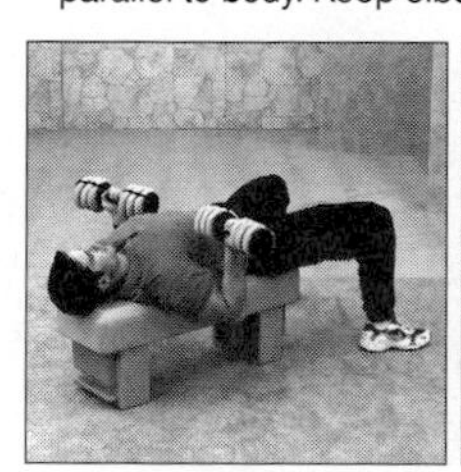

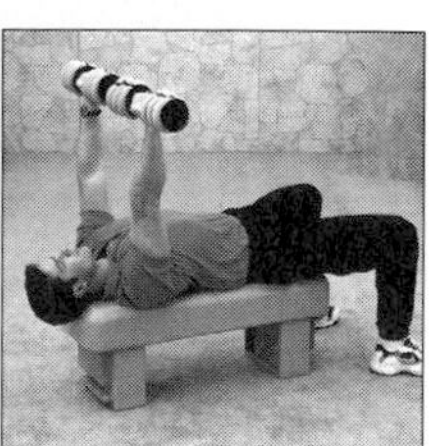

START FINISH

12. Lying Dumbbell Press
20 reps

- Hold weights palms toward knees.
- Relax abdomen.
- Lower weights until even with chest.

THE CAMPITELLI ADVANCED 10 MINUTE EXERCISE METHOD

WOMEN'S WORKOUT #8• PAGE 1

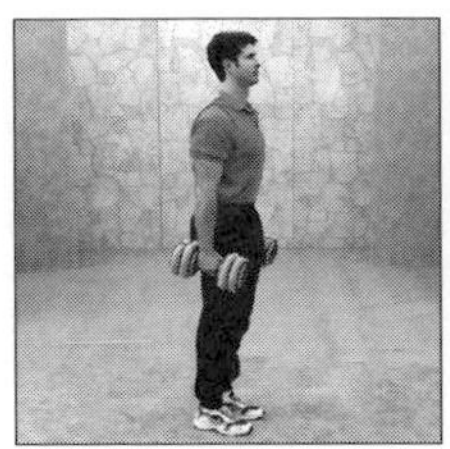
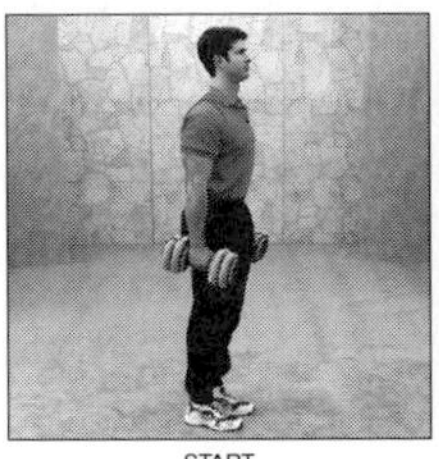

START FINISH

1. Dumbbell Squats
15 reps

- Feet 4-8 inches apart. DBs at side.
- Place weight evenly on heels and ball of feet.
- Back straight. Head up. Push with heels.

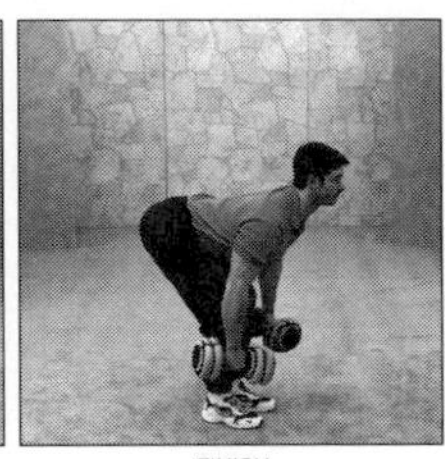

START FINISH

2. Dumbbell Deadlift
15 reps

- Knees slightly bent with feet slightly apart
- Keep low back locked with upper torso. Head up.
- Bend at hips, not at waist. Chest out. Back is flat.

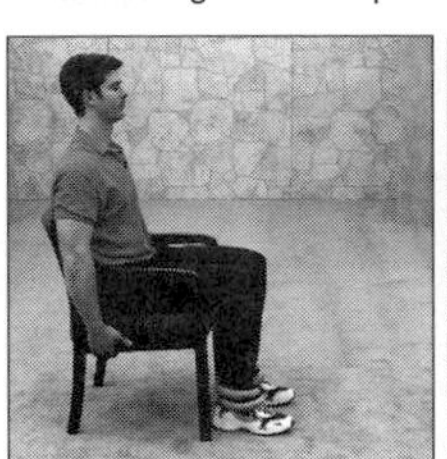
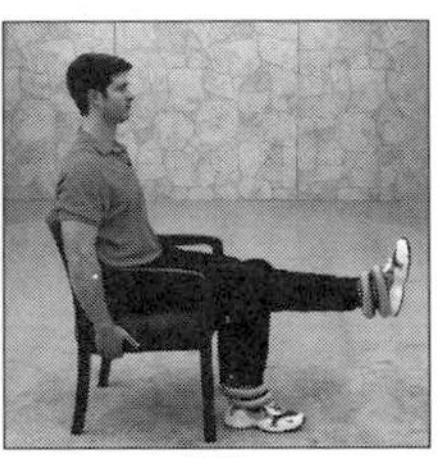

START FINISH

3. Seated Leg Extensions w/Ankle Weights
15 reps Right/Left

- Extend foot out with weights, hold leg straight for a brief pause and then return.

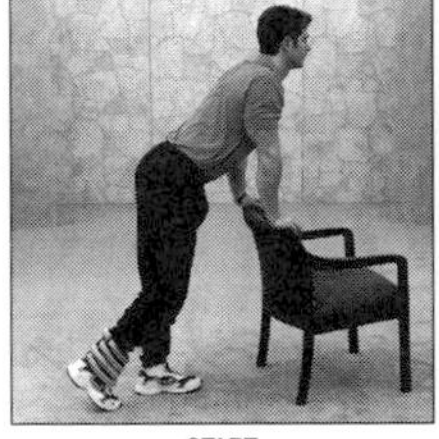
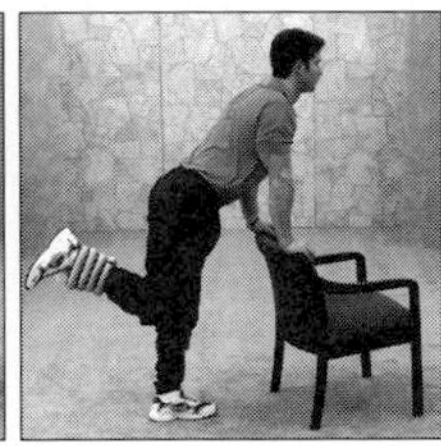

START FINISH

4. Standing Leg Curls w/Ankle Weights
15 reps Right/Left

- Raise leg bending knee.
- Use chair for balance.
- Keep toe pointed down.
- Hold briefly at top position.

THE CAMPITELLI ADVANCED 10 MINUTE EXERCISE METHOD

WOMEN'S WORKOUT #8 • PAGE 2

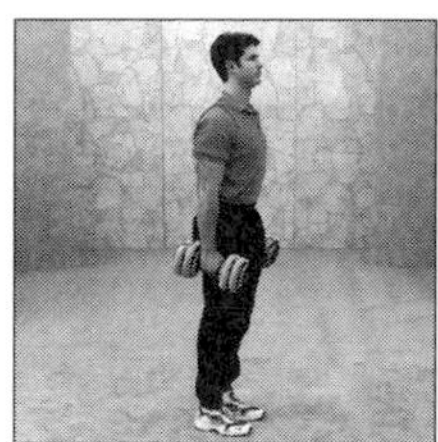

START FINISH

5. Dumbbell Squats
15 reps

- Feet 4-8 inches apart. DBs at side.
- Place weight evenly on heels and balls of feet.
- Back straight. Head up. Push with heels.

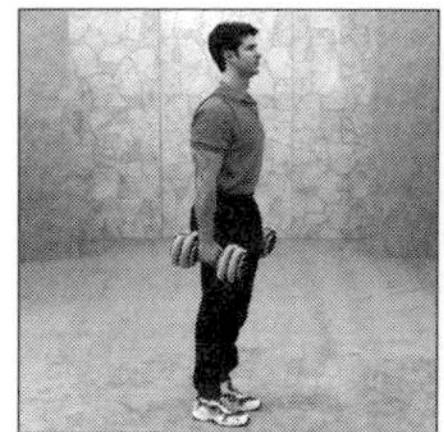

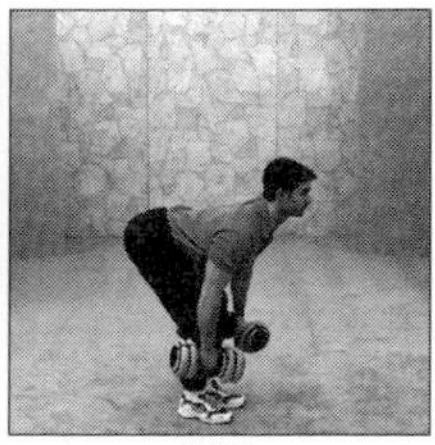

START FINISH

6. Dumbbell Deadlift
15 reps

- Knees slightly bent with feet slightly apart.
- Keep low back locked with upper torso.
- Bend at hips, not at waist. Head up/chest out.
- Back is flat.

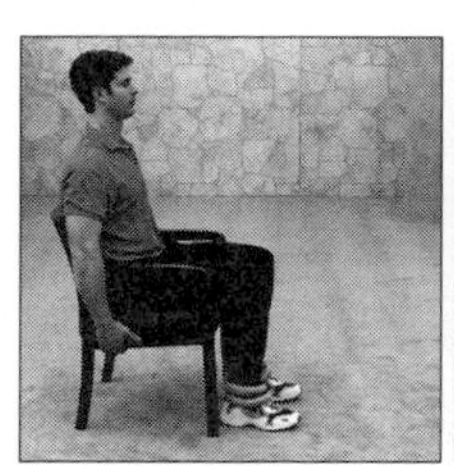

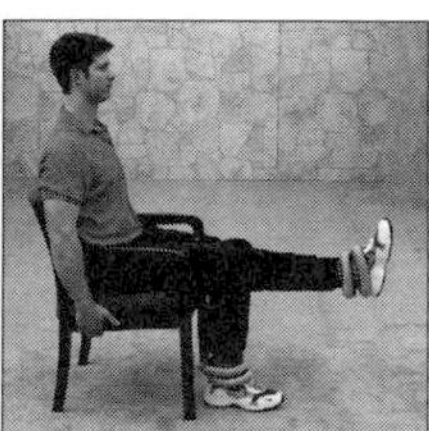

START FINISH

7. Seated Leg Extensions w/Ankle Weights
15 reps Right/Left

- Extend foot out with weights, hold leg straight for a brief pause and then return.

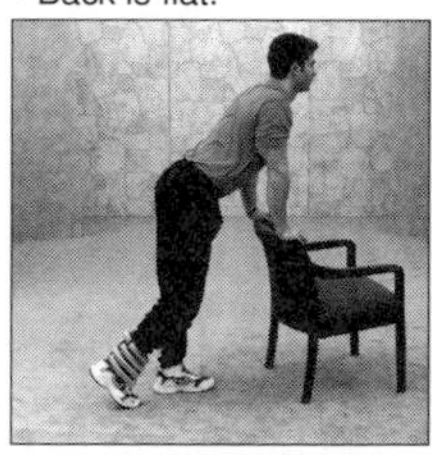

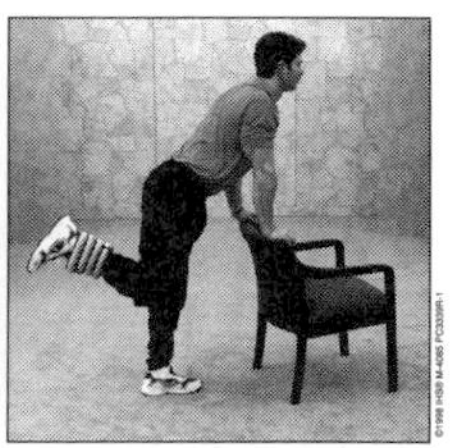

START FINISH

8. Standing Leg Curls w/Ankle Weights
15 reps Right/Left

- Raise leg bending knee.
- Use chair for balance.
- Keep toe pointed down.
- Hold briefly at top position.

THE CAMPITELLI ADVANCED 10 MINUTE EXERCISE METHOD

WOMEN'S WORKOUT #9 • PAGE 1

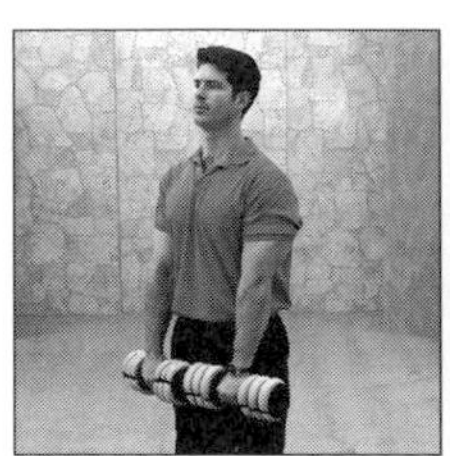

START FINISH

1. Upright row

10 reps

- Pull weights to chin.
- Elbows should be higher than weights at finish.

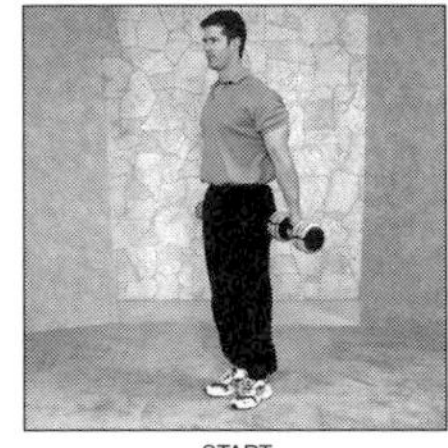

START

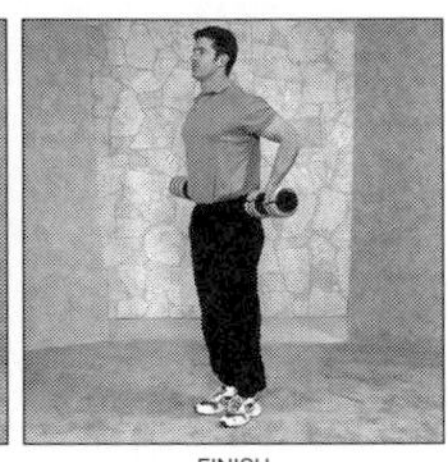

FINISH

2. Rear Dumbbell Row

10 reps

- Stand with DBs palms forward.
- Pull DBs up with elbow to the rear.
- Pinky fingers to armpit. Elbows high as they will go.

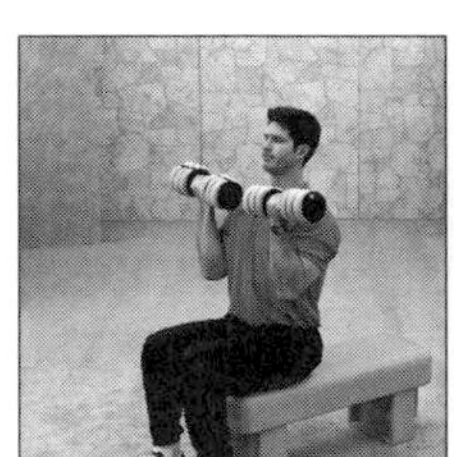

START

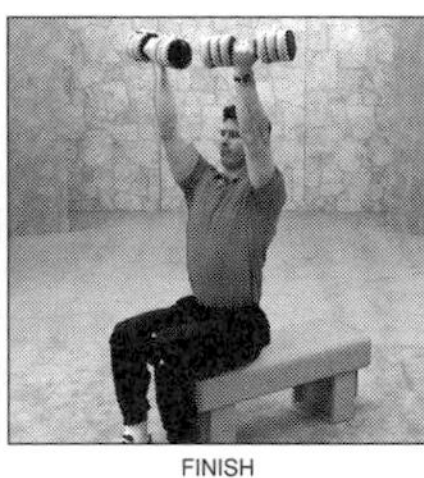

FINISH

3. Arnold Press

10 reps

- DBs in front of neck.
- Palms back.
- Press over head keeping elbows in front.

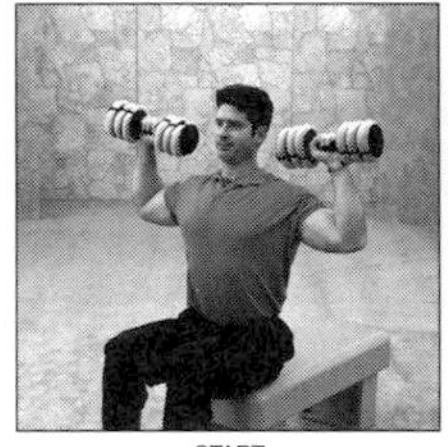

START

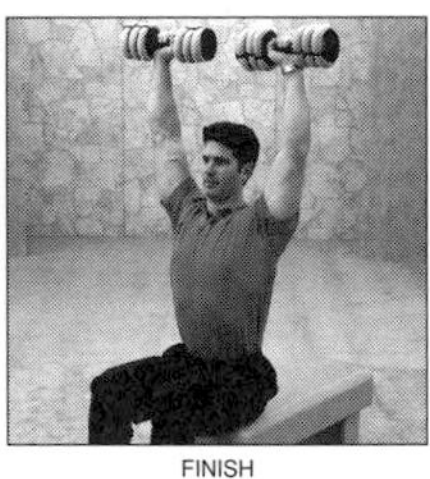

FINISH

4. Shoulder Press

10 reps

- Press weights with elbows out from sides.
- Palms facing forward.

THE CAMPITELLI ADVANCED 10 MINUTE EXERCISE METHOD

WOMEN'S WORKOUT #9 • PAGE 2

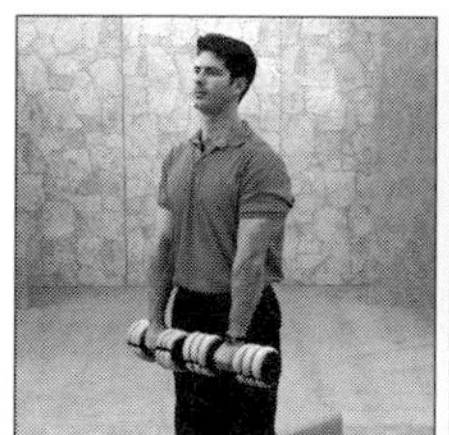

START FINISH

5. Reverse Curl
10 reps

- Palms down.
- Elbows at side.
- Don't swing.

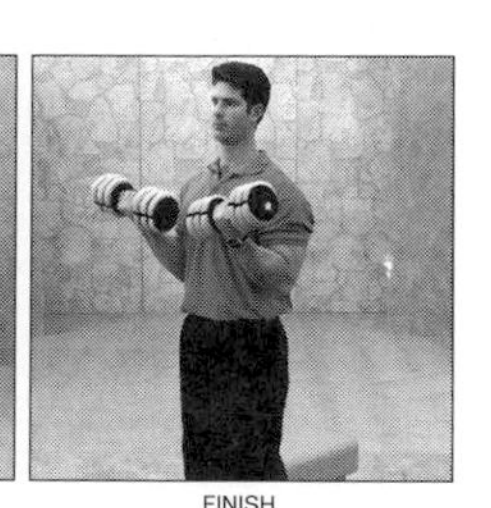

START FINISH

6. Regular Curl
10 reps

- Palms up.
- Elbows at side.
- Don't swing.

START FINISH

7. Lying Tricep extension
10 reps

- Elbows pointed straight up.
- Hands in "thumbs up position."
- Weights come back to ears.

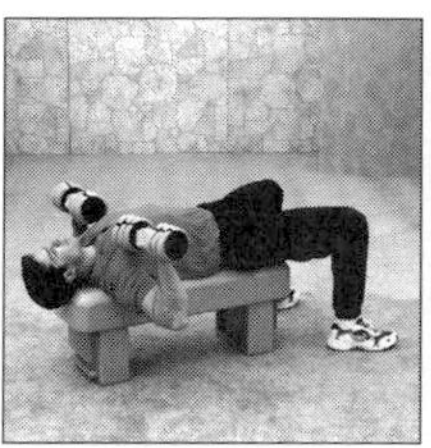

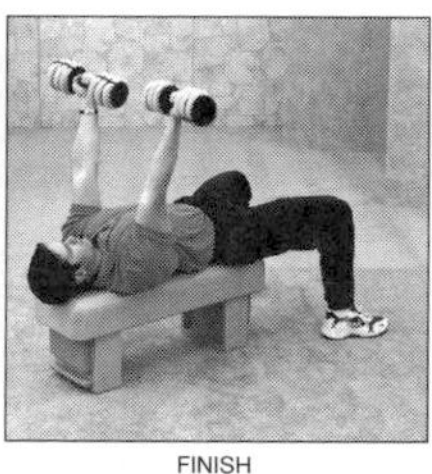

START FINISH

8. Reverse Tricep Press
10 reps

- Hands in "palms up position."
- Elbows stay close to body.
- Lower to side of chest.

REPEAT ENTIRE SEQUENCE (1 THRU 8) FOR A TOTAL OF THREE TIMES

THE CAMPITELLI ADVANCED 10 MINUTE EXERCISE METHOD

WOMEN'S WORKOUT #10 • PAGE 1

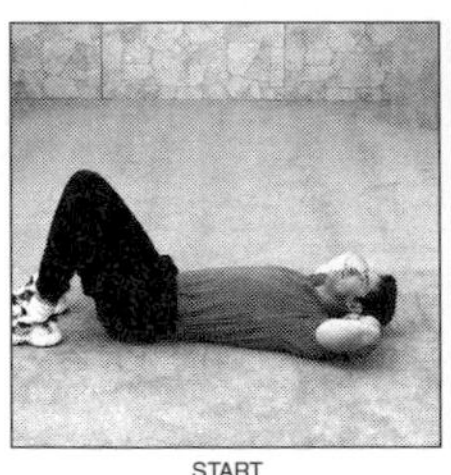

START FINISH

1. Crunch
20 reps

- Push lower back into floor.
- Focus on ceiling, not knees.
- Breathe out as you go up.

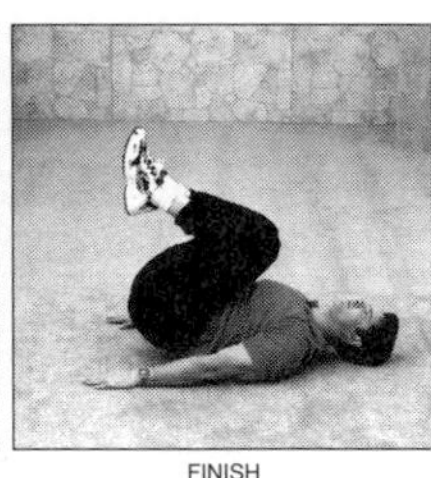

START FINISH

2. Tucks
20 reps

- Knees stay bent.
- Curl up until glutes come off floor.
- Exhale as knees come toward head.

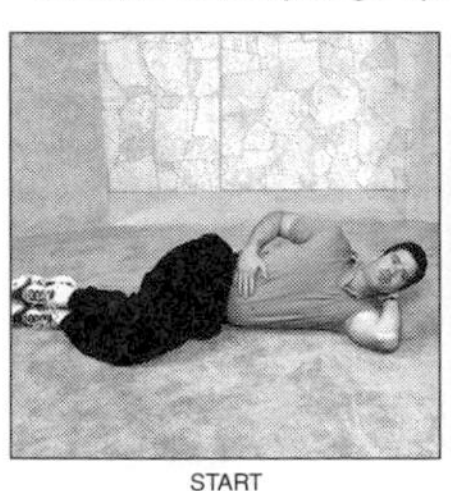
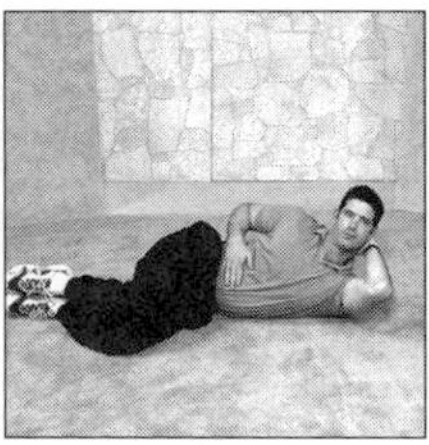

START FINISH

3. Side Crunch
20 reps Right/Left

- Contract top side to pull shoulder to hip.
- Try to lift bottom shoulder off ground.

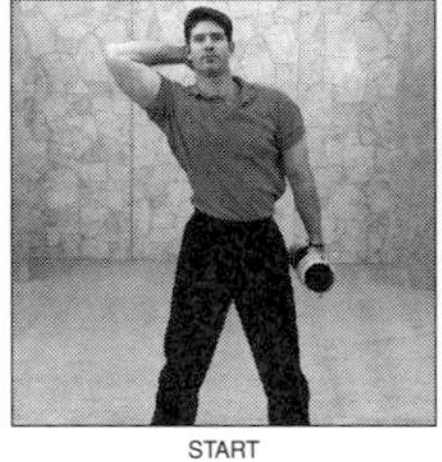
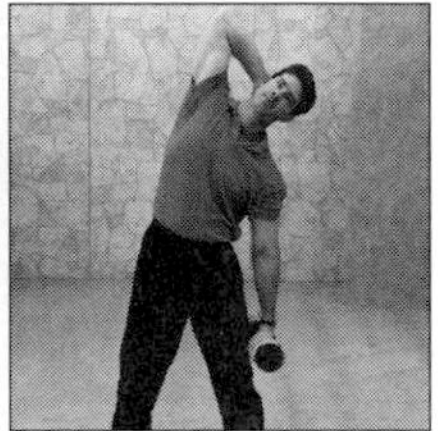

START FINISH

4. Side Bends with Dumbbell
20 reps Right/Left

- Feet shoulder width apart.
- Pull DB up the side of leg.
- Keep shoulders, back and chest out.

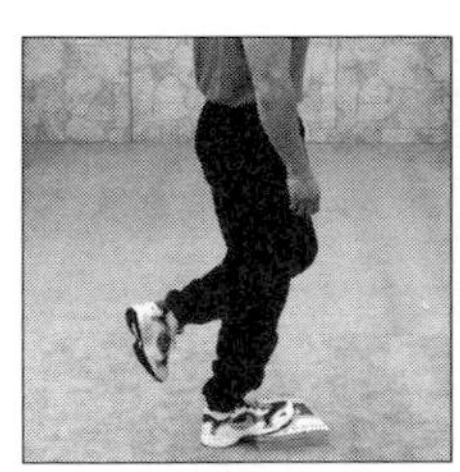
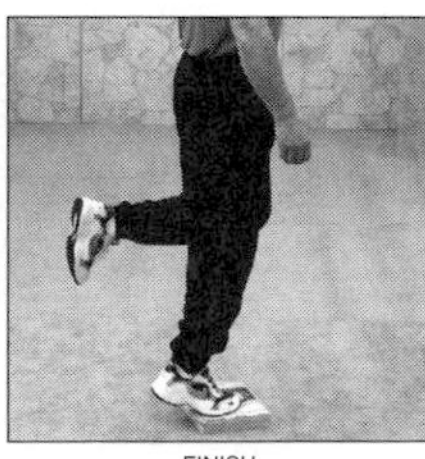

START FINISH

5. Standing Calve Raise
20 reps Right/Left

- Use step or book for elevation.
- Raise heel up.
- Keep knees straight during movement.

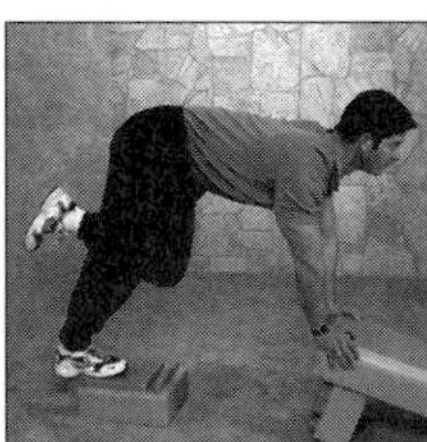
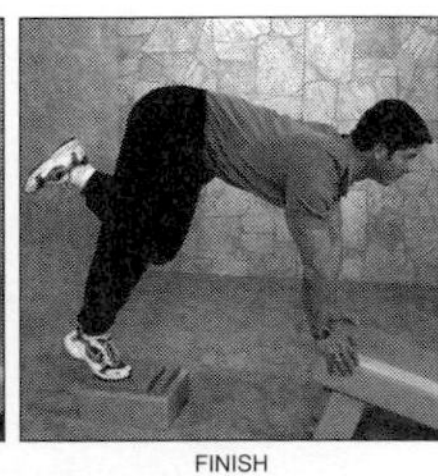

START FINISH

6. Donkey Calf Raise
10 reps Right/Left

- Place ball of foot on step or book and raise heal.
- Keep knee straight.

THE CAMPITELLI ADVANCED 10 MINUTE EXERCISE METHOD

WOMEN'S WORKOUT #10 • PAGE 2

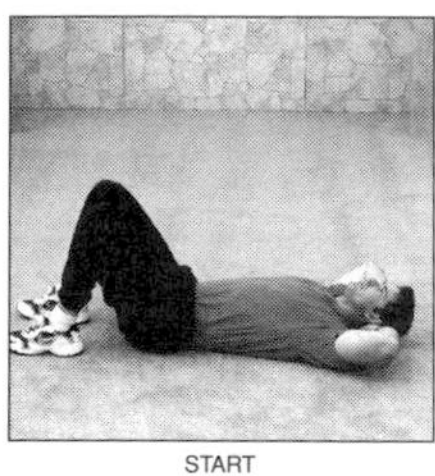

START FINISH

7. Crunch
15 reps

- Push lower back into floor.
- Focus on ceiling, not knees.
- Breathe out as you go up.

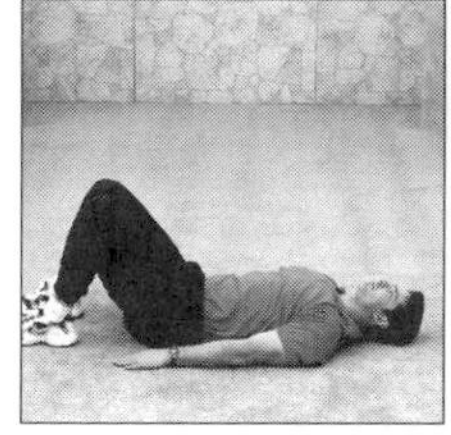
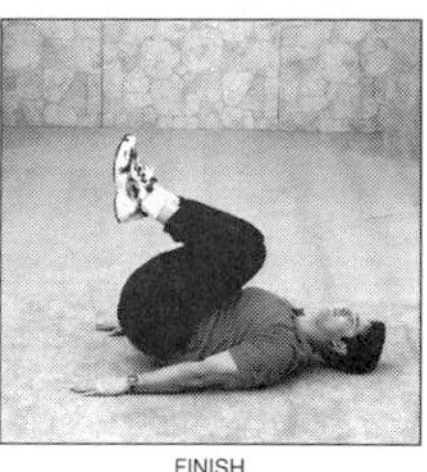

START FINISH

8. Tucks
15 reps

- Knees stay bent.
- Curl up until glutes come off floor.
- Exhale as knees come toward head.

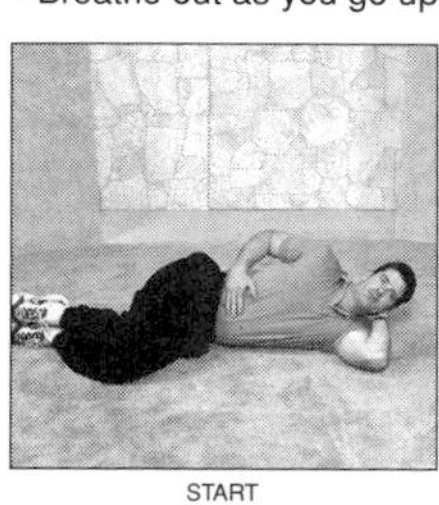
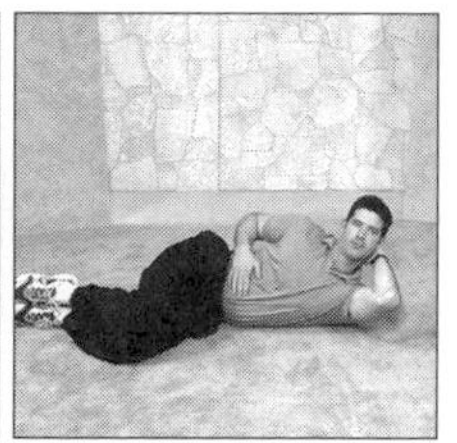

START FINISH

9. Side Crunch
15 reps Right/Left

- Contract top side to pull shoulder to hip.
- Try to lift bottom shoulder off ground.

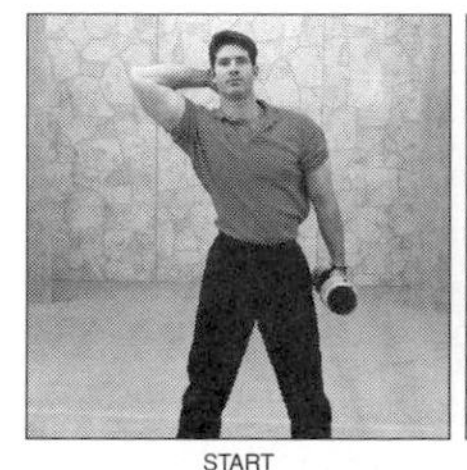
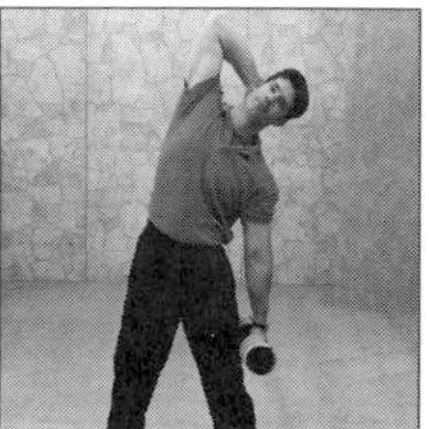

START FINISH

10. Side Bends with Dumbbell
15 reps Right/Left

- Feet shoulder width apart.
- Pull DB up the side of leg.
- Keep shoulders, back and chest out.

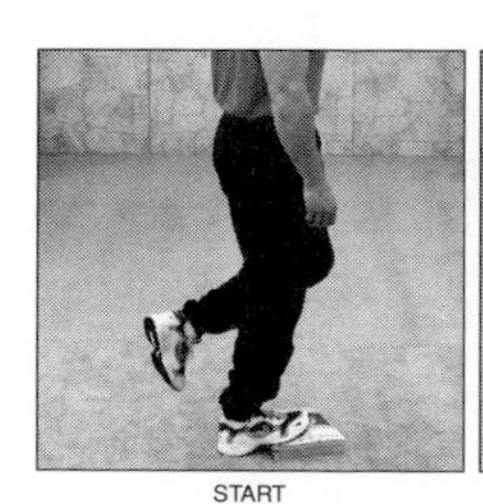
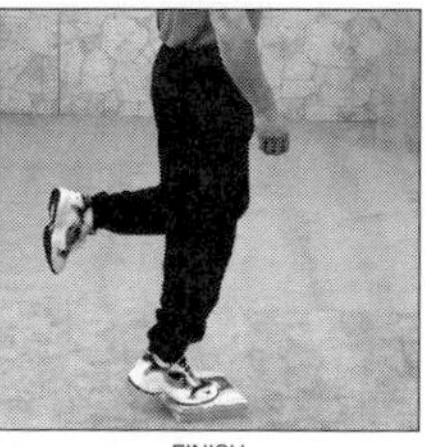

START FINISH

11. Standing Calve Raise
10 reps Right/Left

- Use step or book for elevation.
- Raise heel up.
- Keep knees straight during movement.

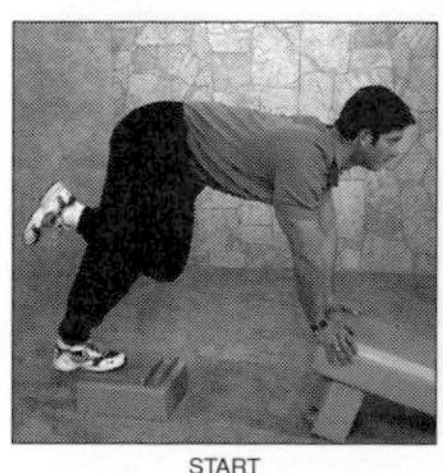
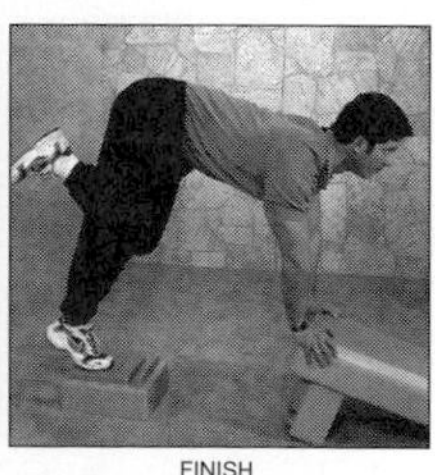

START FINISH

12. Donkey Calf Raise
10 reps Right/Left

- Place ball of foot on step or book and raise heal.
- Keep knee straight.

THE CAMPITELLI ADVANCED 10 MINUTE EXERCISE METHOD

WOMEN'S WORKOUT #11 • PAGE 1

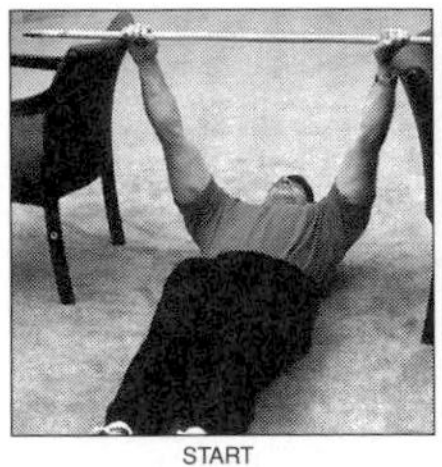

START FINISH

1. Overhand Pullup

10 reps

- Keep body straight.
- Hands out to edge of chair for bar stability.
- Pull chest to bar. Pull up as far as you can.

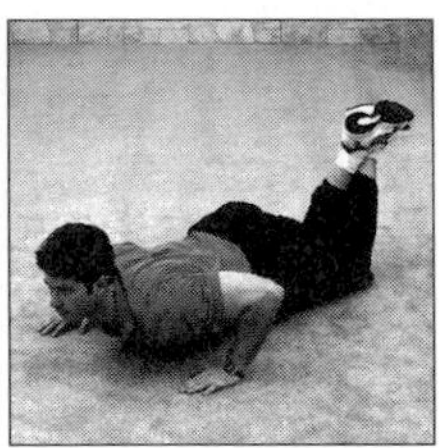

START FINISH

2. Modified Pushup

10 reps

- Heads up. Body straight.
- Hands are slightly wider than shoulders.
- Lower body and chest 2-3 inches from floor.

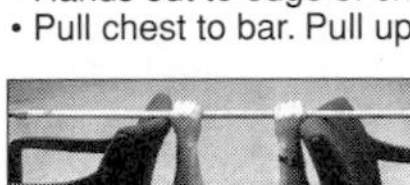

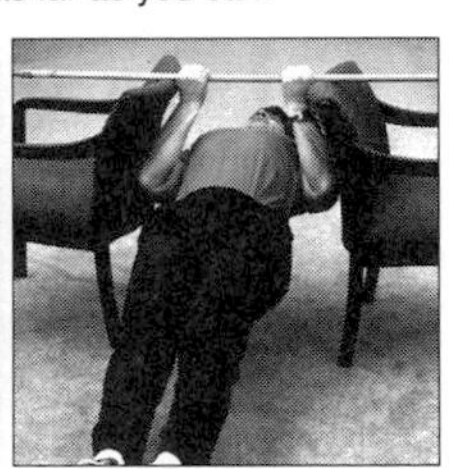

START FINISH

3. Underhand Grip Pullup

10 reps

- Move chairs into shoulder width.
- Keep body straight.
- Pull chest to bar. Pull up as far as you can.

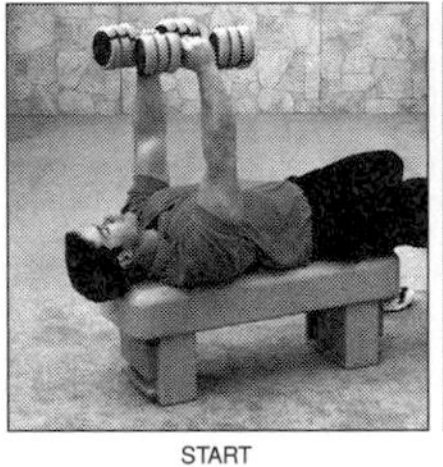

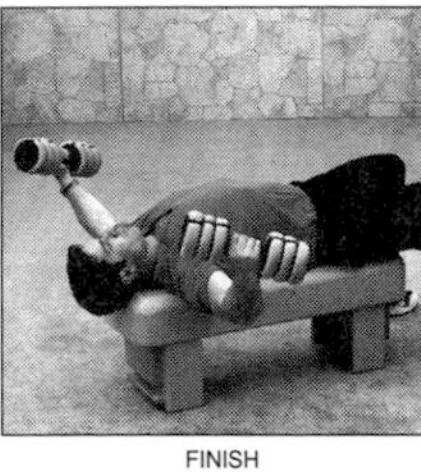

START FINISH

4. Dumbbell Fly

15 reps

- Elbows slightly bent with palms facing each other.
- Lower weights out to the side of body until weight is parallel to body. Keep elbow slightly bent.

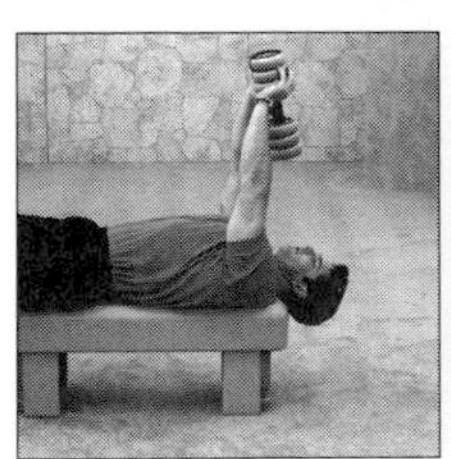

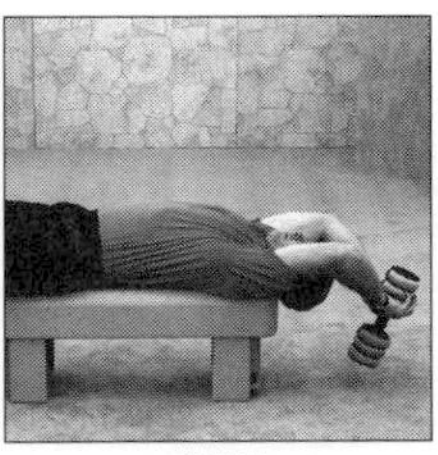

START FINISH

5. Dumbbell Pullover

15 reps

- Relax Abdomen. Keep elbows in toward body.
- Inhale as weight goes over head. Exhale as it goes up.

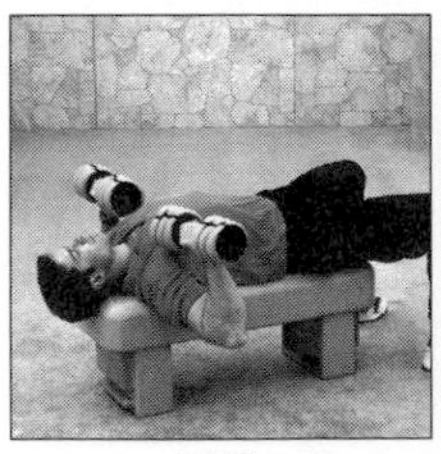

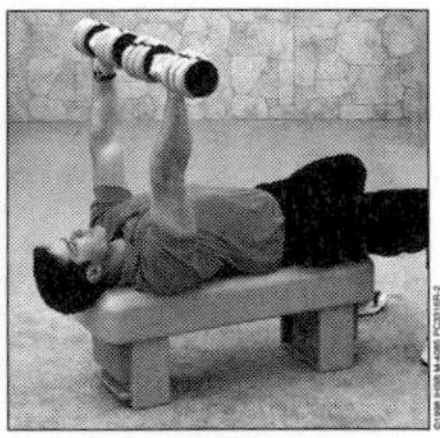

START FINISH

6. Dumbbell Press

15 reps

- Hold weights palms toward knees. Relax abdomen.
- Lower weights until even with chest.

REPEAT ENTIRE SEQUENCE (1 THRU 6) TWO MORE TIMES. END OF ROUTINE. NO PAGE 2.

THE CAMPITELLI ADVANCED 10 MINUTE EXERCISE METHOD

WOMEN'S WORKOUT #12 • PAGE 1

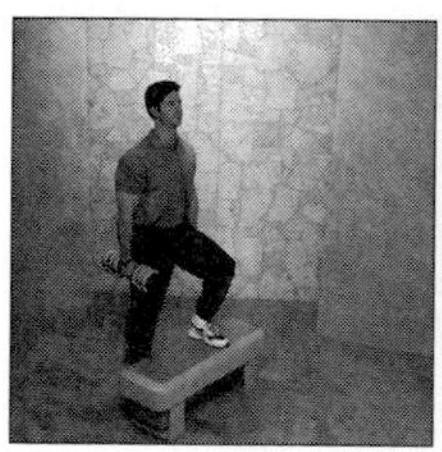
START

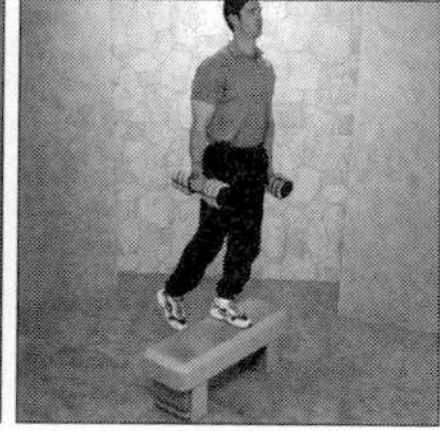
FINISH

1. Step Up With Weights
10 reps Right/Left

- Place entire foot on bench or step.
- Use top leg to push only.
- Look up. Shoulders back.

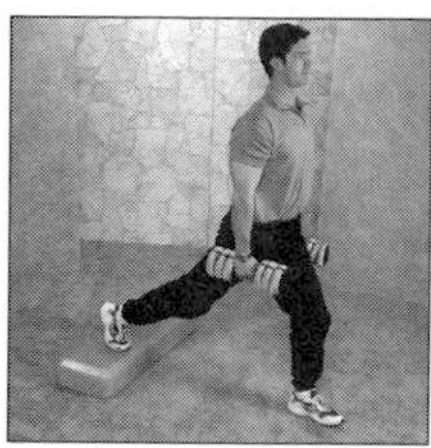
START

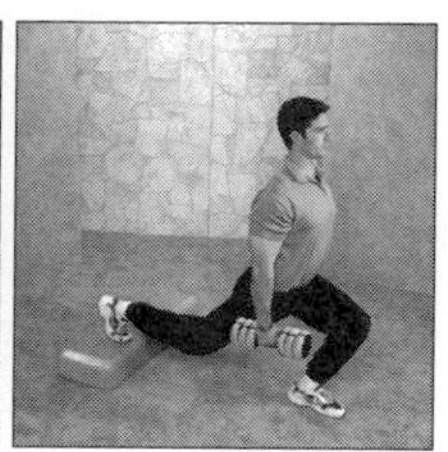
FINISH

2. Dumbbell Lunge with foot on bench
10 reps Right/Left

- Same as regular lunge with DB in one hand.
- Use chair for support and balance.

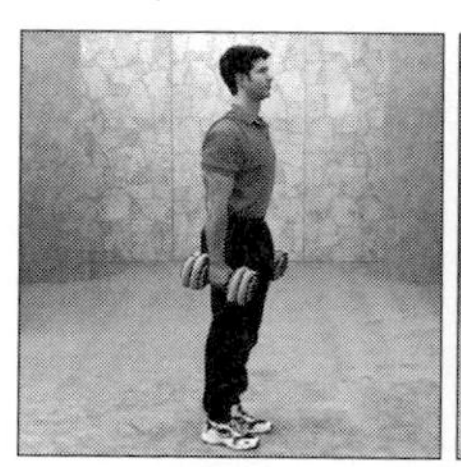
START

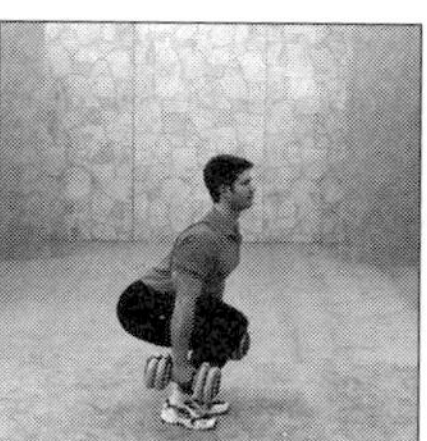
FINISH

3. Dumbbell Squat
10 reps

- Feet 4-8 inches apart. DBs at side.
- Place weight evenly on heels and balls of feet.
- Back straight. Head up. Push with heels.

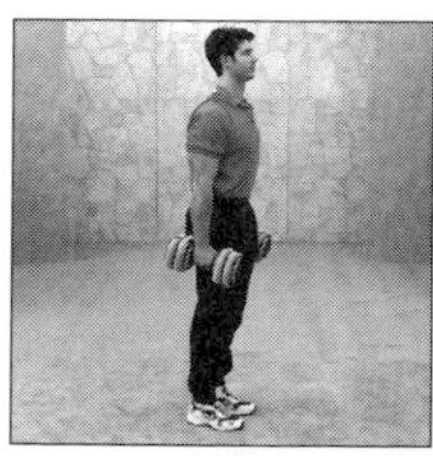
START

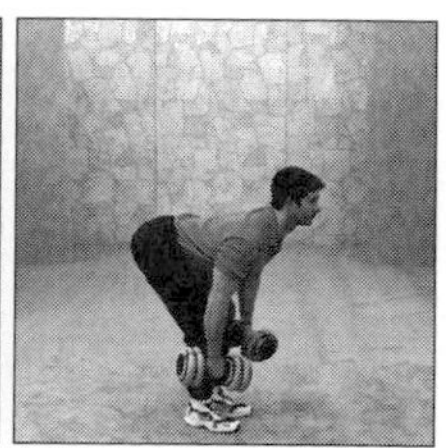
FINISH

4. Dumbbell Deadlift
10 reps

- Knees slightly bent with feet slightly apart.
- Keep low back locked with upper torso.
- Bend at hips, not at waist. Head up/chest out. Back is flat.

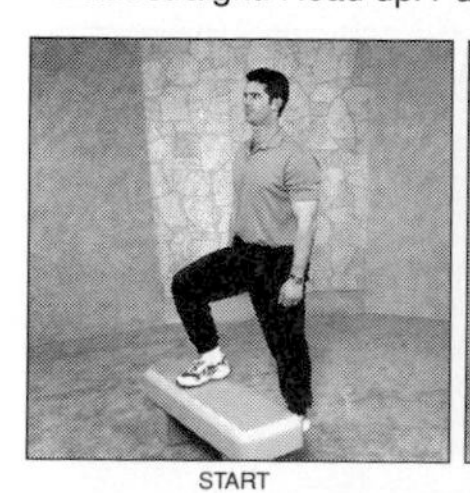
START

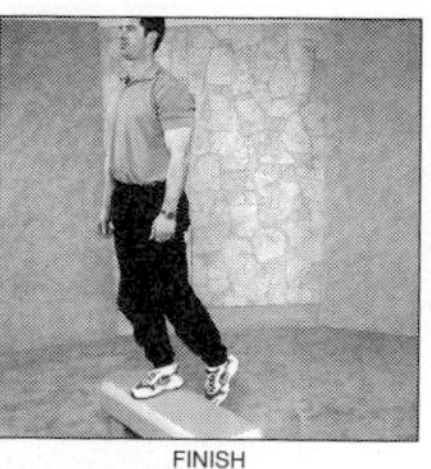
FINISH

5. Step-up without Weights
10 reps Right/Left

- Place whole foot on bench or step. Use top leg to push only. Use wall or chair with free hand for balance.
- Look up. Shoulders back.

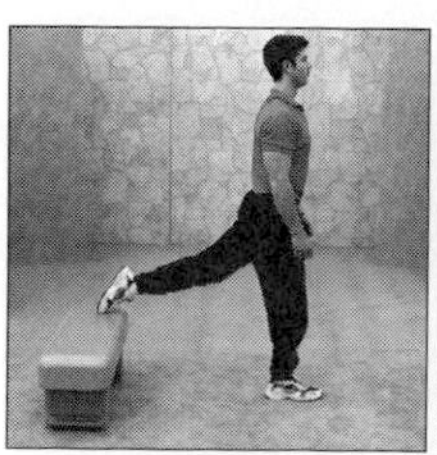
START

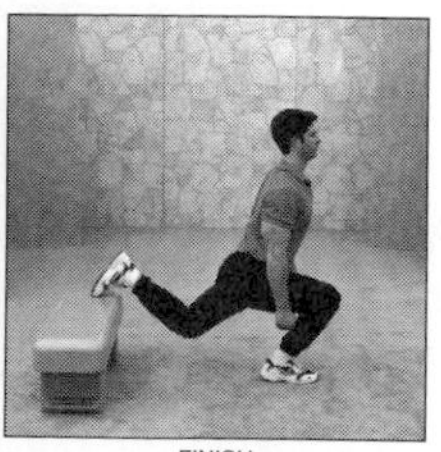
FINISH

6. Lunge with foot on bench - No Weights
10 reps Right/Left

- Same as regular lunge.
- Use chair for support and balance.

THE CAMPITELLI ADVANCED 10 MINUTE EXERCISE METHOD

WOMEN'S WORKOUT #12 • PAGE 2

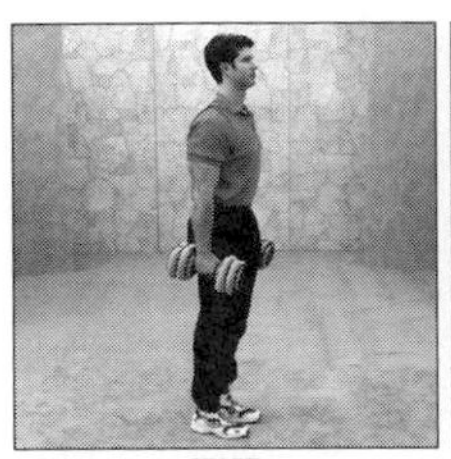

START FINISH

7. Dumbbell Squat

10 reps

- Feet 4-8 inches apart. DBs at side.
- Place weight evenly on heels and balls of feet.
- Back straight. Head up. Push with heels.

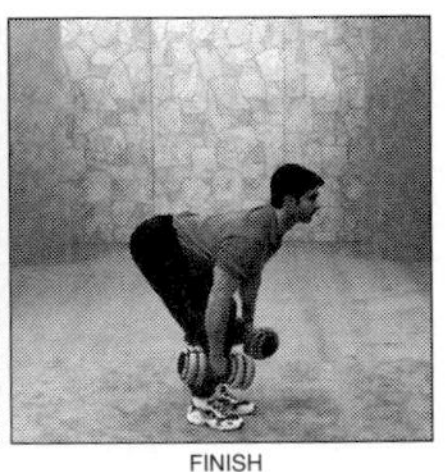

START FINISH

8. Dumbbell deadlift

10 reps

- Knees slightly bent with feet slightly apart.
- Keep low back locked with upper torso.
- Bend at hips, not at waist. Head up/chest out. Back is flat.

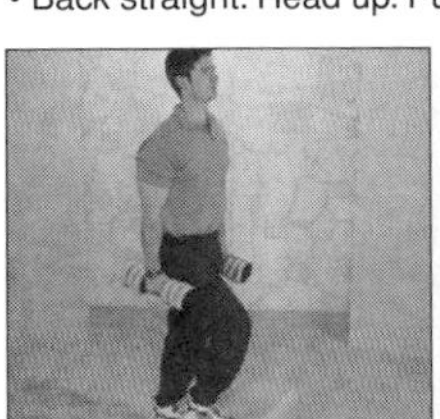

START FINISH

9. Step-up with Weights - Low Bench

10 reps Right/Left

- Place entire foot on bench or step.
- Use top leg to push only.
- Look up. Shoulders back.

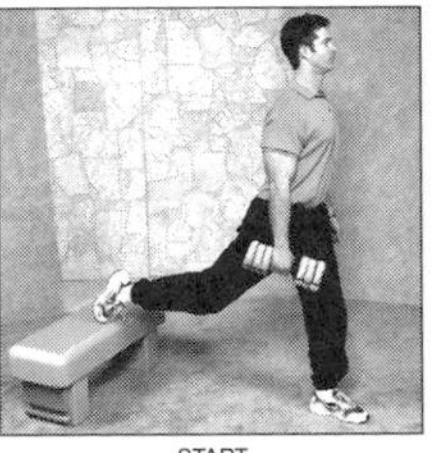

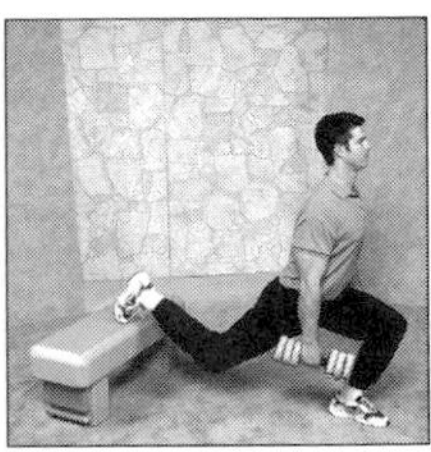

START FINISH

10. Dumbbell Lunge - Low Step

10 reps Right/Left

- Same as regular lunge with DB.

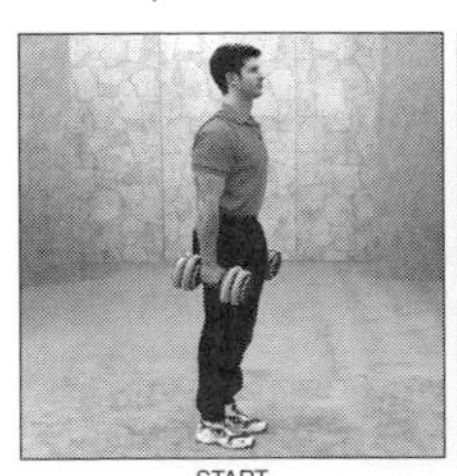

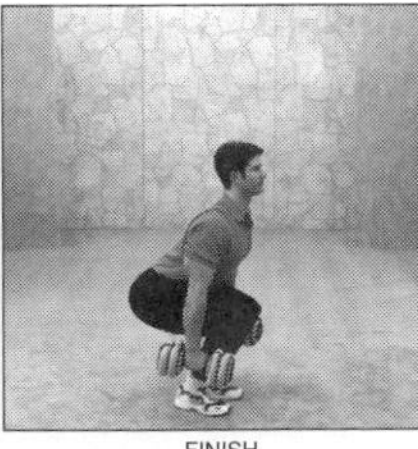

START FINISH

11. Dumbbell Squat

10 reps

- Feet 4-8 inches apart. DB's at side.
- Place weight evenly on heels and balls of feet.
- Back straight. Head up. Push with heels.

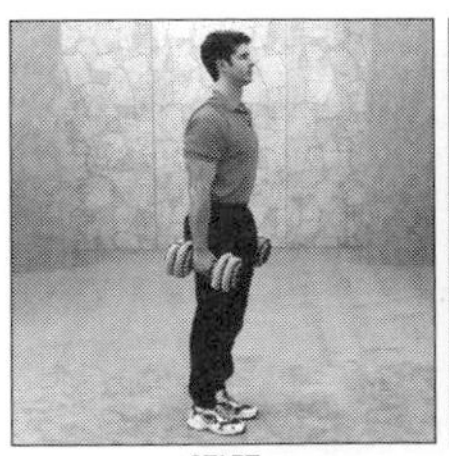

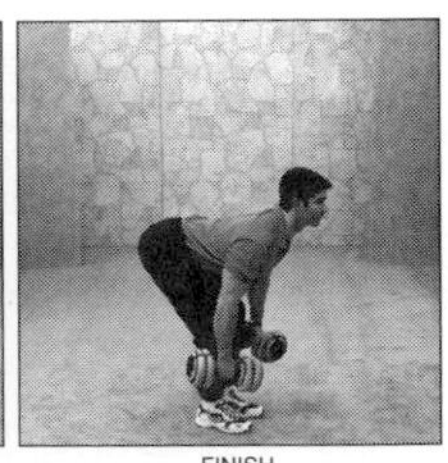

START FINISH

12. Dumbbell Deadlift

10 reps

- Knees slightly bent with feet slightly apart
- Keep low back locked with upper torso.
- Bend at hips, not at waist. Head up/chest out.
- Back is flat.

THE CAMPITELLI ADVANCED 10 MINUTE EXERCISE METHOD

WOMEN'S WORKOUT #13 • PAGE 1

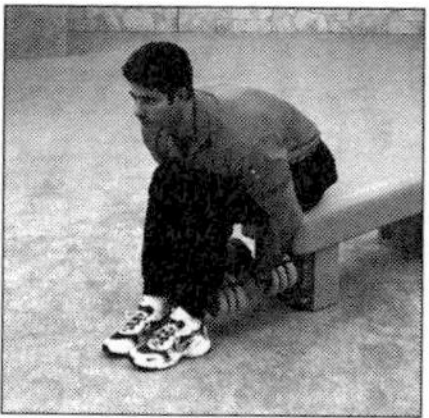

START

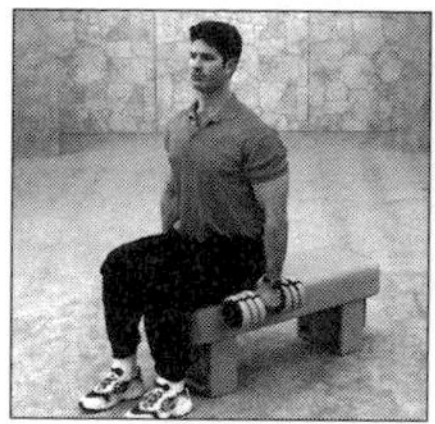

FINISH

1. Rear Lateral Raise
15 reps

- Lean forward keeping head up.
- Raise DB away from body. Elbows up. Palms down.
- Return DBs behind calves. Sit on very edge of bench.

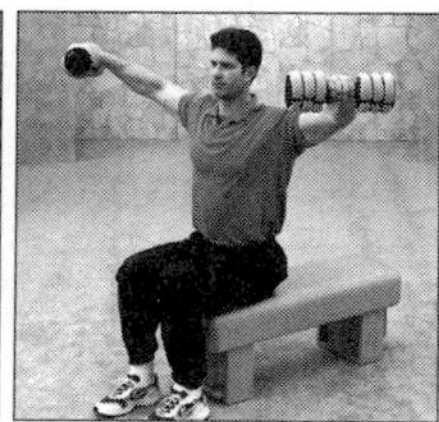

START

FINISH

2. Side Lateral Raise
15 reps

- Raise DBs out to the side keeping palms down.
- Concentrate on raising your elbows, not the DBs.

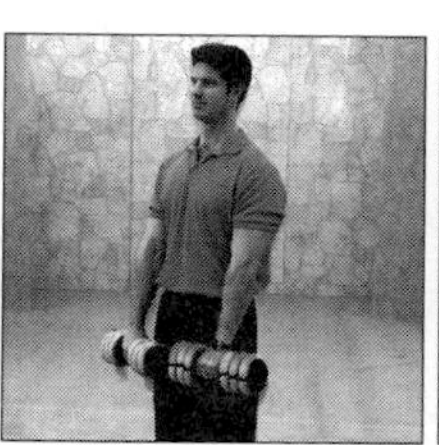

START

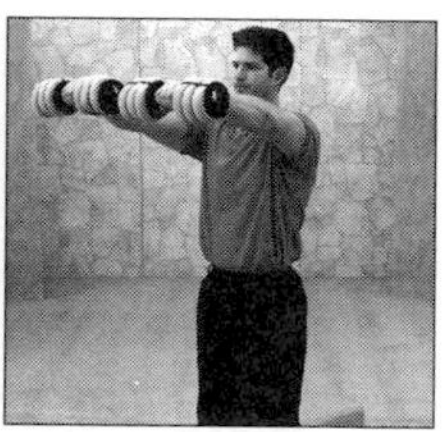

FINISH

3. Frontal Raise
15 reps

- Raise DB to eye level with palms down.
- Return to front of thigh. Don't swing.
- Offset foot stance for good balance.

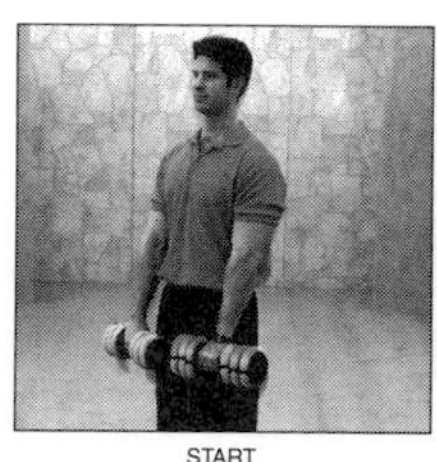

START

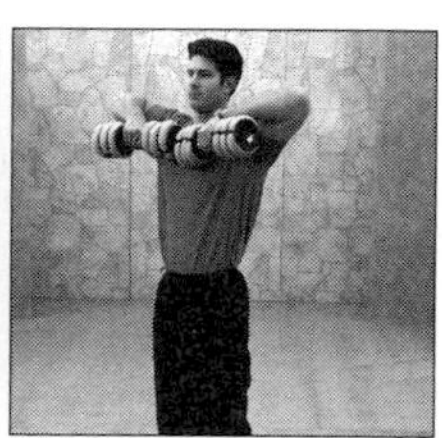

FINISH

4. Upright Row
15 reps

- Pull weights to chin.
- Elbows should be higher than weights at finish.

THE CAMPITELLI ADVANCED 10 MINUTE EXERCISE METHOD

WOMEN'S WORKOUT #13 • PAGE 2

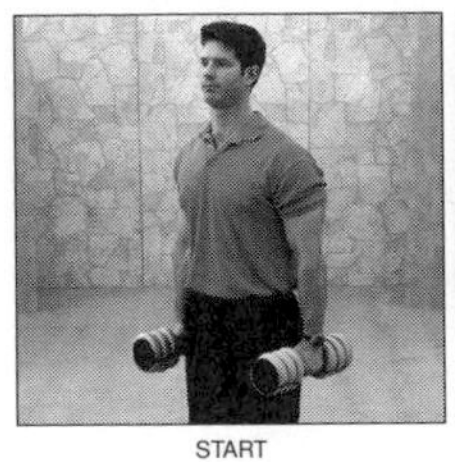

START FINISH

5. Bicep Curl
15 reps

- Palms up.
- Elbows at side.
- Don't swing.

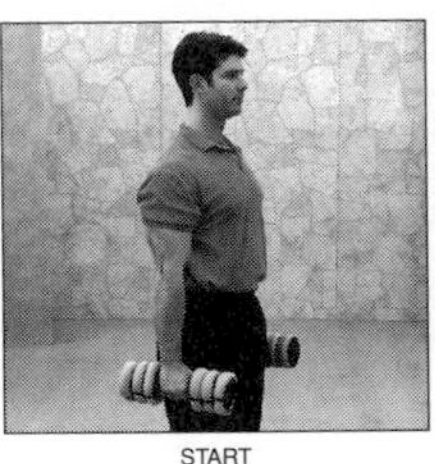

START

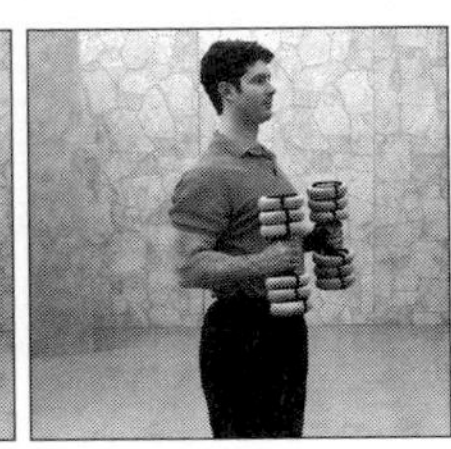

FINISH

6. Hammer Curl
15 reps

- Hands in "thumbs up position."
- Elbows stay at sides.
- Don't swing.

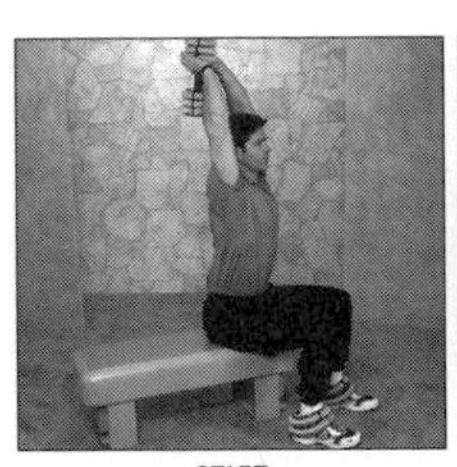

START

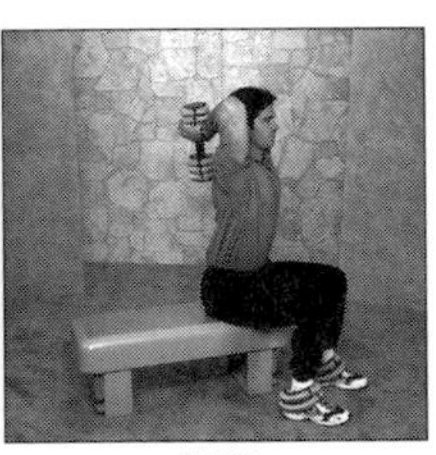

FINISH

7. Overhead Tricep Extension
15 reps

- Extend weight over head.
- Keep elbows up and close to head.

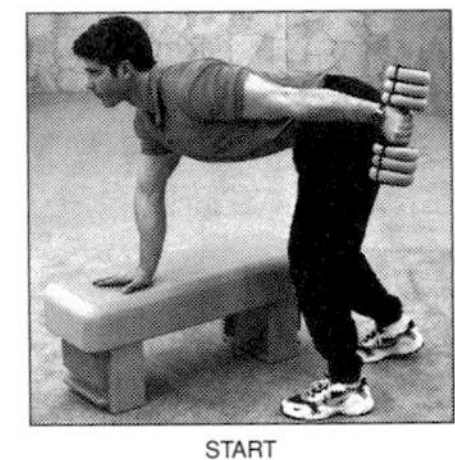

START

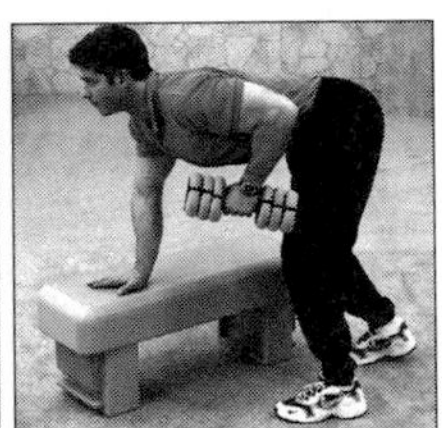

FINISH

8. Tricep Kick Back
15 reps

- Support upper body with non working arm.
- Extend arm until parallel to floor and pause.
- Don't swing weight at bottom.

REPEAT (1 THRU 8) AGAIN AT 15 REPS EACH. THEN REPEAT (1 THRU 8) AT 10 REPS EACH.

THE CAMPITELLI ADVANCED 10 MINUTE EXERCISE METHOD

WOMEN'S WORKOUT #14 • PAGE 1

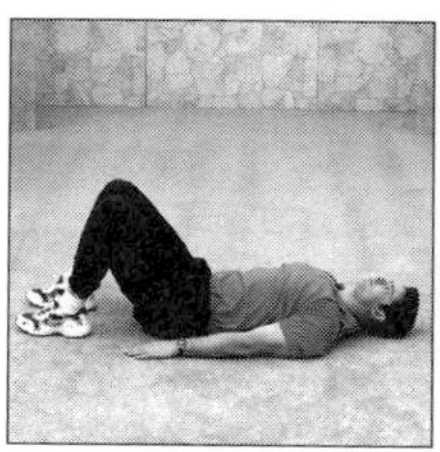
START

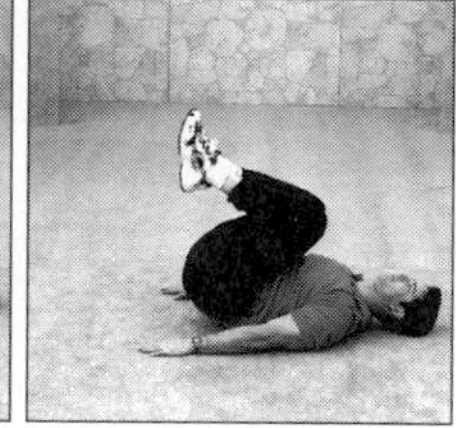
FINISH

1. Tucks with Ankle Weights
15 reps

- Place weights on ankles.
- Draw knees to chest.
- Exhale as knees come up.

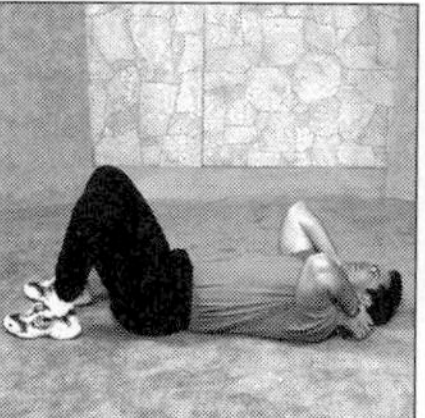
START

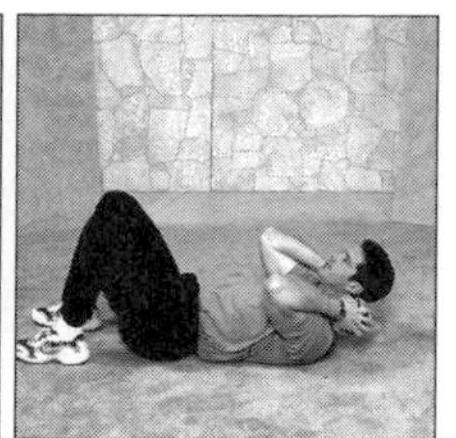
FINISH

2. Crunch with Dumbbell
15 reps

- Place weights behind neck. Hold with both hands.
- Push lower back into floor.
- Focus on ceiling, not knees.
- Breathe out as you go up.

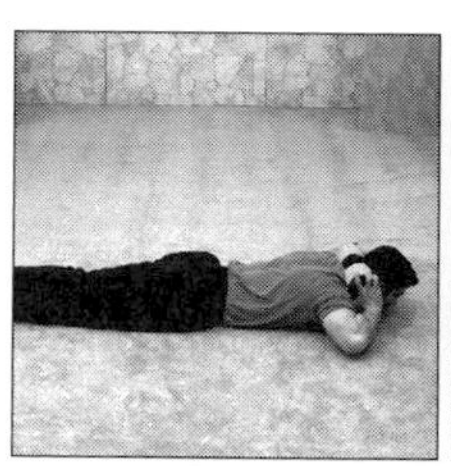
START

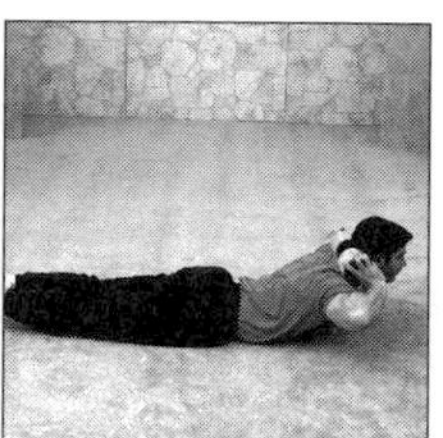
FINISH

3. Hyper Extension with Dumbbell
10 reps

- Place weight behind neck holding with both hands.
- Raise upper body off floor feeling contraction in mid to low back.

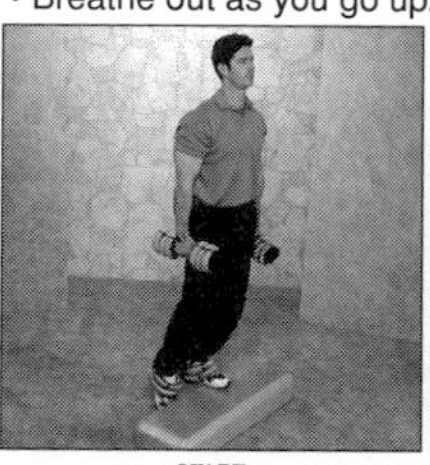
START

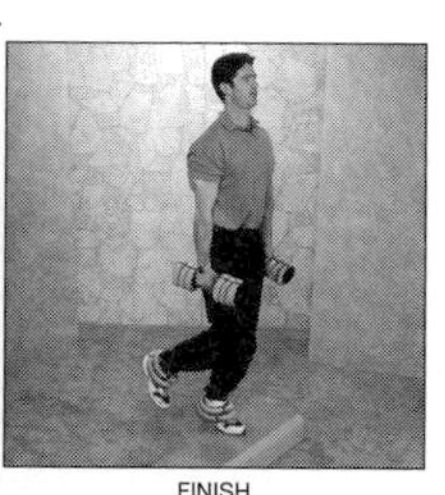
FINISH

4. Calf Raises with Ankle Weights and Dumbbell
20 reps Right/Left/Both

- Use step or book for elevation.
- Use DB for extra resistance.
- Raise heel up. Keep knee straight during movement.

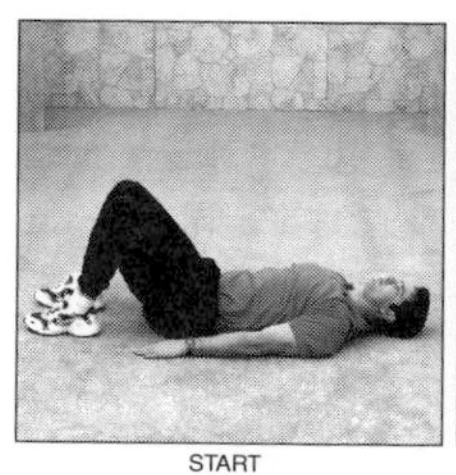
START

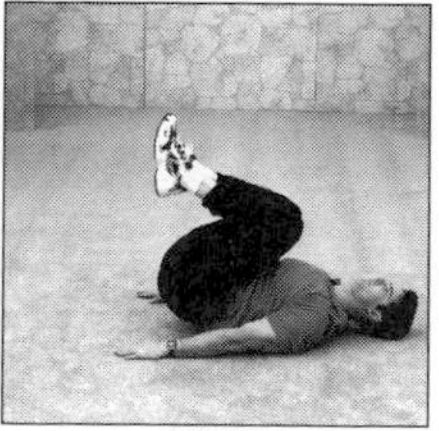
FINISH

5. Tucks with Ankle Weights
15 reps

- Place weights on ankles.
- Draw knees to chest.
- Exhale as knees come up.

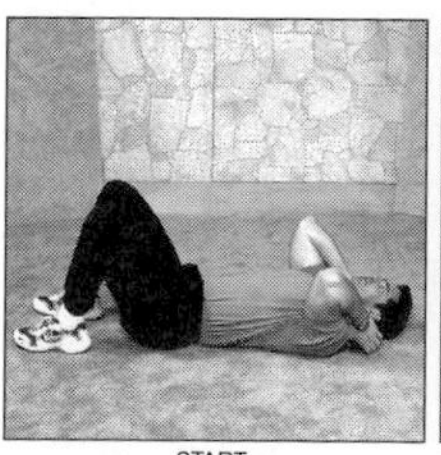
START

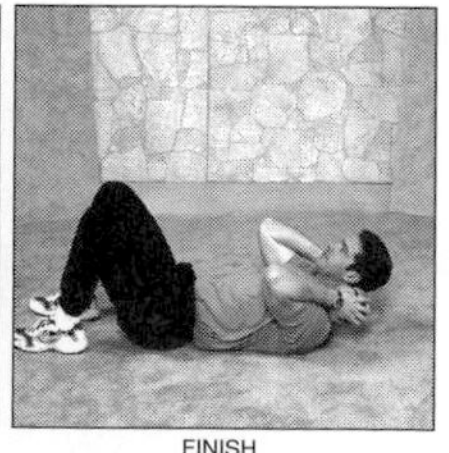
FINISH

6. Crunch with Dumbbell
15 reps

- Place weights behind neck. Hold with both hands.
- Push lower back into floor.
- Focus on ceiling, not knees. Breathe out as you go up.

THE CAMPITELLI ADVANCED 10 MINUTE EXERCISE METHOD

WOMEN'S WORKOUT #14 • PAGE 2

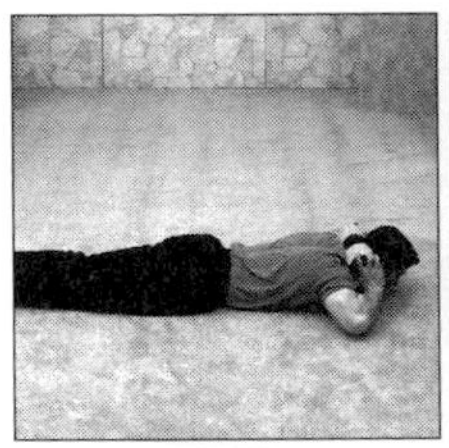

START FINISH

7. Hyper Extension with Dumbbell
10 reps

- Place weight behind neck holding with both hands.
- Raise upper body off floor feeling contraction in mid to low back.

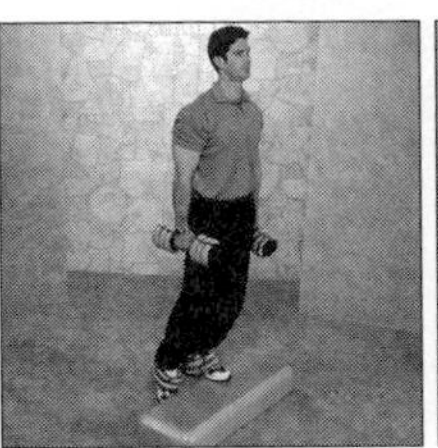
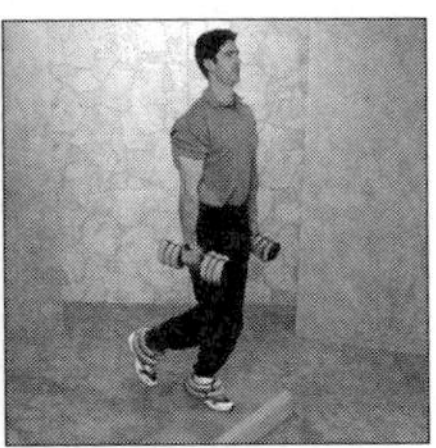

START FINISH

8. Calf Raises with Ankle Weights and Dumbbell
20 reps Right/Left/Both

- Use step or book for elevation.
- Use DB for extra resistance.
- Raise heel up. Keep knee straight during movement.

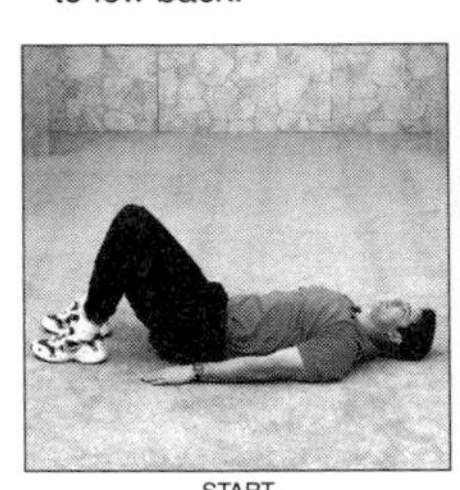
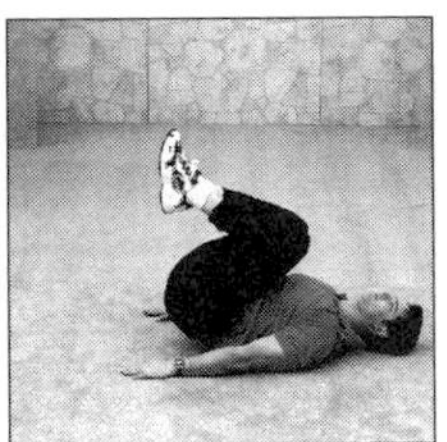

START FINISH

9. Tucks with Ankle Weights
15 reps

- Place weights on ankles.
- Draw knees to chest.
- Exhale as knees come up.

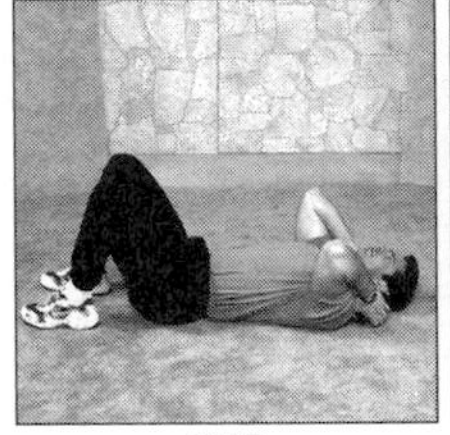
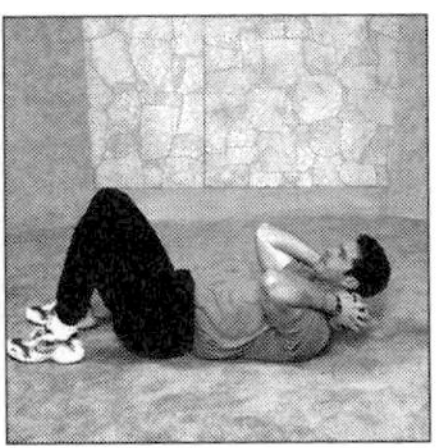

START FINISH

10. Crunch with Dumbbell
15 reps

- Place weights behind neck. Hold with both hands.
- Push lower back into floor.
- Focus on ceiling, not knees. Breathe out as you go up.

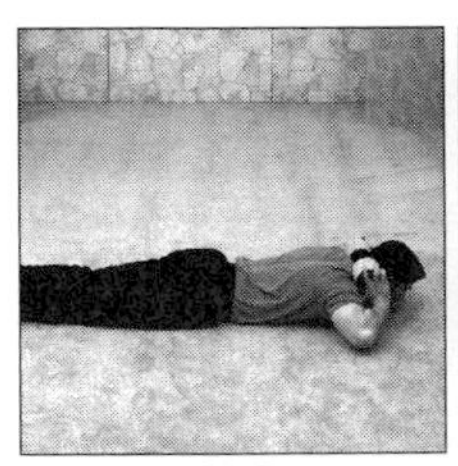
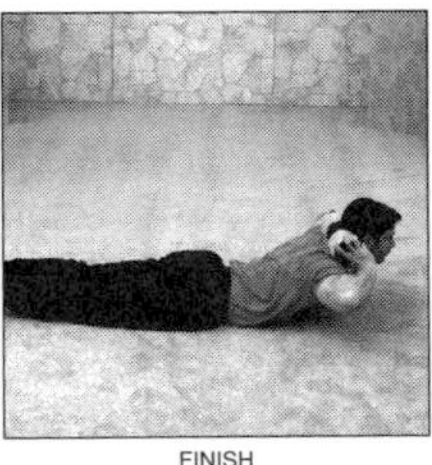

START FINISH

11. Hyper Extension with Dumbbell
10 reps

- Place weight behind neck holding with both hands.
- Raise upper body off floor feeling contraction in mid to low back.

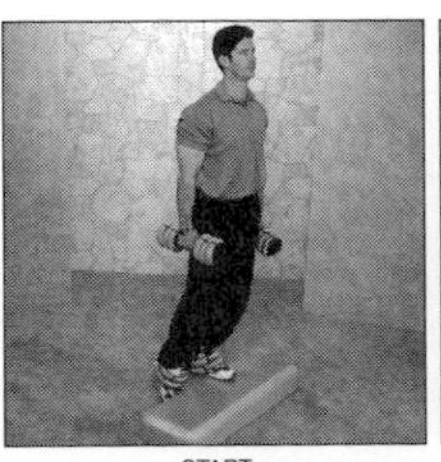
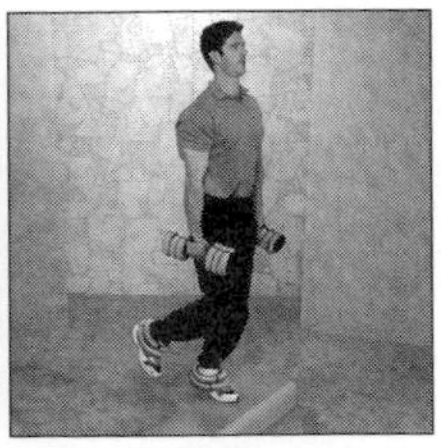

START FINISH

12. Calf Raises with Ankle Weights and Dumbbell
20 reps Right/Left/Both

- Use step or book for elevation.
- Use DB for extra resistance.
- Raise heel up. Keep knee straight during movement.

THE CAMPITELLI ADVANCED 10 MINUTE EXERCISE METHOD

WOMEN'S WORKOUT #15 • PAGE 1

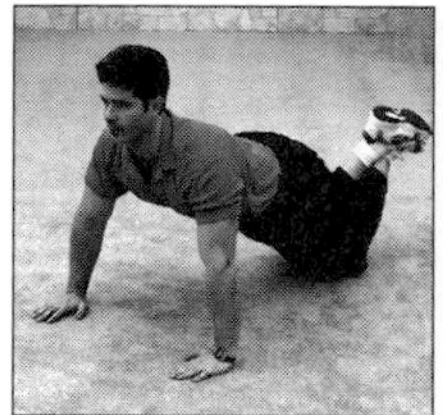
START

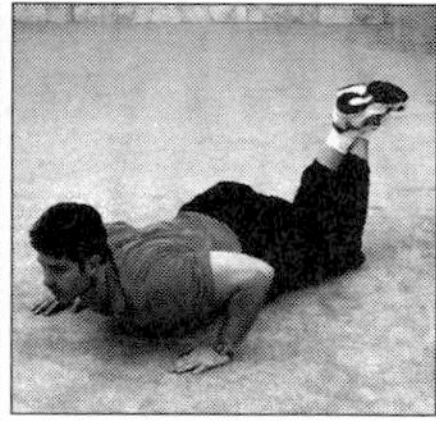
FINISH

1. Modified Pushup
15 reps

- Start from knees
- Hands shoulder width
- Head up.

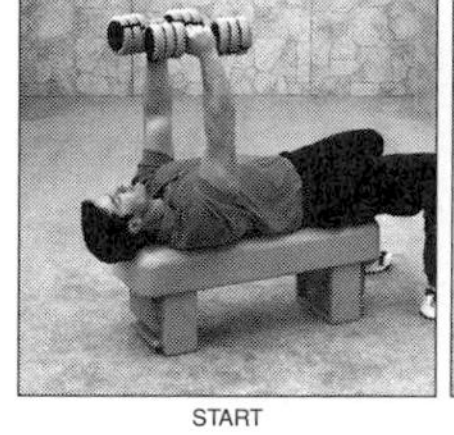
START

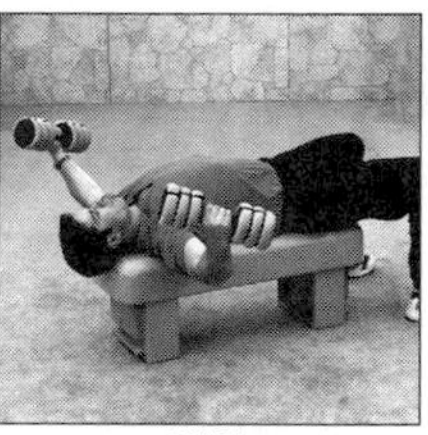
FINISH

2. Dumbbell Fly
15 reps

- Elbows slightly bent with palms facing each other.
- Lower weights out to the side of body until weight is parallel to body.
- Keep elbow slightly bent.

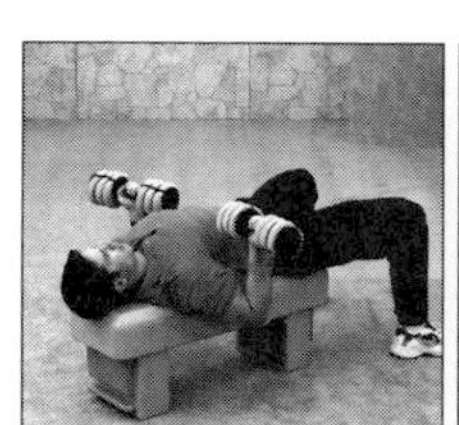
START

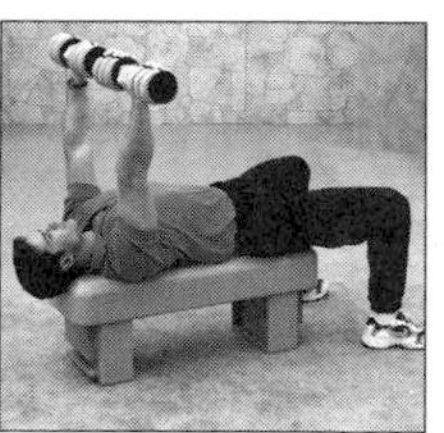
FINISH

3. Dumbbell Press
15 reps

- Hold weights palms toward knees.
- Relax abdomen.
- Lower weights until even with chest.

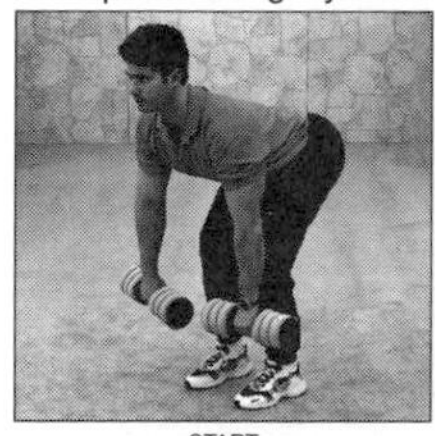
START

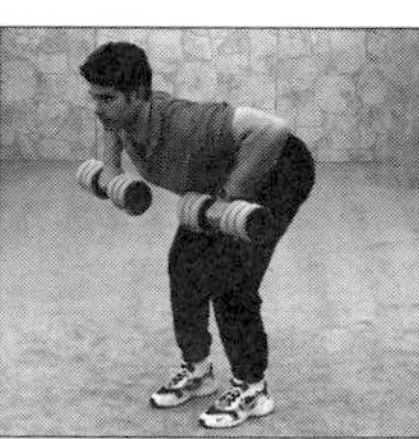
FINISH

4. Dumbbell Row Wide Grip
15 reps

- DBs in "over-hand" position.
- Chest out and head up.
- Knees bent. Back straight.

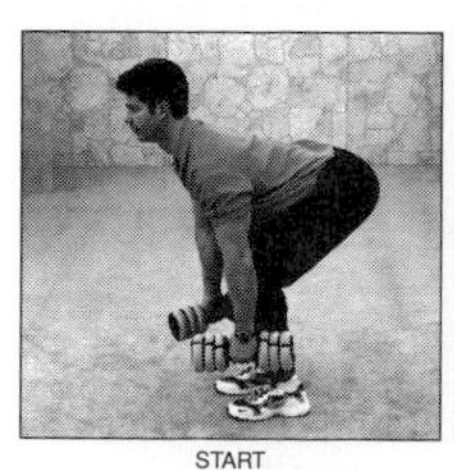
START

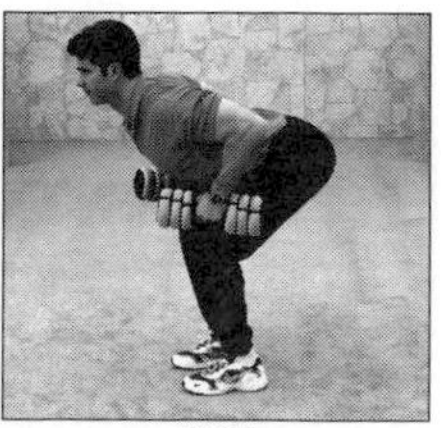
FINISH

5. Dumbbell Row Close Grip
15 reps

- Feet together. Bend at hips, not at waist.
- Back straight. Chest out and head up.
- Pull weights with elbows close to body.

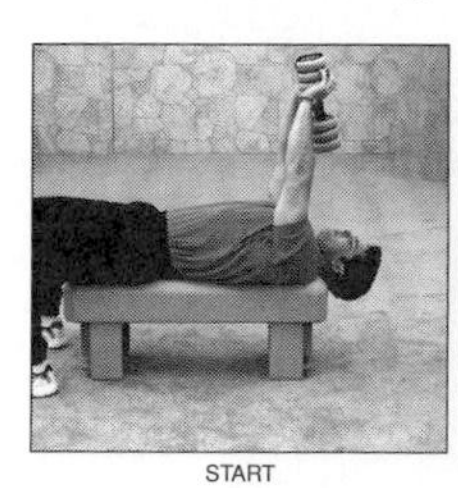
START

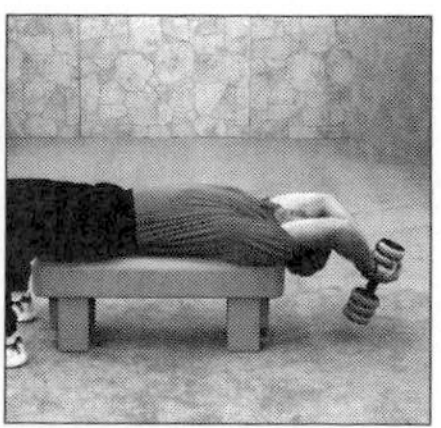
FINISH

6. Dumbbell Pullover
15 reps

- Relax abdomen. Keep elbows in toward body.
- Inhale as weight goes over head.
- Exhale as weight is pulled up.

THE CAMPITELLI ADVANCED 10 MINUTE EXERCISE METHOD

WOMEN'S WORKOUT #15 • PAGE 2

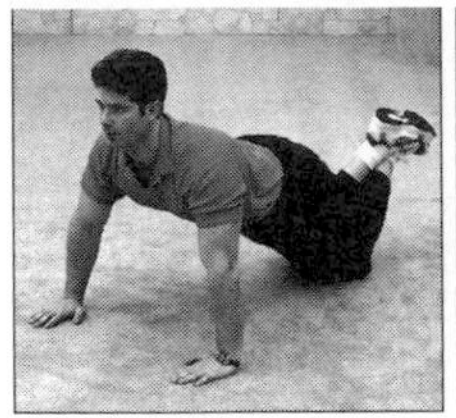
START

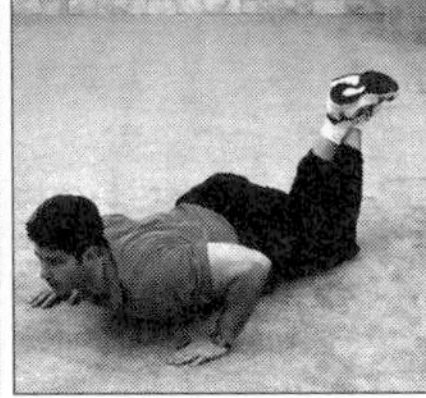
FINISH

7. Modified Pushup
15 reps

- Start from knees
- Hands shoulder width
- Head up.

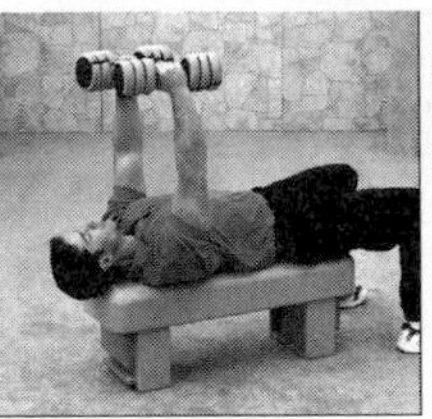
START

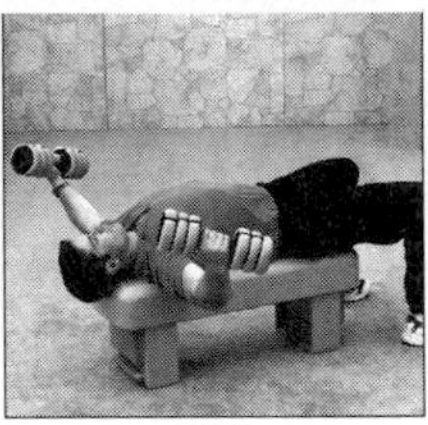
FINISH

8. Dumbbell Fly
15 reps

- Elbows slightly bent with palms facing each other.
- Lower weights out to the side of body until weight is parallel to body.
- Keep elbow slightly bent.

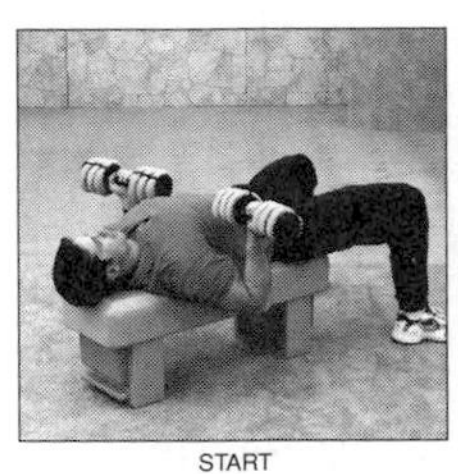
START

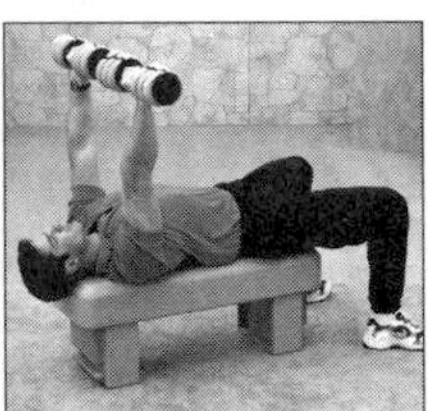
FINISH

9. Dumbbell Press
15 reps

- Hold weights palms toward knees.
- Relax abdomen.
- Lower weights until even with chest.

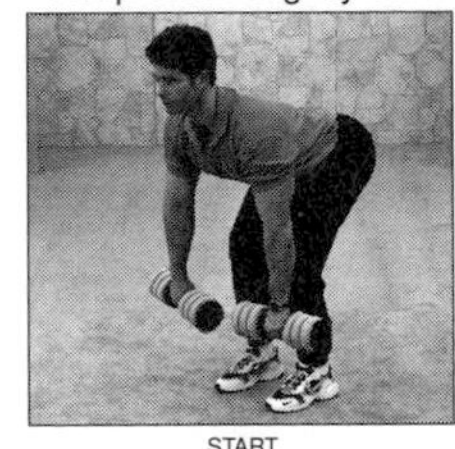
START

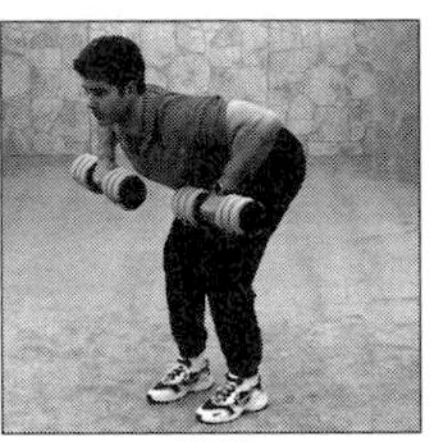
FINISH

10. Dumbbell Row Wide Grip
15 reps

- DBs in "over-hand" position.
- Chest out and head up.
- Knees bent. Back straight.

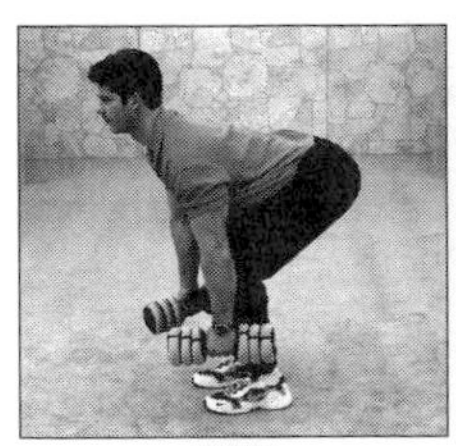
START

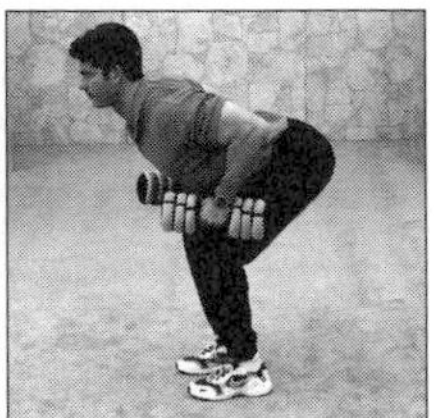
FINISH

11. Dumbbell Row Close Grip
15 reps

- Feet together. Bend at hips, not at waist.
- Back straight. Chest out and head up.
- Pull weights with elbows close to body.

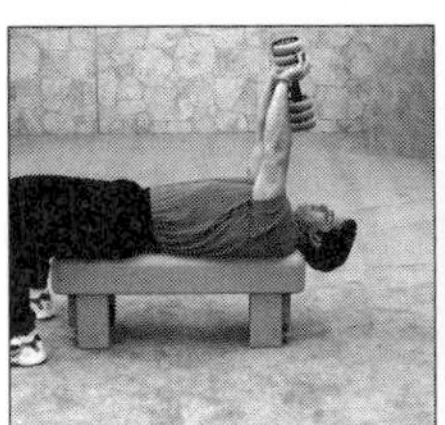
START

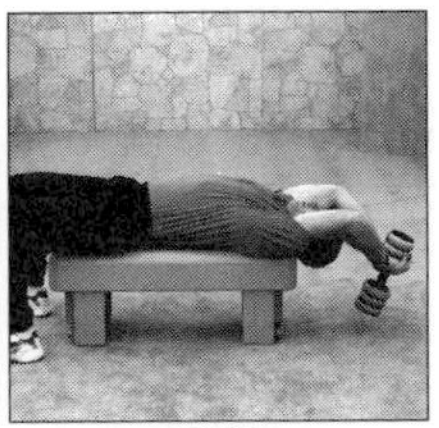
FINISH

12. Dumbbell Pullover
15 reps

- Relax abdomen. Keep elbows in toward body.
- Inhale as weight goes over head.
- Exhale as weight is pulled up.

THE CAMPITELLI ADVANCED 10 MINUTE EXERCISE METHOD

WOMEN'S WORKOUT #16 • PAGE 1

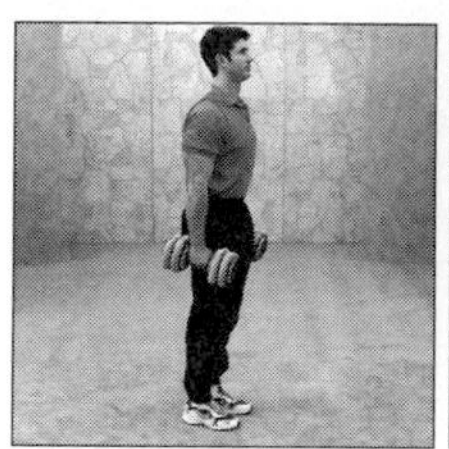

START

FINISH

1. Dumbbell Squat
10 reps Right/Left

- Feet 4-8 inches apart. DBs at side.
- Place weight evenly on heels and balls of feet.
- Back straight. Head up.
- Push with heels.

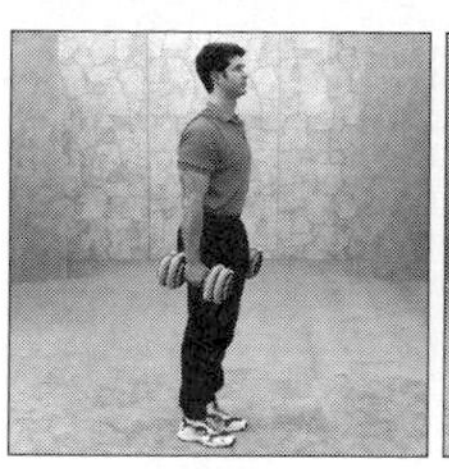

START

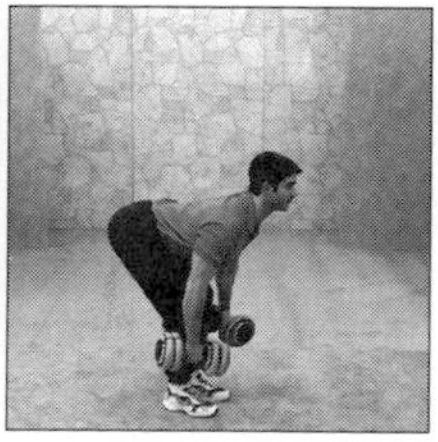

FINISH

2. Dumbbell Deadlift
10 reps

- Knees slightly bent with feet slightly apart.
- Keep low back locked with upper torso.
- Bend at hips, not at waist.
- Head up/chest out. Back is flat.

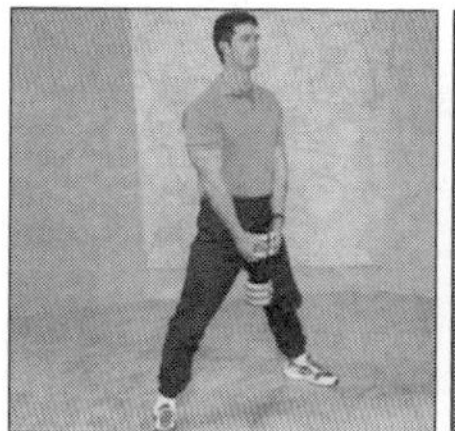

START

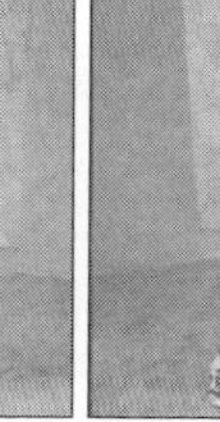

FINISH

3. Wide Stance Squat
10 reps

- Hold DB between legs with both hands.
- Wide stance. Toes out slightly.
- Lower torso. Knees go out over toes.

REPEAT ENTIRE SEQUENCE (1 THRU 3) TWO MORE TIMES BEFORE MOVING ON TO PAGE 2.

THE CAMPITELLI ADVANCED 10 MINUTE EXERCISE METHOD

WOMEN'S WORKOUT #16 • PAGE 2

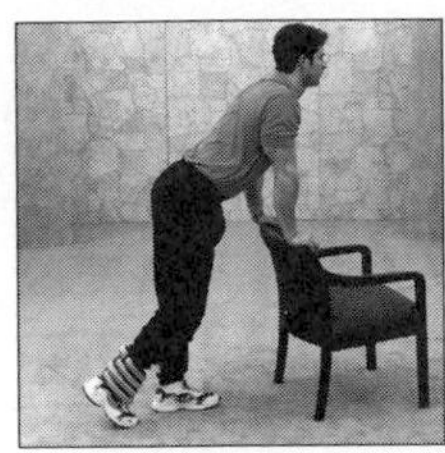

START FINISH

4. Leg Curl with Ankle Weights
10 reps. Right/Left

- Raise leg bending knee.
- Use chair for balance. Keep toe pointed down.
- Hold briefly at top position.

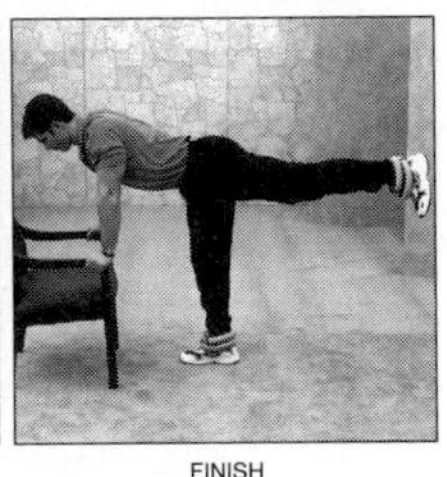

START FINISH

5. Hip Extension with Ankle Weights
10 reps Right/Left

- Support & Balance upper body with chair or wall.
- Raise legs to rear.
- Keep knee straight.

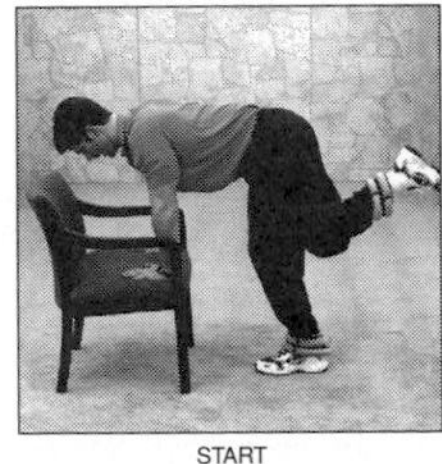

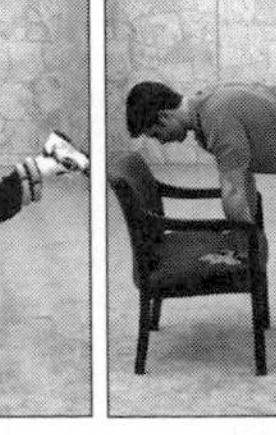

START FINISH

6. Hip Kick with Ankle Weights
10 reps Right/Left

- Support & balance upper body with chair or wall.
- Bend knee.
- Push heel to ceiling.

REPEAT ENTIRE SEQUENCE (4 THRU 6) TWO MORE TIMES.

THE CAMPITELLI ADVANCED 10 MINUTE EXERCISE METHOD

WOMEN'S WORKOUT #17 • PAGE 1

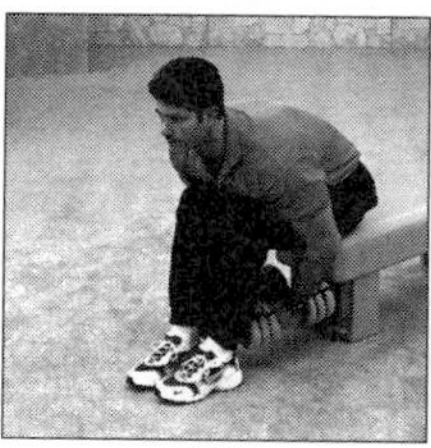
START

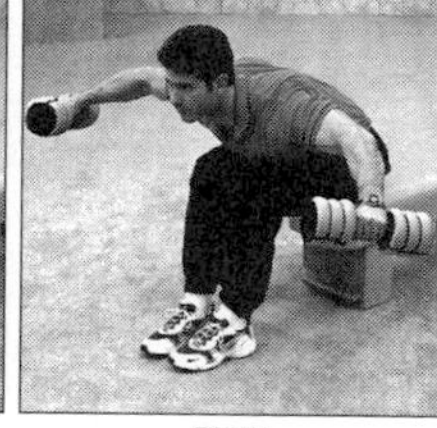
FINISH

1. Rear Lateral Raise
10 reps

- Lean forward keeping head up.
- Raise DB away from body. Elbows up. Palms down.
- Return DBs behind calves. Sit on very edge of bench.

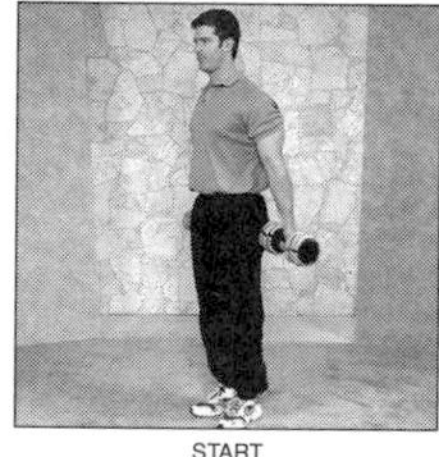
START

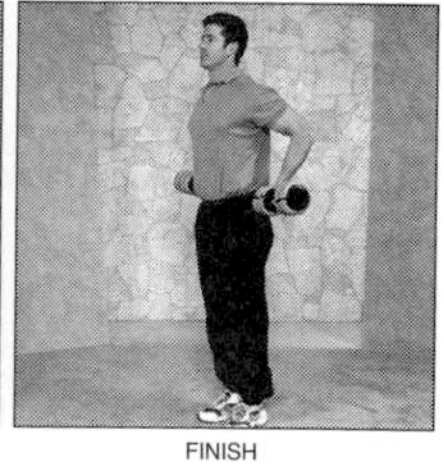
FINISH

2. Rear Row
10 reps

- Stand with DB's palms forward.
- Pull DBs up with elbow to the rear.
- Pinky fingers to armpit.
- Elbows high as they will go.

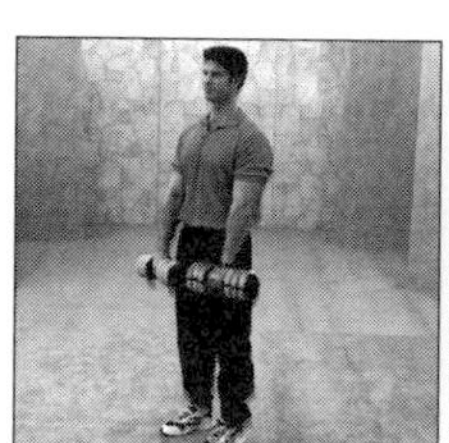
START

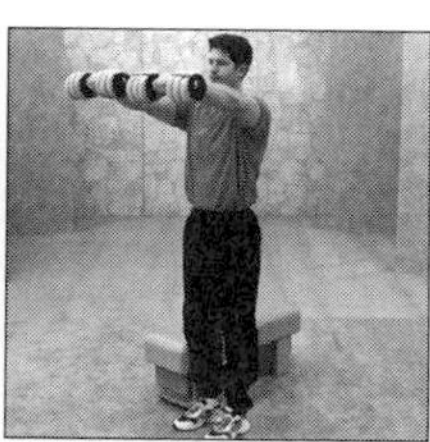
FINISH

3. Frontal Raise
10 reps

- Raise DB with palms down to eye level.
- Return to front of thigh.
- Don't swing.
- Offset foot stance for good balance.

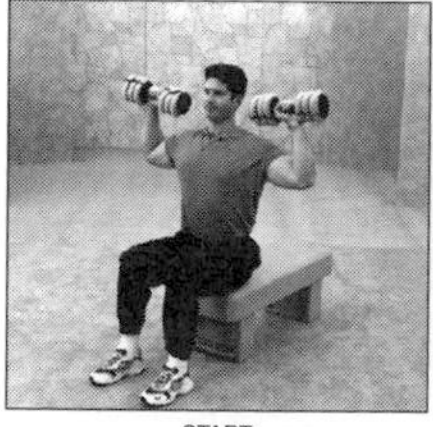
START

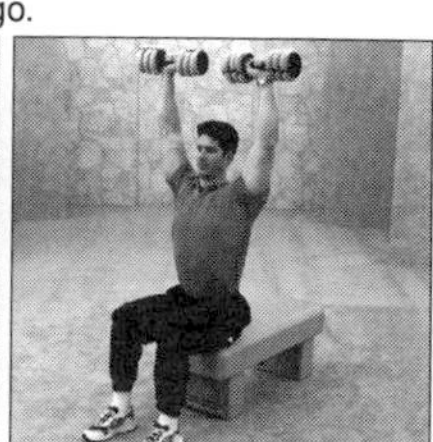
FINISH

4. Shoulder Press
10 reps

- Press weights with elbows out from sides.
- Palms facing forward.

THE CAMPITELLI ADVANCED 10 MINUTE EXERCISE METHOD

WOMEN'S WORKOUT #17 • PAGE 2

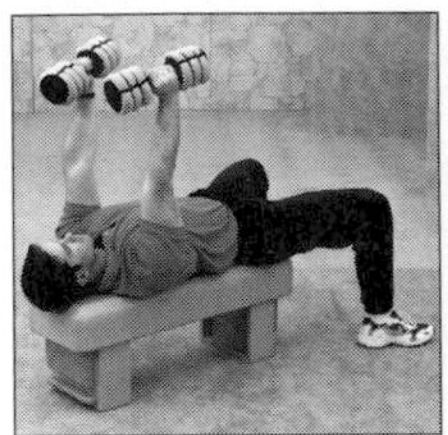
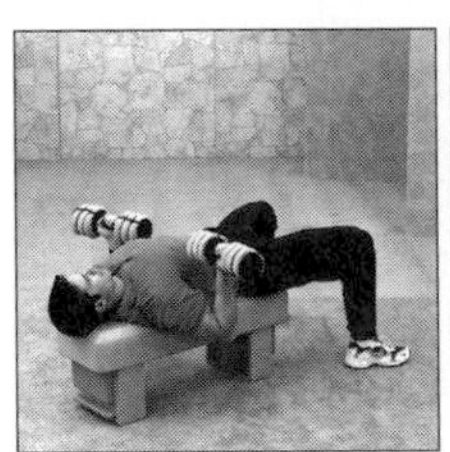

START FINISH

5. Lying Tricep Extension

10 reps

- Elbows pointed straight up.
- Hands in "thumbs up position."
- Weights come back to ears.

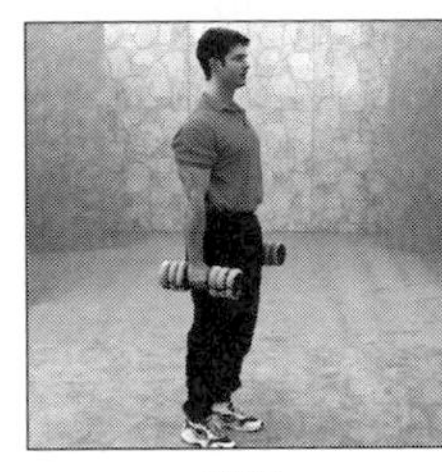
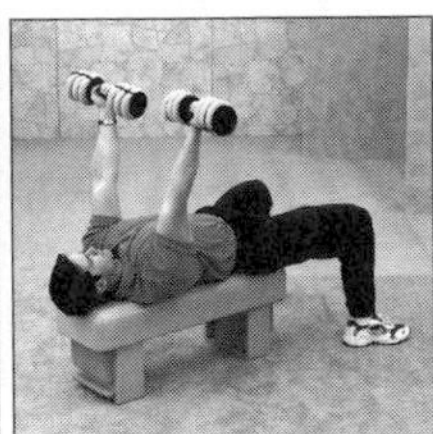

START FINISH

6. Reverse Tricep Press

10 reps

- Hands in "palms up position."
- Elbows stay close to body.
- Lower to side of chest.

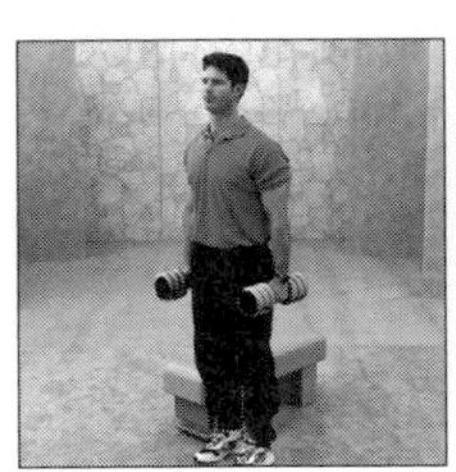
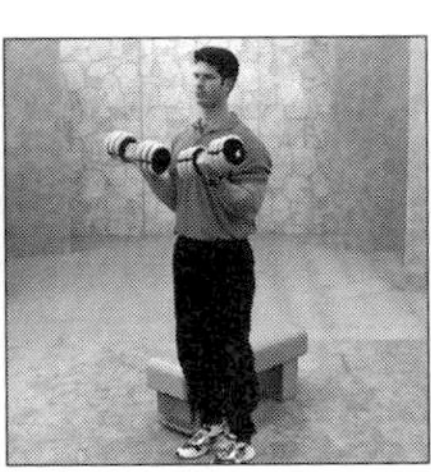

START FINISH

7. Regular Curl

10 reps

- Palms up.
- Elbows at side.
- Don't swing.

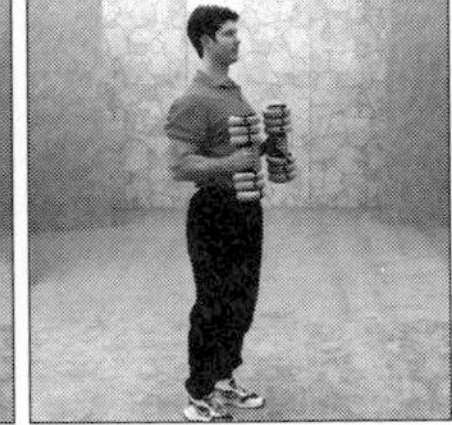

START FINISH

8. Hammer Curl

10 reps

- Hands in "thumbs up position."
- Elbows stay at sides.
- Don't swing.

THE CAMPITELLI ADVANCED 10 MINUTE EXERCISE METHOD

WOMEN'S WORKOUT #18 • PAGE 1

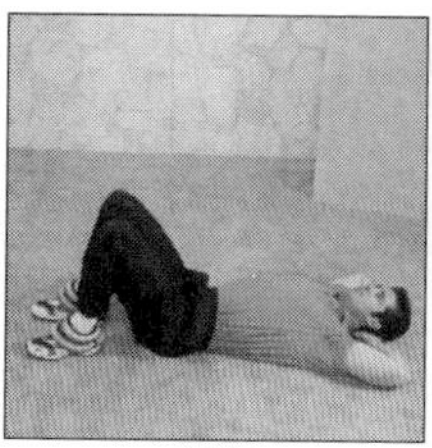
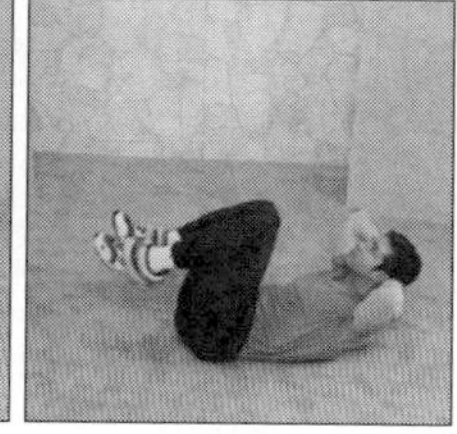

START FINISH

1. V-Crunch with Ankle Weights
20 reps

- Perform V-Crunch as before with addition of ankle weights for more resistance.

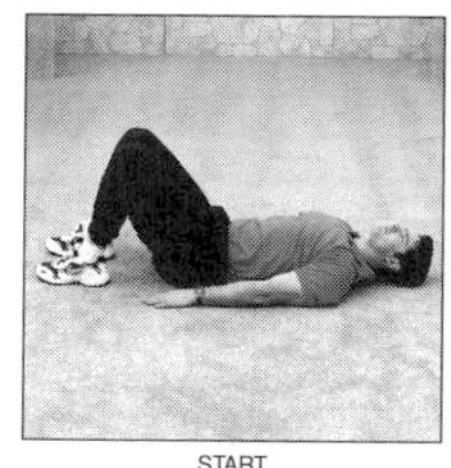
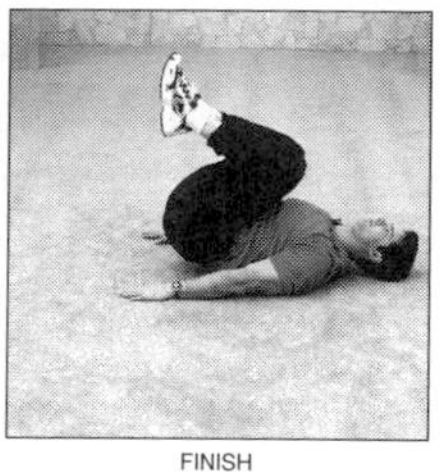

START FINISH

2. Tucks with Ankle Weights
20 reps

- Place weights on ankles.
- Draw knees to chest
- Exhale as knees come up.

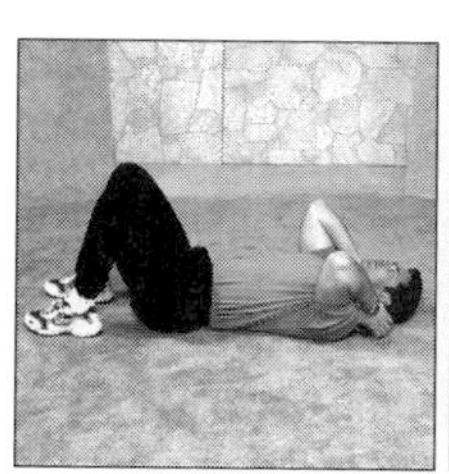
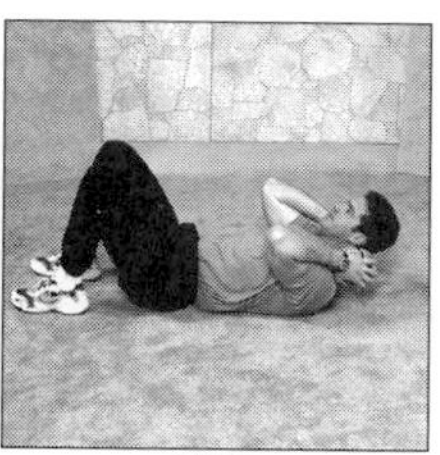

START FINISH

3. Crunch with Dumbbell
20 reps

- Place weights behind neck. Hold with both hands.
- Push lower back into floor.
- Focus on ceiling, not knees. Breathe out as you go up.

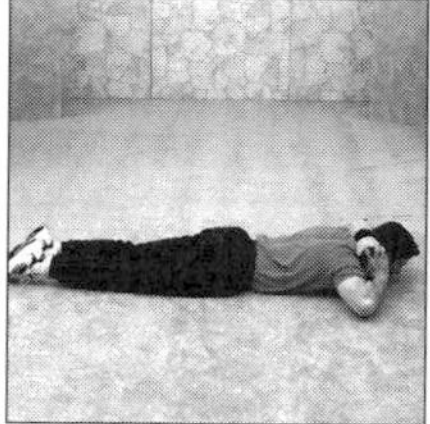
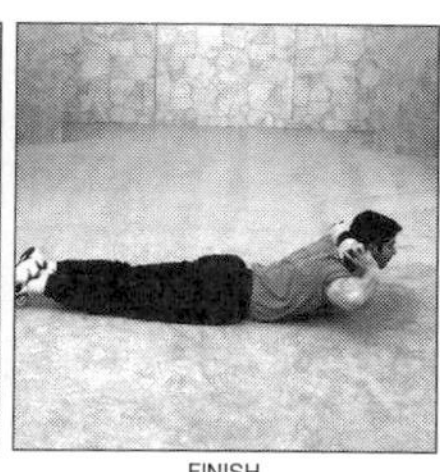

START FINISH

4. Hyper Extension with Dumbbell
10 reps

- Place weight behind neck holding with both hands.
- Raise upper body off floor feeling contraction in mid to low back.

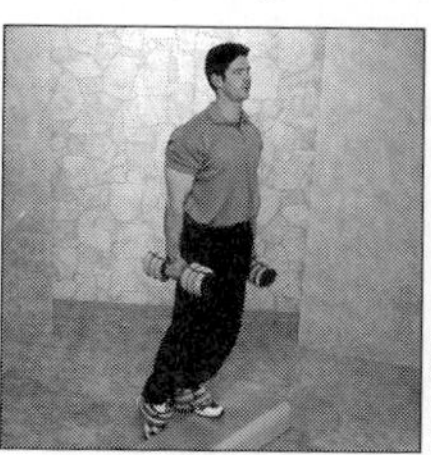
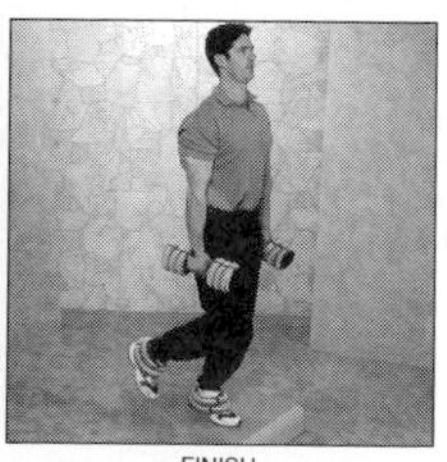

START FINISH

5. Calf Raise w/ Ankle Weights & Dumbbell
10 reps Right/Left/Both

- Use chair or wall for balance.
- Knees stay straight.
- Use ankle weights & DB for additional resistance.

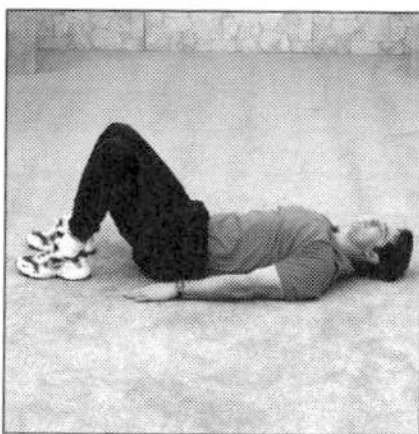
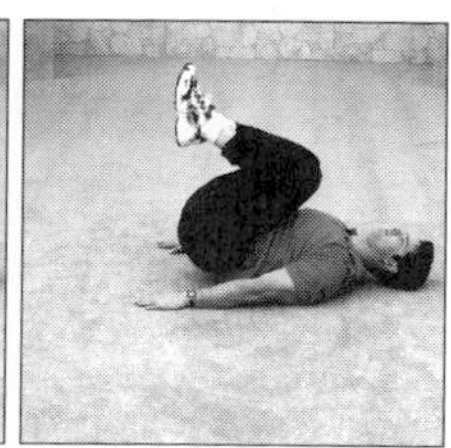

START FINISH

6. Tucks with Ankle Weights
20 reps

- Place weights on ankles.
- Draw knees to chest.
- Exhale as knees come up.

THE CAMPITELLI ADVANCED 10 MINUTE EXERCISE METHOD

WOMEN'S WORKOUT #18 • PAGE 2

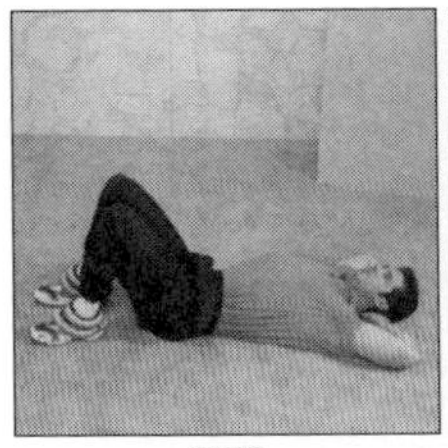

START FINISH

7. V-Crunch with Ankle Weights

20 reps

- Perform V-Crunch as before with addition of ankle weights for more resistance.

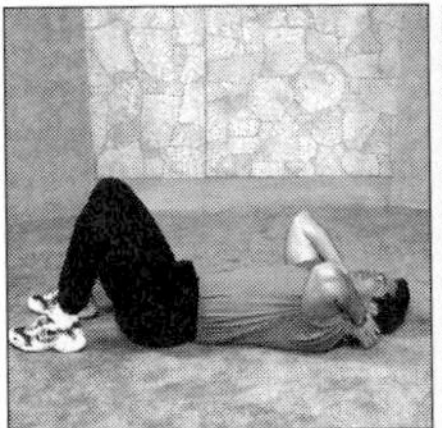

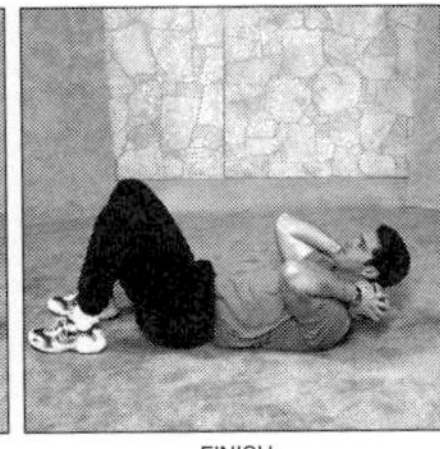

START FINISH

8. Crunch with Dumbbell

20 reps

- Place dumbbell behind head.
- Draw knees to chest.
- Exhale as knees come up.

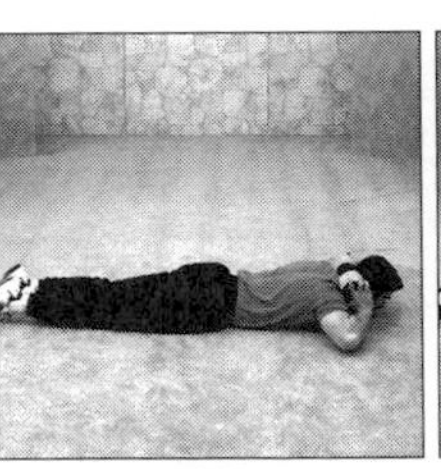

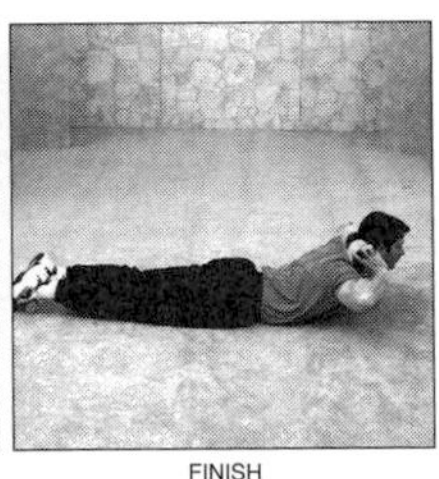

START FINISH

9. Hyper Extension with Dumbbell

10 reps

- Place weight behind neck holding with both hands.
- Raise upper body off floor feeling contraction in mid to low back.

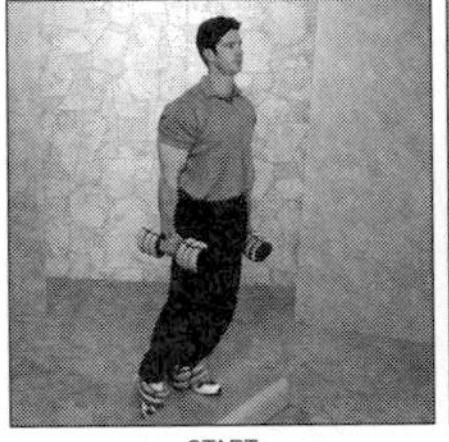

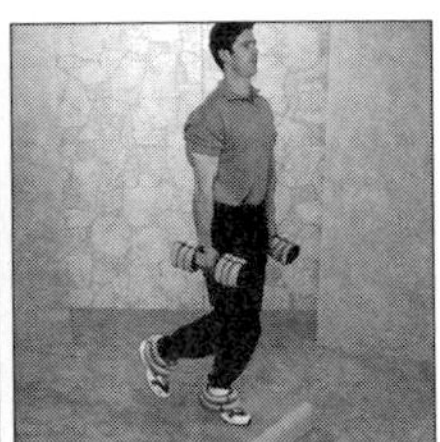

START FINISH

10. Calf Raise with Ankle Weights & Dumbell

10 reps Right/Left/Both

- Use chair or wall for balance.
- Knees stay straight.
- Use ankle weights & DB for additional resistance.

REPEAT EXERCISES (6 THRU 10) ONE MORE TIME AT TEN REPS.

THE CAMPITELLI ADVANCED 10 MINUTE EXERCISE METHOD

WOMEN'S WORKOUT #19 • PAGE 1

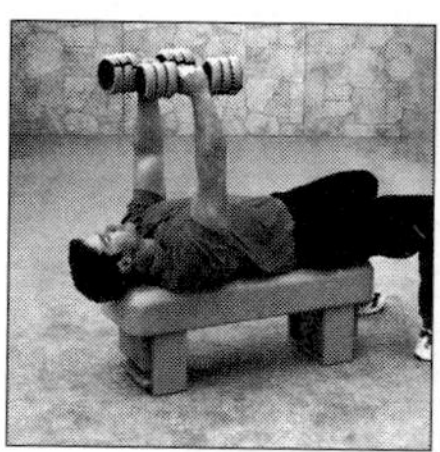
START

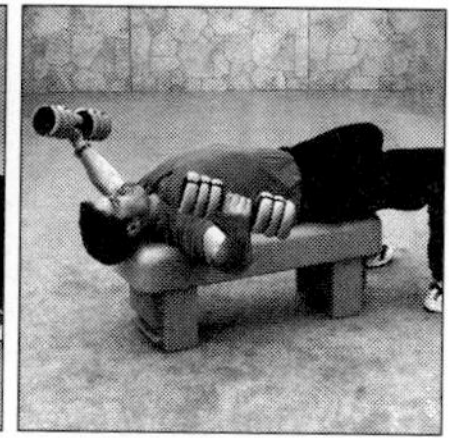
FINISH

1. Dumbbell Fly
10 reps

- Elbows slightly bent with palms facing each other.
- Lower weights out to the side of body until weight is parallel to body. Keep elbow slightly bent.

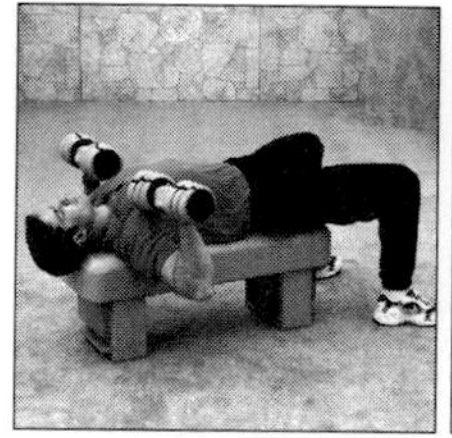
START

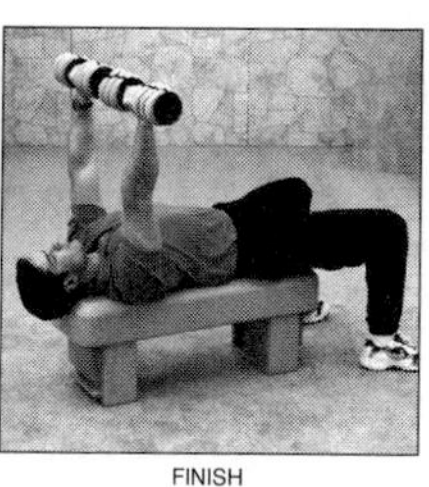
FINISH

2. Dumbbell Press
10 reps

- Hold weights palms toward knees.
- Relax abdomen.
- Lower weights until even with chest.

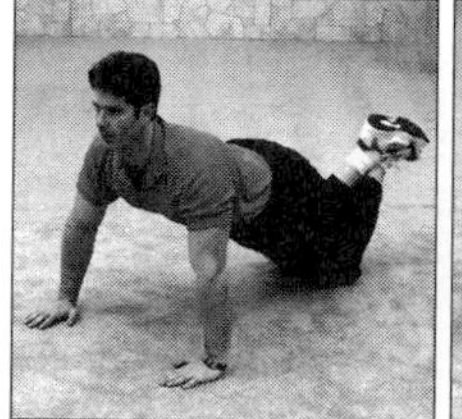
START

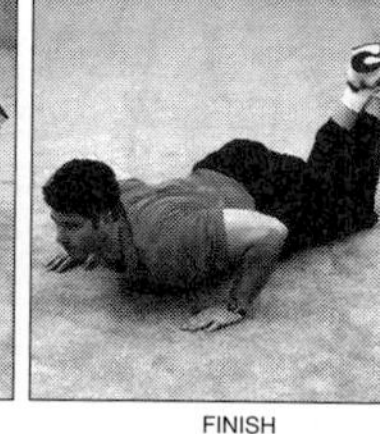
FINISH

3. Modified Pushup
10 reps

- Start from knees
- Hands shoulder width
- Head up.

REPEAT SEQUNCE (1 THRU 3) FOR A TOTAL OF THREE TIMES REDUCING WEIGHT EACH TIME BEFORE MOVING ON TO PAGE 2.

THE CAMPITELLI ADVANCED 10 MINUTE EXERCISE METHOD

WOMEN'S WORKOUT #19 • PAGE 2

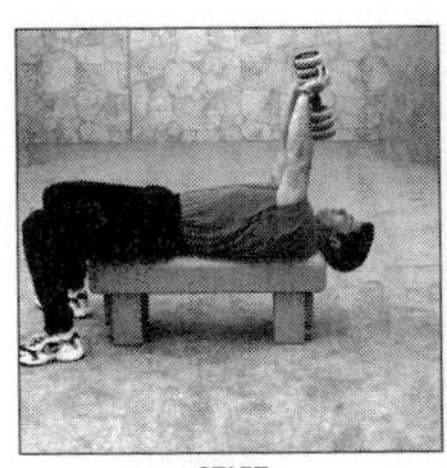

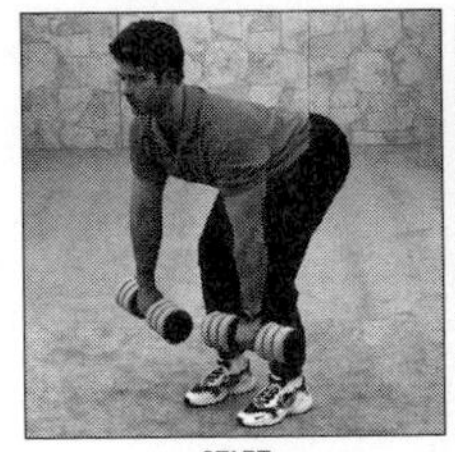

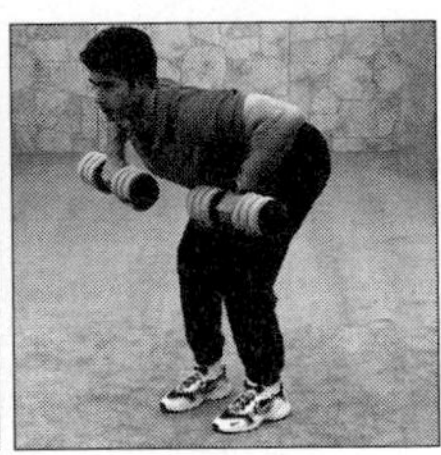

START FINISH

4. Dumbbell Pullover
10 reps

- Relax abdomen. Keep elbows in toward body.
- Inhale as weight goes over head.
- Exhale as weight ispulled up.

START FINISH

5. Dumbbell Row Wide Grip
10 reps

- DBs in "over-hand" position.
- Head up. Chest out.
- Knees bent. Back straight.

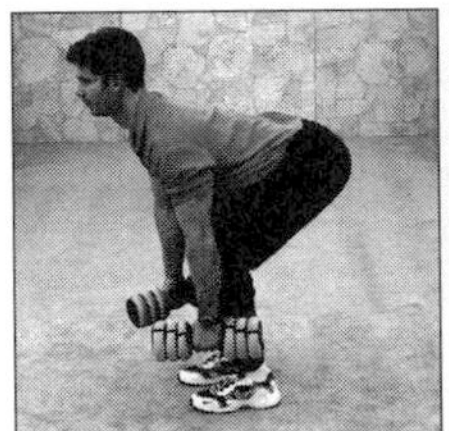

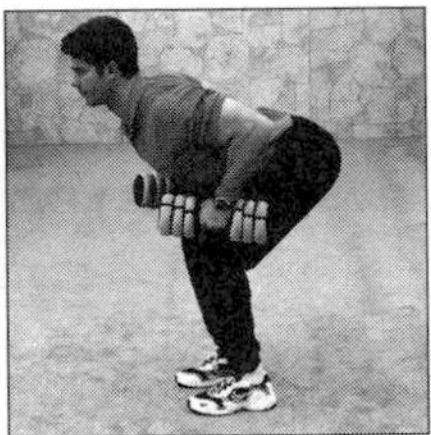

START FINISH

6. Dumbbell Row Close Grip
10 reps

- Feet together.
- Bend at hips, not at waist. Back straight.
- Chest out. Head up.
- Pull weights with elbows close to body.

REPEAT SEQUENCE (4 THRU 6) TWO MORE TIMES REDUCING WEIGHT EACH TIME.

THE CAMPITELLI ADVANCED 10 MINUTE EXERCISE METHOD

WOMEN'S WORKOUT #20 • PAGE 1

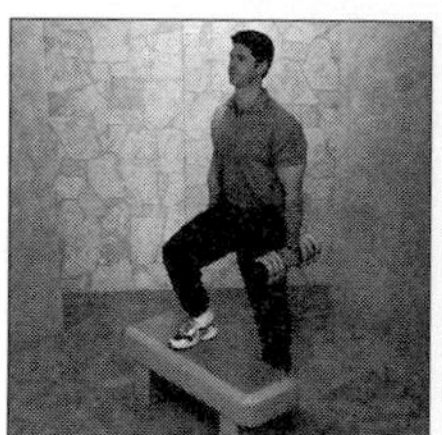

START FINISH

1. Stepup with Dumbbell
10 reps Right Leg

- Place entire foot on bench or step.
- Use top leg to push only.
- Look up. Shoulders back.

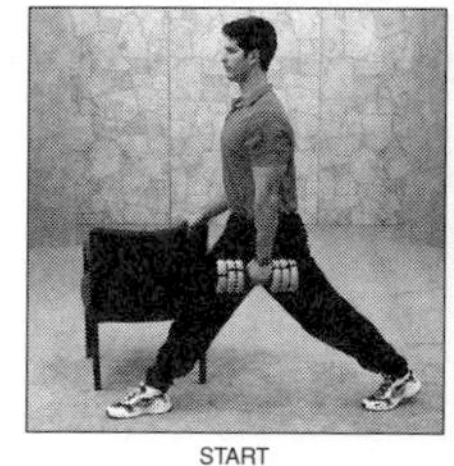

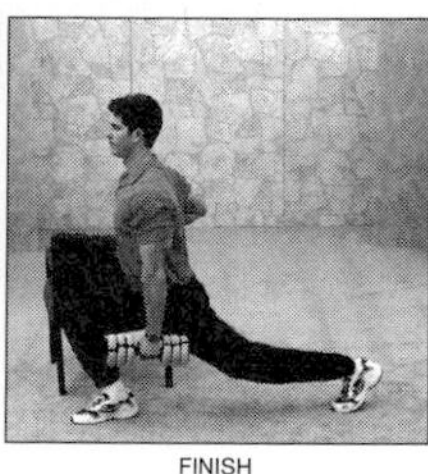

START FINISH

2. Lunge with Dumbbell
10 reps Right Leg

- Same as regular lunge with DB in one hand.
- Use chair for support and balance.

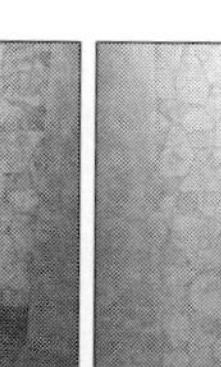

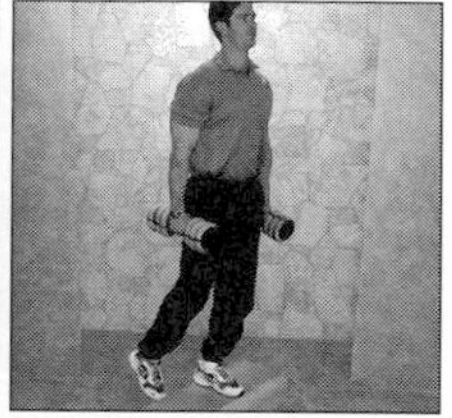

START FINISH

3. Stepup with Dumbbell
10 reps Left Leg

- Place entire foot on bench or step.
- Use top leg to push only.
- Look up. Shoulders back.

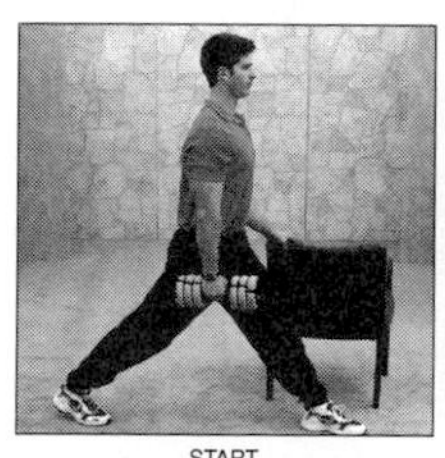

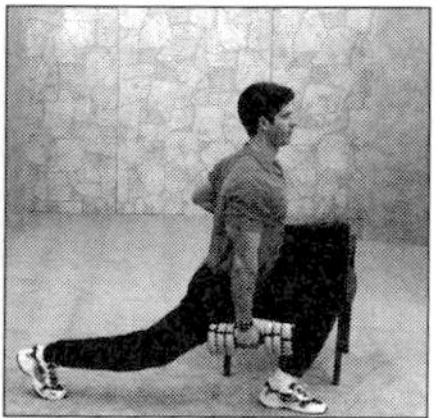

START FINISH

4. Lunge with Dumbbell
10 reps Left Leg

- Same as regular lunge with DB in one hand.
- Use chair for support and balance.

REPEAT SEQUENCE (1 THRU 4) TWO MORE TIMES REDUCING WEIGHT EACH TIME BEFORE PROCEEDING TO "DUMBBELL SQUAT" & "DEADLIFT" ON OTHER SIDE.

THE CAMPITELLI ADVANCED 10 MINUTE EXERCISE METHOD

WOMEN'S WORKOUT #20 • PAGE 2

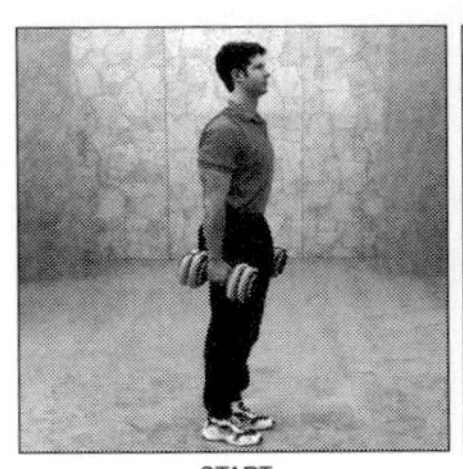

START

FINISH

5. Dumbbell Squat
10 reps

- Feet 4-8 inches apart.
- DBs at side.
- Place weight evenly on heels and balls of feet.
- Back straight. Head up. Push with heels.

START

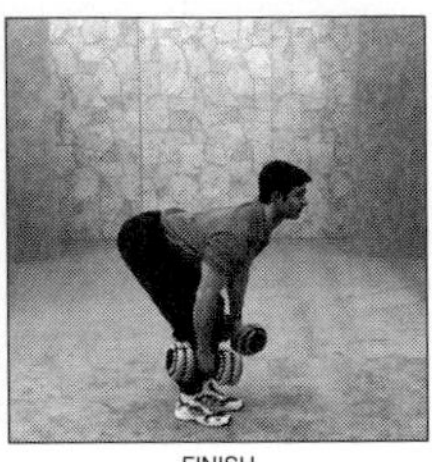

FINISH

6. Dumbbell Deadlift
10 reps

- Knees slightly bent with feet slightly apart.
- Keep low back locked with upper torso.
- Bend at hips, not at waist.
- Head up/chest out. Back is flat.

REPEAT ABOVE EXERCISES ROUTINE (5 THRU 6) TWO MORE TIMES REDUCING WEIGHT EACH TIME.

THE CAMPITELLI ADVANCED 10 MINUTE EXERCISE METHOD

MEN'S WORKOUT #1 • PAGE 1

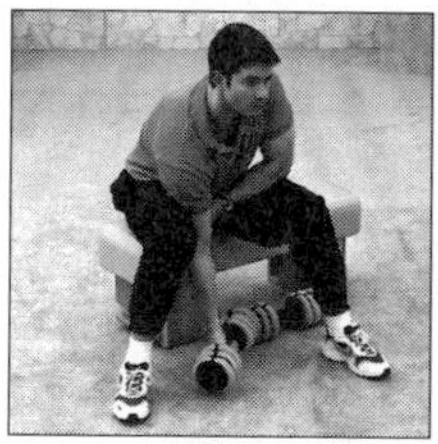

START

FINISH

1. Concentration Curl

20 reps Right/Left

- Brace curling arm inside thigh for support.
- Use other hand for additional support.

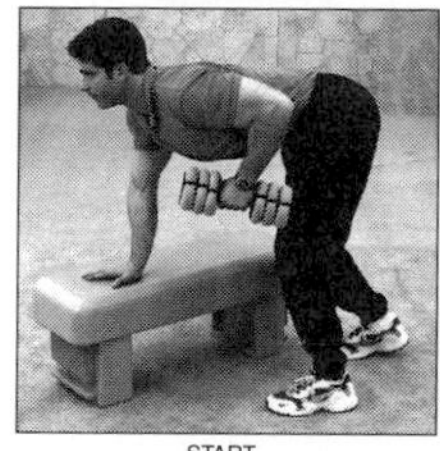
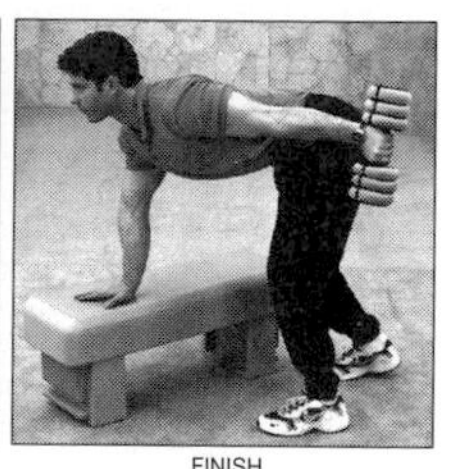

START

FINISH

2. Tricep Kick Back

20 reps Right/Left

- Support upper body with non-working arm.
- Extend arm until parallel to floor and hold.
- Don't swing weight at bottom.

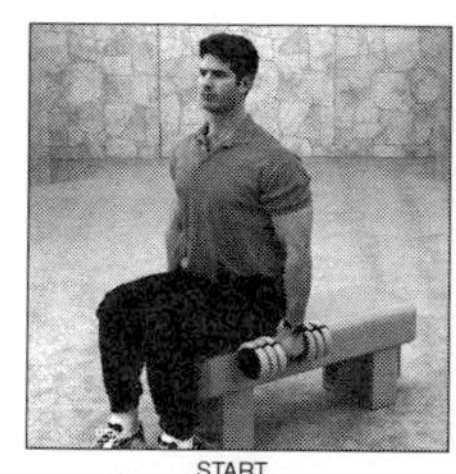
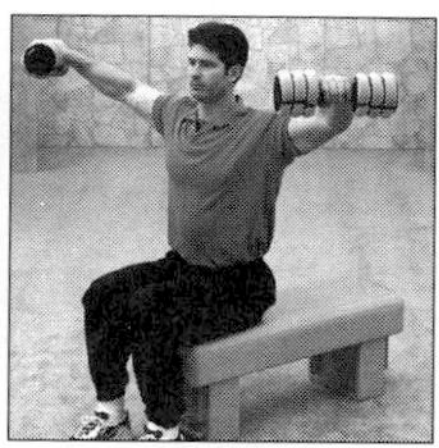

START

FINISH

3. Lateral Raise

20 reps

- Raise DBs out to the side keeping palms down.
- Concentrate on raising your elbows, not the DBs.

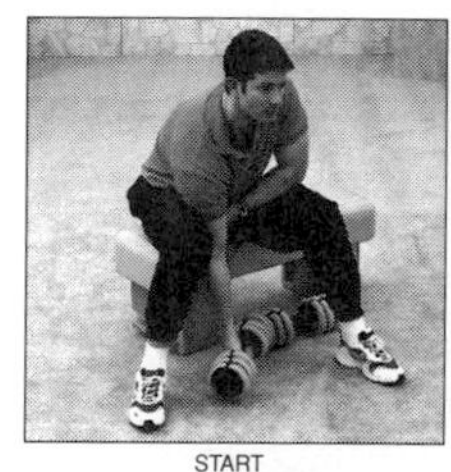
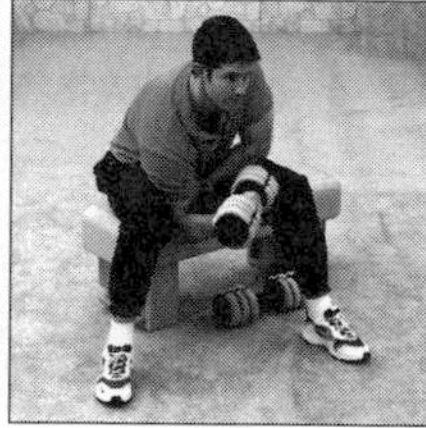

START

FINISH

4. Concentration Curl

15 reps Right/Left

- Brace curling arm inside thigh for support.
- Use other hand for additional support.

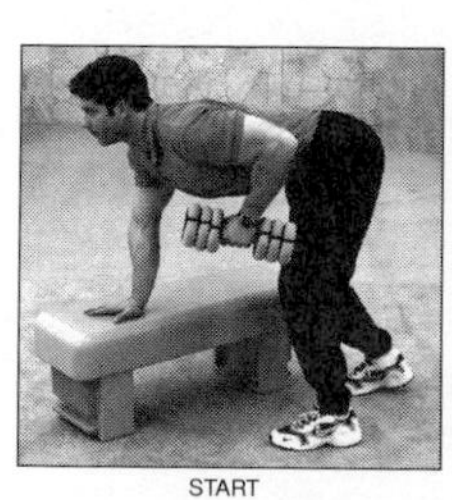
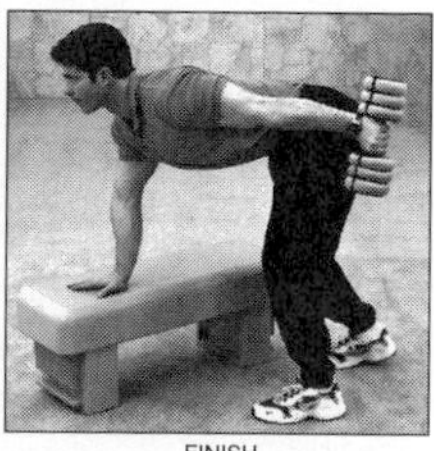

START

FINISH

5. Tricep Kickback

15 reps Right/Left

- Support upper body with non-working arm.
- Extend arm until parallel to floor and hold.
- Don't swing weight at bottom.

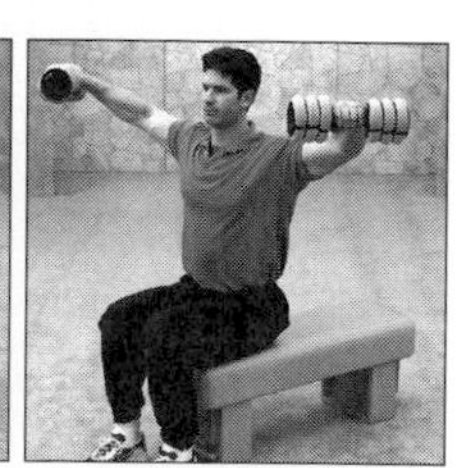

START

FINISH

6. Lateral Raise

15 reps Both Arms

- Raise DBs out to the side keeping palms down.
- Concentrate on raising your elbows, not the DBs.

END OF ROUTINE. NO PAGE 2.

THE CAMPITELLI ADVANCED 10 MINUTE EXERCISE METHOD

MEN'S WORKOUT #2 • PAGE 1

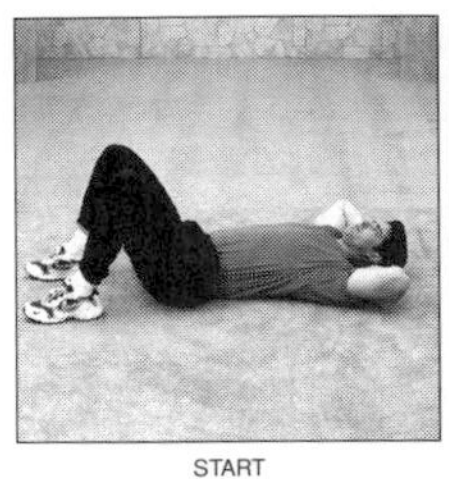

START FINISH

1. Crunch
20 reps

- Push lower back into floor.
- Focus on ceiling, not knees.
- Breathe out as you go up.

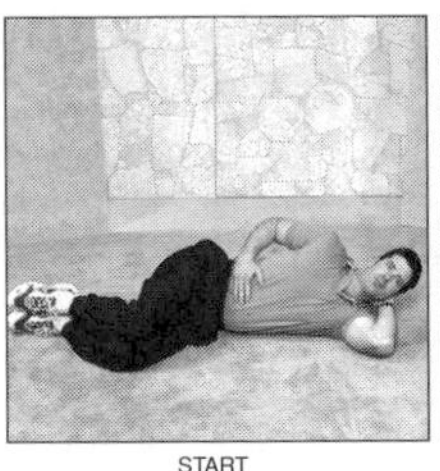

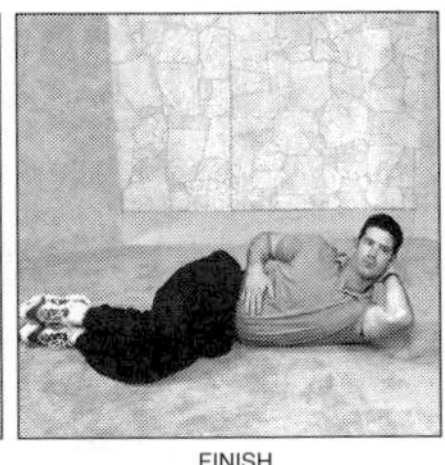

START FINISH

2. Side Crunches
20 reps Right/Left

- Contract top side to pull shoulder to hip.
- Try to lift bottom shoulder off ground.

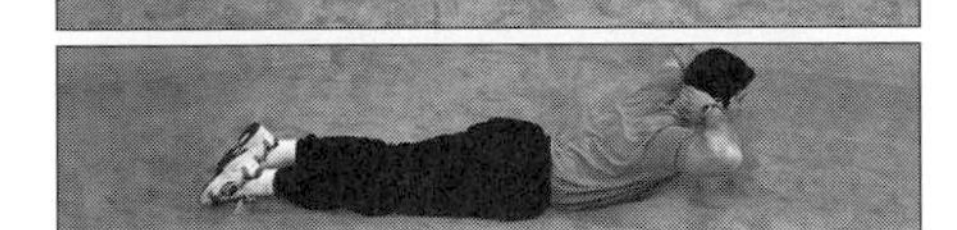

START FINISH

3. Hyper Extension
20 reps

- Raise upper body off floor feeling contraction in mid to low back.

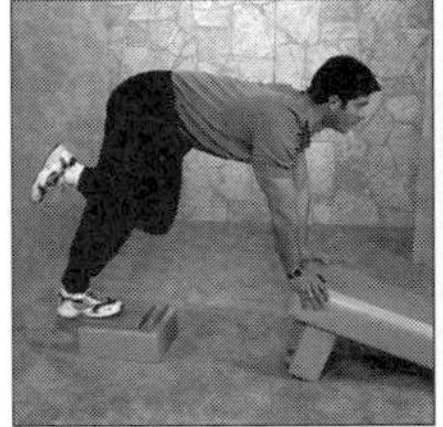

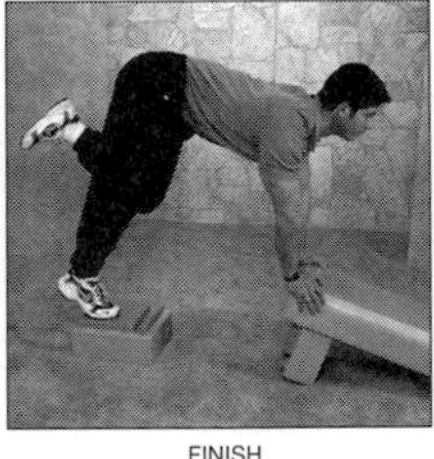

START FINISH

4. Donkey Calf Raise
20 reps Right/Left

- Place ball of foot on step or book and raise heal.
- Keep knee straight.

THE CAMPITELLI ADVANCED 10 MINUTE EXERCISE METHOD

MEN'S WORKOUT #2 • PAGE 2

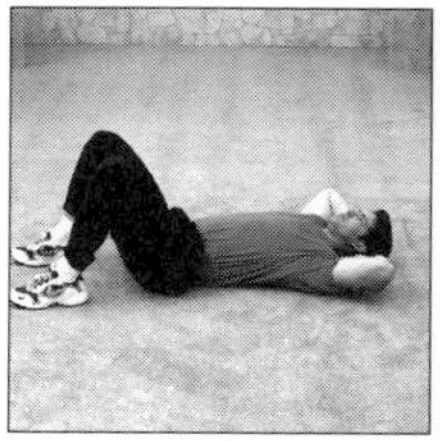

START FINISH

5. Crunch
20 reps

- Push lower back into floor.
- Focus on ceiling, not knees.
- Breathe out as you go up.

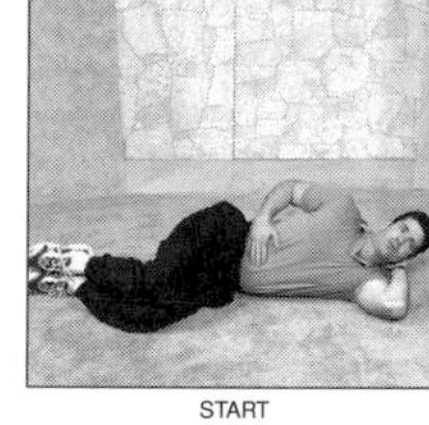

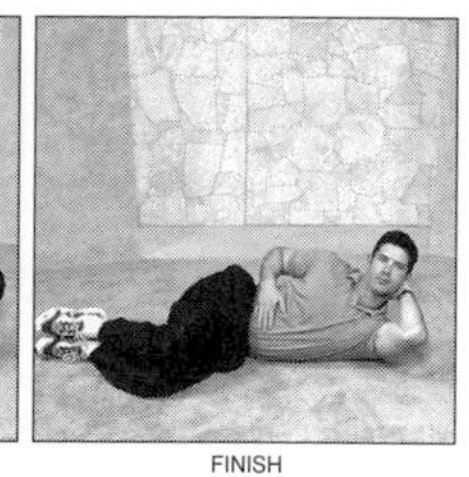

START FINISH

6. Side Crunches
20 reps Right/Left

- Contract top side to pull shoulder to hip.
- Try to lift bottom shoulder off ground.

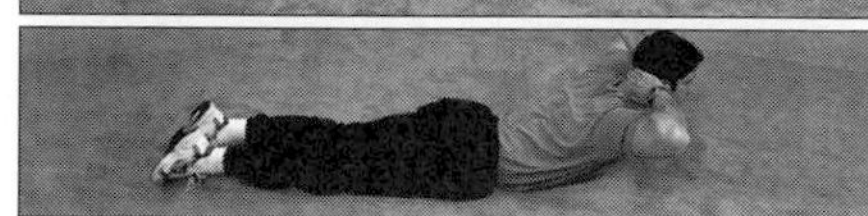

START FINISH

7. Hyper Extension
20 reps

- Raise upper body off floor feeling contraction in mid to low back.

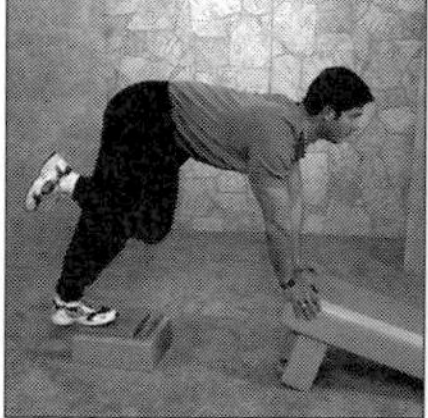

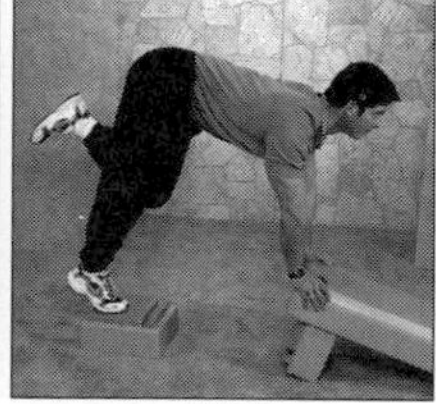

START FINISH

8. Donkey Calf Raise
20 reps Right/Left

- Place ball of foot on step or book and raise heal.
- Keep knee straight.

THE CAMPITELLI ADVANCED 10 MINUTE EXERCISE METHOD

MEN'S WORKOUT #3 • PAGE 1

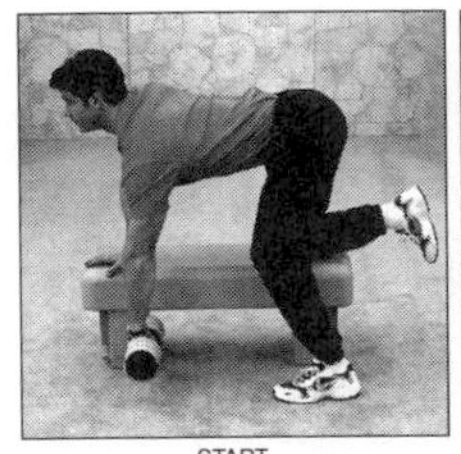

START FINISH

1. Dumbbell Row Wide Grip

10 reps Right/Left

- Pull weight raising elbow away from side.
- Back is arched with chest out.
- Keep non-working hand firmly on bench suppoorting upper body. Head up.

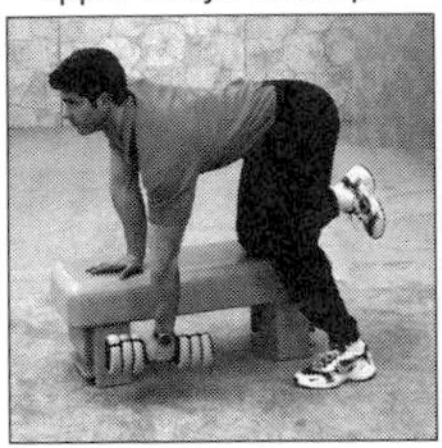

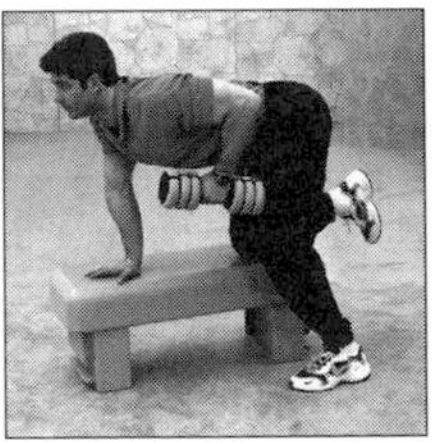

START FINISH

3. Dumbbell Row Close Grip

10 repss Right/Left

- Pull weight raising elbow close to your side.
- Head up. Back is arched with chest out.
- Keep non-working hand firmly on bench supporting upper body.

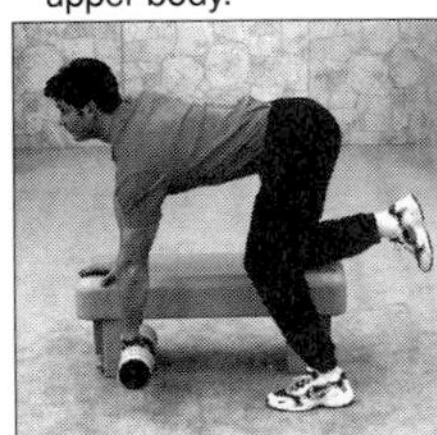

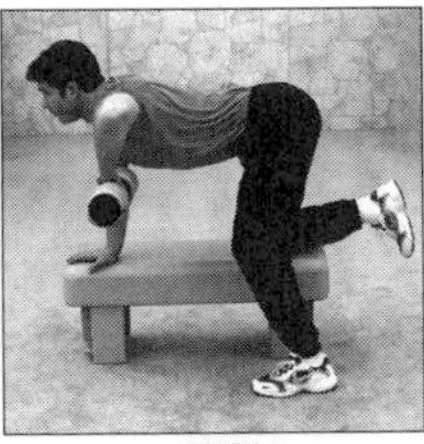

START FINISH

5. Dumbbell Row Wide Grip

10 reps Right/Left

- Pull weight raising elbow away from side.
- Back is arched with chest out.
- Keep non-working hand firmly on bench suppoorting upper body. Head up.

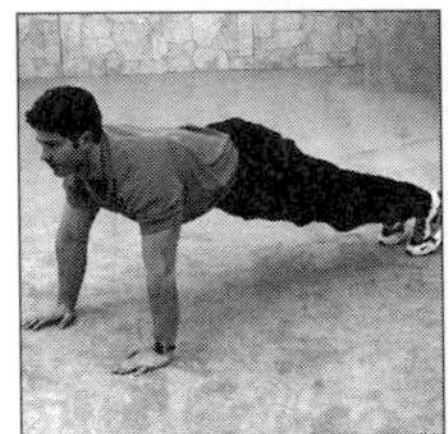

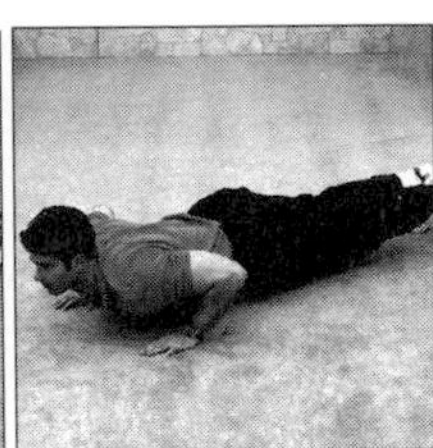

START FINISH

2. Pushup

10 reps

- Head up.
- Body straight.
- Hands are slightly wider than shoulders.
- Lower body and chest 2-3 inches from floor.

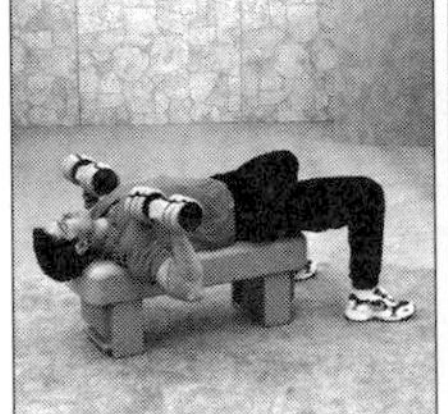

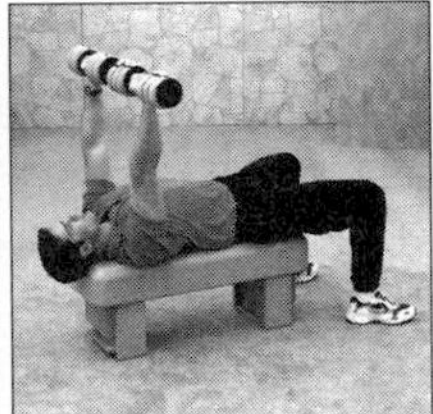

START FINISH

4. Dumbbell Press

10 reps

- Hold weights palms toward knees.
- Relax abdomen.
- Lower weights until even with chest.

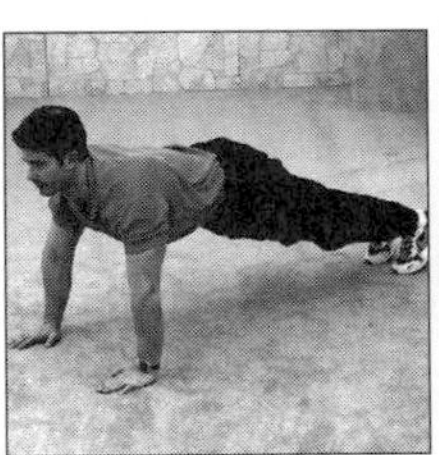

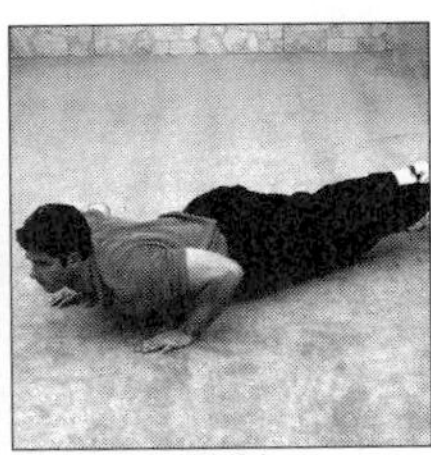

START FINISH

6. Pushup

10 reps

- Head up.
- Body straight.
- Hands are slightly wider than shoulders.
- Lower body and chest 2-3 inches from floor.

THE CAMPITELLI ADVANCED 10 MINUTE EXERCISE METHOD

MEN'S WORKOUT #3 • PAGE 1

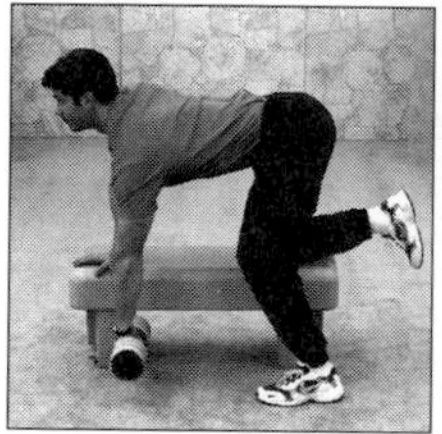

START FINISH

1. Dumbbell Row Wide Grip

10 reps Right/Left

- Pull weight raising elbow away from side.
- Back is arched with chest out.
- Keep non-working hand firmly on bench suppoorting upper body. Head up.

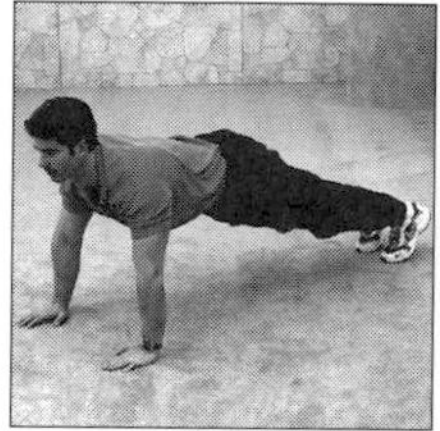
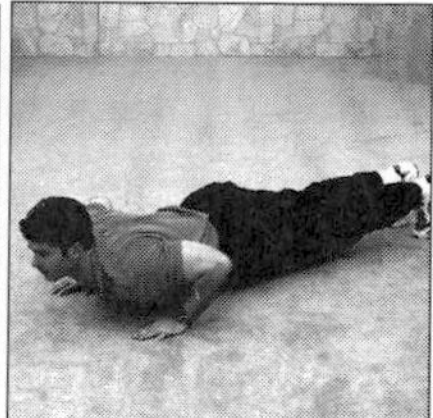

START FINISH

2. Pushup

10 reps

- Head up.
- Body straight.
- Hands are slightly wider than shoulders.
- Lower body and chest 2-3 inches from floor.

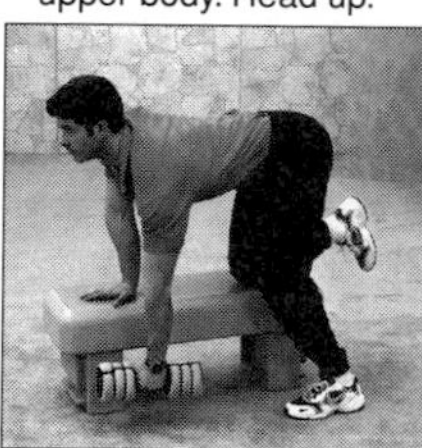
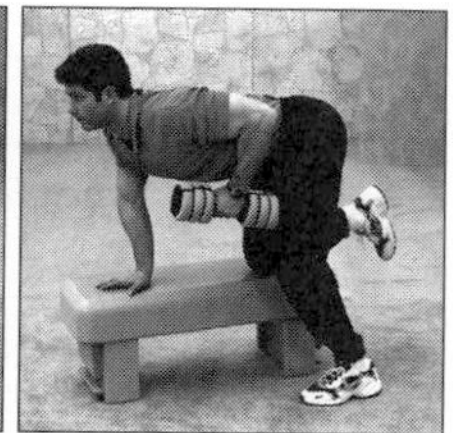

START FINISH

3. Dumbbell Row Close Grip

10 repss Right/Left

- Pull weight raising elbow close to your side.
- Head up. Back is arched with chest out.
- Keep non-working hand firmly on bench supporting upper body.

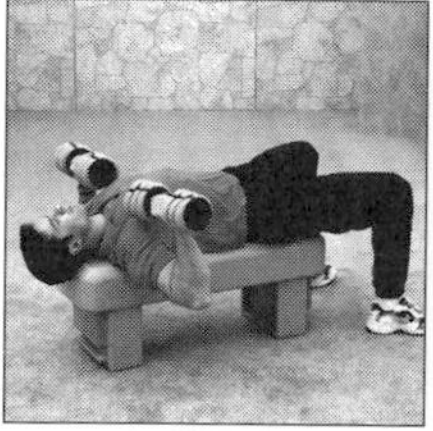
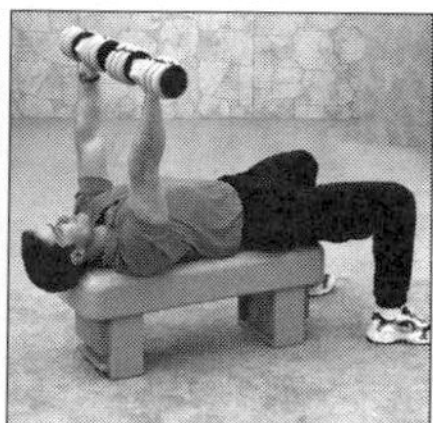

START FINISH

4. Dumbbell Press

10 reps

- Hold weights palms toward knees.
- Relax abdomen.
- Lower weights until even with chest.

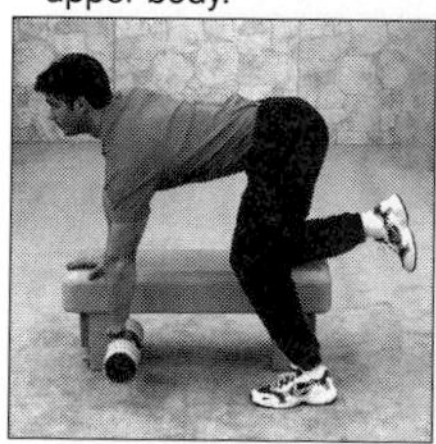
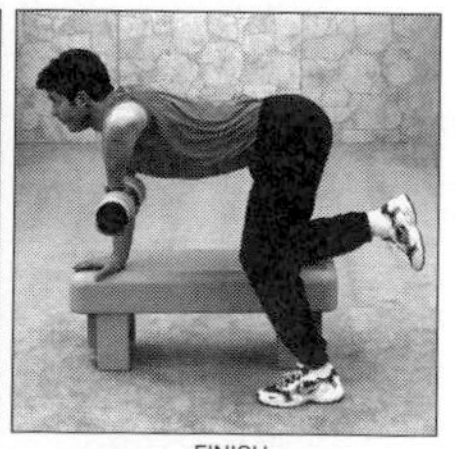

START FINISH

5. Dumbbell Row Wide Grip

10 reps Right/Left

- Pull weight raising elbow away from side.
- Back is arched with chest out.
- Keep non-working hand firmly on bench suppoorting upper body. Head up.

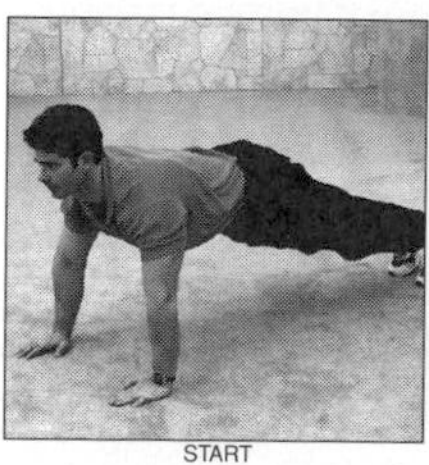
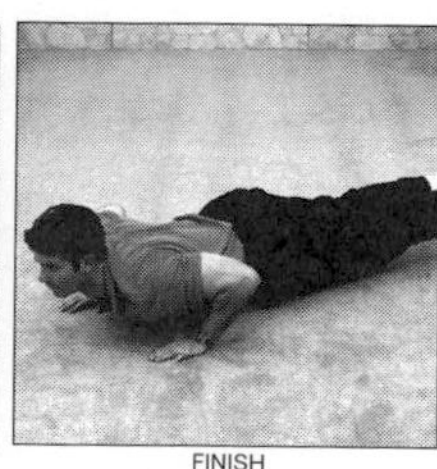

START FINISH

6. Pushup

10 reps

- Head up.
- Body straight.
- Hands are slightly wider than shoulders.
- Lower body and chest 2-3 inches from floor.

THE CAMPITELLI ADVANCED 10 MINUTE EXERCISE METHOD

MEN'S WORKOUT #3 • PAGE 2

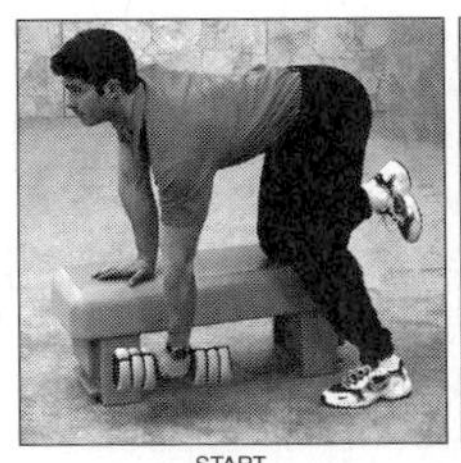
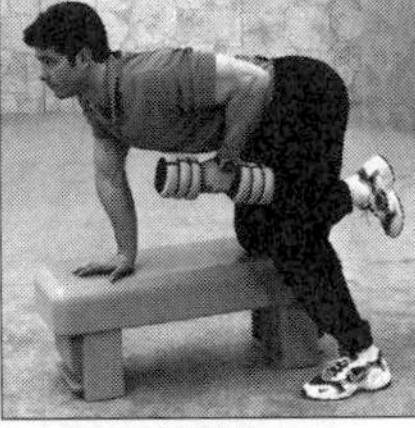

START FINISH

7. Dumbbell Row Close Grip
10 repss Right/Left

- Pull weight raising elbow close to your side.
- Head up. Back is arched with chest out.
- Keep non-working hand firmly on bench supporting upper body.

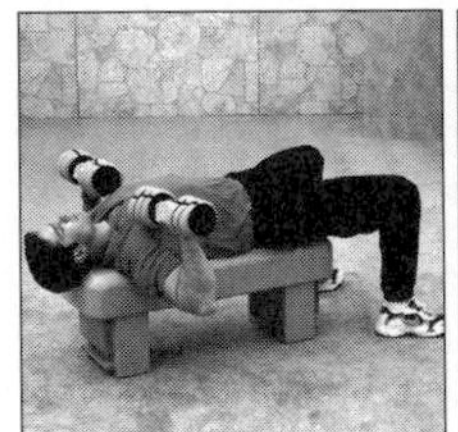
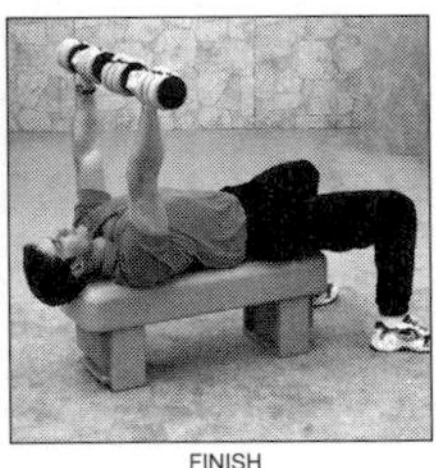

START FINISH

8. Dumbbell Press
10 reps

- Hold weights palms toward knees.
- Relax abdomen.
- Lower weights until even with chest.

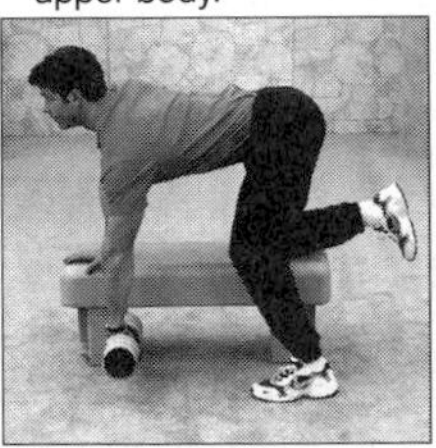
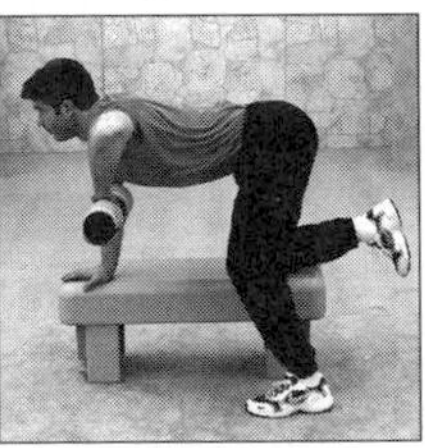

START FINISH

9. Dumbbell Row Wide Grip
10 reps Right/Left

- Pull weight raising elbow away from side.
- Back is arched with chest out.
- Keep non-working hand firmly on bench suppoorting upper body. Head up.

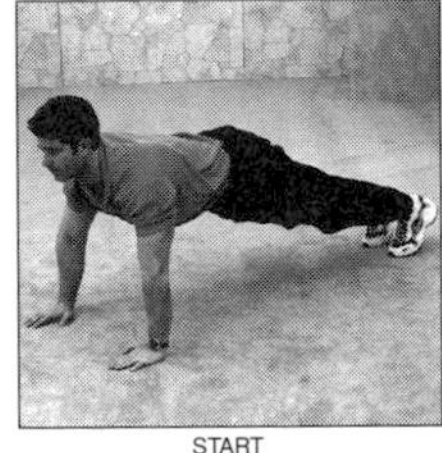
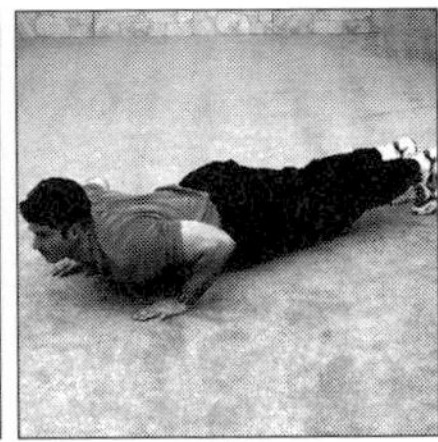

START FINISH

10. Pushup
10 reps

- Head up.
- Body straight.
- Hands are slightly wider than shoulders.
- Lower body and chest 2-3 inches from floor.

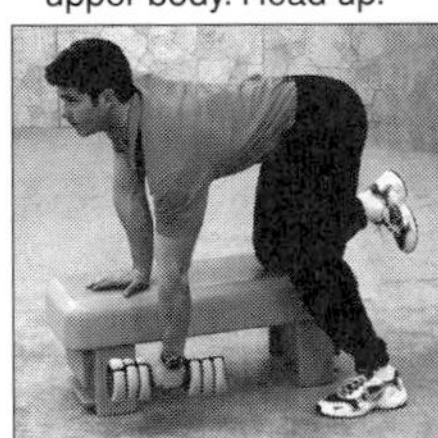
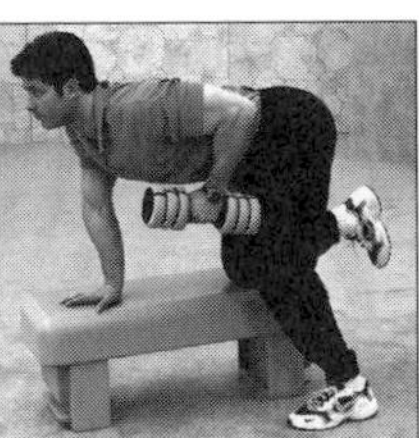

START FINISH

11. Dumbbell Row Close Grip
10 repss Right/Left

- Pull weight raising elbow close to your side.
- Head up. Back is arched with chest out.
- Keep non-working hand firmly on bench supporting upper body.

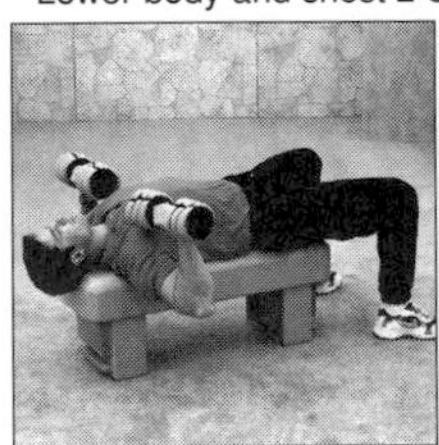
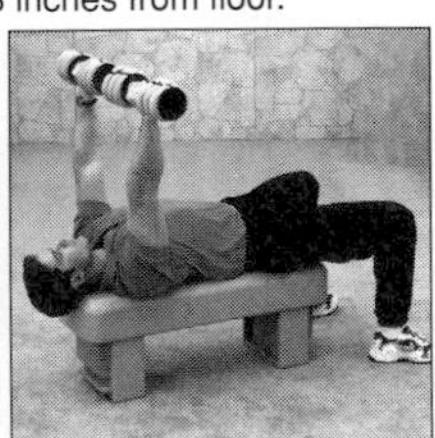

START FINISH

12. Dumbbell Press
10 reps

- Hold weights palms toward knees.
- Relax abdomen.
- Lower weights until even with chest.

THE CAMPITELLI ADVANCED 10 MINUTE EXERCISE METHOD

MEN'S WORKOUT #4 • PAGE 1

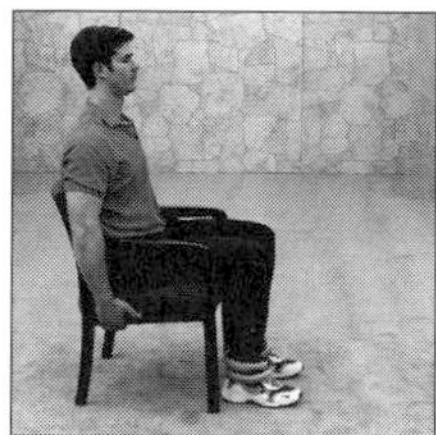

START FINISH

1. Leg Extension with Ankle Weights

10 reps Right/Left

- Extend foot out with weights and hold leg straight for a brief pause and then return.

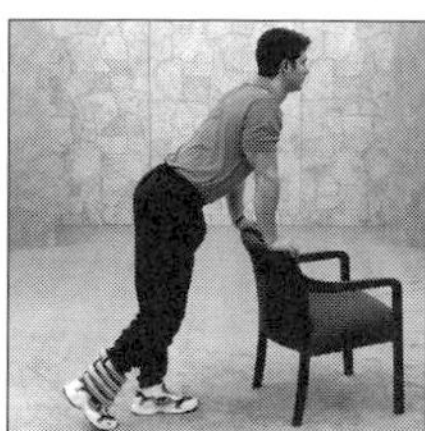

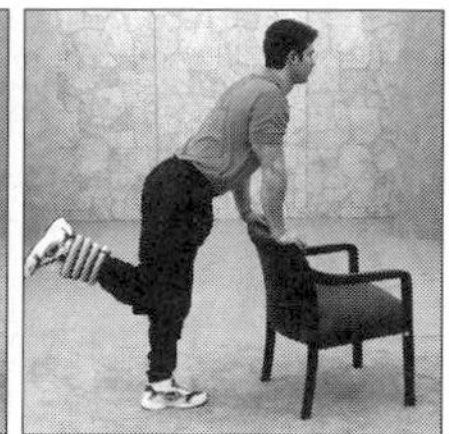

START FINISH

2. Leg Curl with Ankle Weights

10 reps Right/Left

- Raise leg bending knee.
- Use chair for balance.
- Keeptoe pointed down.
- Hold briefly at top position.

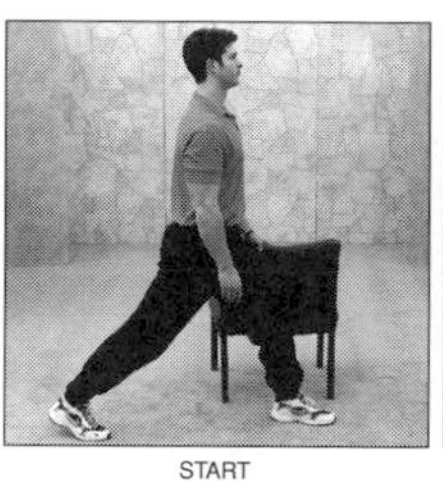

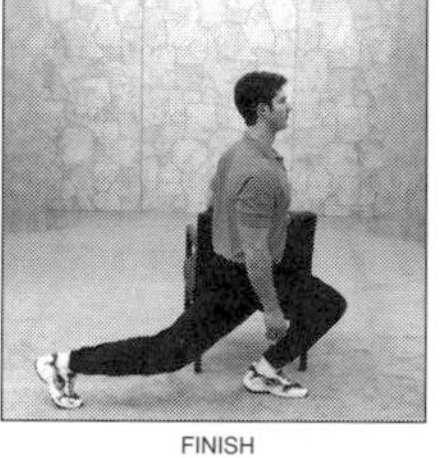

START FINISH

3. Lunges

15 reps Right/Left

- Use chair for balance.
- Back straight. Chest out.
- Push with heal of front leg.

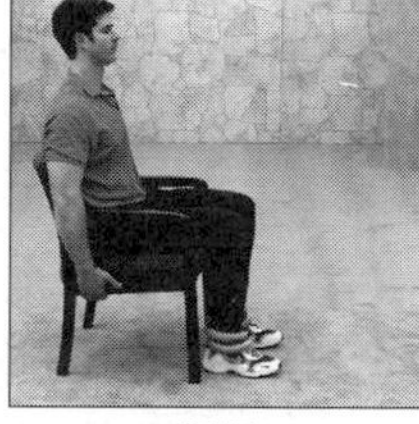

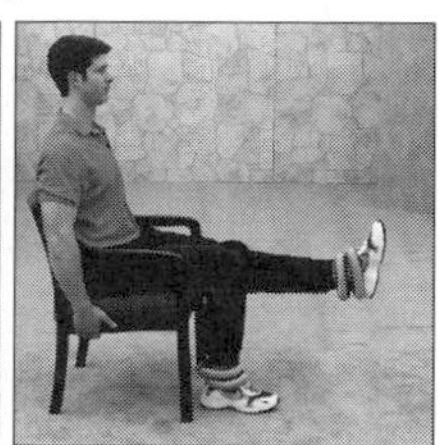

START FINISH

4. Leg Extension with Ankle Weights

10 reps Right/Left

- Extend foot out with weights and hold leg straight for a brief pause and then return.

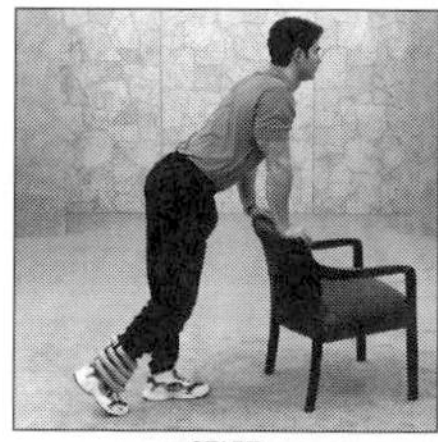

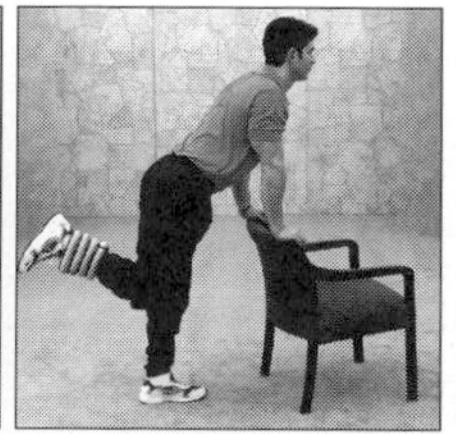

START FINISH

5. Leg Curl with Ankle Weights

10 reps Right/Left

- Raise leg bending knee.
- Use chair for balance.
- Keeptoe pointed down.
- Hold briefly at top position.

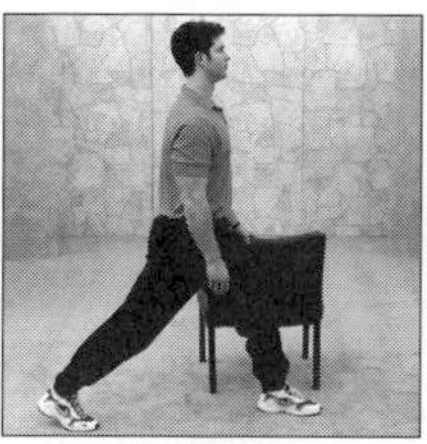

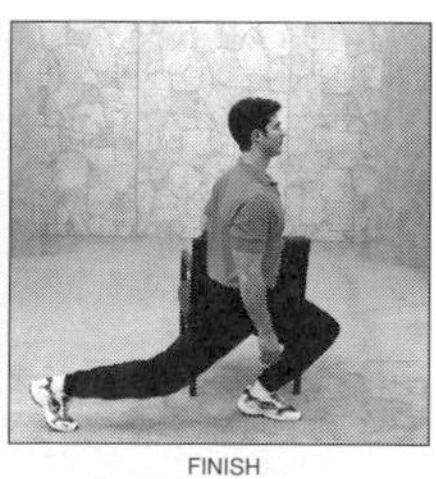

START FINISH

6. Lunges

15 reps Right/Left

- Use chair for balance.
- Back straight. Chest out.
- Push with heal of front leg.

THE CAMPITELLI ADVANCED 10 MINUTE EXERCISE METHOD

MEN'S WORKOUT #4 • PAGE 2

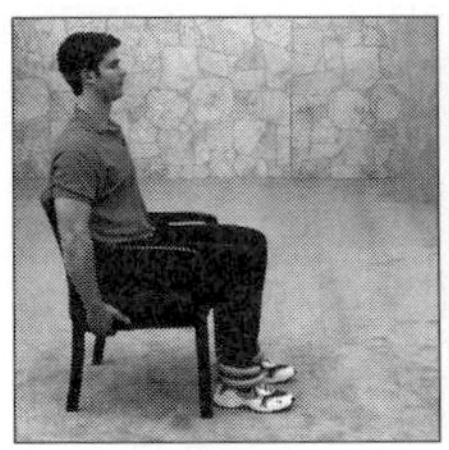

START

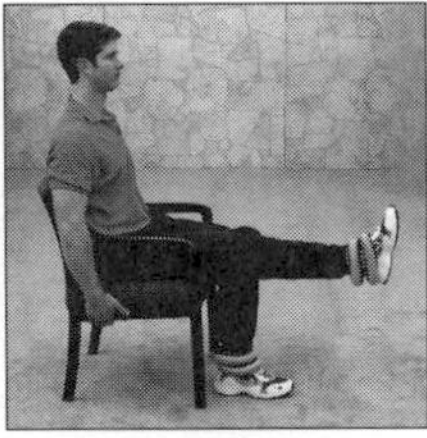

FINISH

7. Leg Extension with Ankle Weights
10 reps Right/Left

- Extend foot out with weights and hold leg straight for a brief pause and then return.

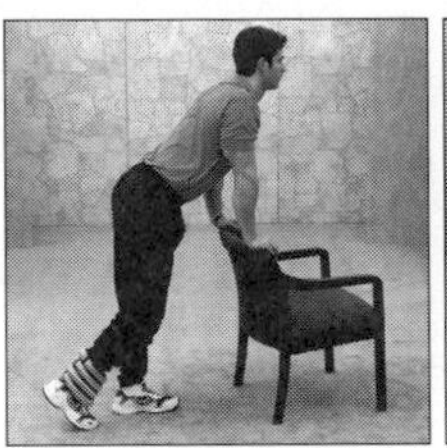

START

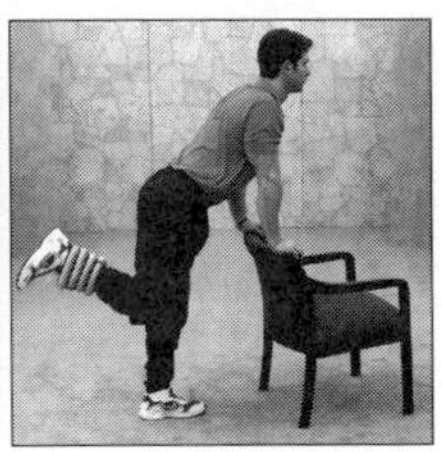

FINISH

8. Leg Curl with Ankle Weights
10 reps Right/Left

- Raise leg bending knee.
- Use chair for balance.
- Keeptoe pointed down.
- Hold briefly at top position.

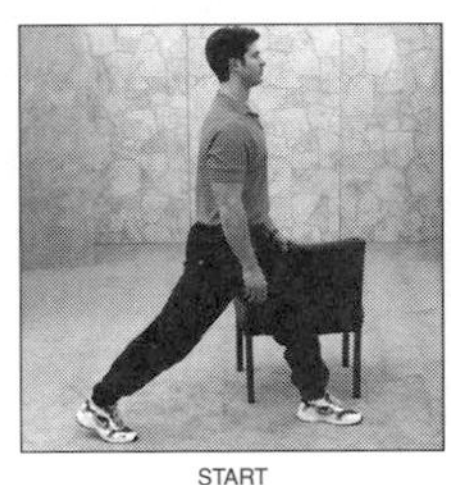

START

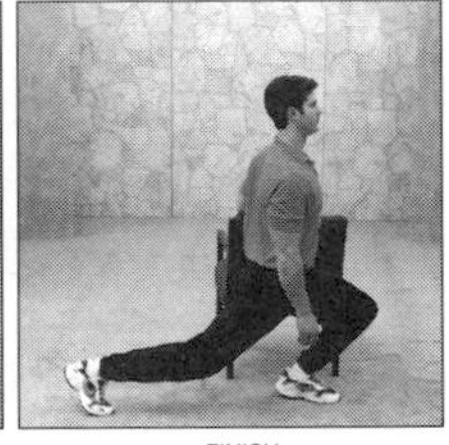

FINISH

9. Lunges
15 reps Right/Left

- Use chair for balance.
- Back straight. Chest out.
- Push with heal of front leg.

THE CAMPITELLI ADVANCED 10 MINUTE EXERCISE METHOD

MEN'S WORKOUT #5 • PAGE 1

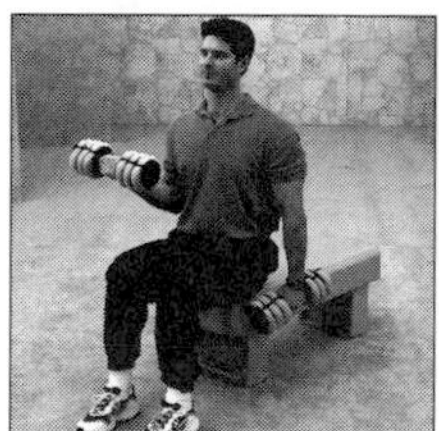

START FINISH

1. Alternating Dumbbell Curl
10 reps

- Chest out and shoulders back.
- Keep elbows to your side.
- Palms up at top.
- Don't swing weights.

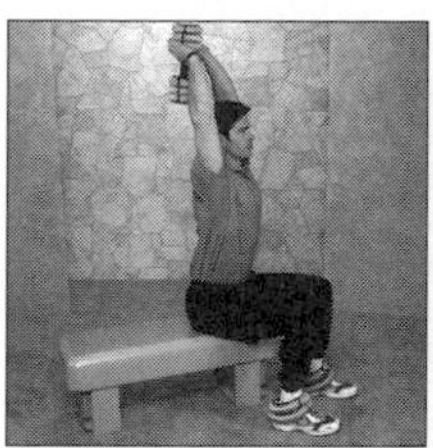
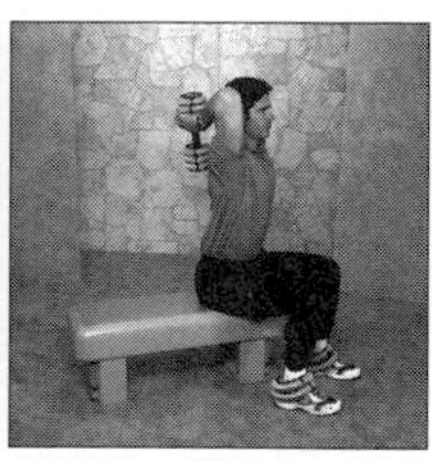

START FINISH

2. Overhead Tricep Extension
10 reps

- Extend weight over head.
- Keep elbows up and close to head.

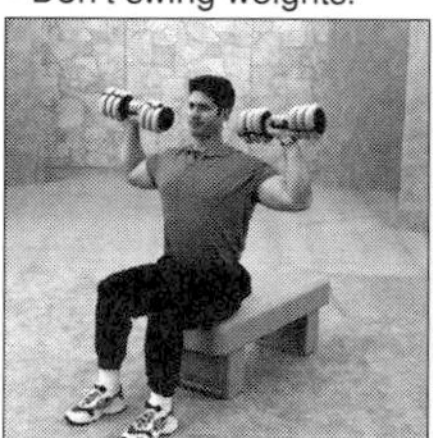
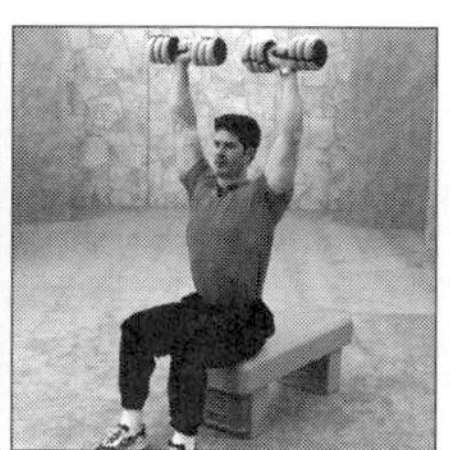

START FINISH

3. Shoulder Press
10 reps

- Press weights with elbows out from sides.
- Palms facing forward.

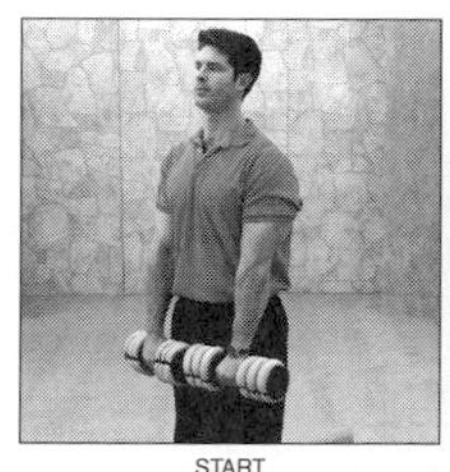
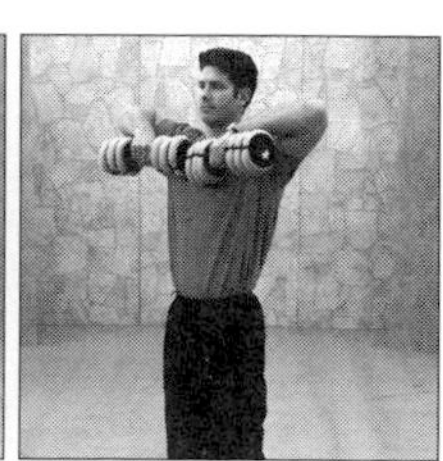

START FINISH

4. Upright Rows
10 reps

- Pull weights to chin.
- Elbows should be higher than weights at finish.

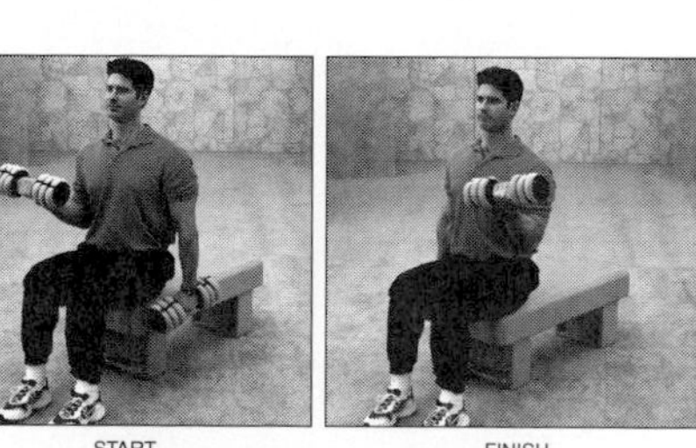

START FINISH

5. Alternating Dumbbell Curl
10 reps

- Chest out and shoulders back.
- Keep elbows to your side.
- Palms up at top. Don't swing weights.

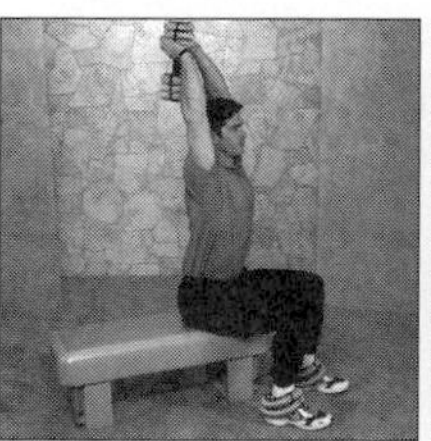
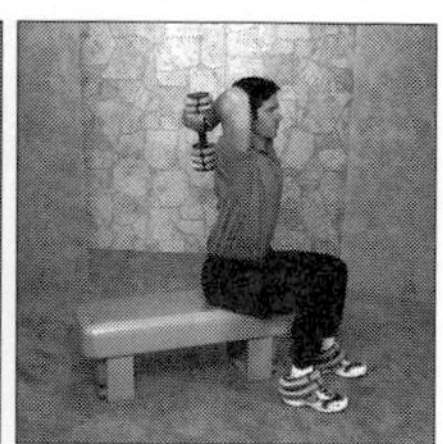

START FINISH

6. Overhead Tricep Extension
10 reps

- Extend weight over head.
- Keep elbows up and close to head.

THE CAMPITELLI ADVANCED 10 MINUTE EXERCISE METHOD

MEN'S WORKOUT #5 • PAGE 2

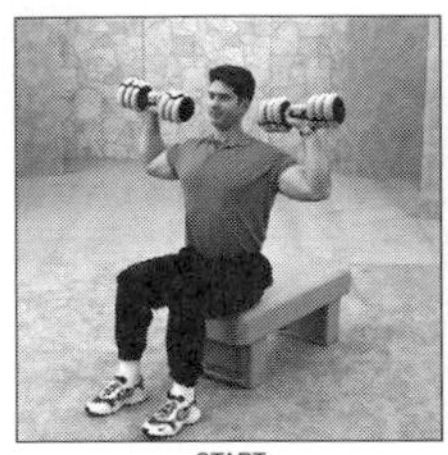

START FINISH

7. Shoulder Press
10 reps

- Press weights with elbows out from sides.
- Palms facing forward.

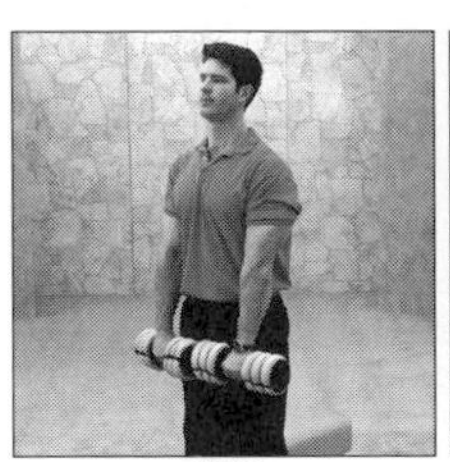

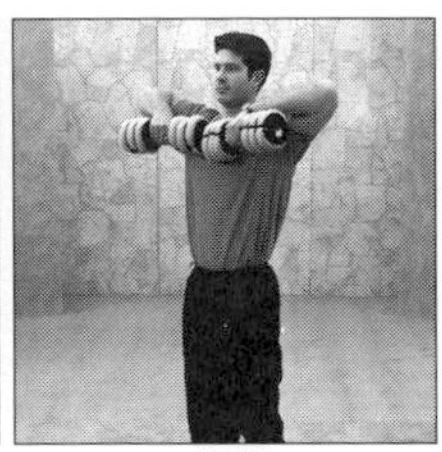

START FINISH

8. Upright Rows
10 reps

- Pull weights to chin.
- Elbows should be higher than weights at finish.

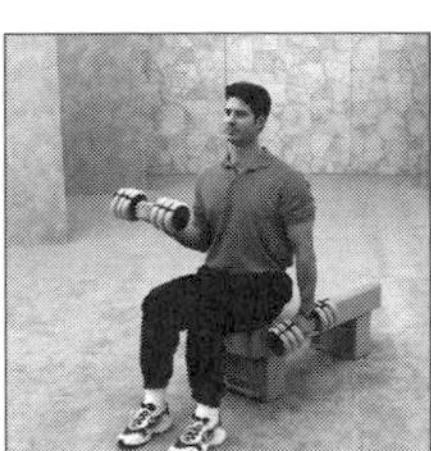

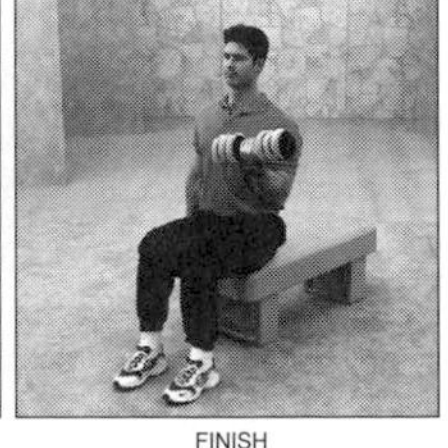

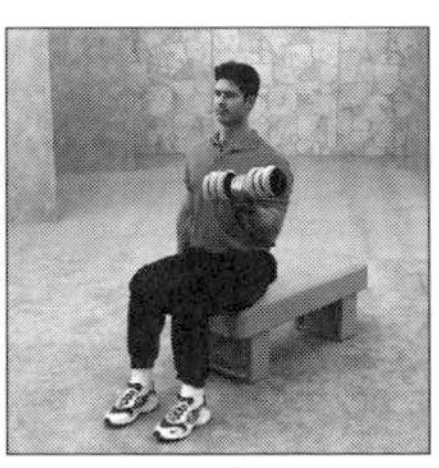

START FINISH

9. Alternating Dumbbell Curl
10 reps

- Chest out and shoulders back.
- Keep elbows to your side.
- Palms up at top.
- Don't swing weights.

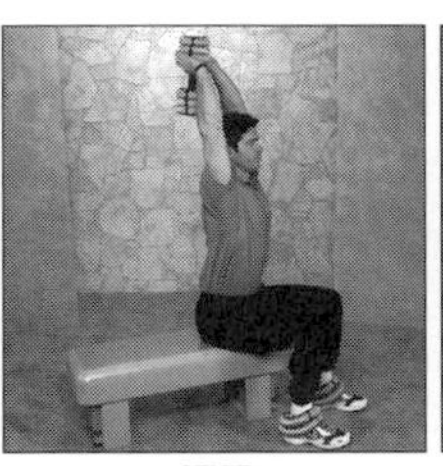

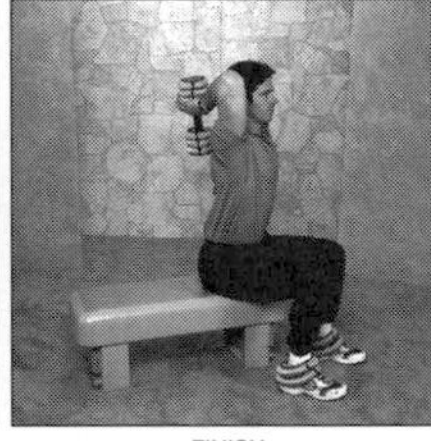

START FINISH

10. Overhead Tricep Extension
10 reps

- Extend weight over head.
- Keep elbows up and close to head.

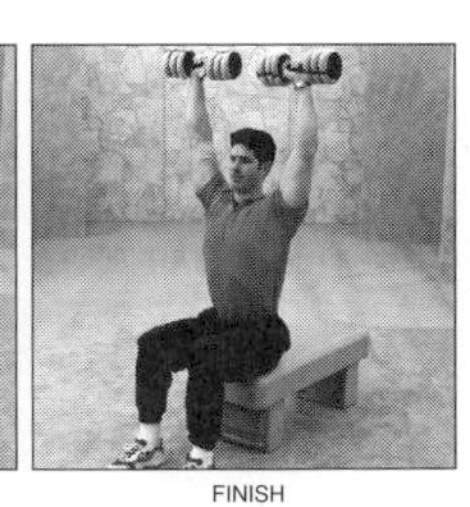

START FINISH

11. Shoulder Press
10 reps

- Press weights with elbows out from sides.
- Palms facing forward.

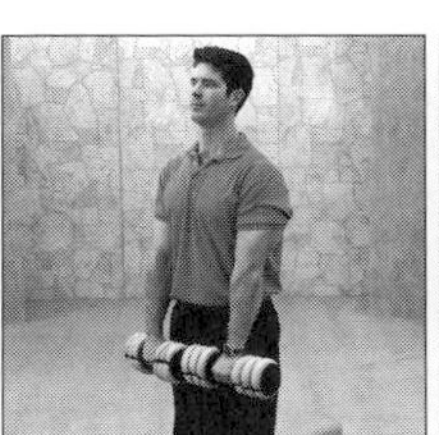

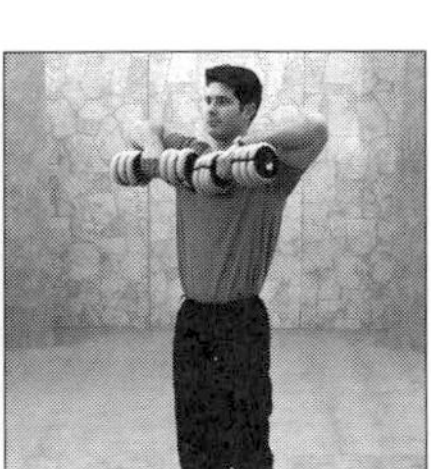

START FINISH

12. Upright Rows
10 reps

- Pull weights to chin.
- Elbows should be higher than weights at finish.

THE CAMPITELLI ADVANCED 10 MINUTE EXERCISE METHOD

MEN'S WORKOUT #6 • PAGE 1

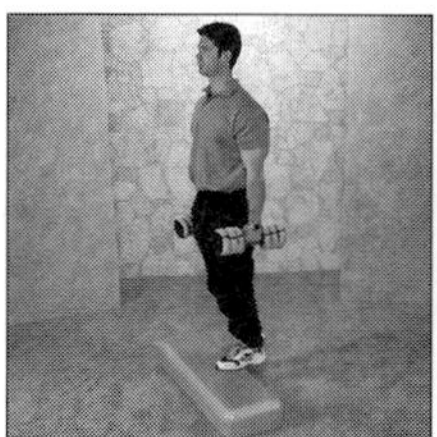
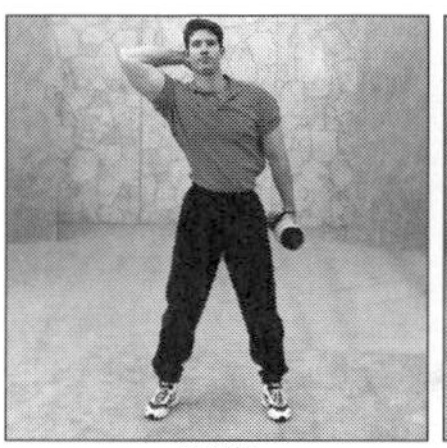
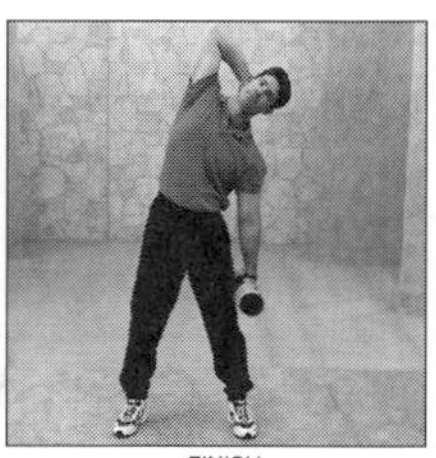

START FINISH

1. Calf Raise with Dumbbell
20 reps Right/Left

- Use step or book for elevation.
- Use DB for extra resistance.
- Raise heel up.
- Keep knees straight during movement.

START FINISH

2. Side Bends with Dumbbell
20 reps Right/Left

- Feet shoulder width apart.
- Pull DB up the side of leg.
- Keep shoulders, back and chest out.

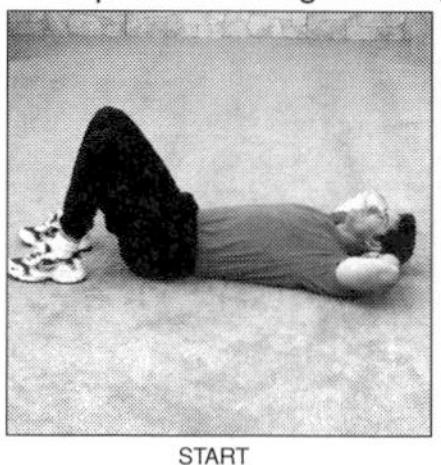
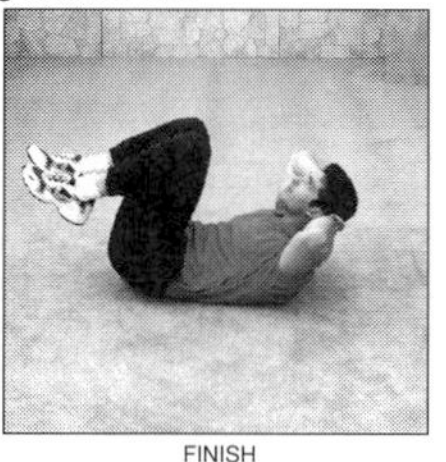

START FINISH

3. V-Crunch
20 reps

- Draw knees to chest as you lift shoulder from the floor.
- Exhale as knees and shoulders come up.

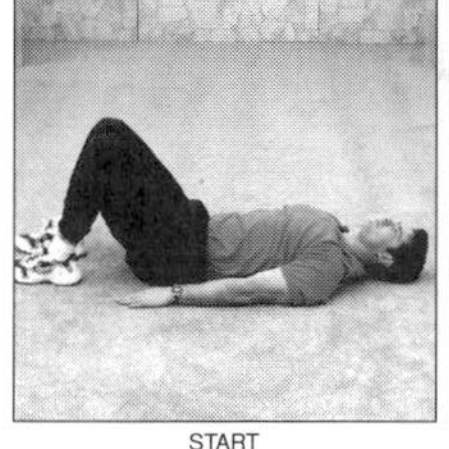
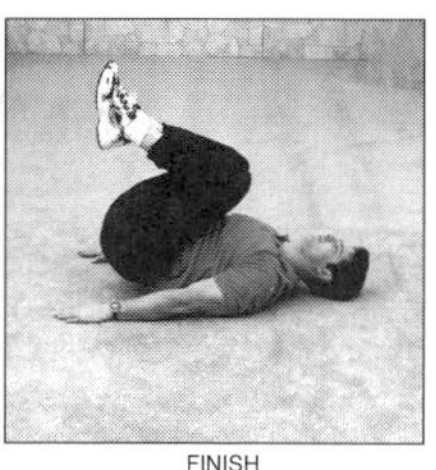

START FINISH

4. Tucks
20 reps

- Knees stay bent.
- Curl up until glutes come off floor.
- Exhale as knees come toward head.

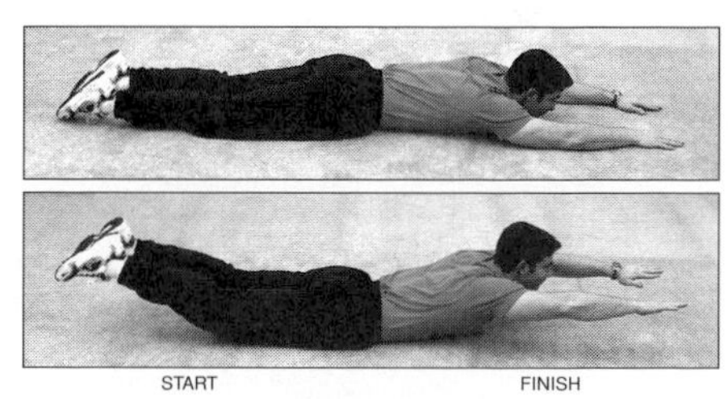

START FINISH

5. Supermans
20 reps

- Raise both hands and legs at the same time.
- Hold briefly at top.

THE CAMPITELLI ADVANCED 10 MINUTE EXERCISE METHOD

MEN'S WORKOUT #6 • PAGE 2

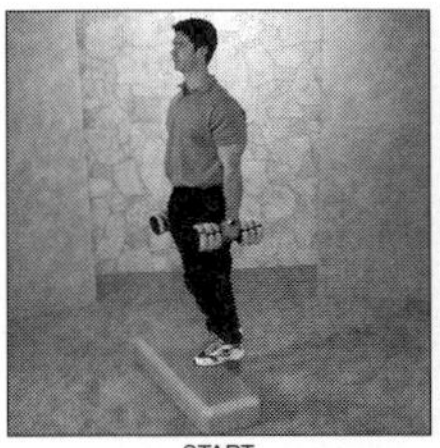 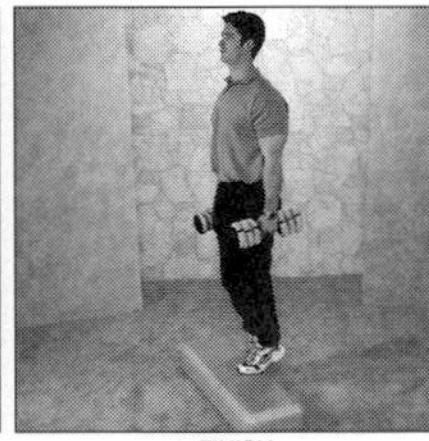

START FINISH

6. Calf Raise with Dumbbell

20 reps Right/Left

- Use step or book for elevation.
- Use DB for extra resistance.
- Raise heel up.
- Keep knees straight during movement.

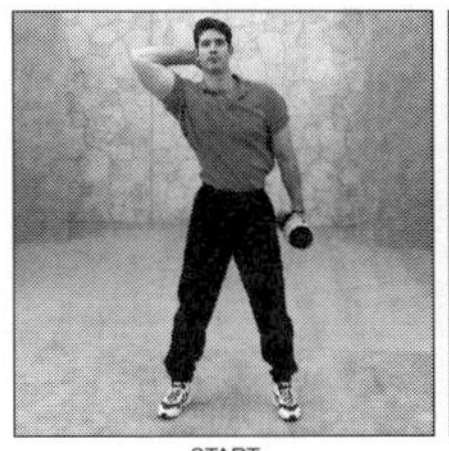 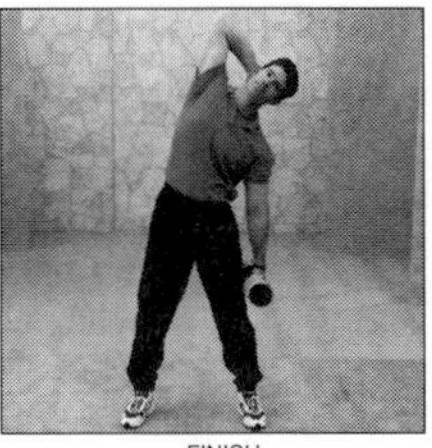

START FINISH

7. Side Bends with Dumbbell

20 reps Right/Left

- Feet shoulder width apart.
- Pull DB up the side of leg.
- Keep shoulders, back and chest out.

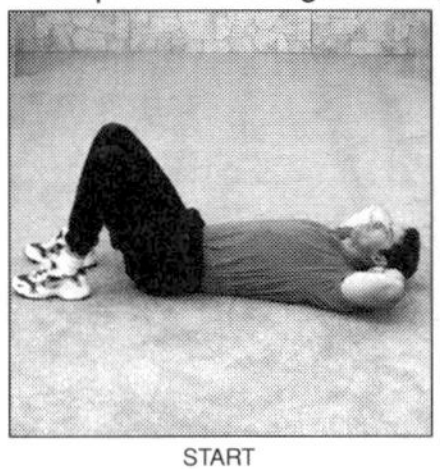 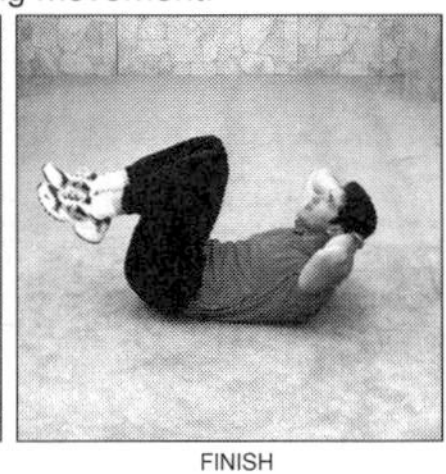

START FINISH

8. V-Crunch

20 reps

- Draw knees to chest as you lift shoulder from the floor.
- Exhale as knees and shoulders come up.

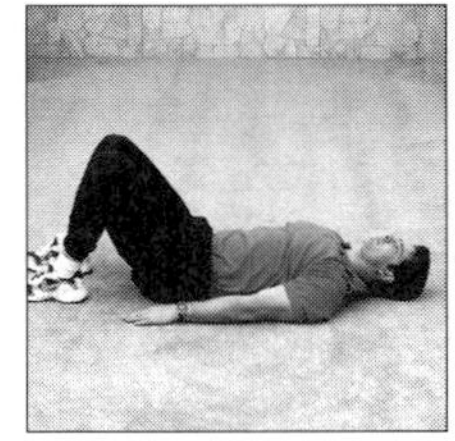 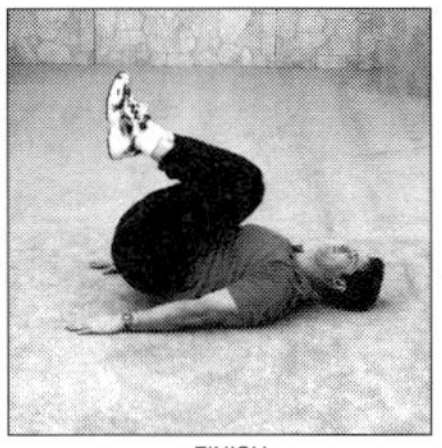

START FINISH

9. Tucks

20 reps

- Knees stay bent.
- Curl up until glutes come off floor.
- Exhale as knees come toward head.

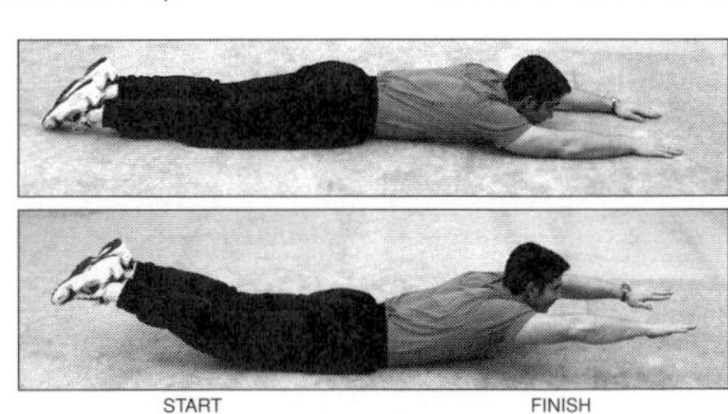

START FINISH

10. Supermans

20 reps

- Raise both hands and legs at the same time.
- Hold briefly at top.

THE CAMPITELLI ADVANCED 10 MINUTE EXERCISE METHOD

MEN'S WORKOUT #7 • PAGE 1

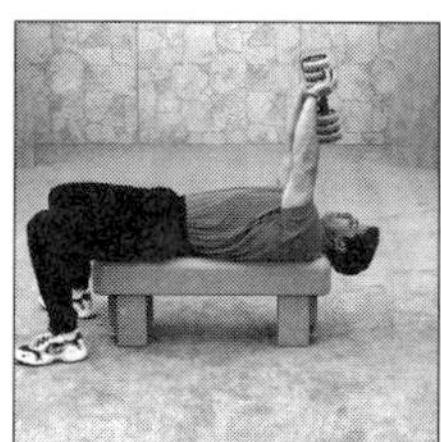
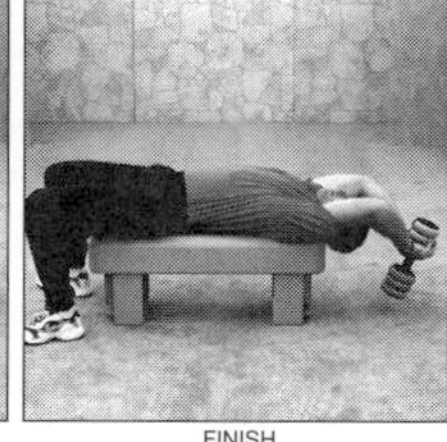

START FINISH

1. Dumbbell Pullover
10 reps

- Relax Abdomen. Keep elbows in toward body.
- Inhale as weight goes over head.
- Exhale as it goes up.

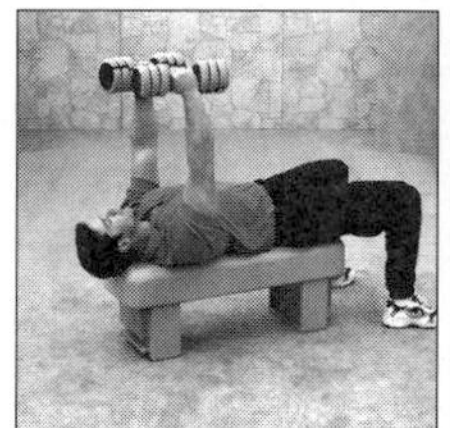
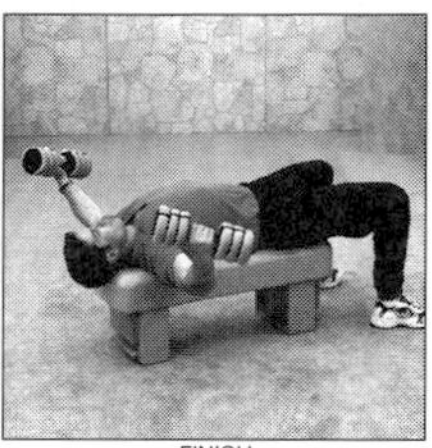

START FINISH

2. Dumbbell Fly
10 reps

- Elbows slightly bent with palms facing each other.
- Lower weights out to the side of body until weight is parallel to body.
- Keep elbow slightly bent.

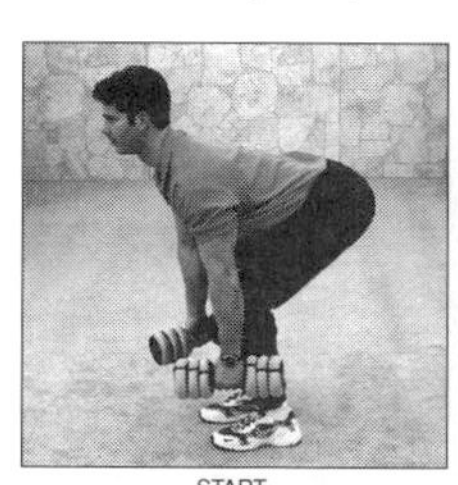
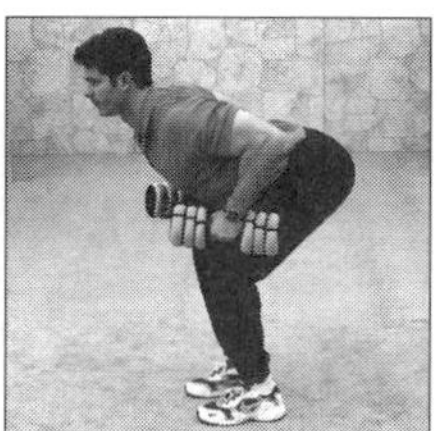

START FINISH

3. Dumbbell Row
10 reps

- Feet together. Bend at hips, not at waist.
- Bach straight. Chest out.
- Head up.
- Pull weights with elbows close to body.

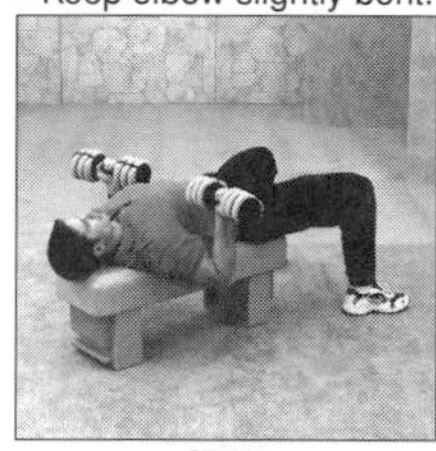
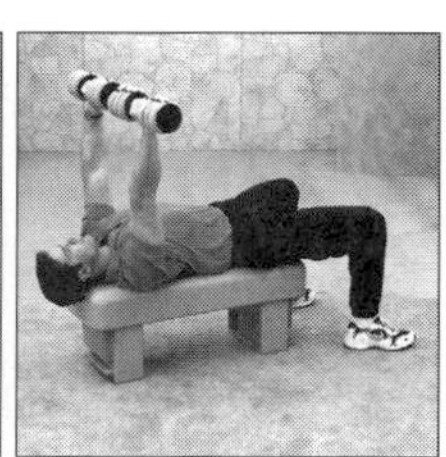

START FINISH

4. Dumbbell Press
10 reps

- Hold weights palms toward knees.
- Relax abdomin.
- Lower weights until even with chest.

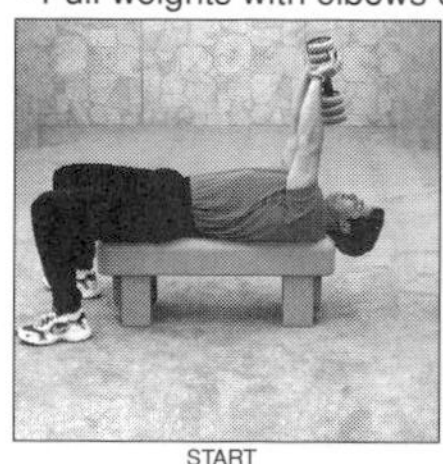
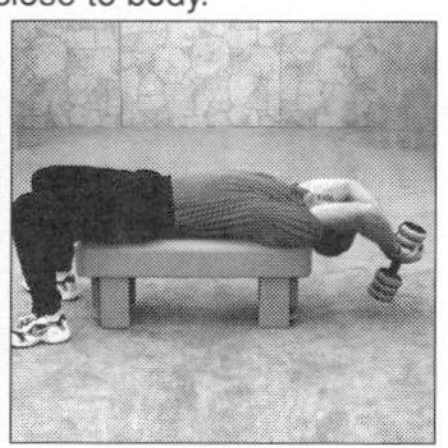

START FINISH

5. Dumbbell Pullover
10 reps

- Relax Abdomen. Keep elbows in toward body.
- Inhale as weight goes over head.
- Exhale as it goes up.

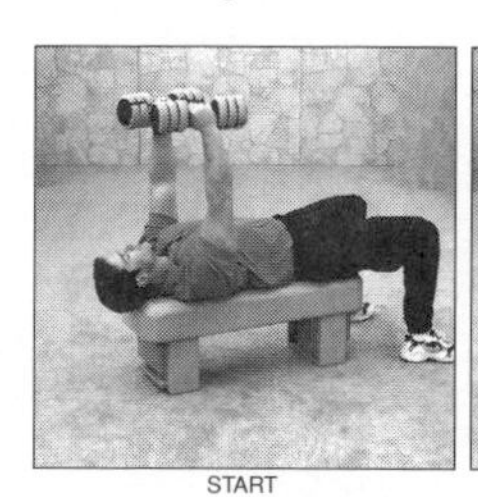
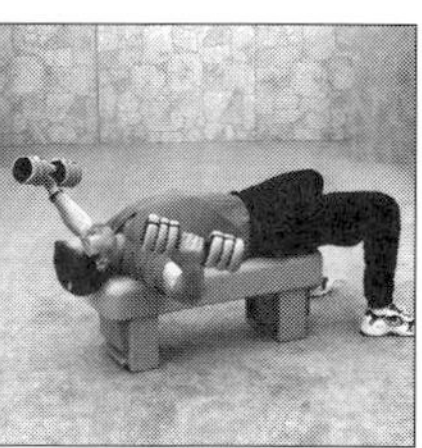

START FINISH

6. Dumbbell Fly
10 reps

- Elbows slightly bent with palms facing each other.
- Lower weights out to the side of body until weight is parallel to body.
- Keep elbow slightly bent.

THE CAMPITELLI ADVANCED 10 MINUTE EXERCISE METHOD

MEN'S WORKOUT #7 • PAGE 2

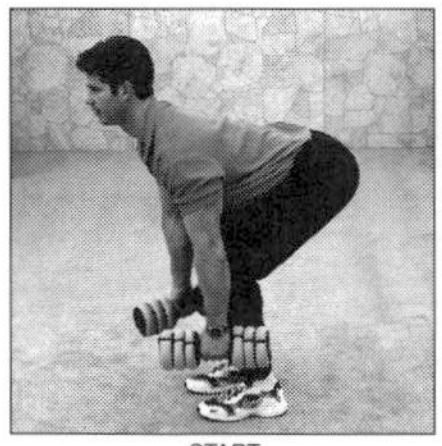

START

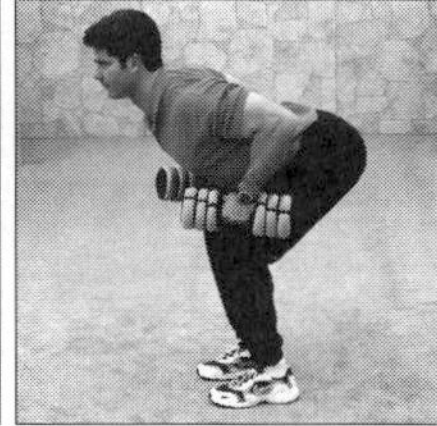

FINISH

7. Dumbbell Row

10 reps

- Feet together. Bend at hips, not at waist.
- Bach straight. Chest out.
- Head up.
- Pull weights with elbows close to body.

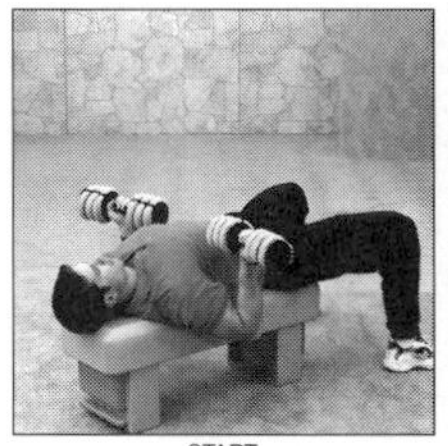

START

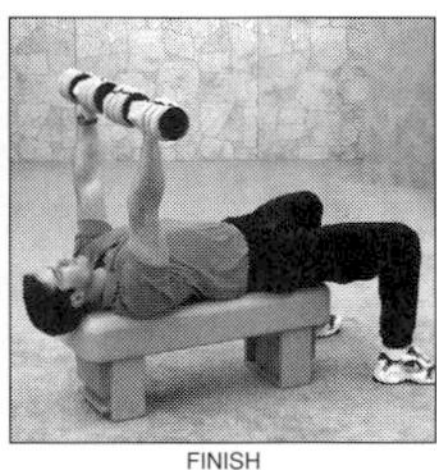

FINISH

8. Dumbbell Press

10 reps

- Hold weights palms toward knees.
- Relax abdomin.
- Lower weights until even with chest.

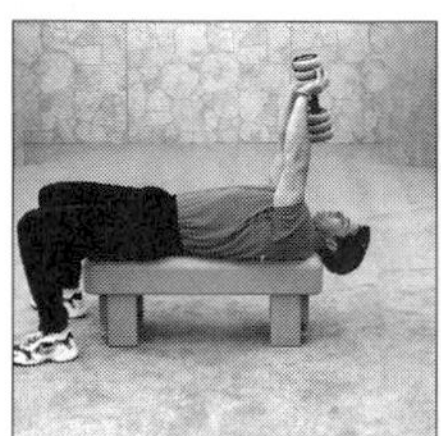

START

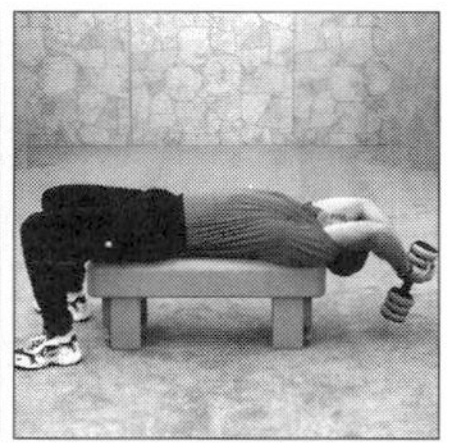

FINISH

9. Dumbbell Pullover

10 reps

- Relax Abdomen. Keep elbows in toward body.
- Inhale as weight goes over head.
- Exhale as it goes up.

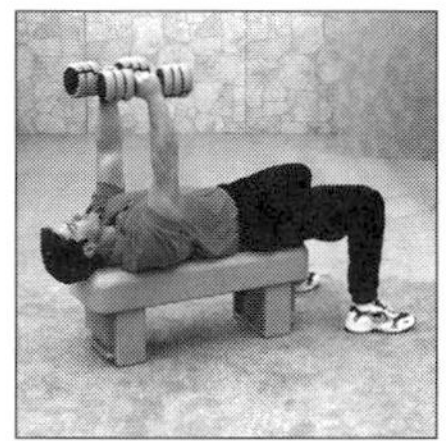

START

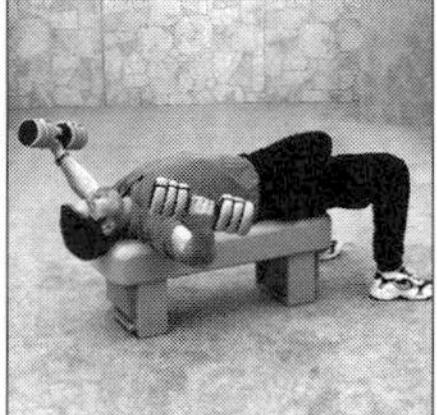

FINISH

10. Dumbbell Fly

10 reps

- Elbows slightly bent with palms facing each other.
- Lower weights out to the side of body until weight is parallel to body.
- Keep elbow slightly bent.

THE CAMPITELLI ADVANCED 10 MINUTE EXERCISE METHOD

MEN'S WORKOUT #8 • PAGE 1

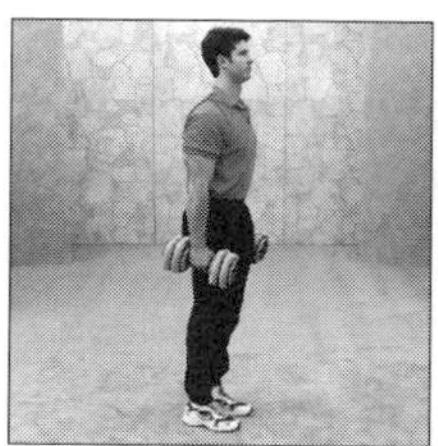
START

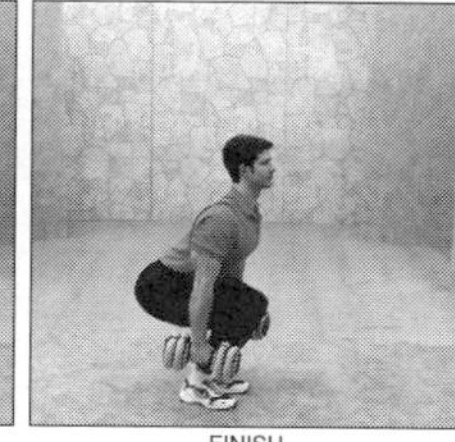
FINISH

1. Dumbbell Squat
10 reps

- Feet 4-8 inches apart. DBs at side.
- Place weight evenly on heels and balls of feet.
- Back straight. Head up.
- Push with heels.

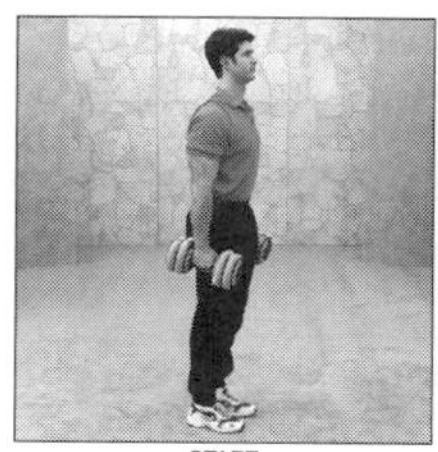
START

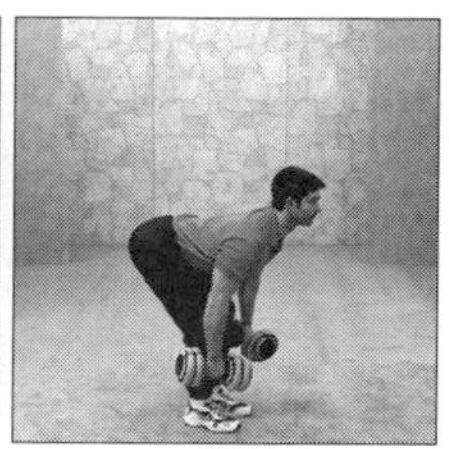
FINISH

2. Dumbbell Deadlift
10 reps

- Knees slightly bent with feet slightly apart
- Keep low back locked with upper torso.
- Bend at hips, not at waist. Head up/chest out.
- Back is flat.

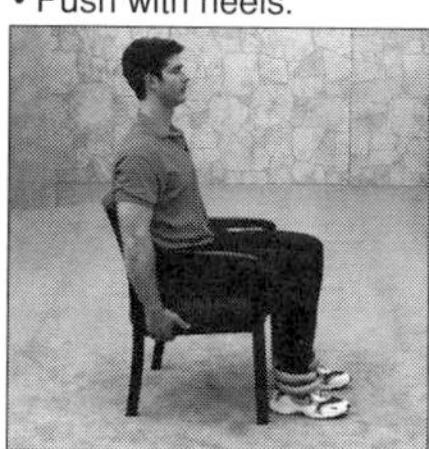
START

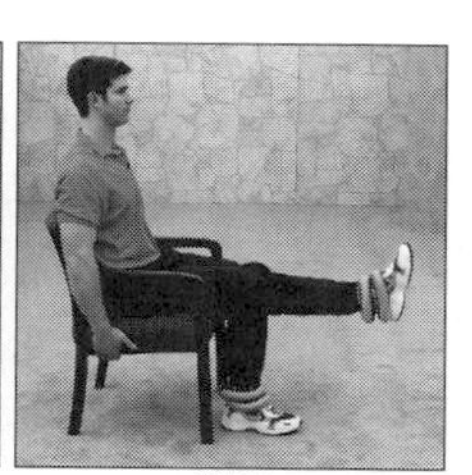
FINISH

3. Seated Leg Extension with Ankle Weights
10 reps Right/Left

- Extend foot out with weights, hold leg straight for a brief pause and then return.

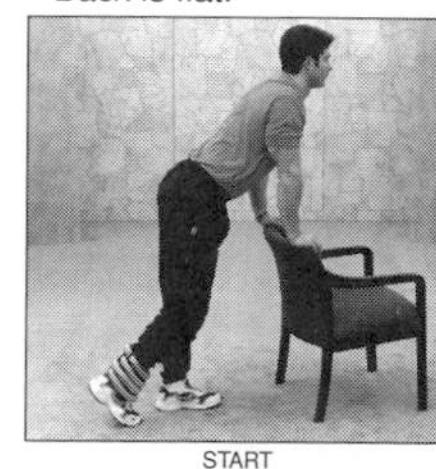
START

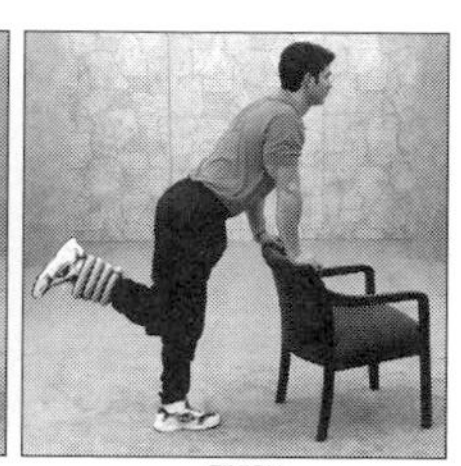
FINISH

4. Leg Curl with Ankle Weights
10 reps Right/Left

- Raise leg bending knee. • Use chair for balance.
- Keep toe pointed down.
- Hold briefly at top position.

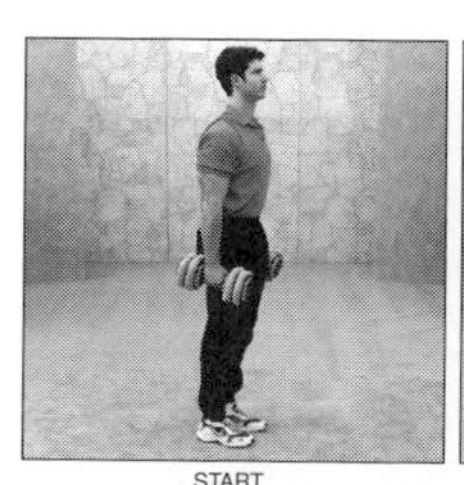
START

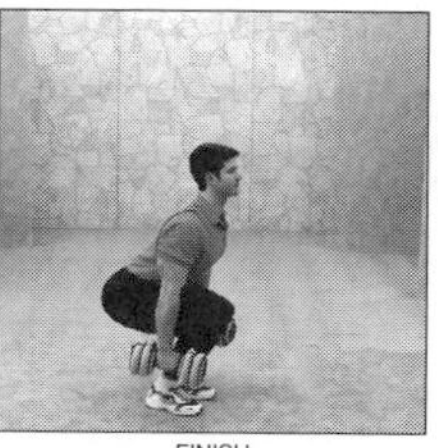
FINISH

5. Dumbbell Squat
10 reps

- Feet 4-8 inches apart. DBs at side.
- Place weight evenly on heels and balls of feet.
- Back straight. Head up.
- Push with heels.

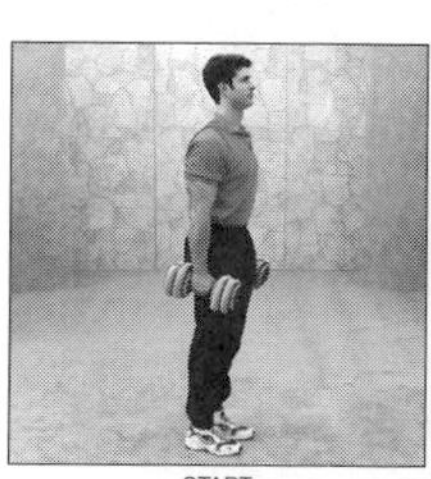
START

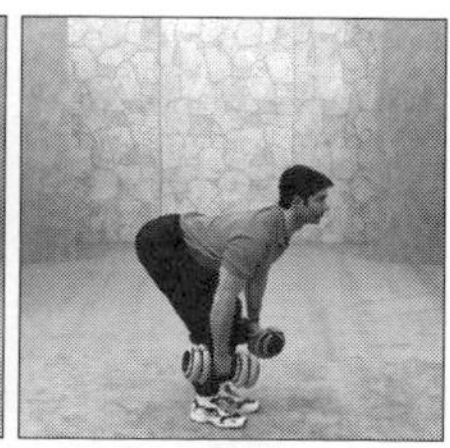
FINISH

6. Dumbbell Deadlift
10 reps

- Knees slightly bent with feet slightly apart
- Keep low back locked with upper torso.
- Bend at hips, not at waist. Head up/chest out.
- Back is flat.

THE CAMPITELLI ADVANCED 10 MINUTE EXERCISE METHOD

MEN'S WORKOUT #8 • PAGE 2

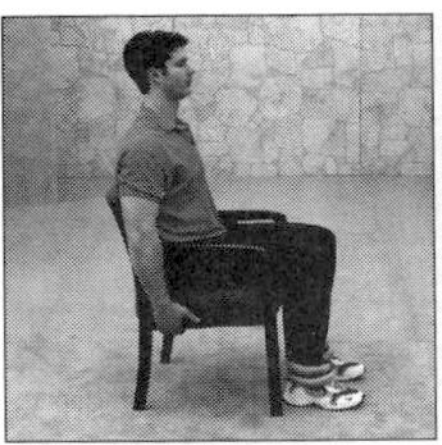

START FINISH

7. Seated Leg Extension with Ankle Weights

10 reps Right/Left

- Extend foot out with weights, hold leg straight for a brief pause and then return.

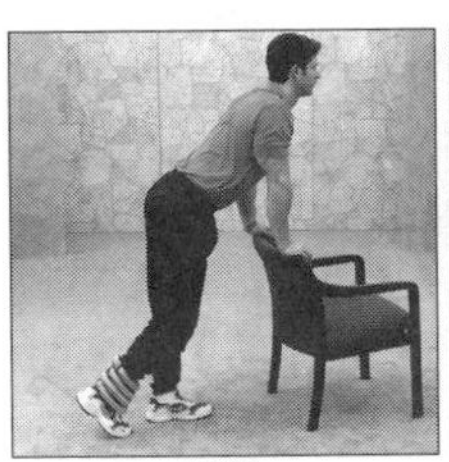

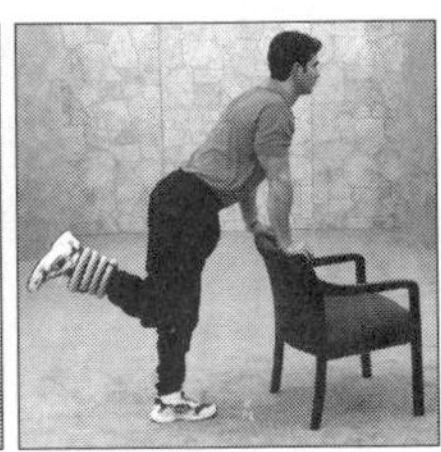

START FINISH

8. Leg Curl with Ankle Weights

10 reps Right/Left

- Raise leg bending knee. Use chair for balance.
- Keep toe pointed down.
- Hold briefly at top position.

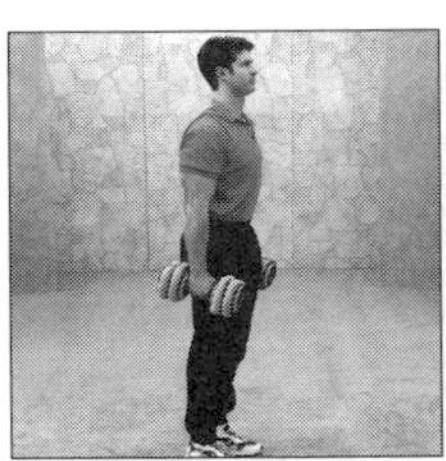

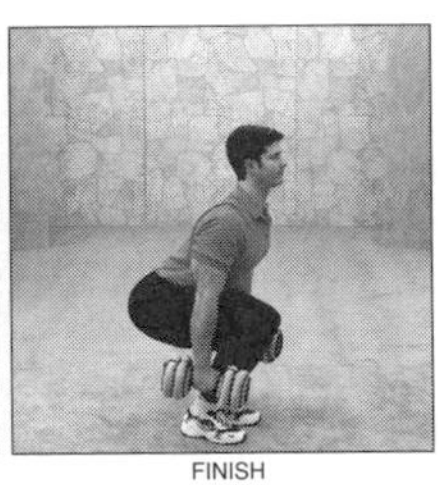

START FINISH

9. Dumbbell Squat

10 reps

- Feet 4-8 inches apart. DBs at side.
- Place weight evenly on heels and balls of feet.
- Back straight. Head up.
- Push with heels.

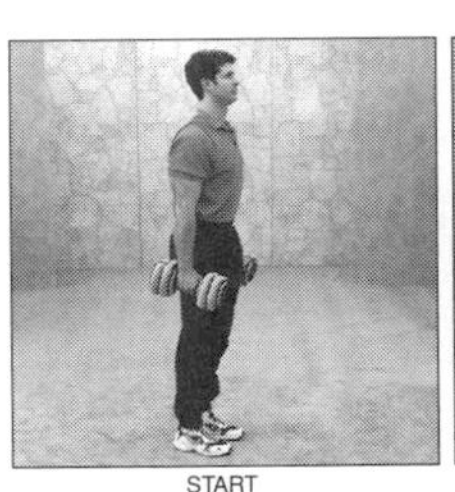

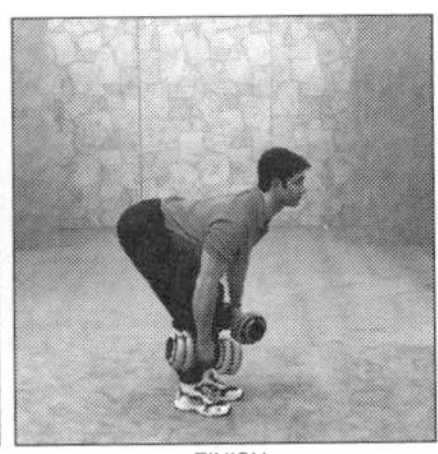

START FINISH

10. Dumbbell Deadlift

10 reps

- Knees slightly bent with feet slightly apart
- Keep low back locked with upper torso.
- Bend at hips, not at waist. Head up/chest out.
- Back is flat.

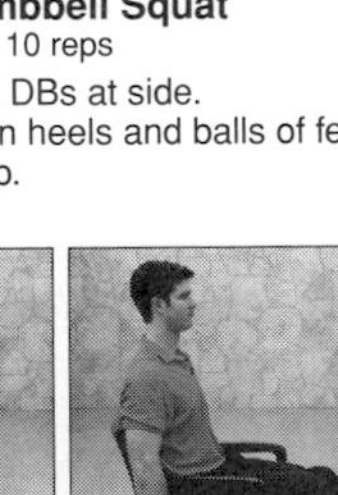

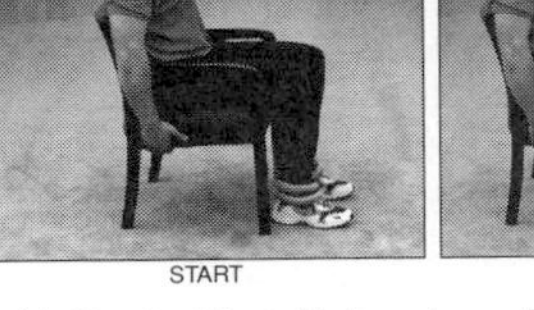

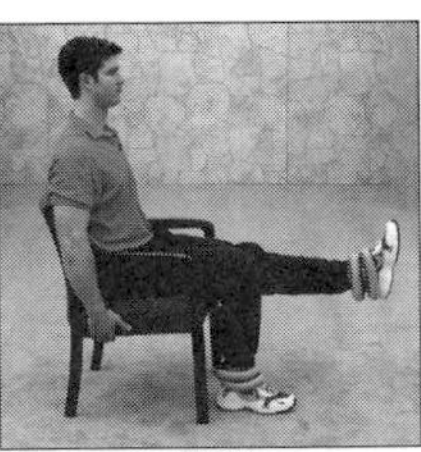

START FINISH

11. Seated Leg Extension with Ankle Weights

10 reps Right/Left

- Extend foot out with weights, hold leg straight for a brief pause and then return.

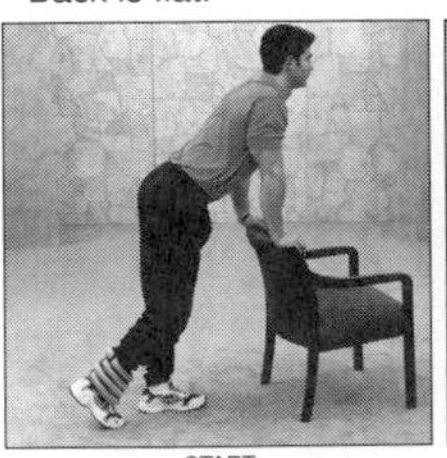

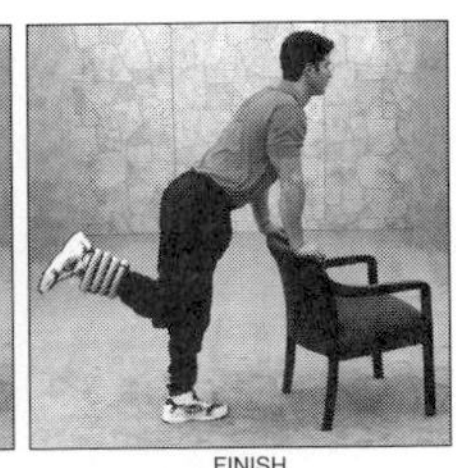

START FINISH

12. Leg Curl with Ankle Weights

10 reps Right/Left

- Raise leg bending knee. Use chair for balance.
- Keep toe pointed down.
- Hold briefly at top position.

THE CAMPITELLI ADVANCED 10 MINUTE EXERCISE METHOD

MEN'S WORKOUT #9 • PAGE 1

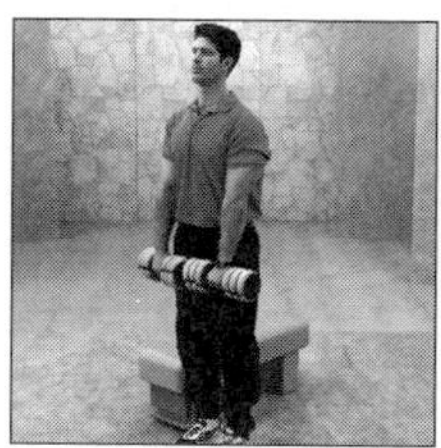
START

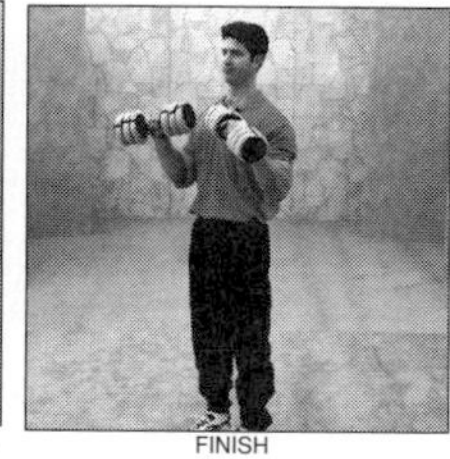
FINISH

1. Reverse Grip Curl
10 reps

- Palms down.
- Elbows at side.
- Don't swing.

START

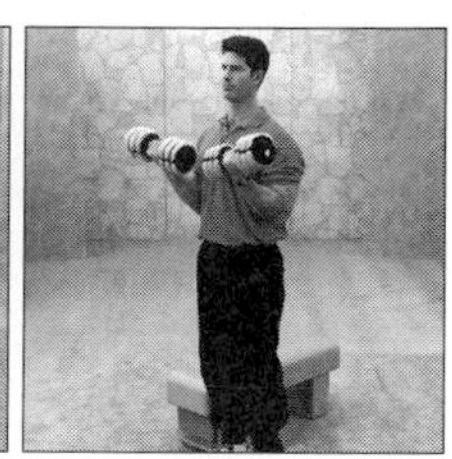
FINISH

2. Regular Curl
10 reps

- Palms up.
- Elbows at side.
- Don't swing.

START

FINISH

3. Tricep Kickback
10 reps

- Support upper body with non working arm
- Extend arm until parallel to floor and hold.
- Don't swing weight at bottom.

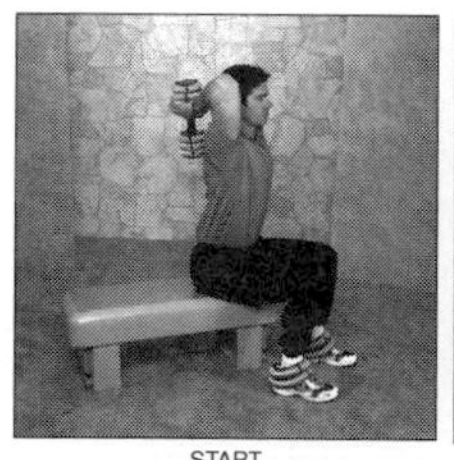
START

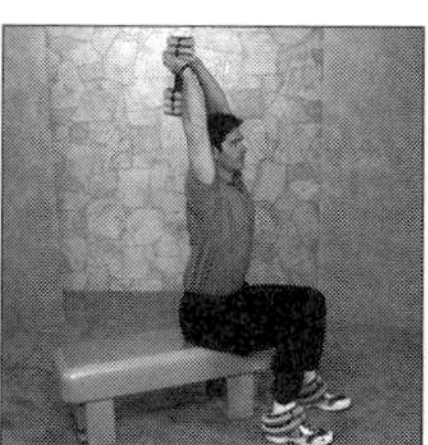
FINISH

4. Overhead Extension
10 reps

- Extend weight over head.
- Keep elbows up and close to head.

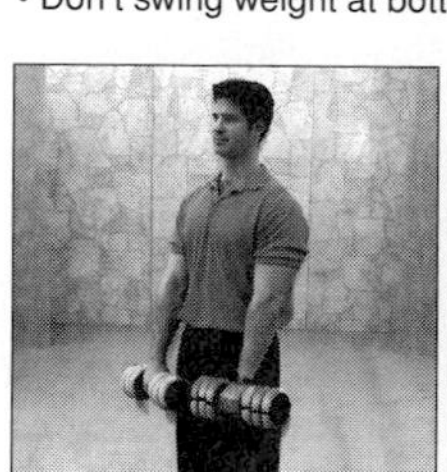
START

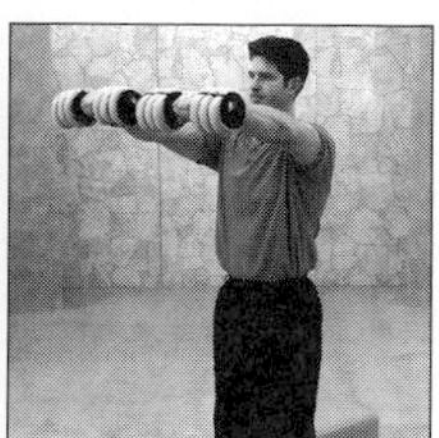
FINISH

5. Frontal Raise
10 reps

- Raise DB with palms down to eye level.
- Return to front of thigh.
- Don't swing.
- Offset foot stance for good balance.

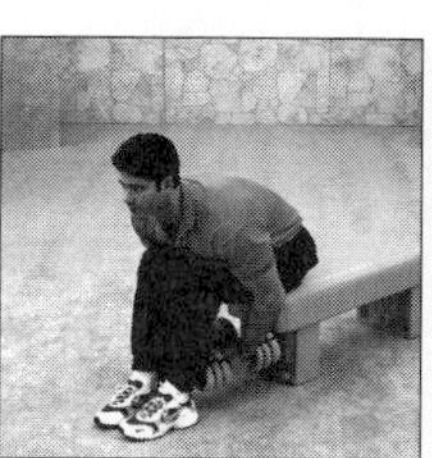
START

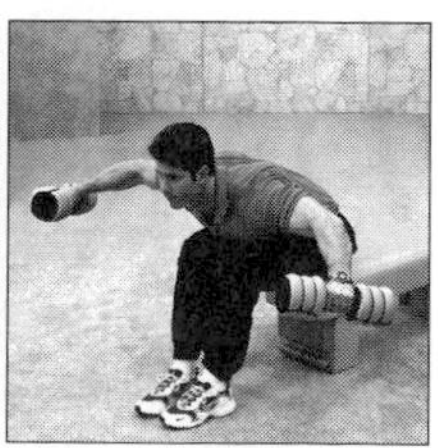
FINISH

6. Rear Lateral Raise
10 reps

- Lean forward keeping head up.
- Raise DB away from body.
- Elbows up. Palms down.
- Return DBs behind calves. • Sit on very edge of bench.

THE CAMPITELLI ADVANCED 10 MINUTE EXERCISE METHOD

MEN'S WORKOUT #9 • PAGE 2

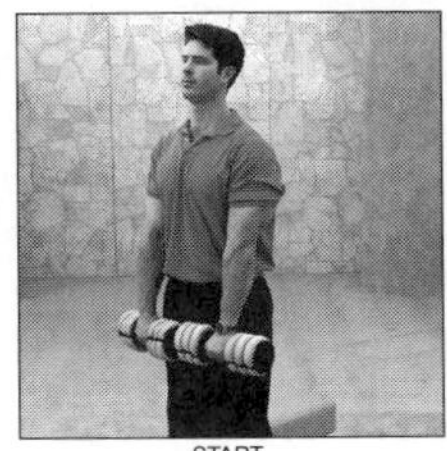
START

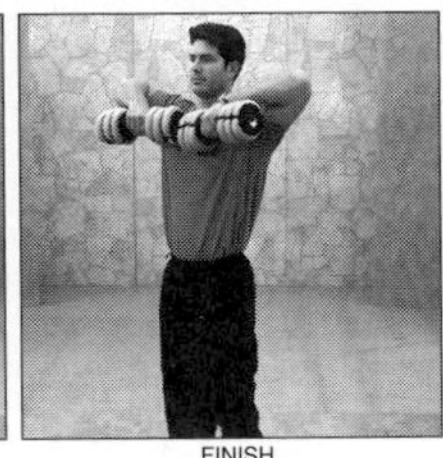
FINISH

7. Upright Row
10 reps

- Pull weights to chin.
- Elbows should be higher than weights at finish.

REPEAT ENTIRE ROUTINE (1 THRU 7) TWO MORE TIMES.

THE CAMPITELLI ADVANCED 10 MINUTE EXERCISE METHOD

MEN'S WORKOUT #10 • PAGE 1

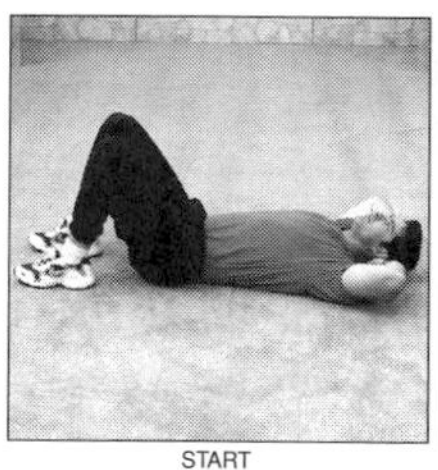
START

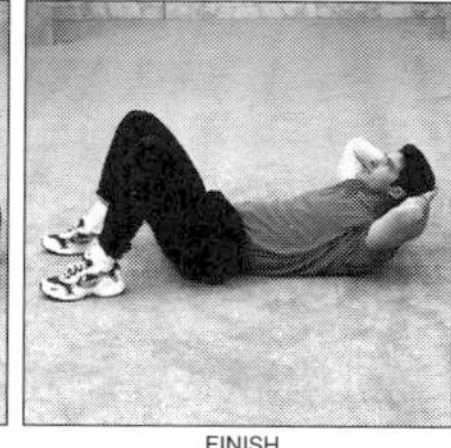
FINISH

1. Crunch
10 reps

- Push lower back into floor.
- Focus on ceiling, not knees.
- Breathe out as you go up.

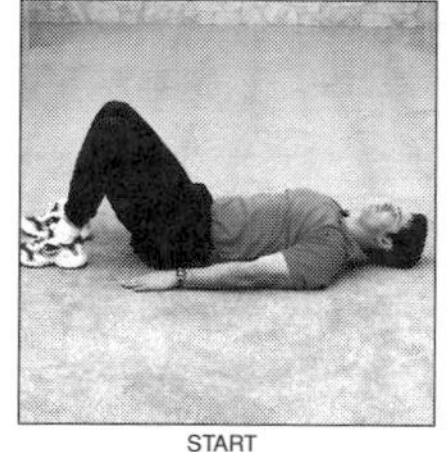
START

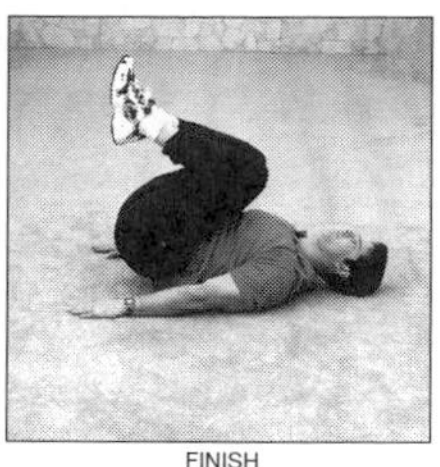
FINISH

2. Tucks
10 reps

- Feet shoulder width apart.
- Pull DB up the side of leg.
- Keep shoulders, back and chest out.

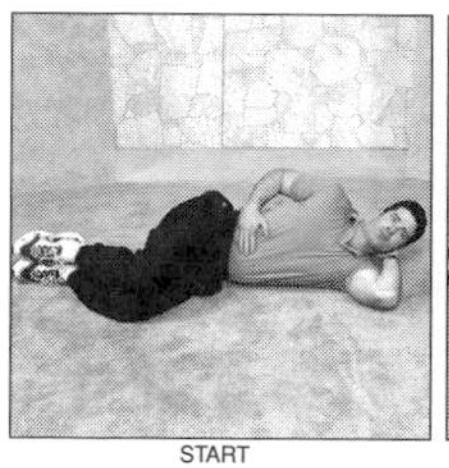
START

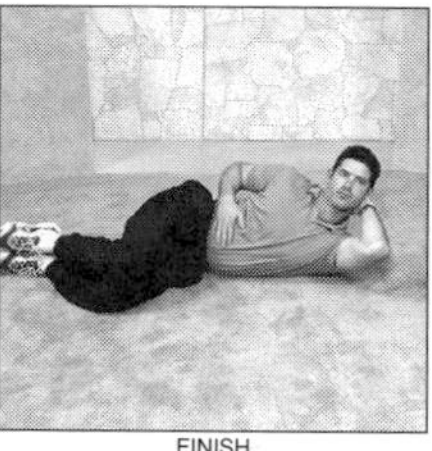
FINISH

3. Side Crunches
10 reps Right/left

- Contract top side to pull shoulder to hip.
- Try to lift bottom shoulder off ground.

START FINISH

4. Hyper Extension
10 reps

- Raise upper body off floor feeling contraction in mid to low back.

THE CAMPITELLI ADVANCED 10 MINUTE EXERCISE METHOD

MEN'S WORKOUT #10 • PAGE 2

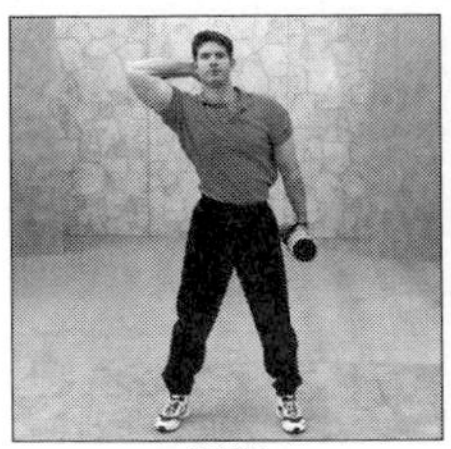

START FINISH

5. Side Bends with Dumbbell

10 reps Right/Left

- Feet shoulder width apart.
- Pull DB up the side of leg.
- Keep shoulders, back and chest out.

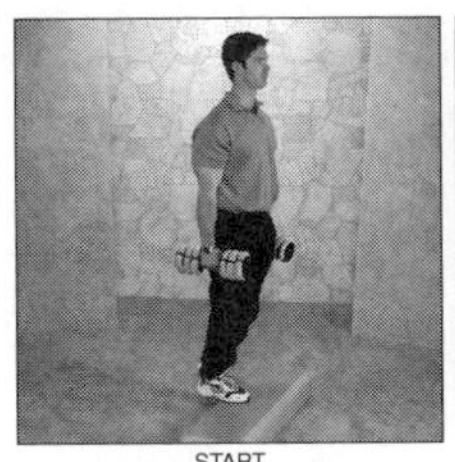

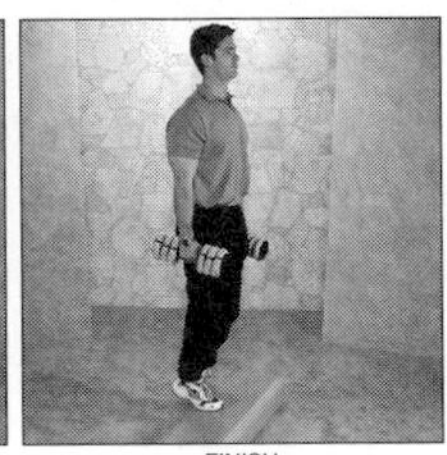

START FINISH

6. Standing Calf Raise with Dumbbell

10 reps Right/Left

- Use step or book for elevation.
- Use DB for extra resistance.
- Raise heel up.
- Keep knees straight during movement.

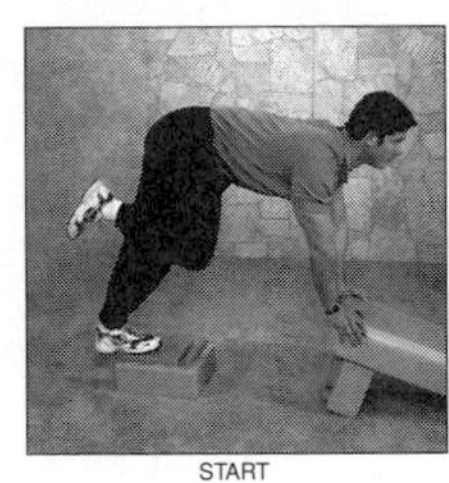

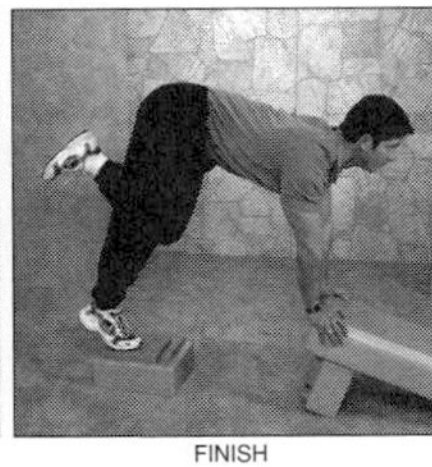

START FINISH

7. Donkey Calf Raise

10 reps Right/Left

- Place ball of foot on step or book and raise heal.
- Keep knee straight.

REPEAT SEQUENCE (1 THRU 7) ONE MORE TIME.

THE CAMPITELLI ADVANCED 10 MINUTE EXERCISE METHOD

MEN'S WORKOUT #11 • PAGE 1

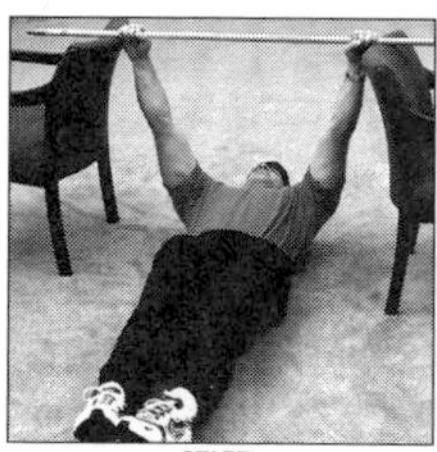

START

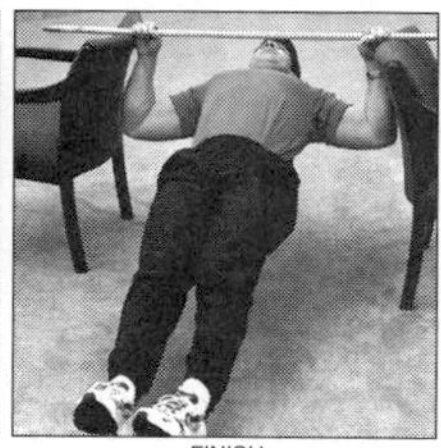

FINISH

1. Overhand Pullup

10 reps

- Keep body straight.
- Hands out to edge of chair for bar stability.
- Pull chest to bar.
- Pull up as far as you can.

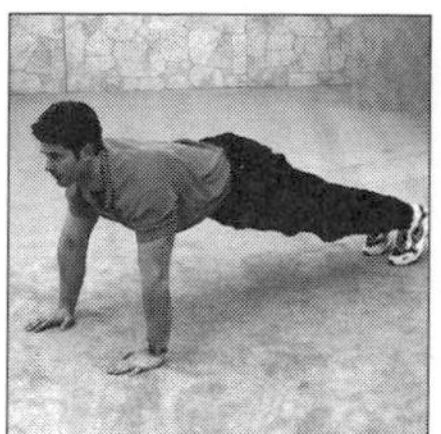

START

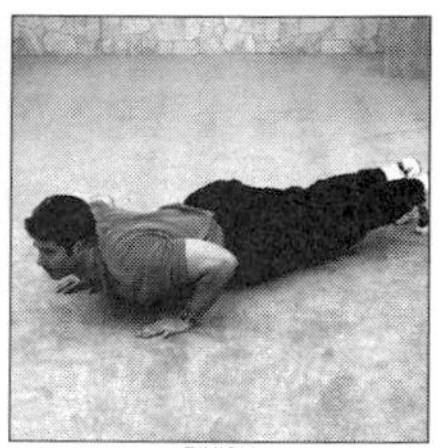

FINISH

2. Pushup

10 reps

- Head up.
- Body straight.
- Hands are slightly wider than shoulders.
- Lower body and chest 2-3 inches from floor.

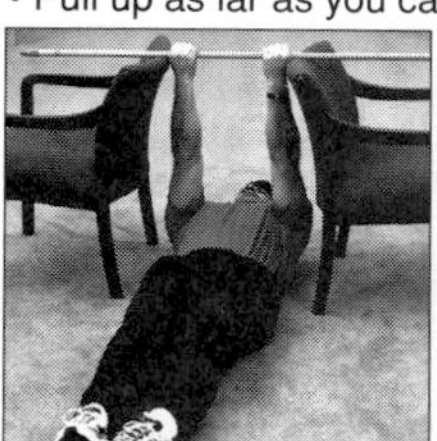

START

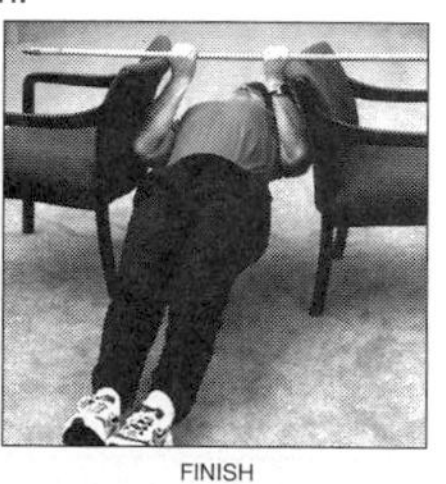

FINISH

3. Underhand Pullup

10 reps

- Move chairs into shoulder width.
- Keep body straight. Pull chest to bar.
- Pull up as far as you can.

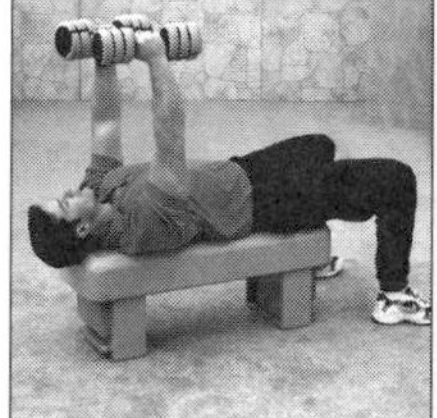

START

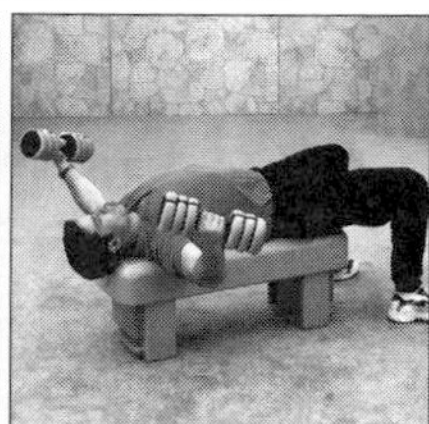

FINISH

4. Dumbbell Fly

10 reps

- Elbows slightly bent with palms facing each other.
- Lower weights out to the side of body until weight is parallel to body.
- Keep elbow slightly bent.

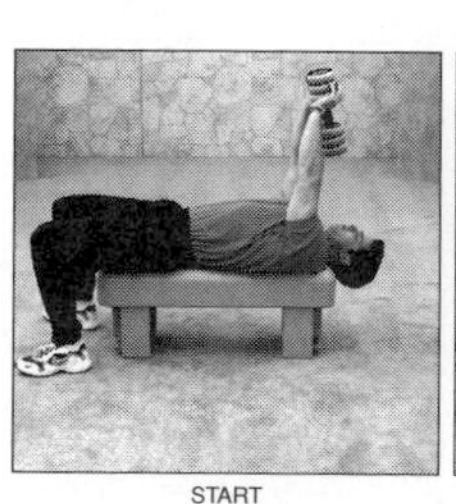

START

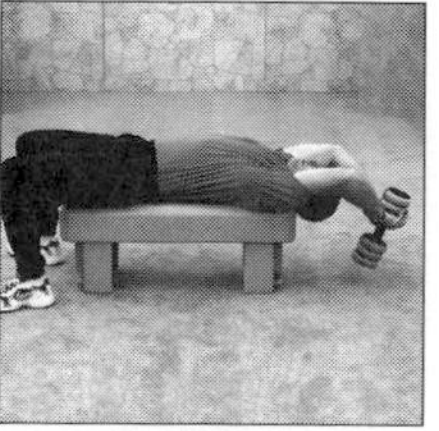

FINISH

5. Dumbbell Pullover

10 reps

- Relax Abdomen. Keep elbows in toward body.
- Inhale as weight goes over head.
- Exhale as it goes up.

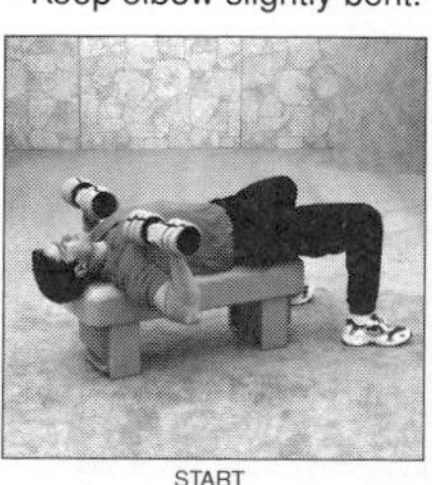

START

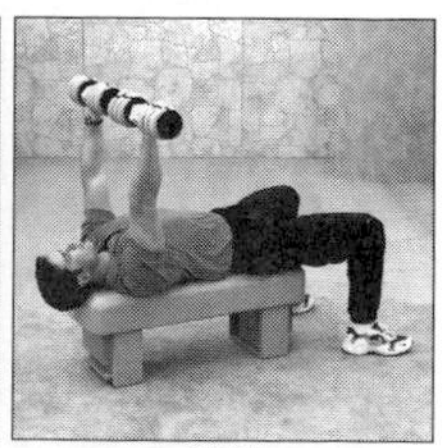

FINISH

6. Dumbbell Press

10 reps

- Hold weights palms toward knees.
- Relax abdomen.
- Lower weights until even with chest.

REPEAT WORKOUT SEQUENCE (1 THRU 6) THREE TIMES THROUGH. END OF ROUTINE. NO PAGE 2.

THE CAMPITELLI ADVANCED 10 MINUTE EXERCISE METHOD

MEN'S WORKOUT #12 • PAGE 1

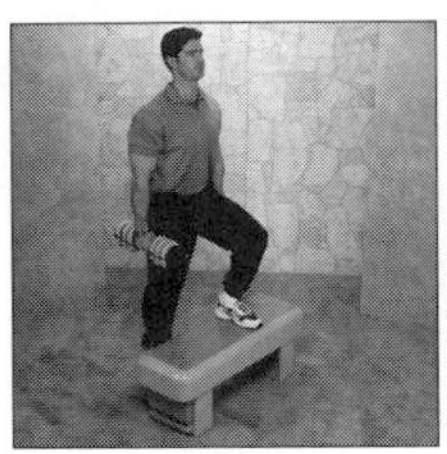

START FINISH

1. Dumbbell Stepup

10 reps Right/Left

- Place whole foot on bench or step.
- Use top leg to push only.
- Look up. Shoulders back.

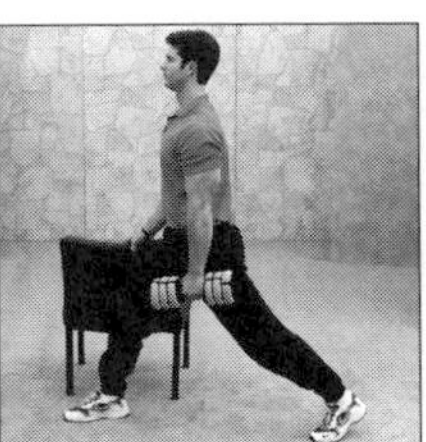

START

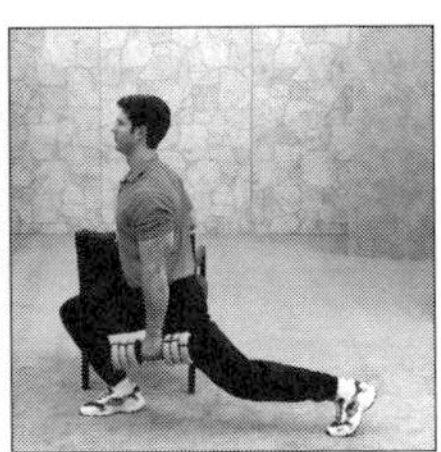

FINISH

2. Dumbbell Lunge

10 reps Right/Left

- Same as regular lunge with DB in one hand.
- Use chair for support and balance.

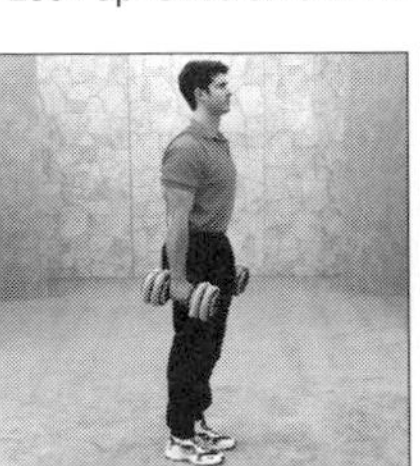

START

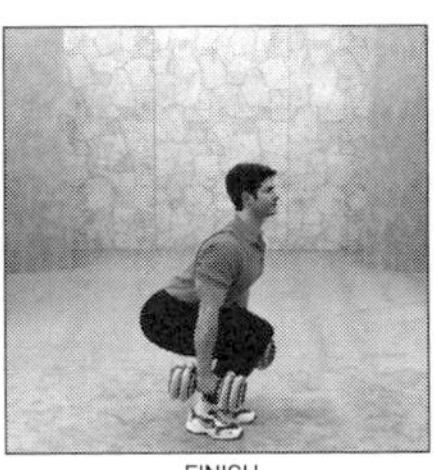

FINISH

3. Dumbbell Squat

10 reps

- Feet 4-8 inches apart. • DB's at side.
- Place weight evenly on heels and balls of feet.
- Back straight. • Head up.
- Push with heels.

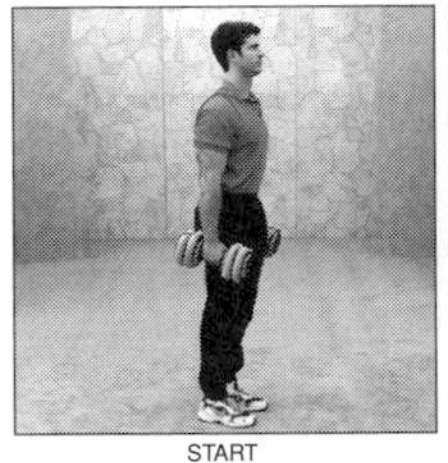

START

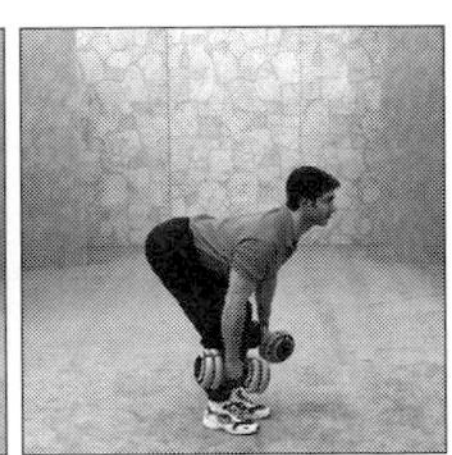

FINISH

4. Dumbbell Deadlift

10 reps

- Knees slightly bent with feet slightly apart.
- Keep low back locked with upper torso.
- Bend at hips, not at waist.
- Head up/chest out. • Back is flat.

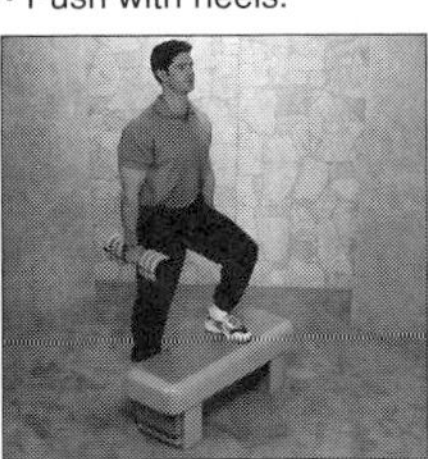

START

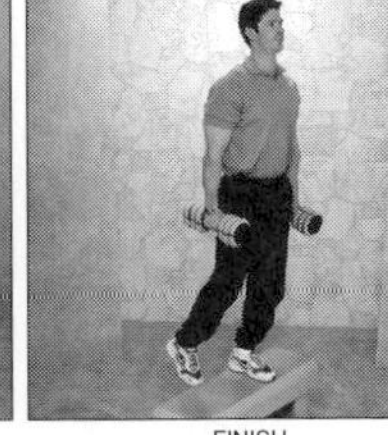

FINISH

5. Dumbbell Stepup

10 reps Right/Left

- Place whole foot on bench or step.
- Use top leg to push only.
- Look up. Shoulders back.

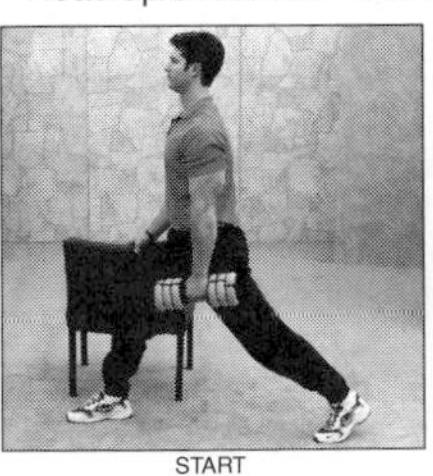

START

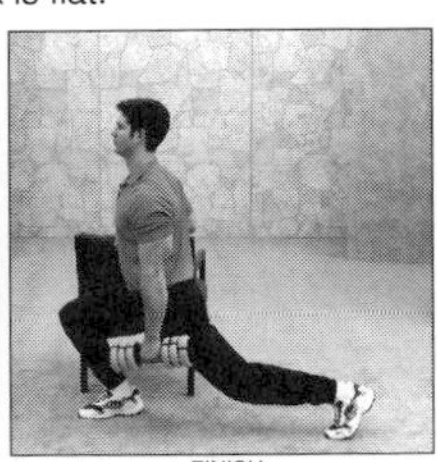

FINISH

6. Dumbbell Lunge

10 reps Right/Left

- Same as regular lunge with DB in one hand.
- Use chair for support and balance.

THE CAMPITELLI ADVANCED 10 MINUTE EXERCISE METHOD

MEN'S WORKOUT #12 • PAGE 2

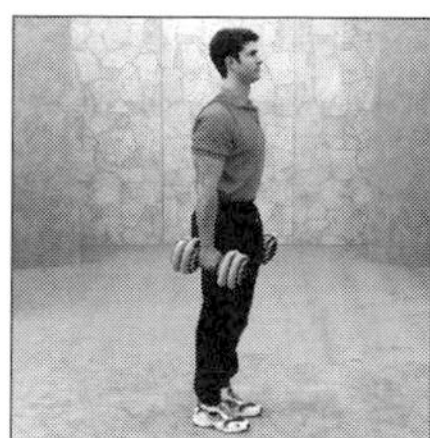

START FINISH

7. Dumbbell Squat

10 reps

- Feet 4-8 inches apart. • DBs at side.
- Place weight evenly on heels and balls of feet.
- Back straight. • Head up.
- Push with heels.

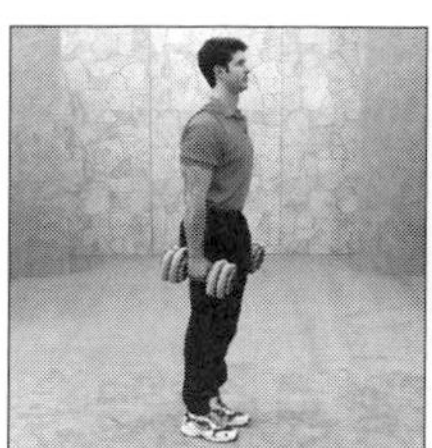
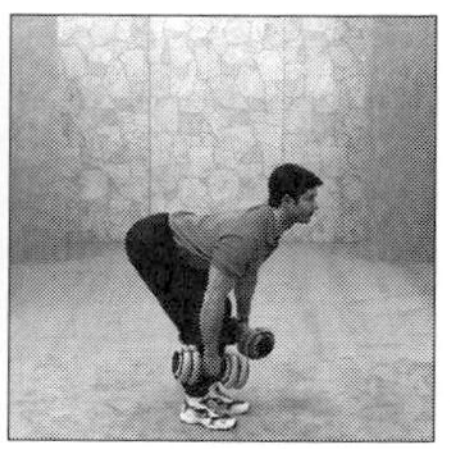

START FINISH

8. Dumbbell Deadlift

10 reps

- Knees slightly bent with feet slightly apart.
- Keep low back locked with upper torso.
- Bend at hips, not at waist.
- Head up/chest out. • Back is flat.

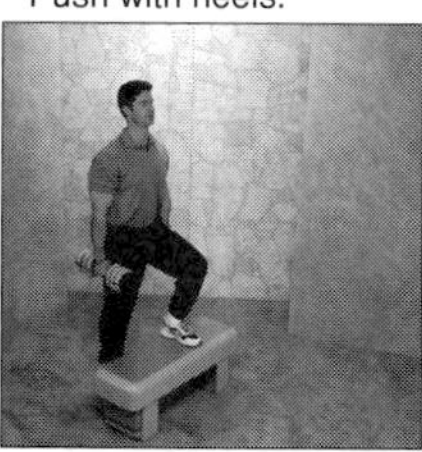
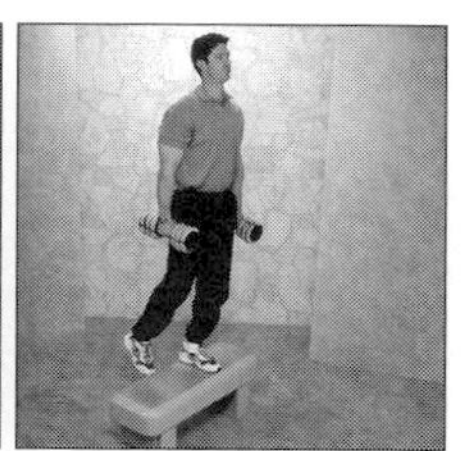

START FINISH

9. Dumbbell Stepup

10 reps Right/Left

- Place whole foot on bench or step.
- Use top leg to push only.
- Look up. Shoulders back.

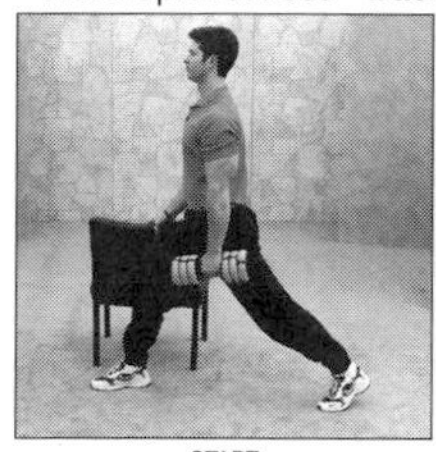
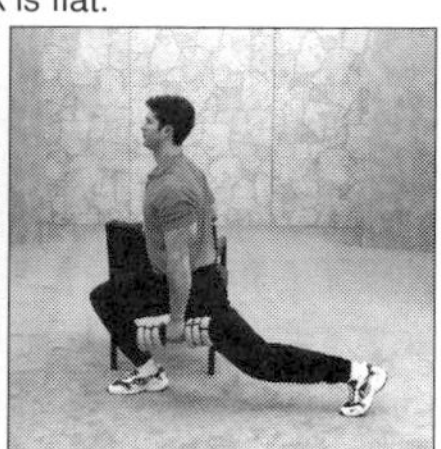

START FINISH

10. Dumbbell Lunge

10 reps Right/Left

- Same as regular lunge with DB in one hand.
- Use chair for support and balance.

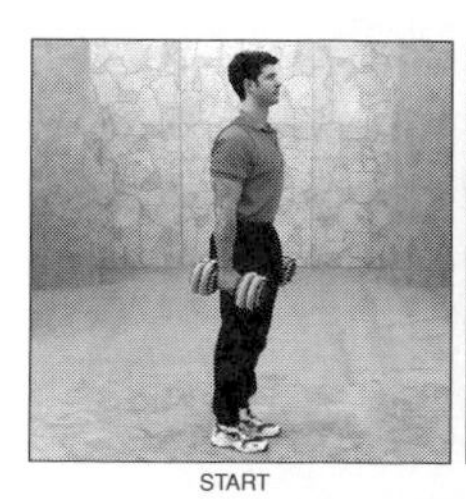
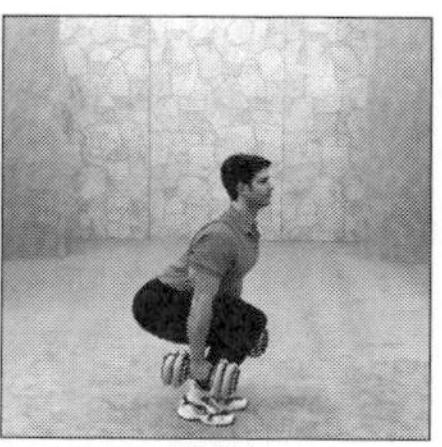

START FINISH

11. Dumbbell Squat

10 reps

- Feet 4-8 inches apart. • DB's at side.
- Place weight evenly on heels and balls of feet.
- Back straight. • Head up.
- Push with heels.

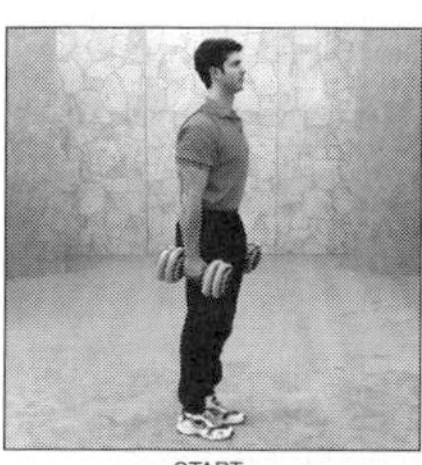
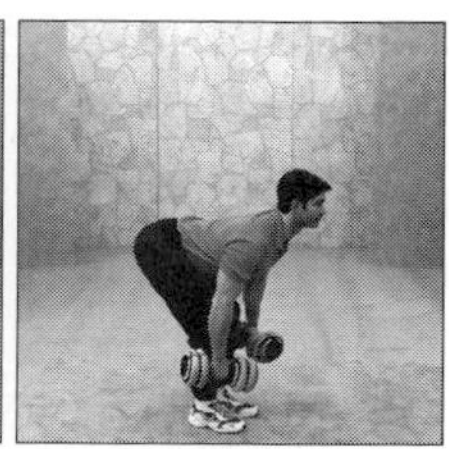

START FINISH

12. Dumbbell Deadlift

10 reps

- Knees slightly bent with feet slightly apart.
- Keep low back locked with upper torso.
- Bend at hips, not at waist.
- Head up/chest out. • Back is flat.

THE CAMPITELLI ADVANCED 10 MINUTE EXERCISE METHOD

MEN'S WORKOUT #13 • PAGE 1

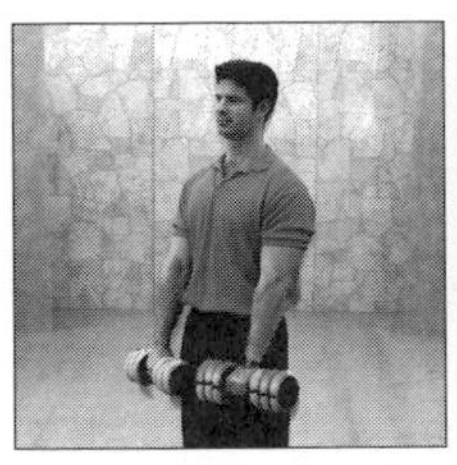

1. Reverse Grip Curl
10 reps

- Palms down.
- Elbows at side. Don't swing.

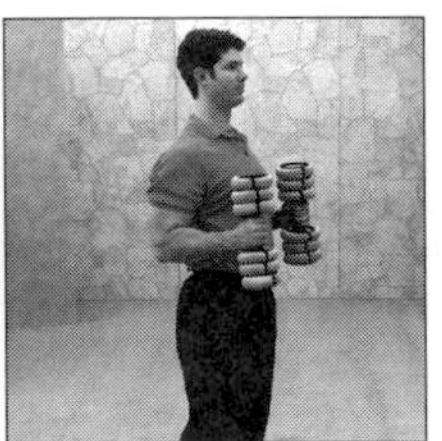

2. Hammer Curl
10 reps

- Hands in "thumbs up position."
- Elbows stay at sides. Don't swing.

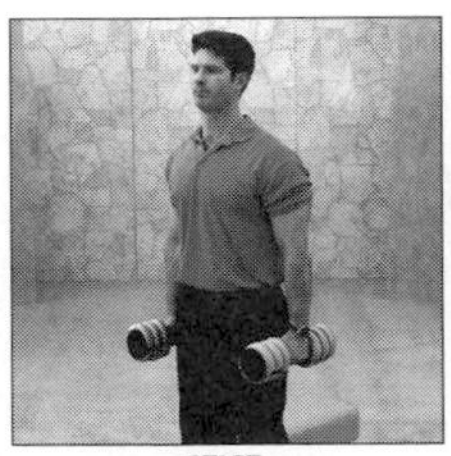

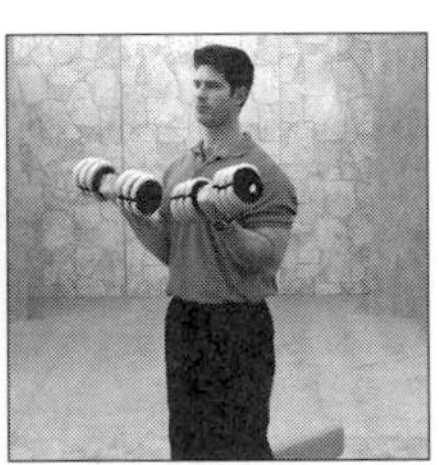

START FINISH

3. Regular Curl
10 reps

- Hands in "palms up position."
- Elbows stay at sides.
- Curl both arms together. Don't swing.

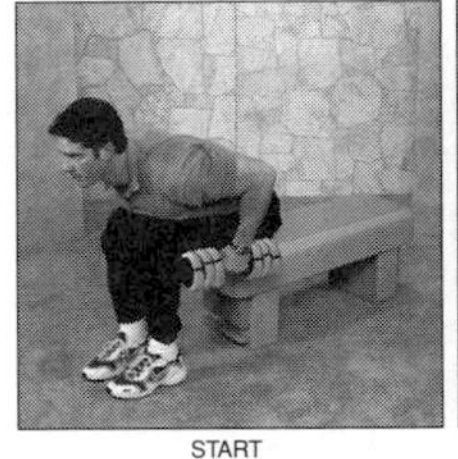

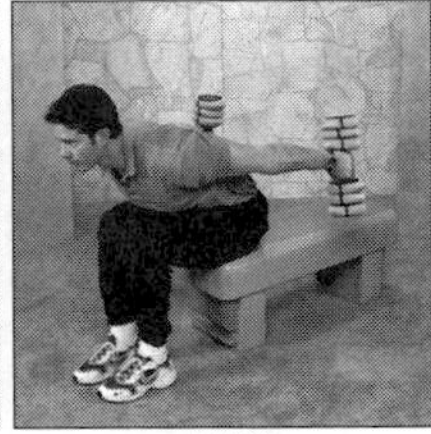

START FINISH

4. Tricep Kick Back
10 reps

- Lean forward in seated position.
- Hold elbows up to side of body.
- Extend forearm back until arm is straight.

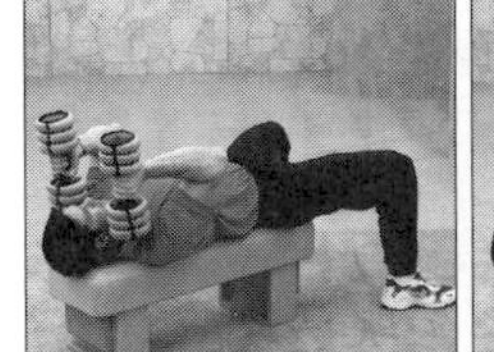

START FINISH

5. Tricep Overhead Extension
10 reps

- Elbows pointed straight up.
- Hands in "thumbs up position."
- Weights come back to ears.

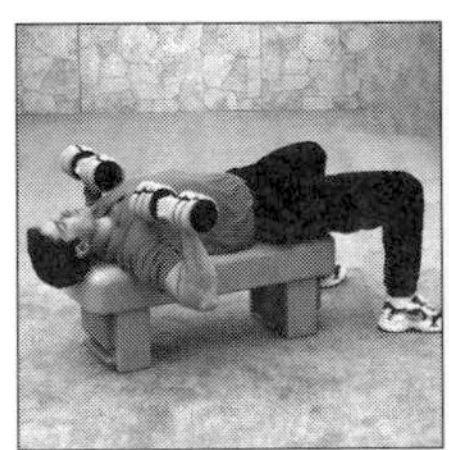

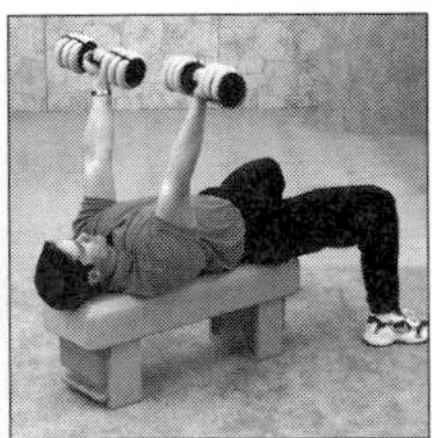

START FINISH

6. Reverse Grip Press
10 reps

- Hands in "palms up position."
- Elbows stay close to body.
- Lower to side of chest.

THE CAMPITELLI ADVANCED 10 MINUTE EXERCISE METHOD

MEN'S WORKOUT #13 • PAGE 2

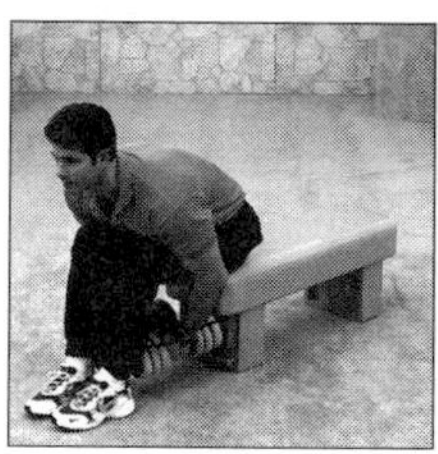
START

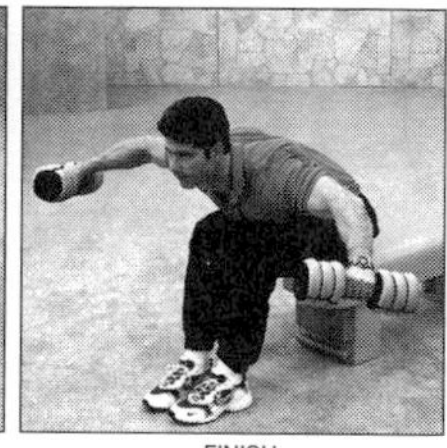
FINISH

7. Rear Lateral Raise
10 reps

- Lean forward keeping head up.
- Raise DB away from body.
- Elbows up. Palms down.
- Return DBs behind calves. Sit on very edge of bench.

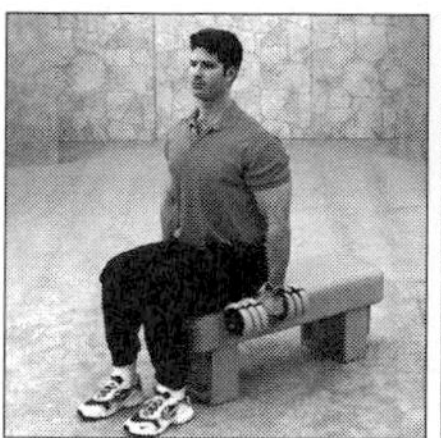
START

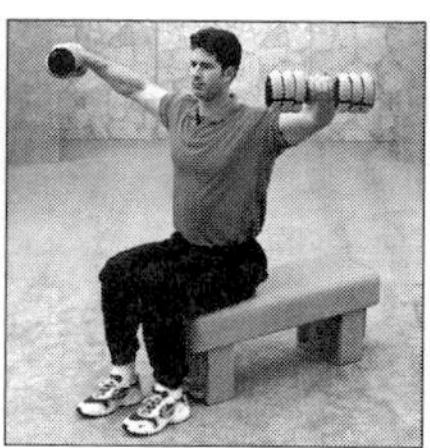
FINISH

8. Side Lateral Raise
10 reps

- Raise DBs out to the side keeping palms down.
- Concentrate on raising your elbows, not the DBs.

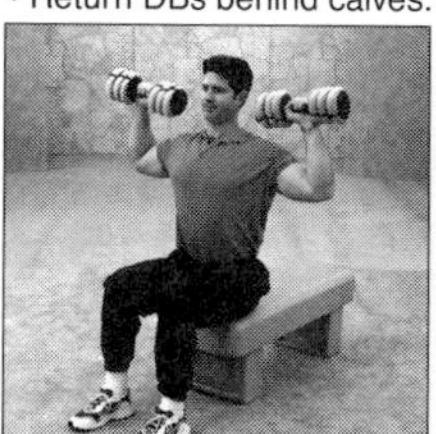
START

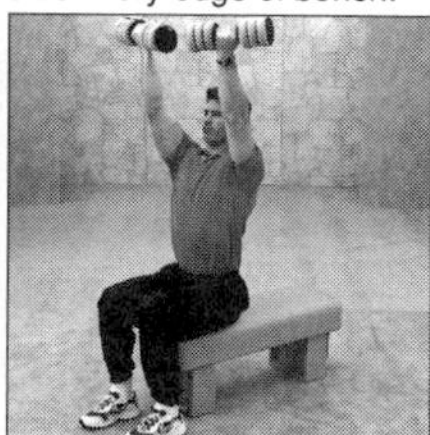
FINISH

9. Shoulder Press
10 reps

- Press weights with elbows out from sides.
- Palms facing forward.

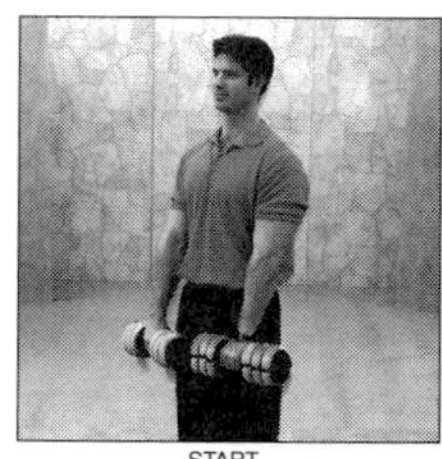
START

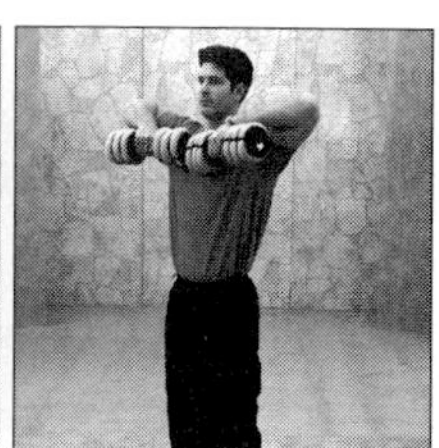
FINISH

10. Upright Row
10 reps

- Pull weights to chin.
- Elbows should be higher than weights at finish.

REPEAT ENTIRE ROUTINE (1 THRU 10) ONE MORE TIME

THE CAMPITELLI ADVANCED 10 MINUTE EXERCISE METHOD

MEN'S WORKOUT #14 • PAGE 1

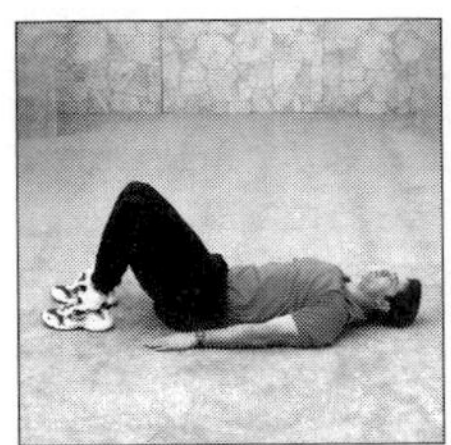
START

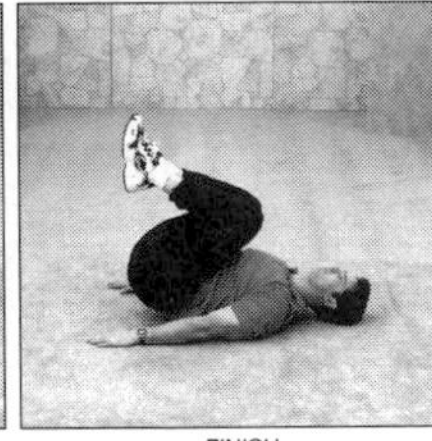
FINISH

1. Tucks with Ankle Weights
15 reps

- Place weights on ankles.
- Draw knees to chest.
- Exhale as knees come up.

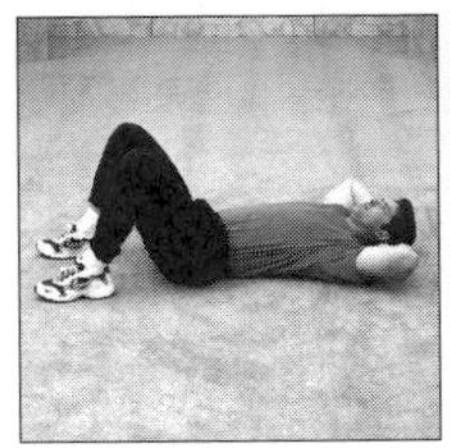
START

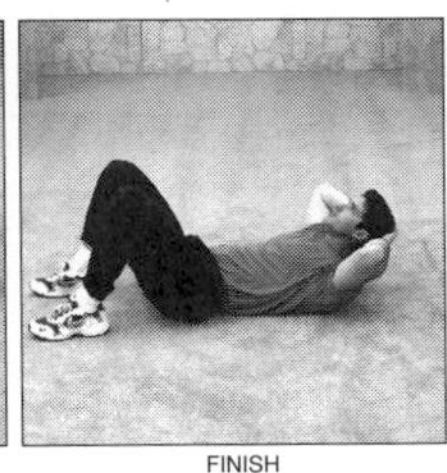
FINISH

2. Crunch with Dumbbell
15 reps

- Place weights behind neck. Hold with both hands.
- Push lower back into floor.
- Focus on ceiling, not knees.
- Breathe out as you go up.

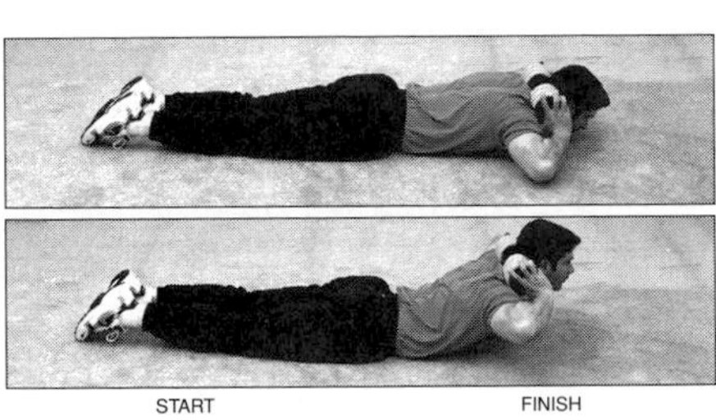
START FINISH

3. Hyper Extension with Dumbbell
10 reps

- Place weight behind neck holding with both hands.
- Raise upper body off floor feeling contraction in mid to low back.

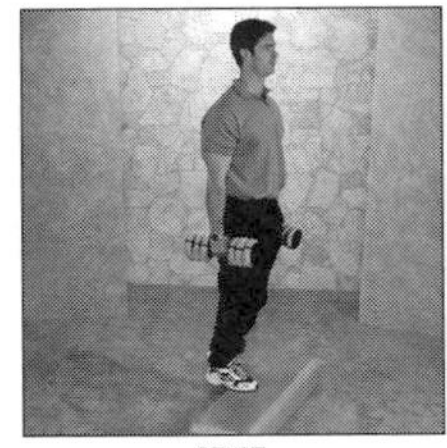
START

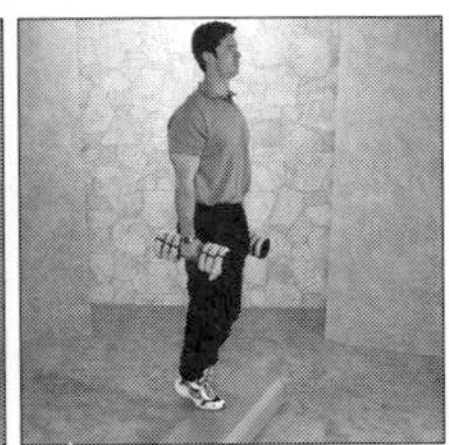
FINISH

4. Standing Calf Raise with Dumbbell
20 reps Right/Left/Both

- Use step or book for elevation.
- Use DB for extra resistance.
- Raise heel up.
- Keep knees straight during movement.

REPEAT ENTIRE SEQUENCE (1 THRU 4) TWO MORE TIMES. END OF ROUTINE. NO PAGE 2.

THE CAMPITELLI ADVANCED 10 MINUTE EXERCISE METHOD

MEN'S WORKOUT #15 • PAGE 1

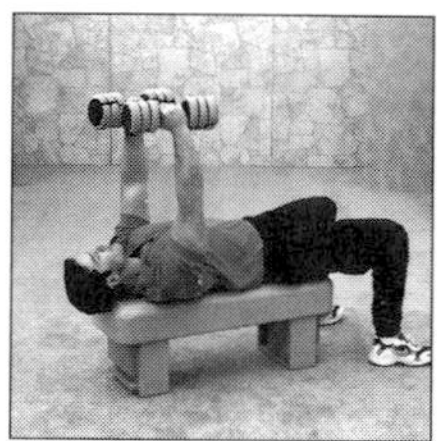

START

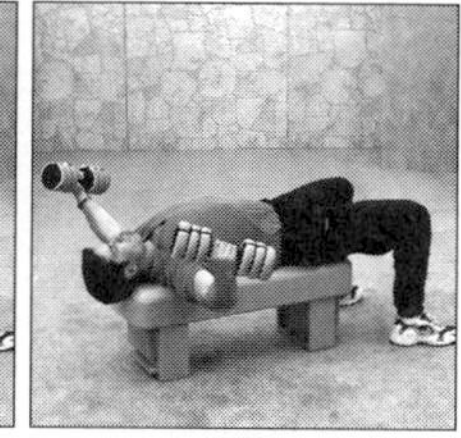

FINISH

1. Dumbbell Fly
10 reps

- Elbows slightly bent with palms facing each other.
- Lower weights out to the side of body until weight is parallel to body. Keep elbow slightly bent.

START

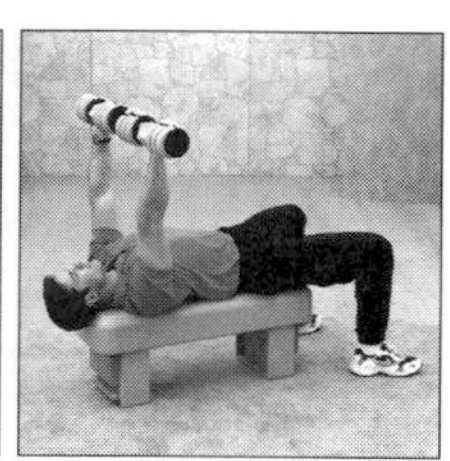

FINISH

2. Dumbbell Press
10 reps

- Hold weights palms toward knees.
- Relax abdomen.
- Lower weights until even with chest.

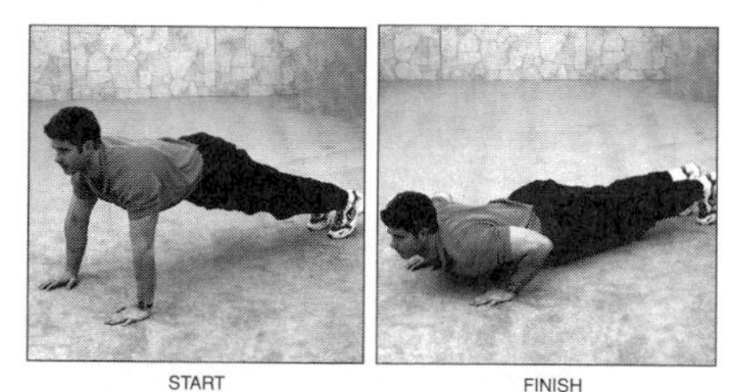

START FINISH

3. Pushup
10 reps

- Heads up.
- Body straight.
- Hands are slightly wider than shoulders.
- Lower body and chest 2-3 inches from floor.

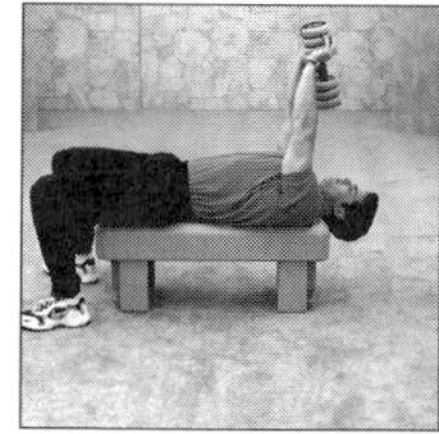

START

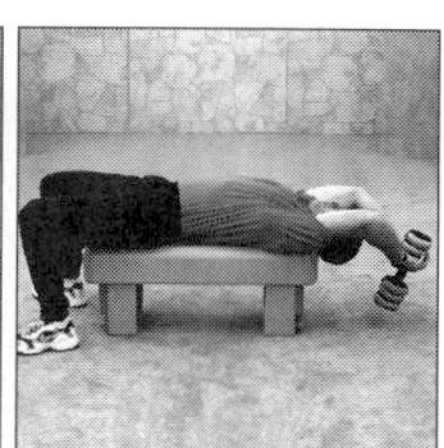

FINISH

4. Dumbbell Pullover
10 reps

- Relax abdomen.
- Keep elbows in toward body.
- Inhale as weight goes over head.
- Exhale as it goes up.

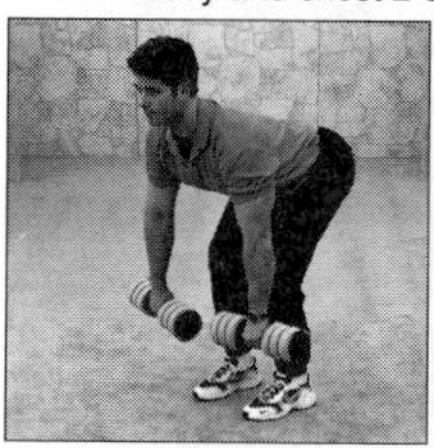

START

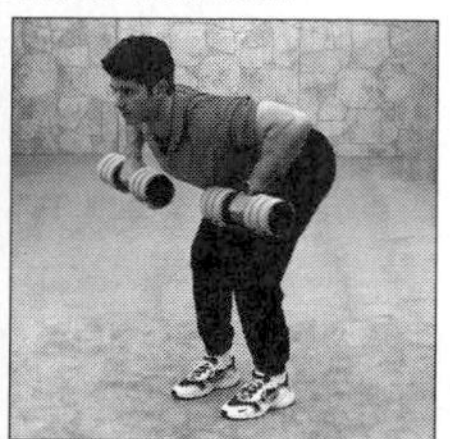

FINISH

5. Dumbbell Row Wide Grip
10 reps

- DBs in "over-hand" position.
- Head up. Chest out.
- Knees bent. Back straight.

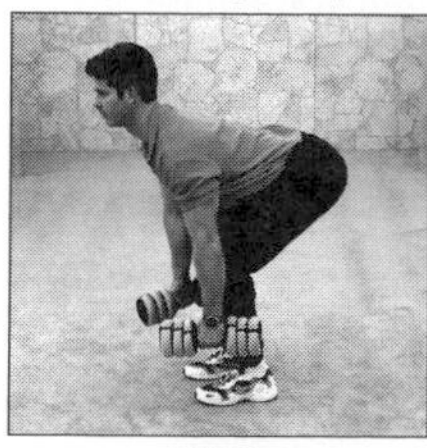

START

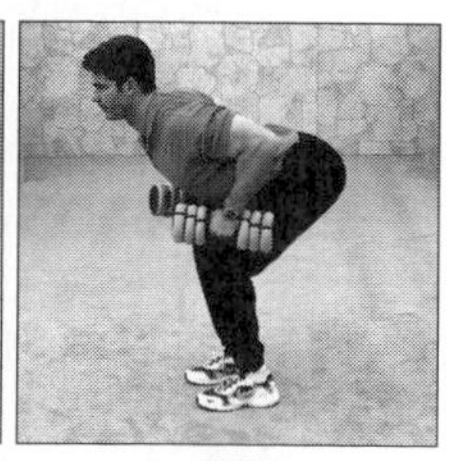

FINISH

6. Dumbbell Row Close Grip
10 reps

- Feet together. Bend at hips, not at waist.
- Bach straight. Chest out.
- Head up. Pull weights with elbows close to body.

REPEAT ENTIRE WORKOUT SEQUENCE (1 THRU 6) THREE TIMES THROUGH. END OF ROUTINE. NO PAGE 2.

THE CAMPITELLI ADVANCED 10 MINUTE EXERCISE METHOD

MEN'S WORKOUT #16 • PAGE 1

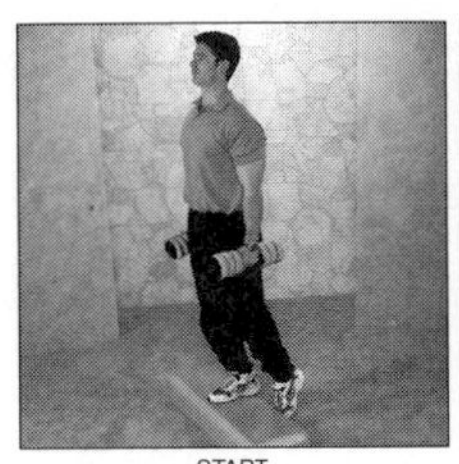

START

FINISH

1. Step-up with Dumbbell and Ankle Weights

10 reps Right/Left

- Place entire foot on bench or step.
- Use top leg to push only.
- Look up. Shoulders back.
- Hold DBs and add ankle weights.

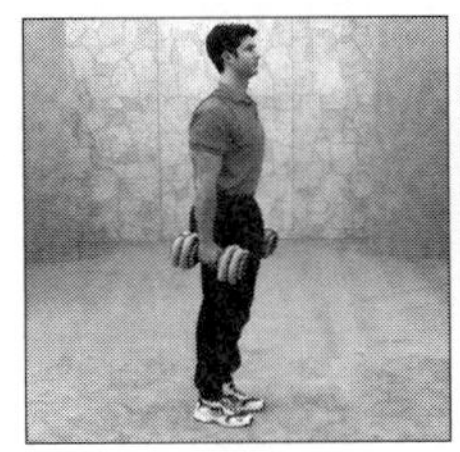

START

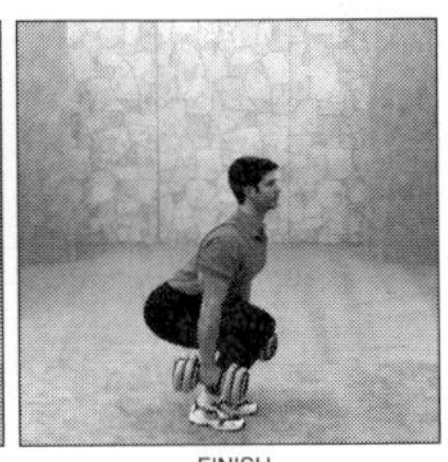

FINISH

2. Dumbbell Squats

10 reps

- Feet 4-8 inches apart. • DBs at side.
- Place weight evenlyeels and ball of feet.
- Back straight. • Head up. • Push with heels.

REPEAT SEQUENCE (1 THRU 2) TWO MORE TIMES, REDUCING WEIGHT EACH TIME, BEFORE MOVING ON TO LEG CURL & DEADLIFT.

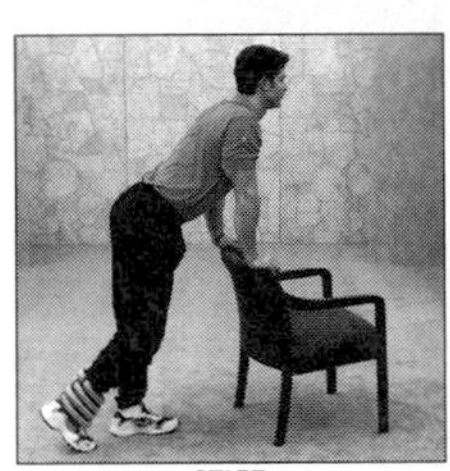

START

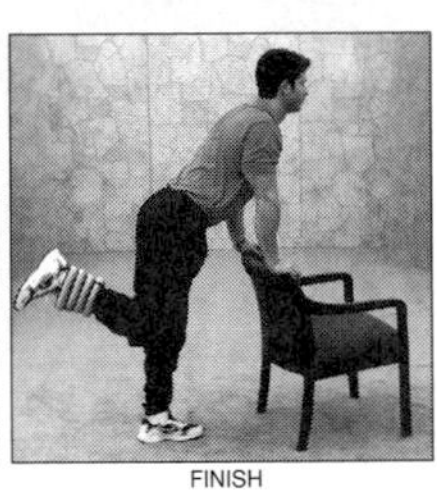

FINISH

3. Leg Curl with Ankle Weights

10 reps Right/Left

- Raise leg bending knee.
- Use chair for balance.
- Keeptoe pointed down.
- Hold breifly at top position.

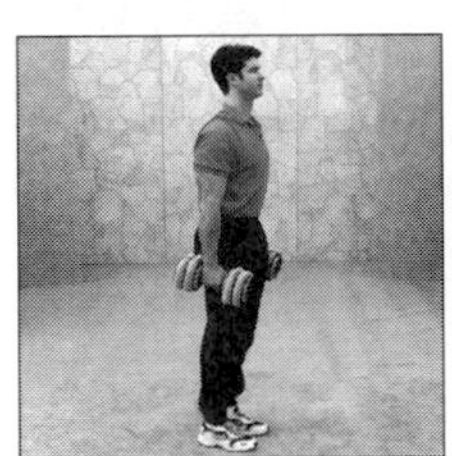

START

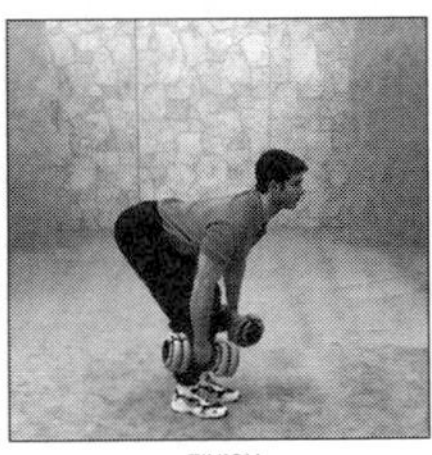

FINISH

4. Dumbbell Dead Lift

10 reps

- Knees slightly bent with feet slightly apart.
- Keep low back locked with upper torso.
- Bend at hips, not at waist.
- Head up/chest out. • Back is flat.

REPEAT SEQUENCE (3 THRU 4) TWO MORE TIMES, REDUCING WEIGHT EACH TIME. END OF ROUTINE. NO PAGE 2.

THE CAMPITELLI ADVANCED 10 MINUTE EXERCISE METHOD

MEN'S WORKOUT #17 • PAGE 1

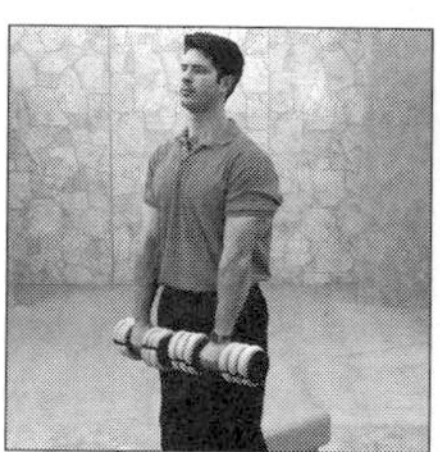

START FINISH

1. Frontal Raise
10 reps

- Raise DB with palms down to eye level.
- Return to front of thigh.
- Don't swing.
- Offset foot stance for good balance.

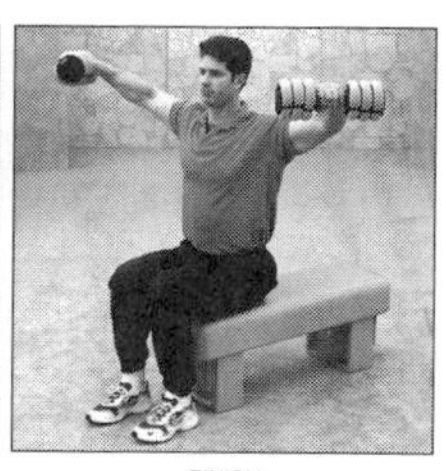

START FINISH

2. Lateral Raise
10 reps

- Raise DBs out to the side keeping palms down.
- Concentrate on raising your elbows, not the DBs.

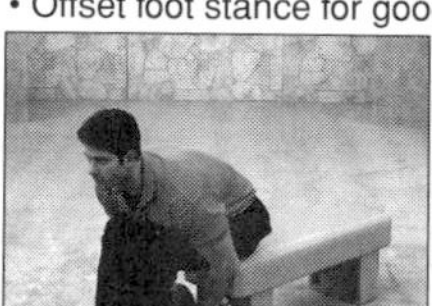

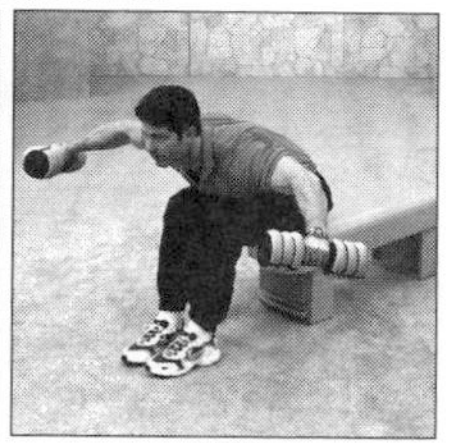

START FINISH

3. Rear Lateral Raise
10 reps

- Sit on very edge of bench.
- Lean forward keeping head up.
- Raise DB away from body. Elbows up. Palms down.
- Return DBs behind calves.

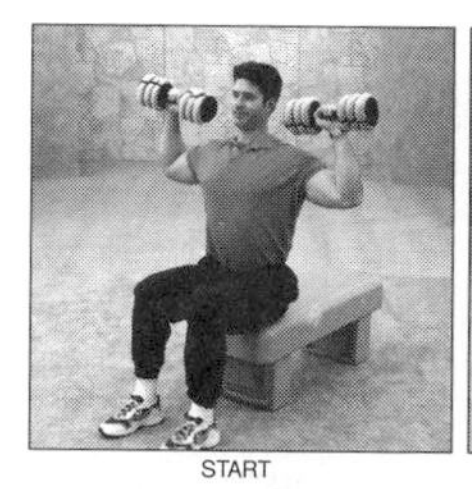

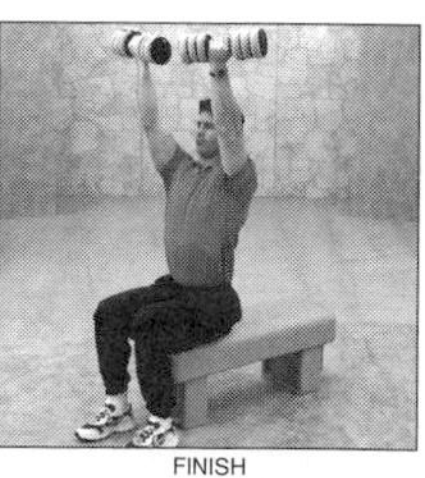

START FINISH

4. Shoulder Press
10 reps

- Press weights with elbows out from sides.
- Palms facing forward.

**REPEAT SEQUENCE (1 THRU 4) ONE MORE TIME
REDUCING WEIGHTS BEFORE MOVING ON TO PAGE TWO.**

THE CAMPITELLI ADVANCED 10 MINUTE EXERCISE METHOD

MEN'S WORKOUT #17 • PAGE 2

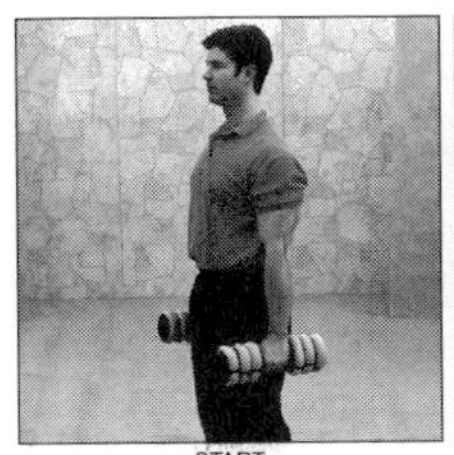
START

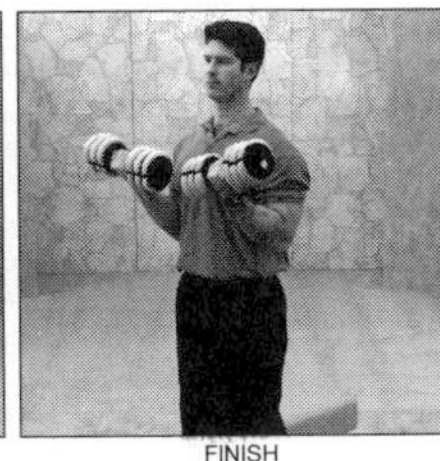
FINISH

5. Regular Dumbbell Curl
10 reps

- Palms up. Elbows at side.
- Don't swing.

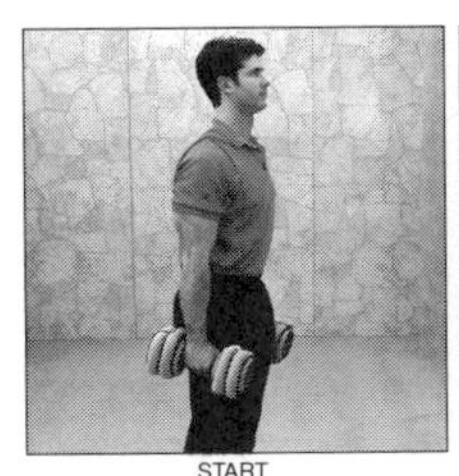
START

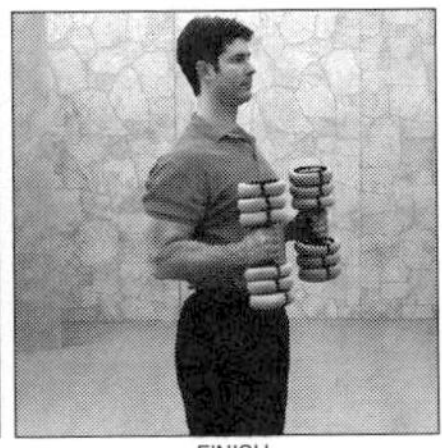
FINISH

6. Hammer Curl
10 reps

- Hands in "thumbs up position."
- Elbows stay at sides.
- Don't swing.

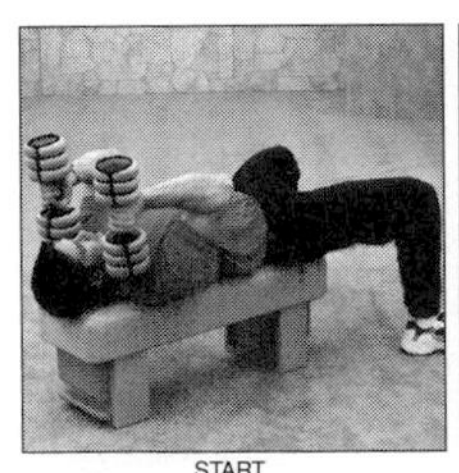
START

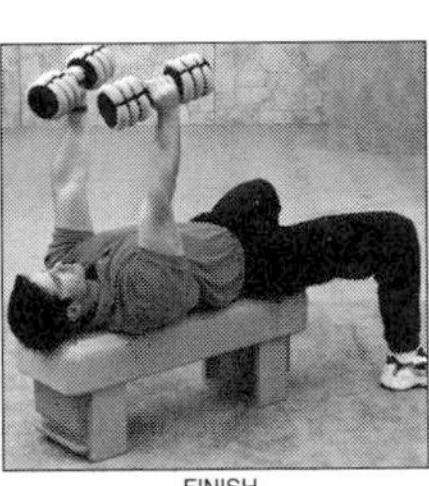
FINISH

7. Tricep Extension
10 reps

- Elbows pointed straight up.
- Hands in "thumbs up position."
- Weights come back to ears.

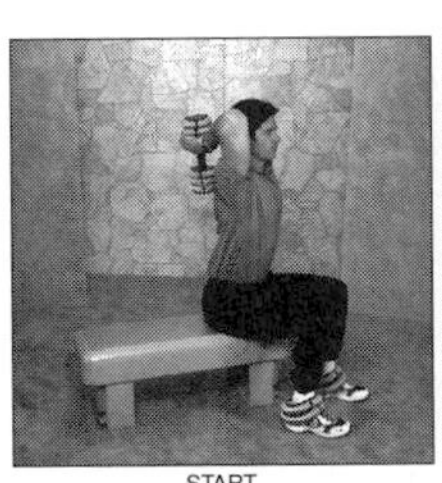
START

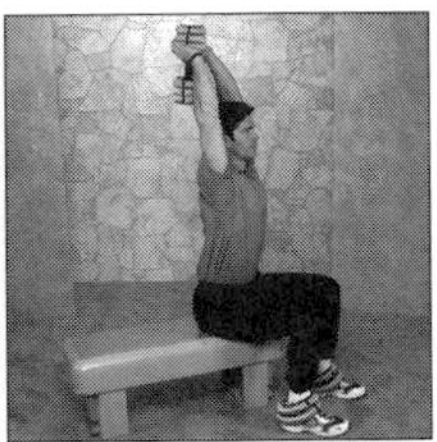
FINISH

8. Overhead Tricep Extension
10 reps

- Extend weight over head.
- Keep elbows up and close to head.

REPEAT SEQUENCE (5 THRU 8) TWO MORE TIMES REDUCING WEIGHTS EACH TIME.

THE CAMPITELLI ADVANCED 10 MINUTE EXERCISE METHOD

MEN'S WORKOUT #18 • PAGE 1

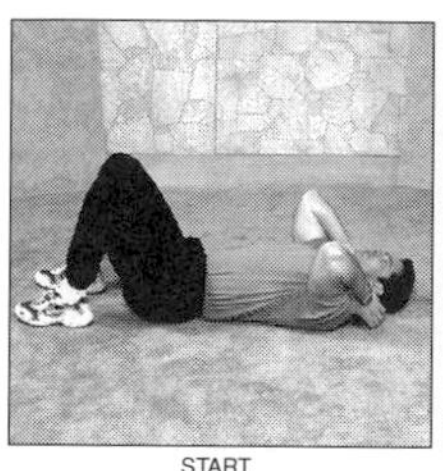 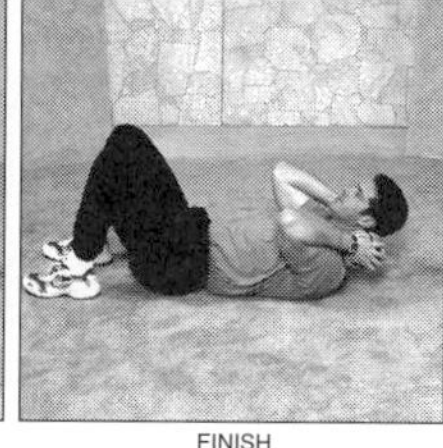

START FINISH

1. Crunch with Dumbbell

20 reps

- Place weights behind neck.
- Hold with both hands.

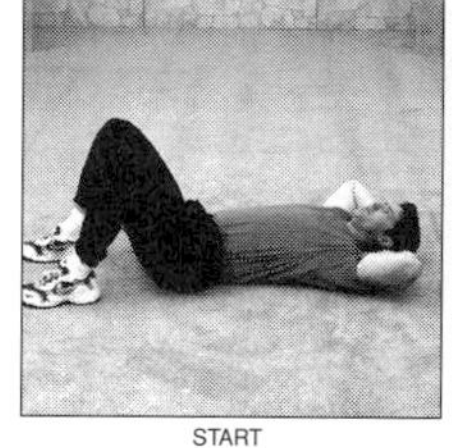 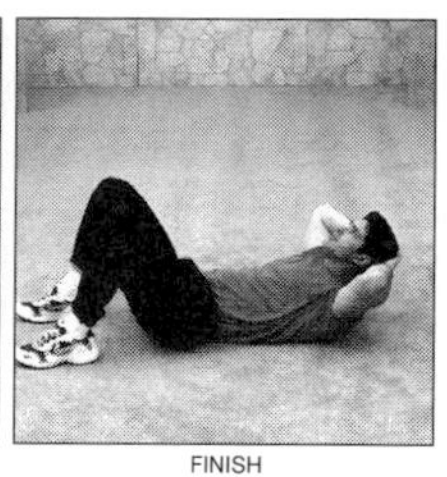

START FINISH

2. Crunches

20 reps

- Push lower back into floor.
- Focus on ceiling, not knees.
- Breathe out as you go up.

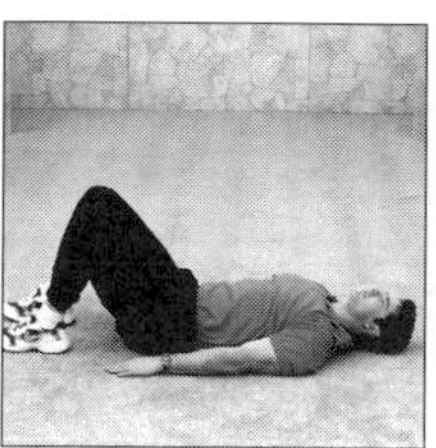 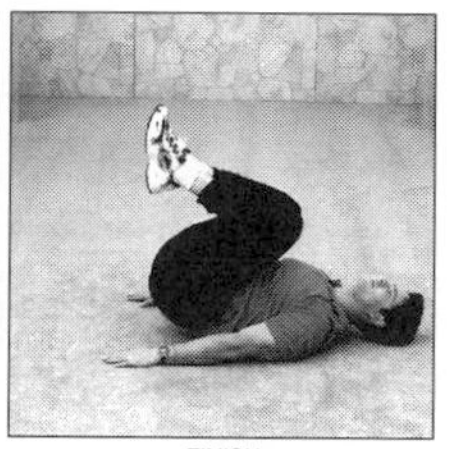

START FINISH

3. Tucks with Ankle Weights

20 reps

- Place weights on ankles.
- Draw knees to chest.
- Exhale as knees come up.

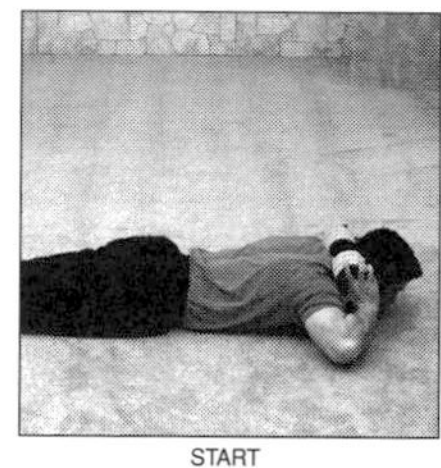 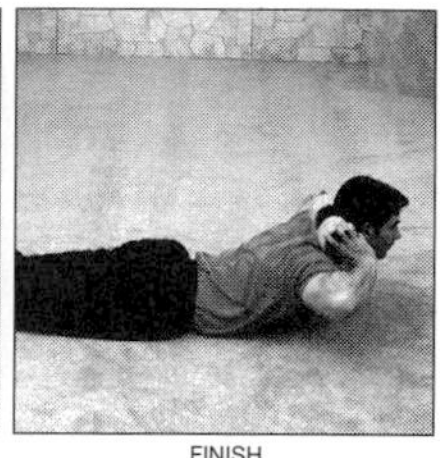

START FINISH

4. Hyper Extension with Dumbell

10 reps

- Raise upper body off floor feeling contraction in mid to low back.
- Place weight behind neck holding with both hands.

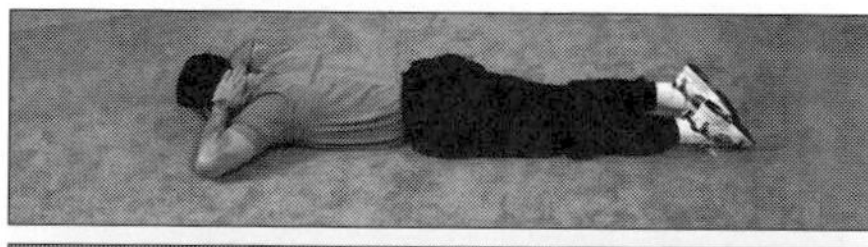

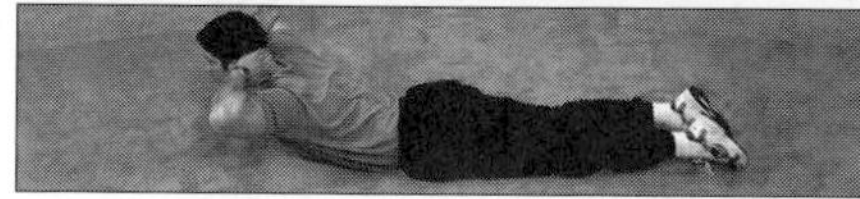

START FINISH

5. Hyper Extension without Dumbbell

10 reps

- Raise upper body off floor feeling contraction in mid to low back.

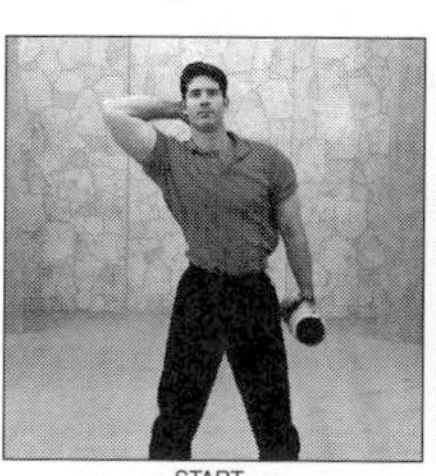 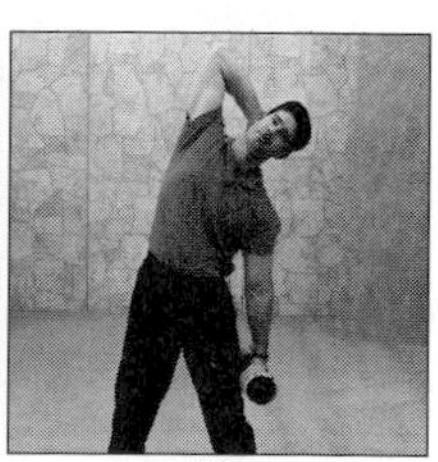

START FINISH

6. Side Bends with Dumbbell

20 reps Right/Left

- Feet shoulder width apart.
- Pull DB up the side of leg.
- Keep shoulders, back and chest out.

THE CAMPITELLI ADVANCED 10 MINUTE EXERCISE METHOD

MEN'S WORKOUT #18 • PAGE 2

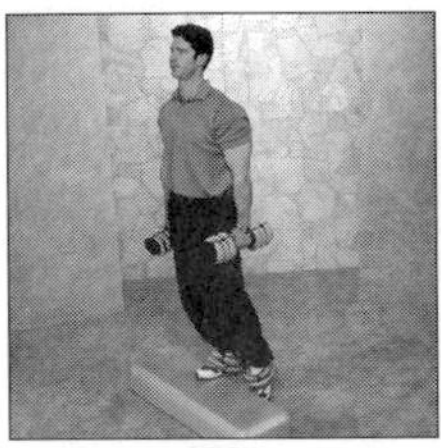

START FINISH

7. Calf Raise with Dumbbell & Ankle Weights

20 reps Right Leg

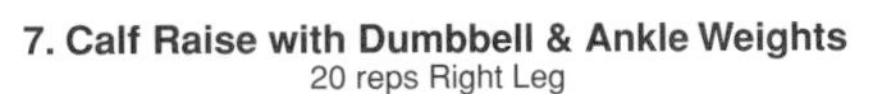

- Use step or book for elevation.
- Use DB for extra resistance.
- Raise heel up.
- Keep knees straight during movement.

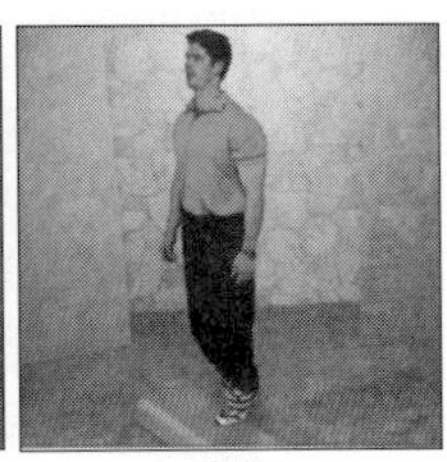

START FINISH

8. Calf Raise without Dumbbell

10 reps Right Leg

- Use step or book for elevation.
- Drop DB to decrease resistance.
- Raise heel up.
- Keep knees straight during movement.

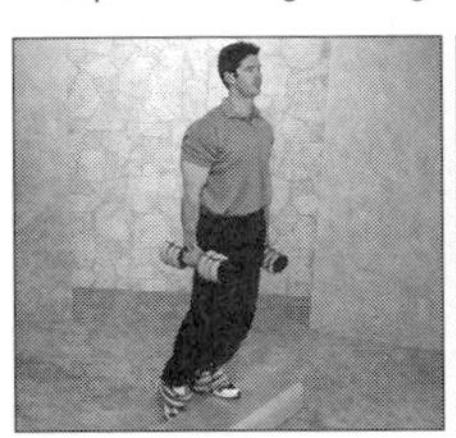

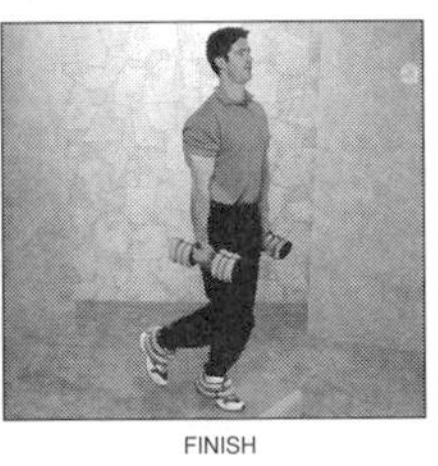

START FINISH

9. Calf Raise with Dumbbell & Ankle Weights

20 reps Left leg

- Use step or book for elevation.
- Use DB for extra resistance.
- Raise heel up.
- Keep knees straight during movement.

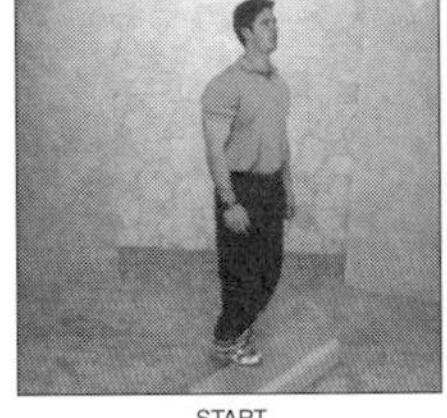

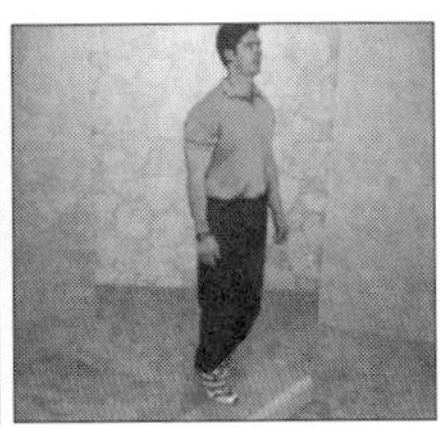

START FINISH

10. Calf Raise without Dumbbell

10 reps Left leg

- Use step or book for elevation.
- Raise heel up.
- Keep knees straight during movement.

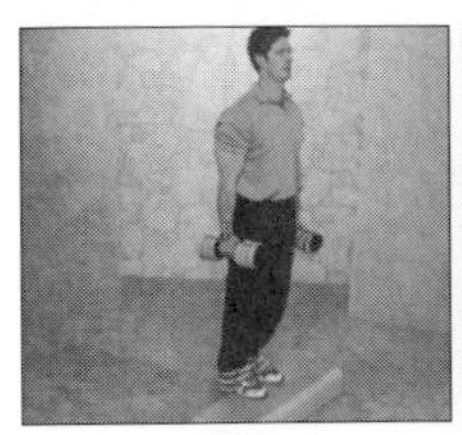

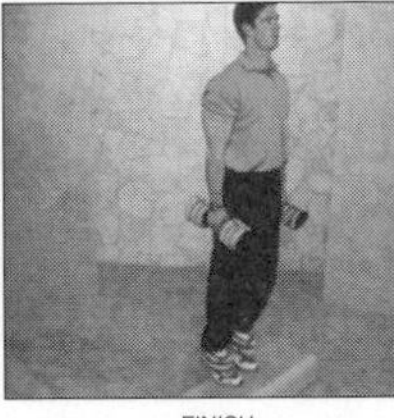

START FINISH

11. Calf Raise with Dumbbell & Ankle Weights

20 reps both legs.

- Use step or book for elevation.
- Use DB for extra resistance.
- Raise heels, knees straight.

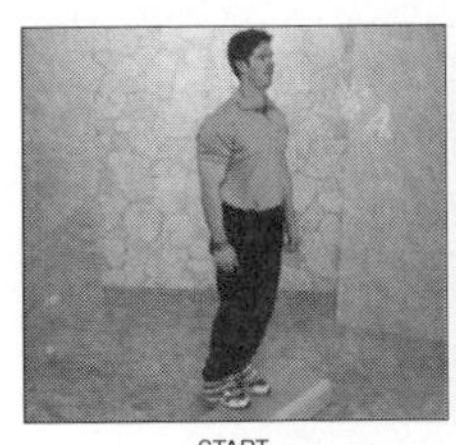

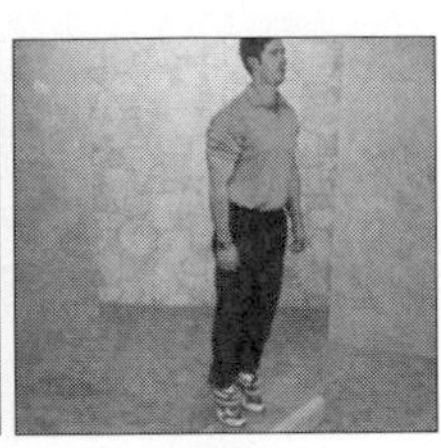

START FINISH

12. Calf Raise without Dumbbell

10 reps both legs.

- Raise heels up.
- Keep knees straight during movement.

REPEAT SEQUENCE (7 THRU 12) ONE MORE TIME.

THE CAMPITELLI ADVANCED 10 MINUTE EXERCISE METHOD

MEN'S WORKOUT #19 • PAGE 1

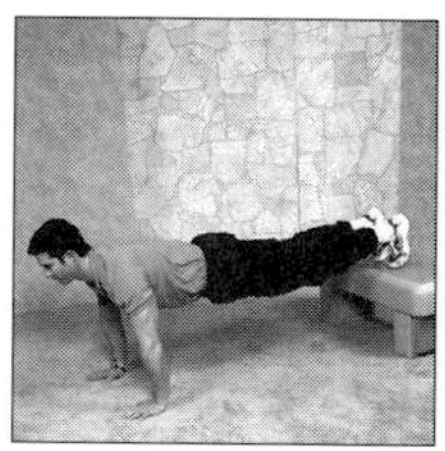
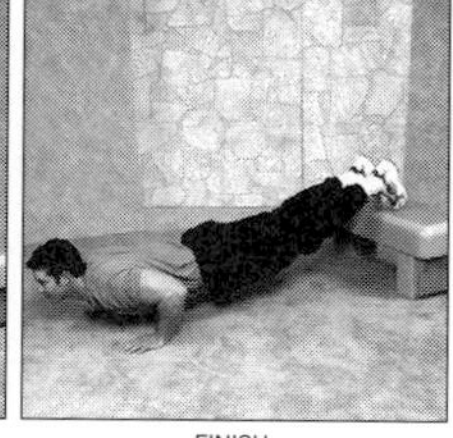

START FINISH

1. Push-up with Feet on Bench
20 reps

- Elevate feet with bench. Head up. Body straight.
- Hands are slightly wider than shoulders.
- Lower body and chest 2-3 inches from floor.

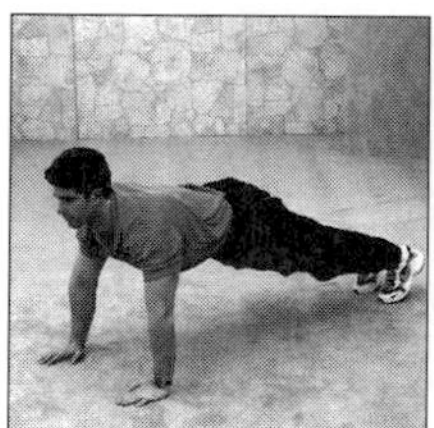
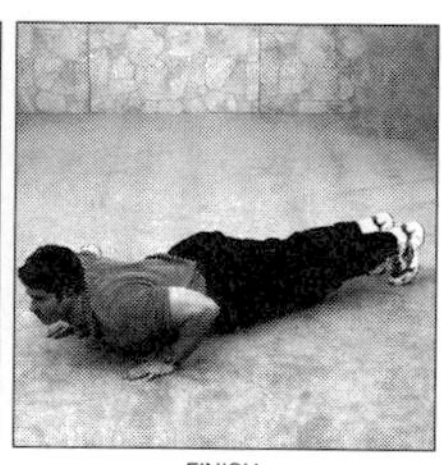

START FINISH

2. Regular Push-up
10 reps

- Head up. Body straight.
- Hands are slightly wider than shoulders.
- Lower body and chest 2-3 inches from floor.

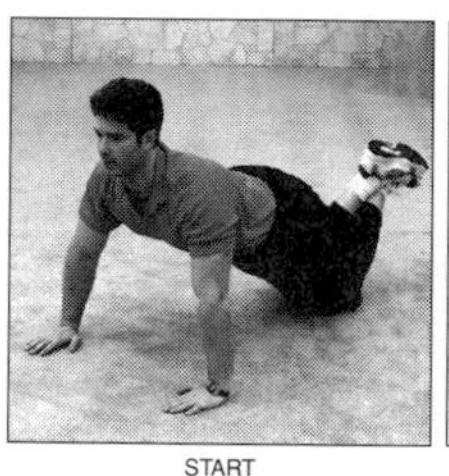
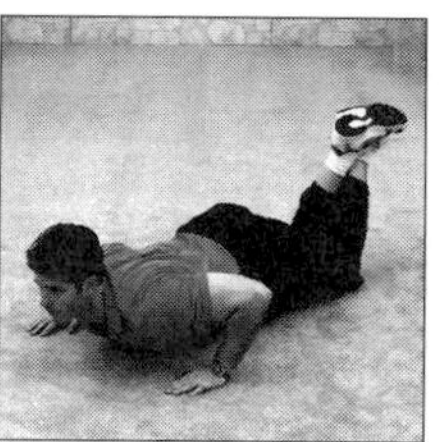

START FINISH

3. Modified Push-up
10 reps

- Start from knees
- Hands shoulder width
- Head up.

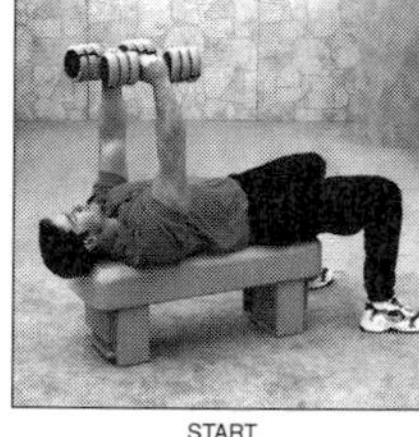
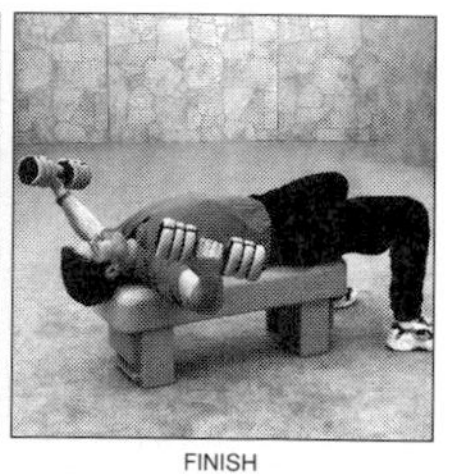

START FINISH

4. Dumbbell Fly
10 reps

- Elbows slightly bent with palms facing each other.
- Lower weights out to the side of body until weight is parallel to body. Keep elbows slightly bent.

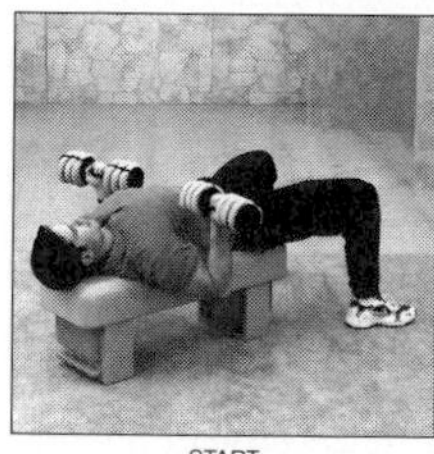
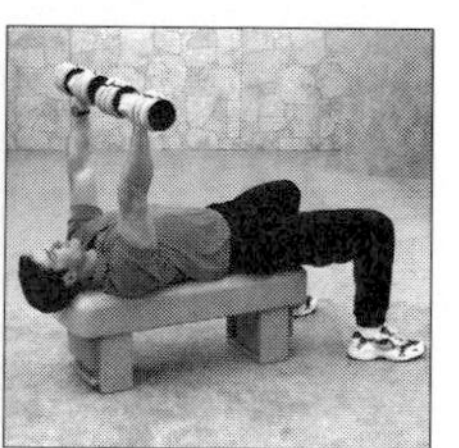

START FINISH

5. Dumbbell Press
10 reps

- Hold weights palms toward knees.
- Relax abdomen.
- Lower weights until even with chest.

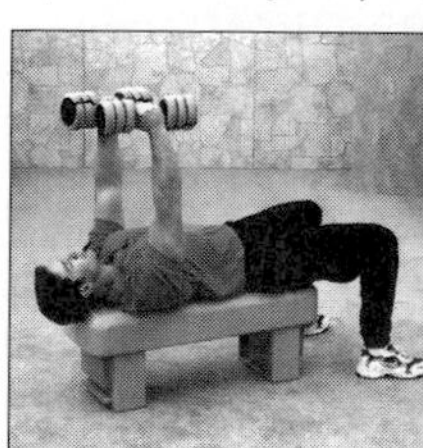
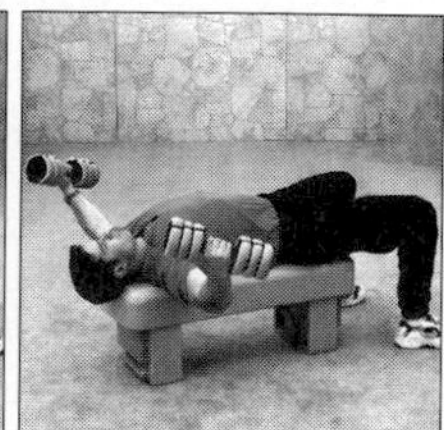

START FINISH

6. Dumbbell Fly
10 reps reduced weight

- Elbows slightly bent with palms facing each other.
- Lower weights out to the side of body until weight is parallel to body. Keep elbow slightly bent.

THE CAMPITELLI ADVANCED 10 MINUTE EXERCISE METHOD

MEN'S WORKOUT #19 • PAGE 2

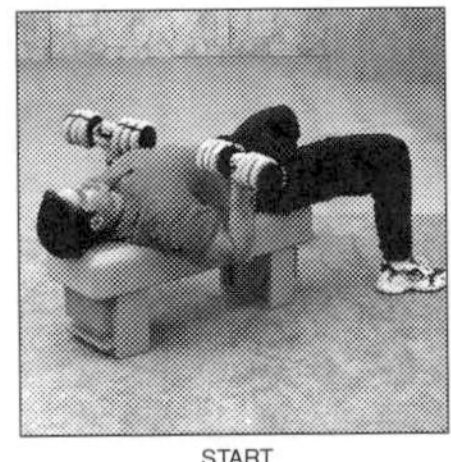

START

FINISH

7. Dumbbell Press
10 reps with reduced weights

- Hold weights palms toward knees.
- Relax abdomen.
- Lower weights until even with chest.

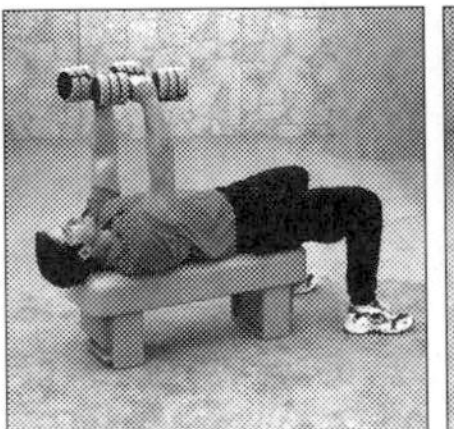

START

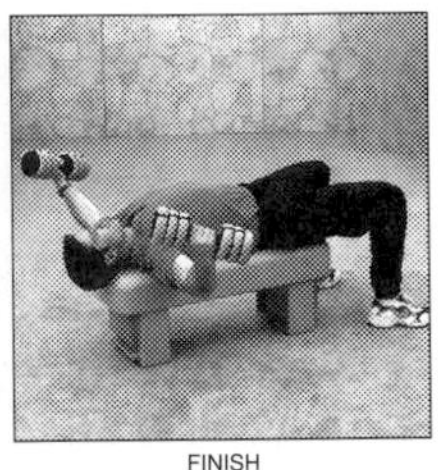

FINISH

8. Dumbbell Fly
10 reps with reduced weights

- Elbows slightly bent with palms facing each other.
- Lower weights out to the side of body until weight is parallel to body. Keep elbows slightly bent.

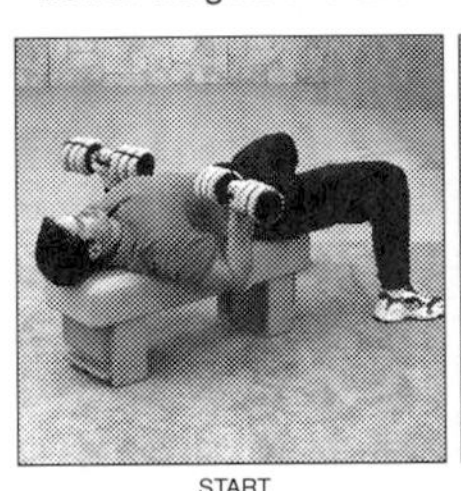

START

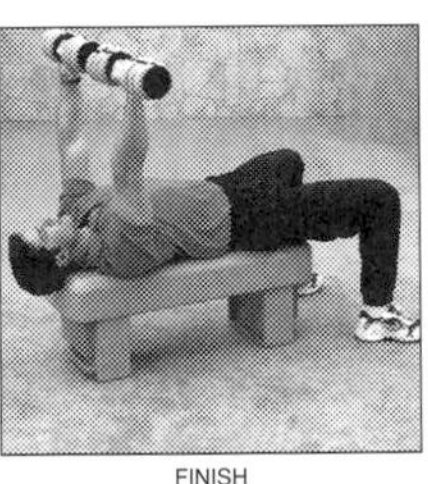

FINISH

9. Dumbbell Press
10 reps with reduced weights

- Hold weights palms toward knees.
- Relax abdomen.
- Lower weights until even with chest.

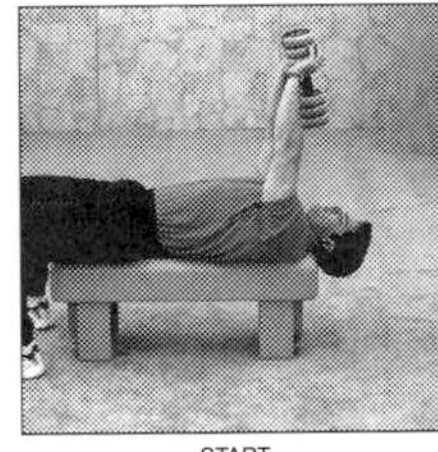

START

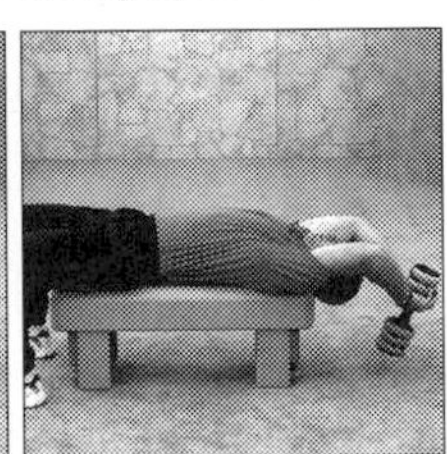

FINISH

10. Dumbbell Pullover
10 reps

- Relax abdomen. Keep elbows in toward body.
- Inhale as weight goes over head.
- Exhale as it goes up.

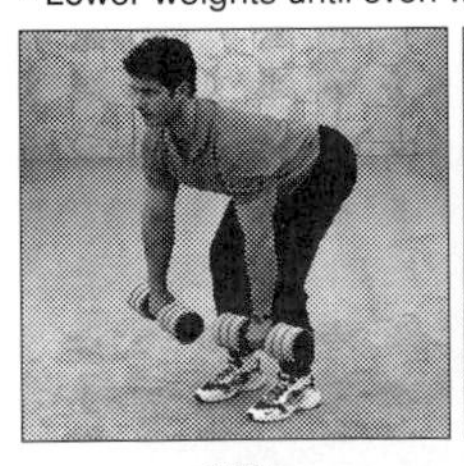

START

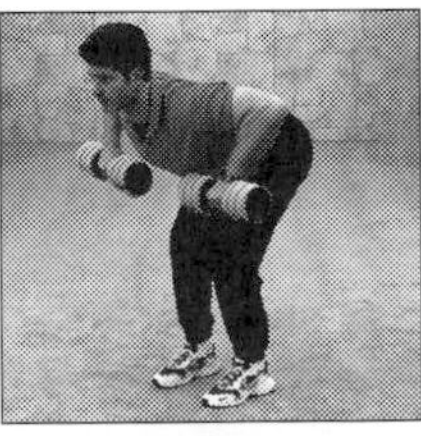

FINISH

11. Dumbbell Row with Wide Grip
10 reps

- DBs in "over-hand" position. Head up. Chest out.
- Knees bent. Back straight.

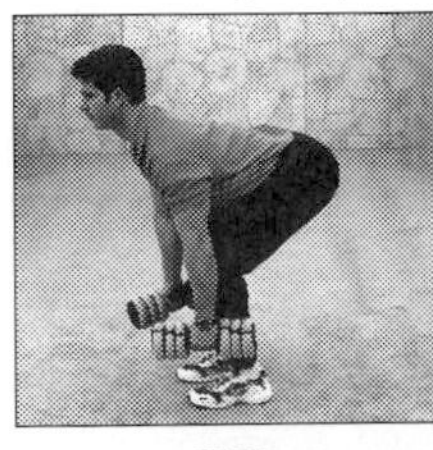

START

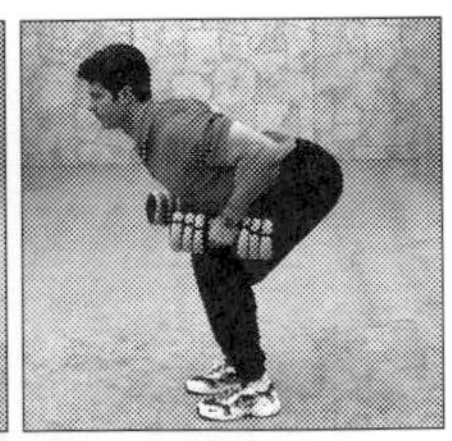

FINISH

12. Dumbbell Row Close Grip
10 reps

- Feet together. Bend at hips, not at waist.
- Back straight. Chest out. Head up. Pull weights with elbows close to body.

REPEAT SEQUENCE (10 THRU 12) FOR A TOTAL OF THREE TIMES REDUCING WEIGHT EACH TIME.

THE CAMPITELLI ADVANCED 10 MINUTE EXERCISE METHOD

MEN'S WORKOUT #20 • PAGE 1

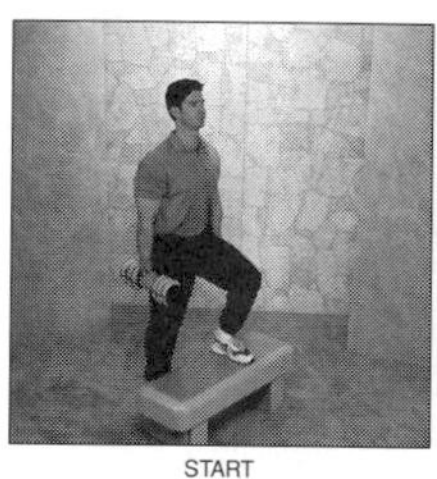
START

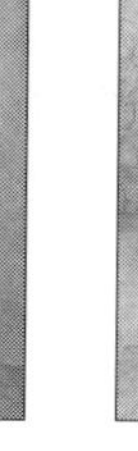
FINISH

1. Dumbbell Stepup
10 reps Right Leg

- Place entire foot on bench or step.
- Use top leg to push only.
- Look up. Shoulders back.

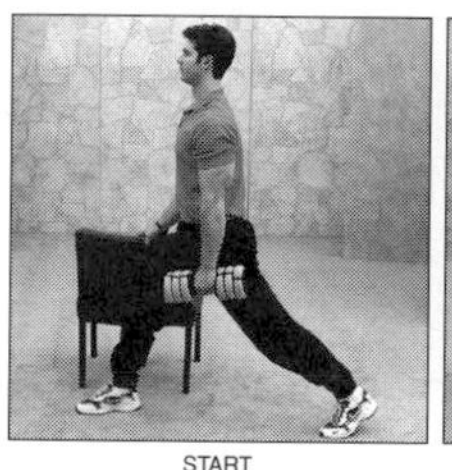
START

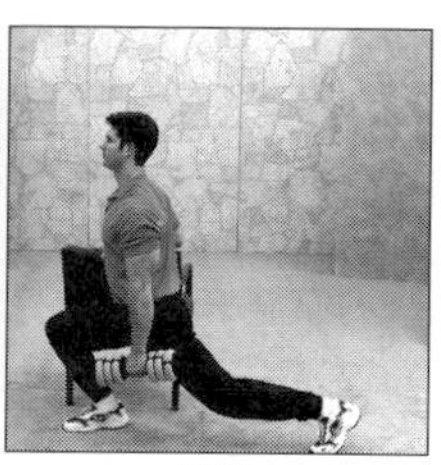
FINISH

2. Lunge with Dumbbell
10 reps Right Leg

- Same as regular lunge with DB in one hand.
- Use chair for support and balance.

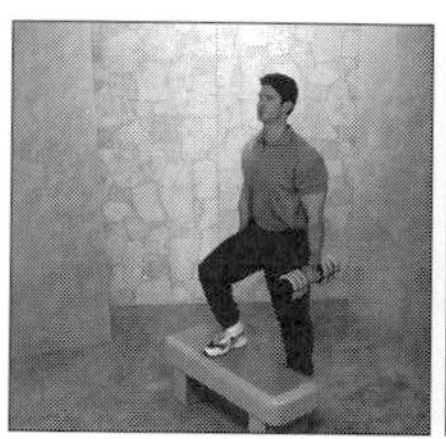
START

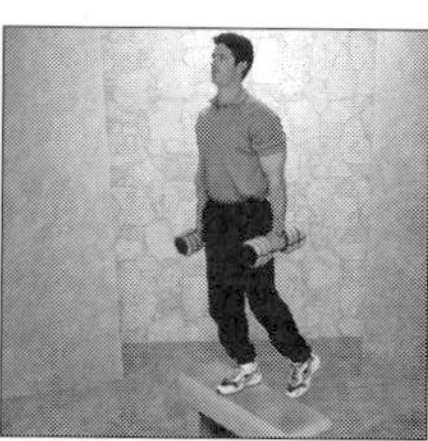
FINISH

3. Dumbbell Stepup
10 reps Left Leg

- Place ENTIRE foot on bench or step.
- Use top leg to push only.
- Look up. Shoulders back.

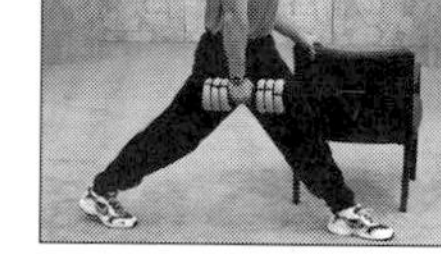
START

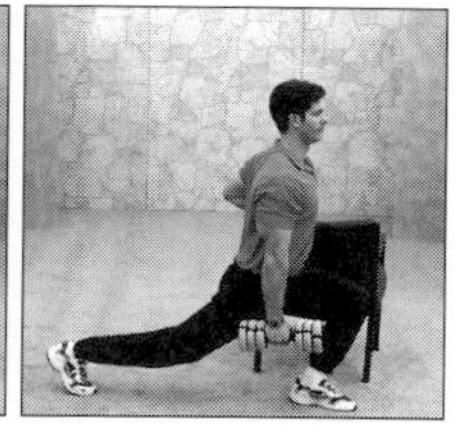
FINISH

4. Lunge with Dumbbell
10 reps Left Leg

- Same as regular lunge with DB in one hand.
- Use chair for support and balance.

REPEAT SEQUENCE (1 THRU 4) TWO MORE TIMES REDUCING WEIGHT EACH TIME BEFORE MOVING ON TO PAGE 2.

THE CAMPITELLI ADVANCED 10 MINUTE EXERCISE METHOD

MEN'S WORKOUT #20 • PAGE 2

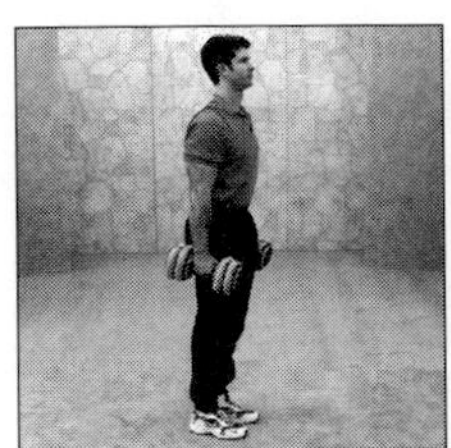

START

FINISH

5. Dumbbell Squat

10 reps

- Feet 4-8 inches apart. DBs at side.
- Place weight even on heels and balls of feet.
- Back straight. Head up. Push with heels.

START

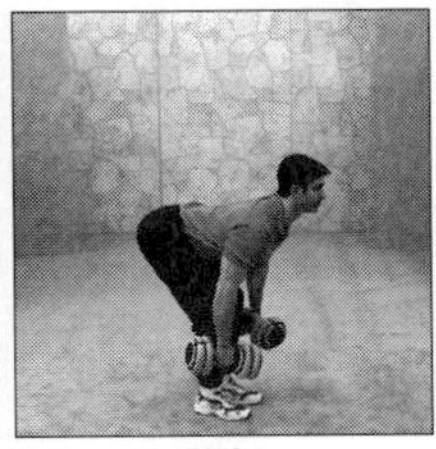

FINISH

6. Dumbell Deadlift

10 reps

- Knees slightly bent with feet slightly apart.
- Keep low back locked with upper torso.
- Bend at hips, <u>not</u> at waist. Head up/chest out.
- Back is flat.

REPEAT SEQUENCE (5 THRU 6) TWO MORE TIMES REDUCING WEIGHT EACH TIME.

17

BIOGENESIS PHASE FOUR PHOTOGRAPHS

PHASE FOUR - SHOULDER EXERCISES

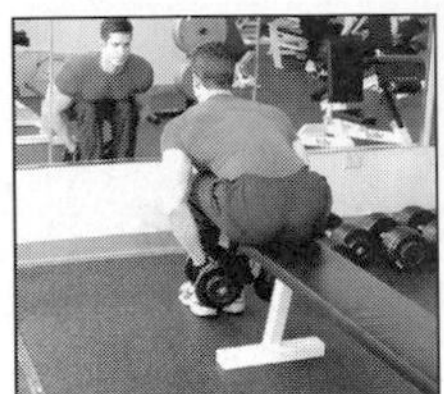

START FINISH

Rear Delts

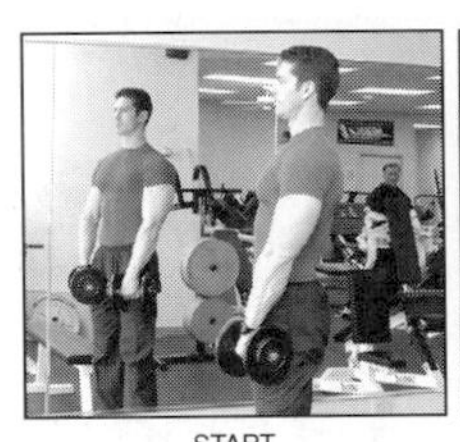
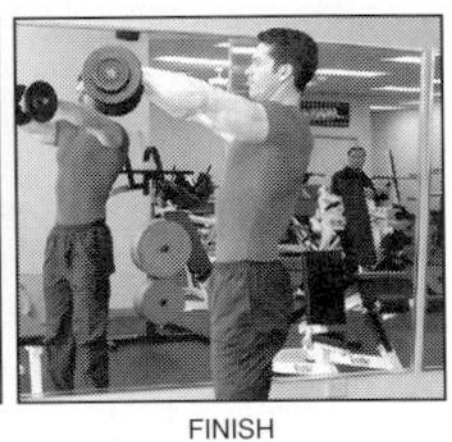

START FINISH

Front Raises

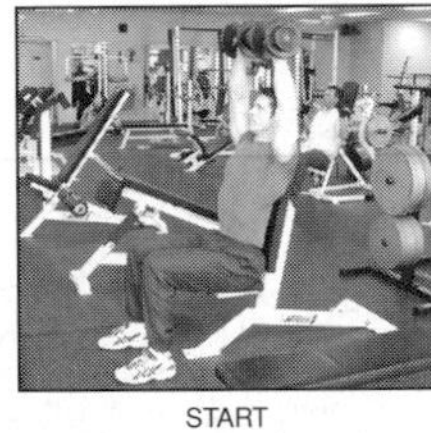
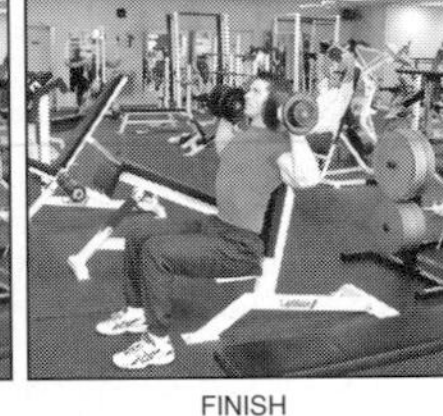

START FINISH

Shoulder Press

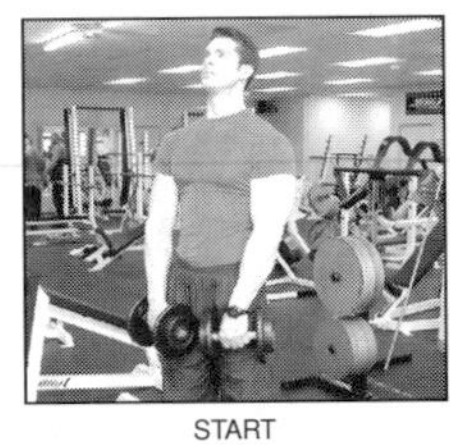
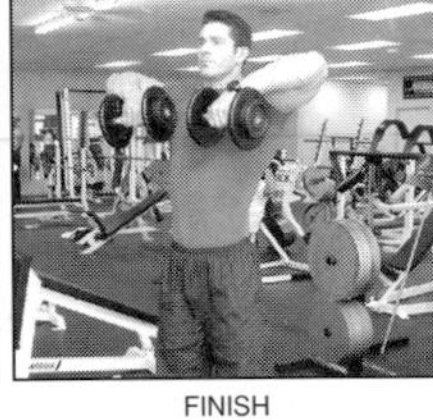

START FINISH

Upright Row

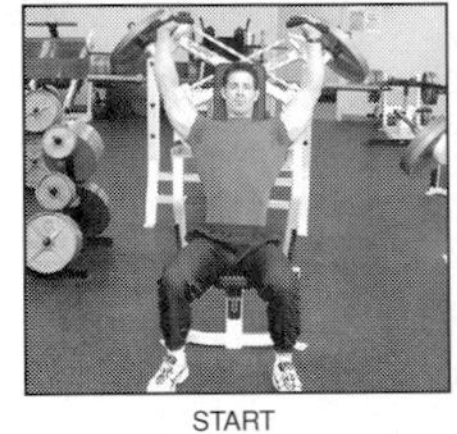
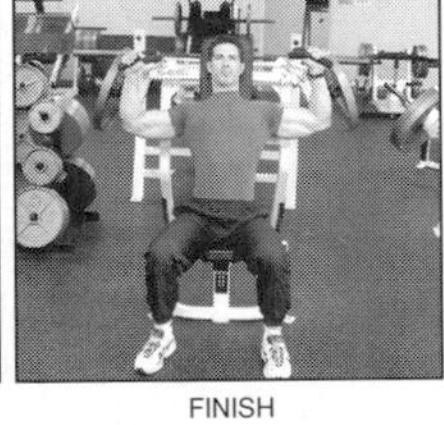

START FINISH

Delt Machine

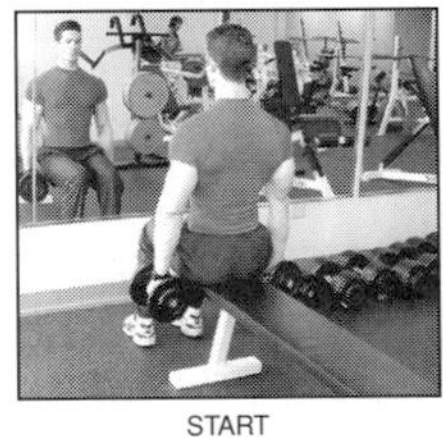
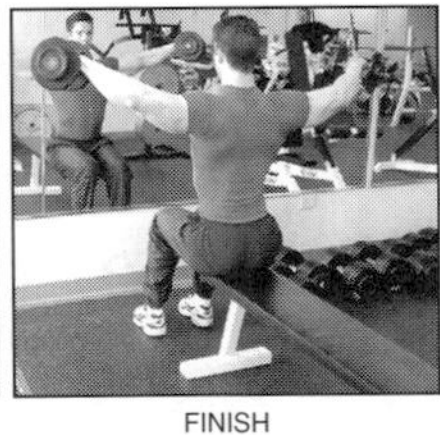

START FINISH

Lateral Raise

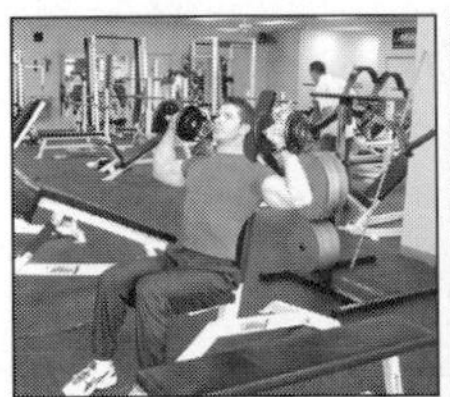
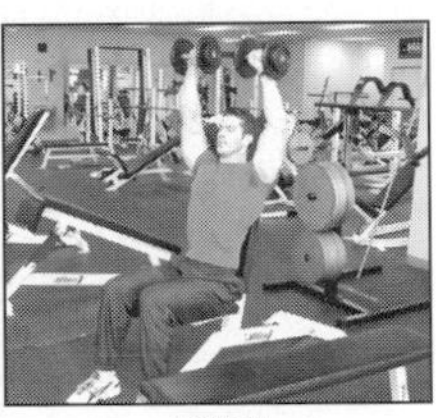

START FINISH

Overhead Dumbbell Press

PHASE FOUR - SHOULDER EXERCISES (continued)

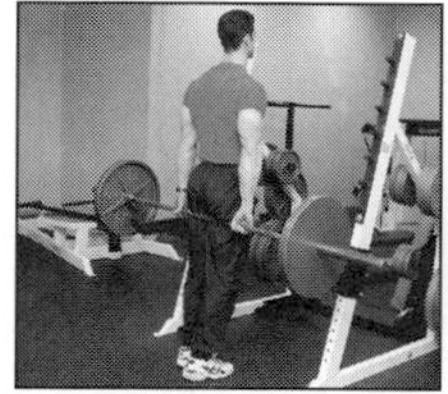
START FINISH

Deltoid Row

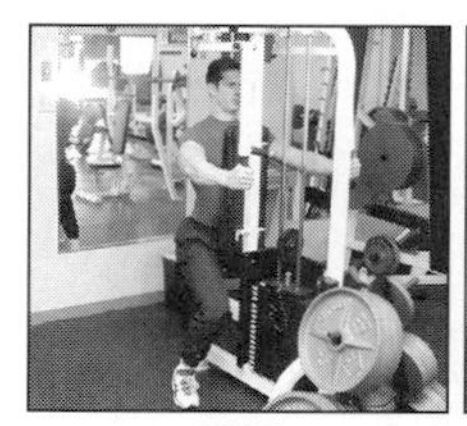
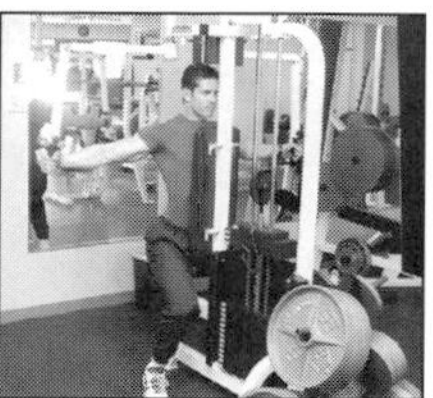
START FINISH

Rear Delt Machine

PHASE FOUR - ABDOMINAL EXERCISES

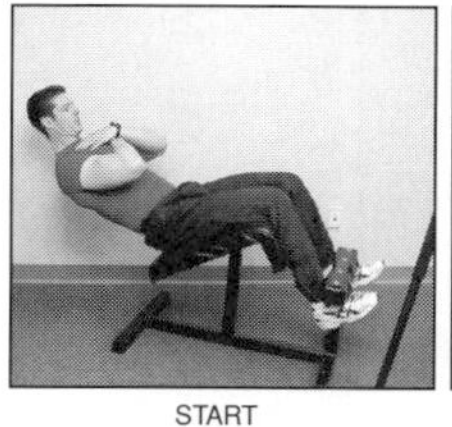
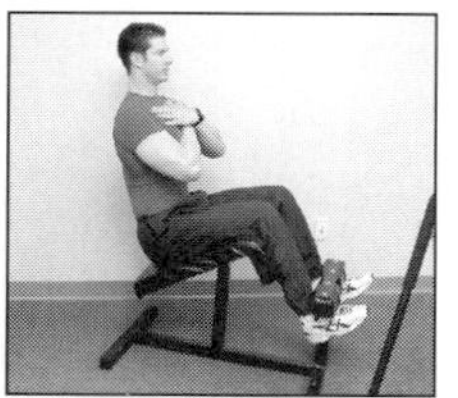
START FINISH

Dumbbell Floor Crunch

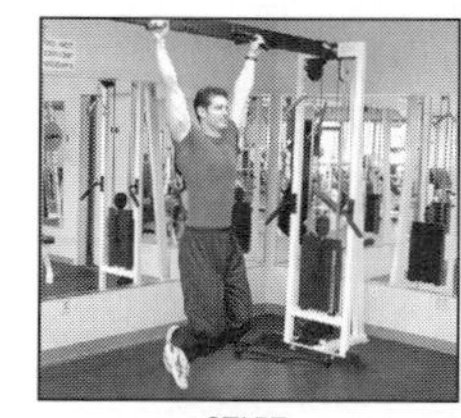
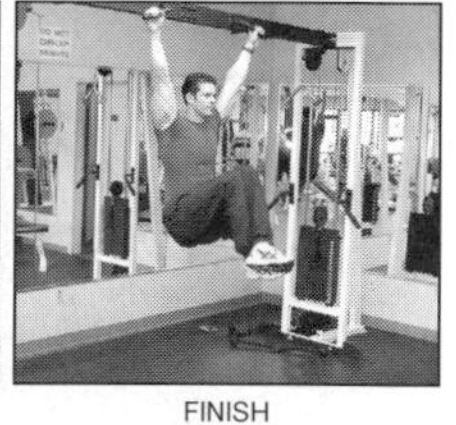
START FINISH

Dumbbell Floor Tuck

PHASE FOUR - BACK EXERCISES

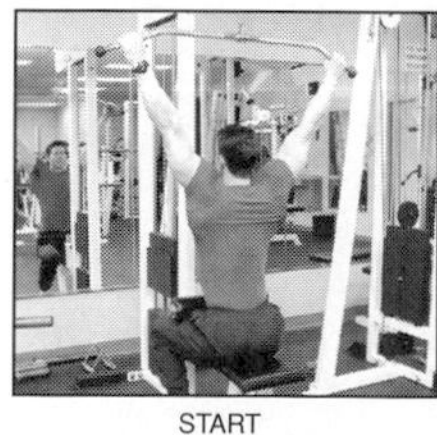
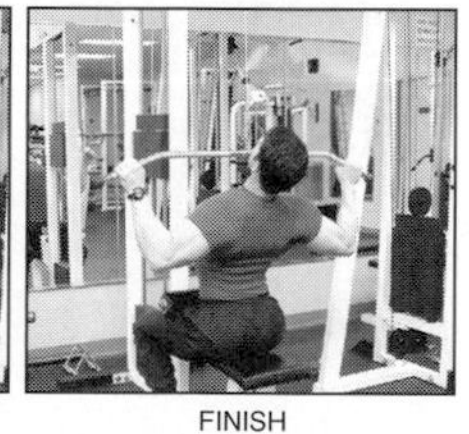
START FINISH

Pull Down Front

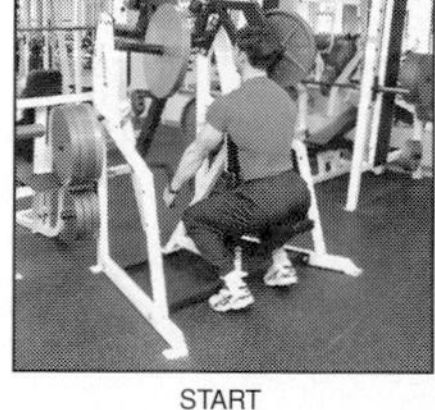
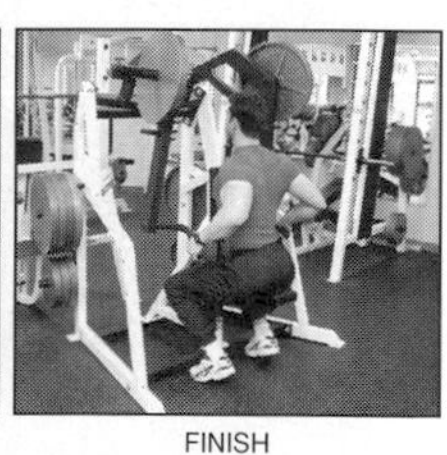
START FINISH

Row Machine

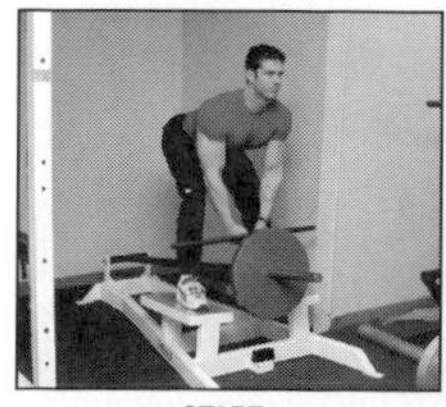
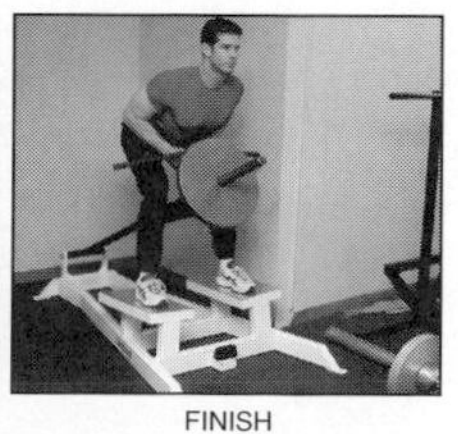
START FINISH

T-Bar Row

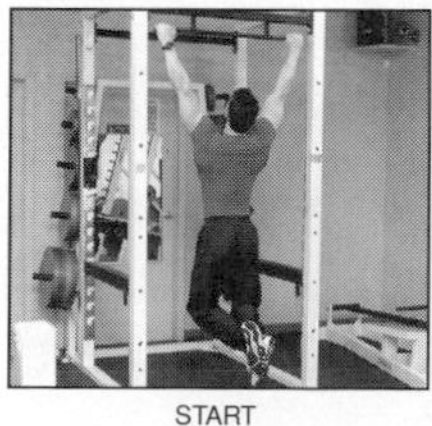
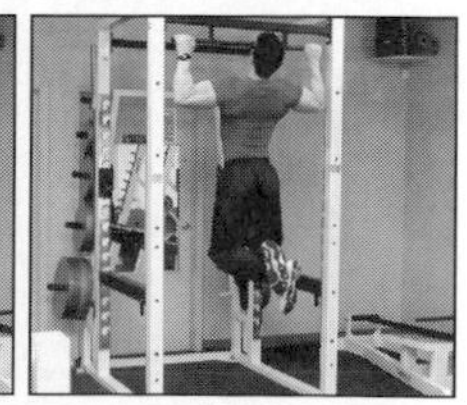
START FINISH

Wide Grip Pull Up

PHASE FOUR - BACK EXERCISES (continued)

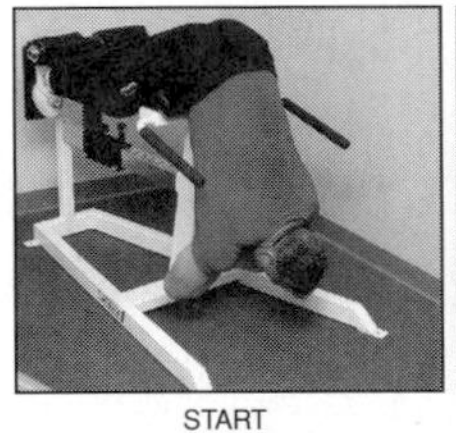

START FINISH

Hyper Extension

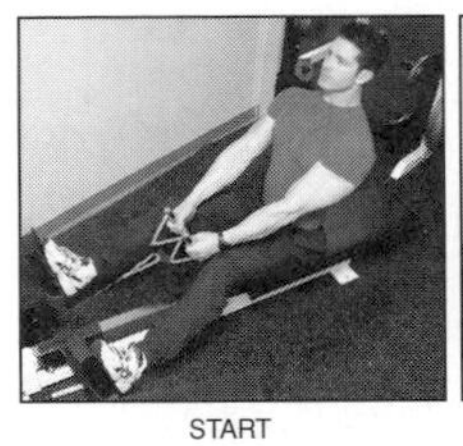
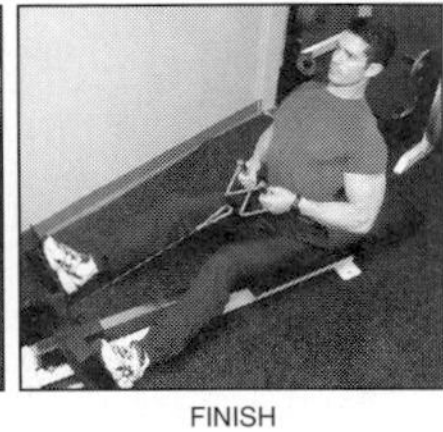

START FINISH

Low Cable Row

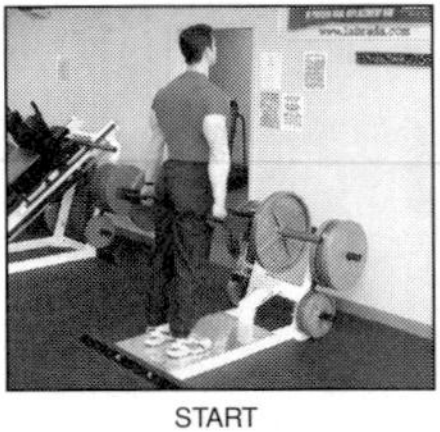
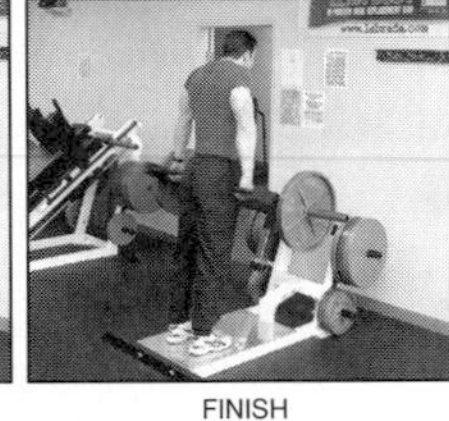

START FINISH

Machine Shrug

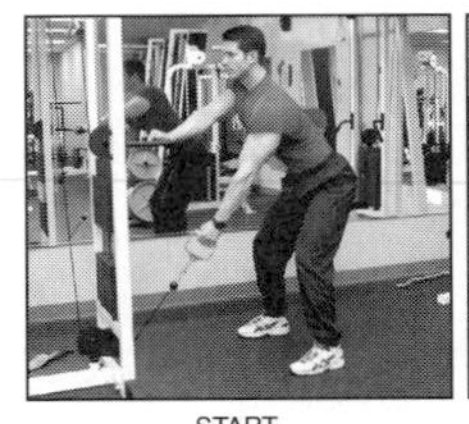
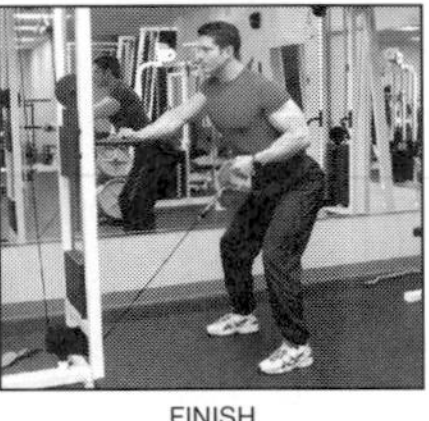

START FINISH

One Arm Cable Row

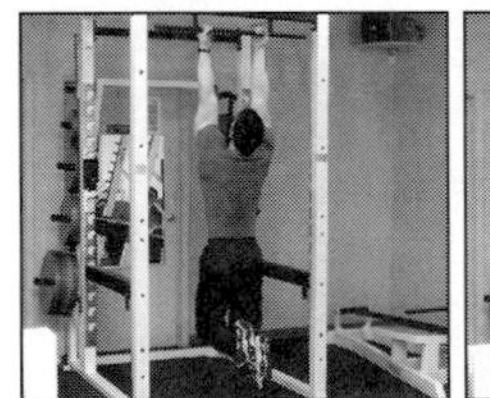
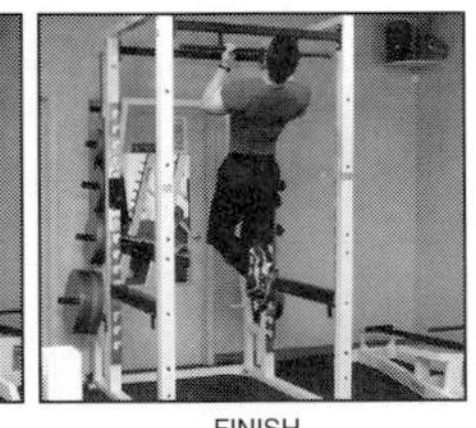

START FINISH

Pull Up

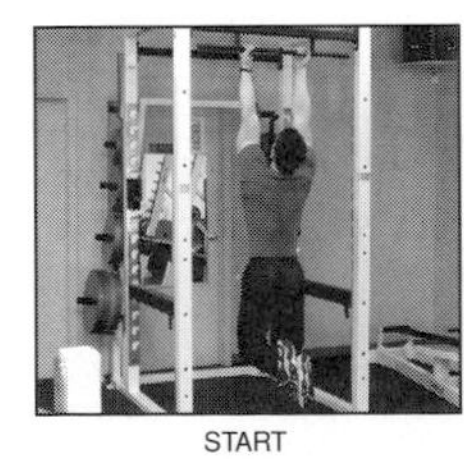
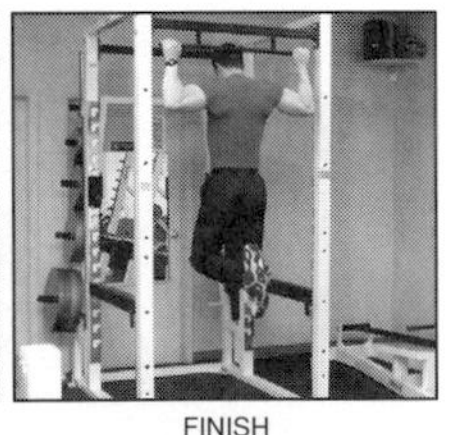

START FINISH

Pull Up Behind Head

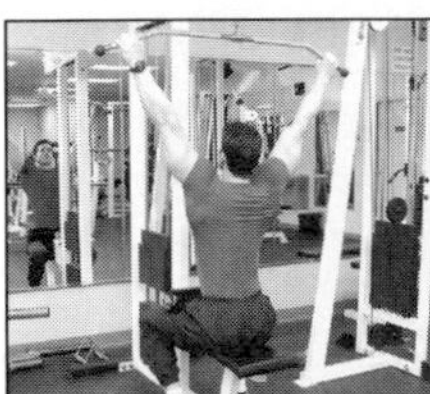
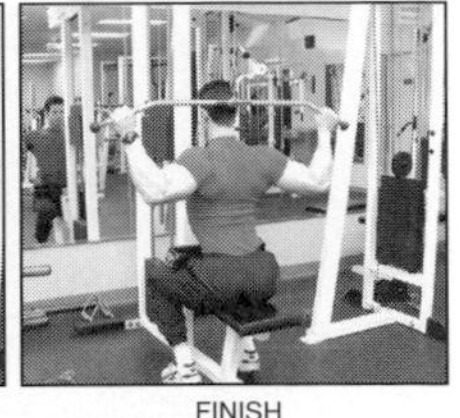

START FINISH

Pull Down Behind Head

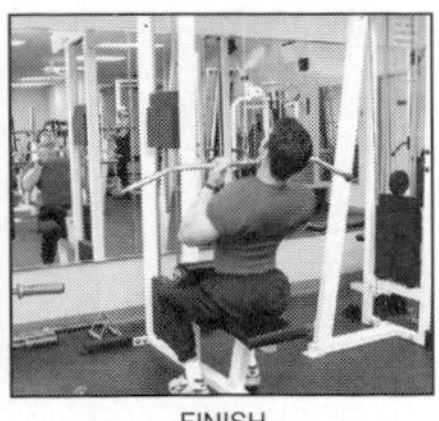

START FINISH

Pull Down Close Grip

PHASE FOUR - BACK EXERCISES (continued)

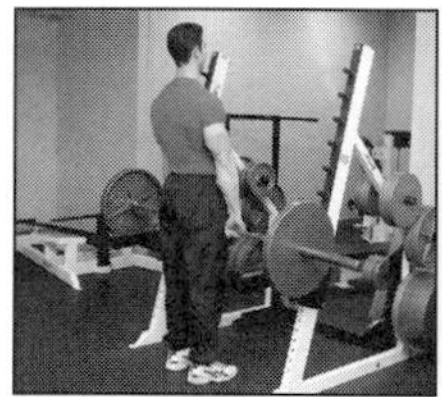

START FINISH

Barbell Shrug

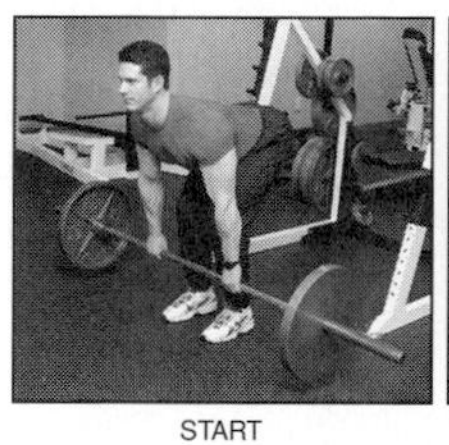
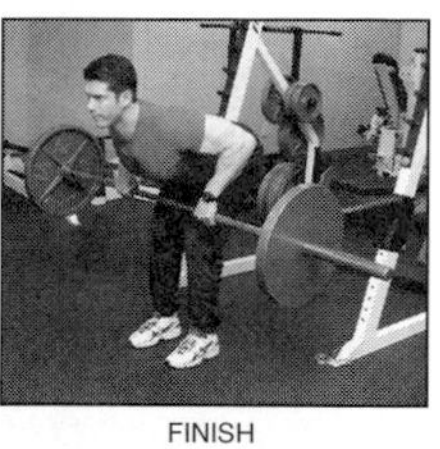

START FINISH

Bent Barbell Row

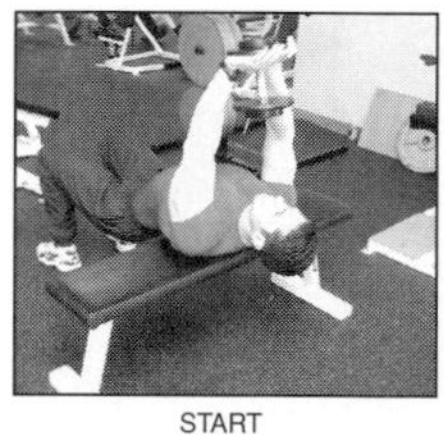
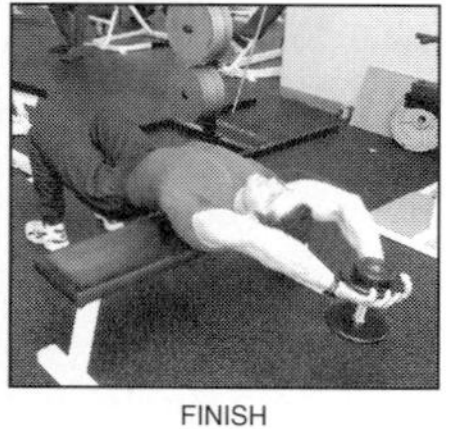

START FINISH

Dumbbell Pull Over

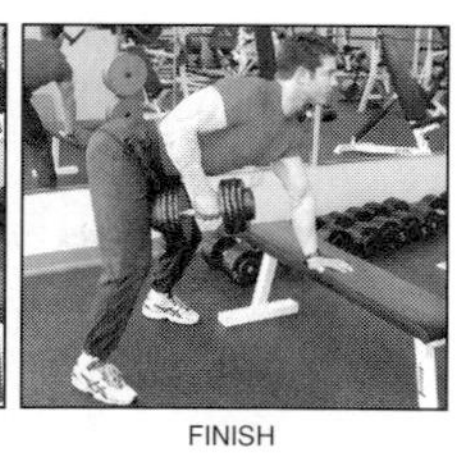

START FINISH

Dumbbell Row

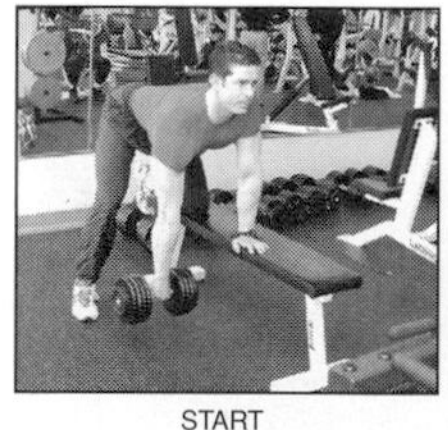
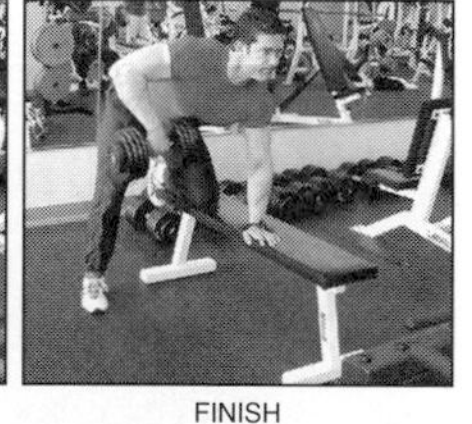

START FINISH

Dumbbell Row Wide

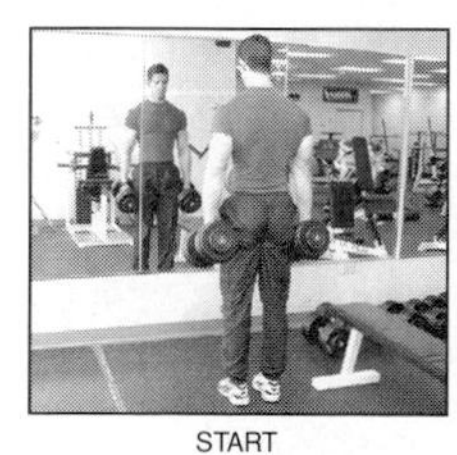
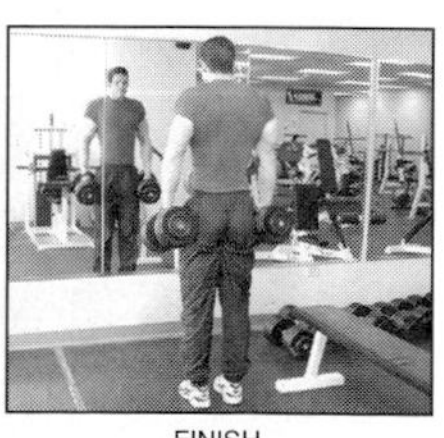

START FINISH

Dumbbell Shrug

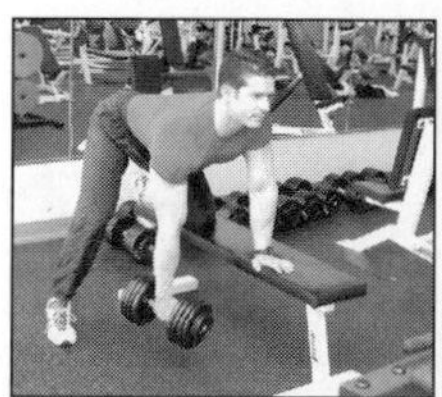
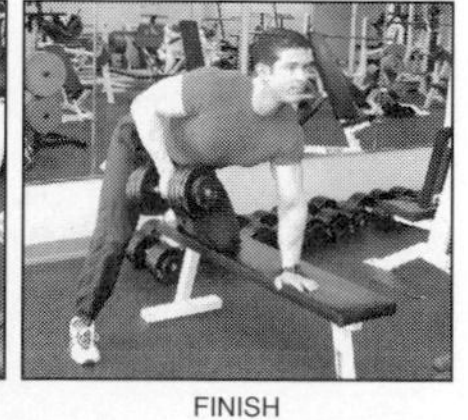

START FINISH

Dumbbell Row

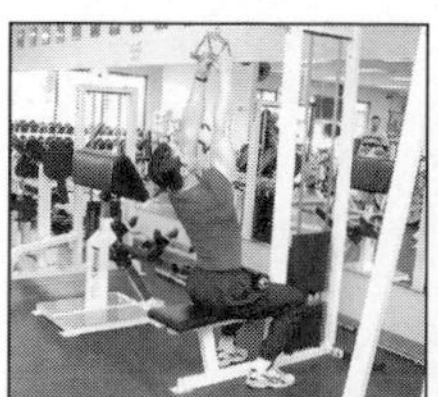
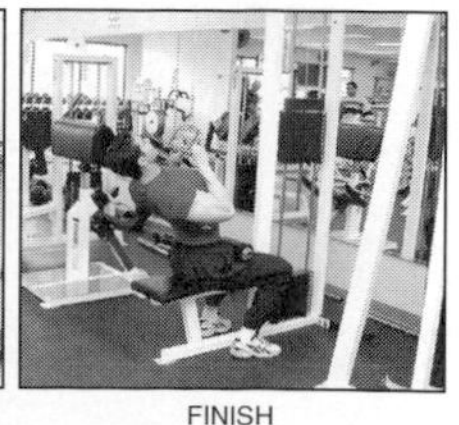

START FINISH

High Cable Row

PHASE FOUR - CHEST EXERCISES

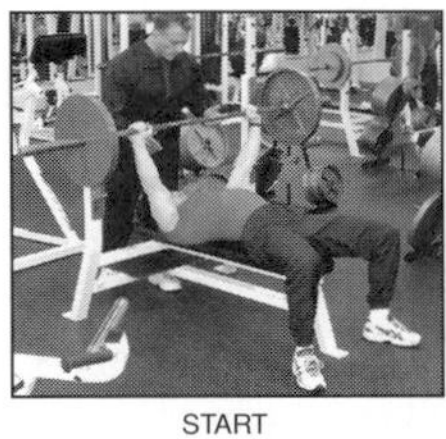

START FINISH

Bench

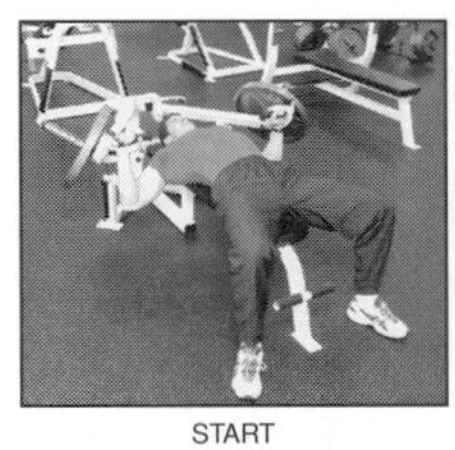

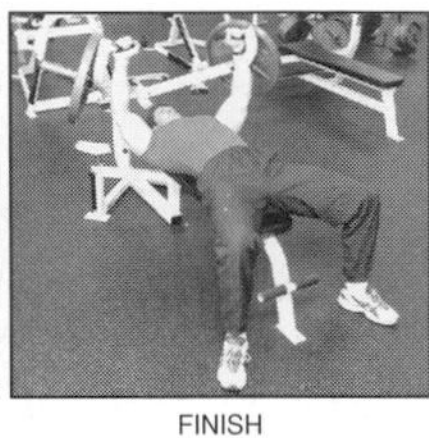

START FINISH

Bench Machine

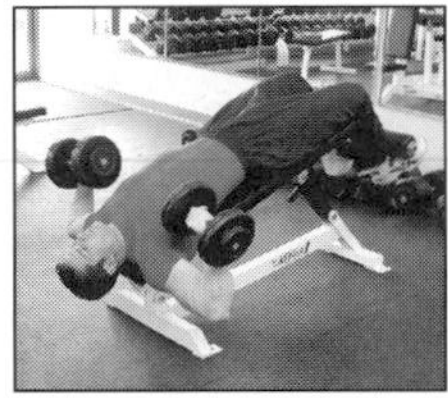

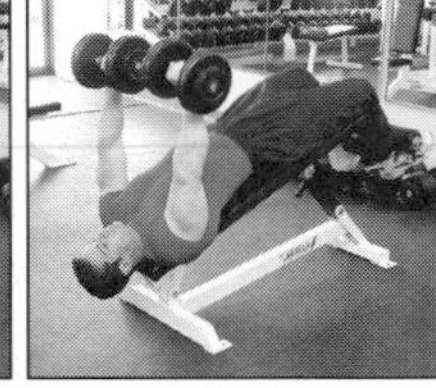

START FINISH

Decline Dumbbell Press

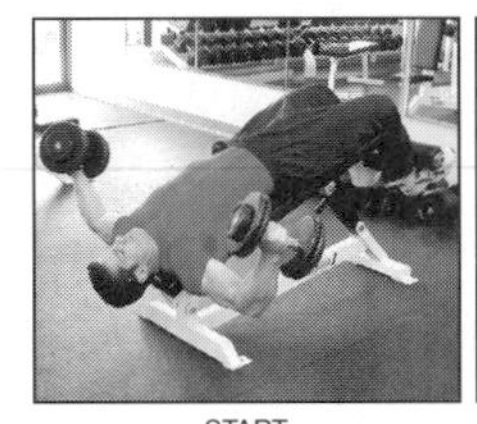

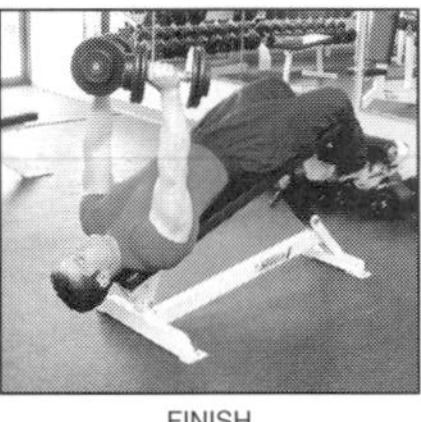

START FINISH

Decline Dumbbell Fly

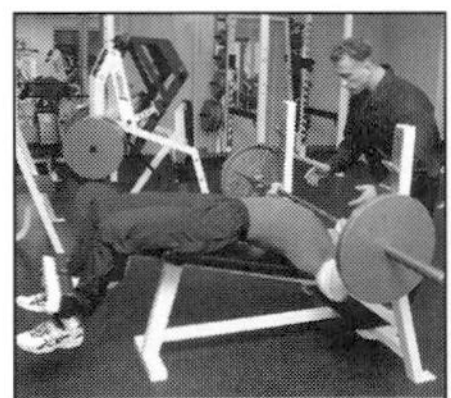

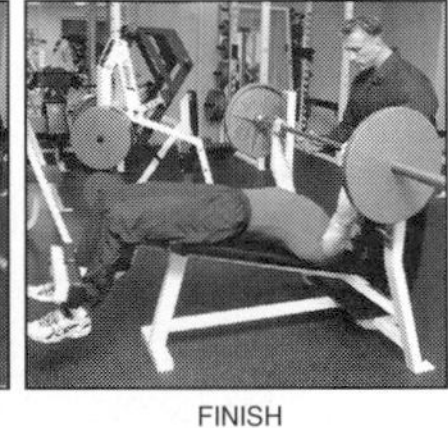

START FINISH

Decline Barbell Press

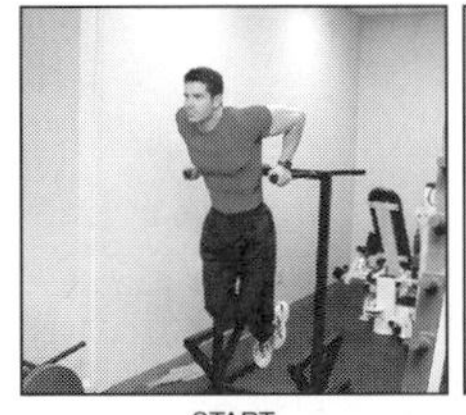

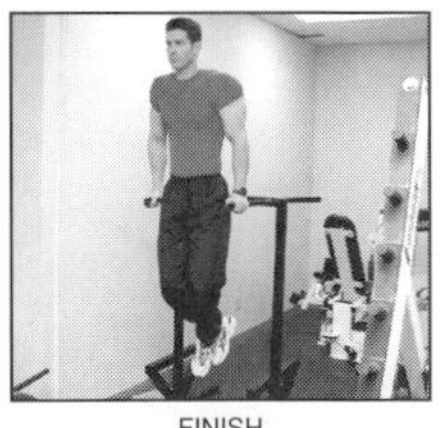

START FINISH

Dip

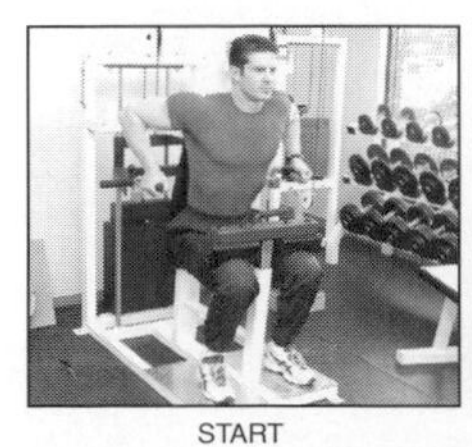

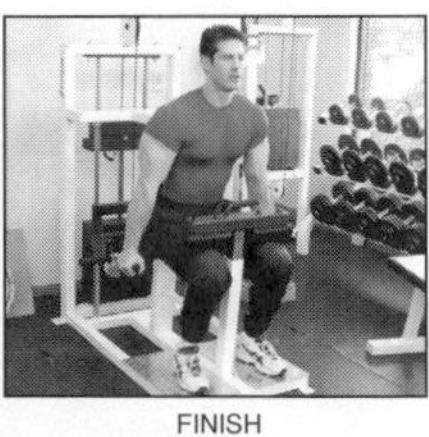

START FINISH

Dip Machine

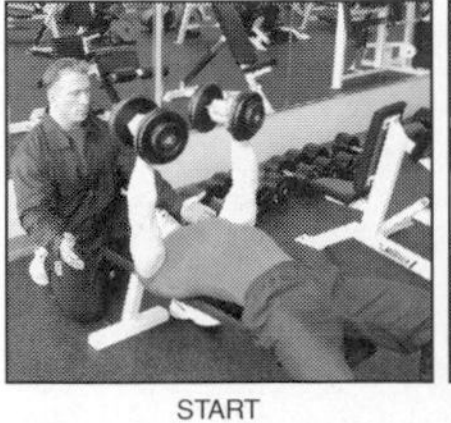

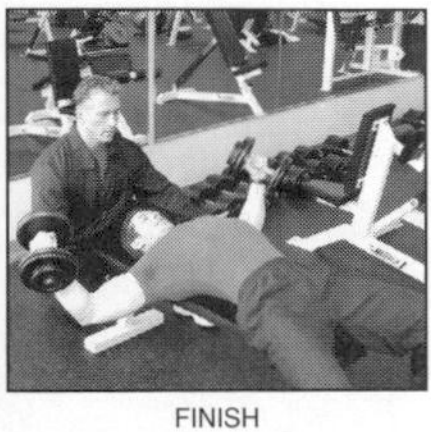

START FINISH

Dumbbell Fly

PHASE FOUR - CHEST EXERCISES (continued)

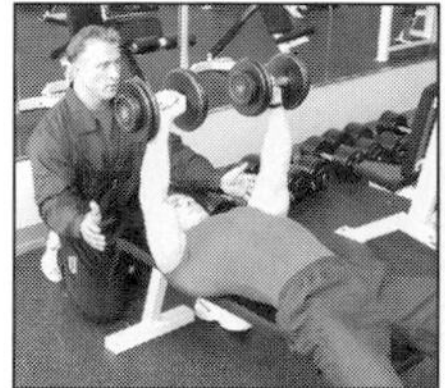

START FINISH

Dumbbell Press

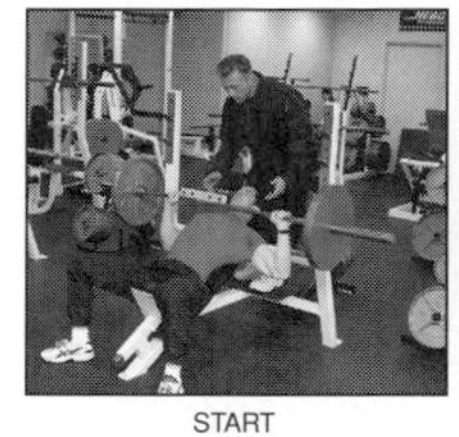
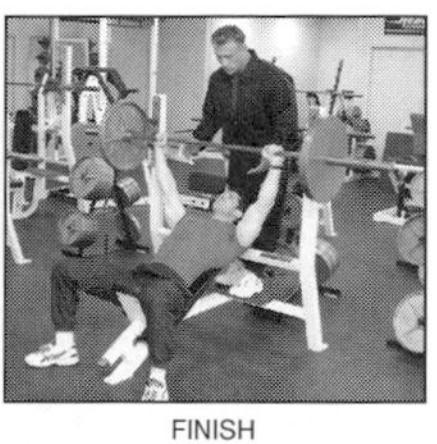

START FINISH

Incline Bench Press

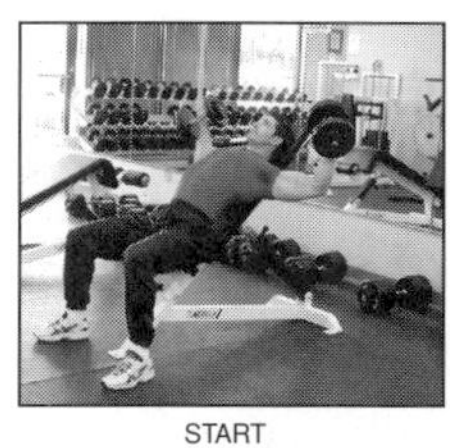
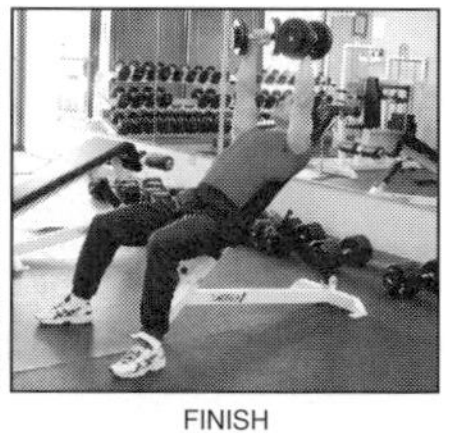

START FINISH

Incline Dumbbell Fly

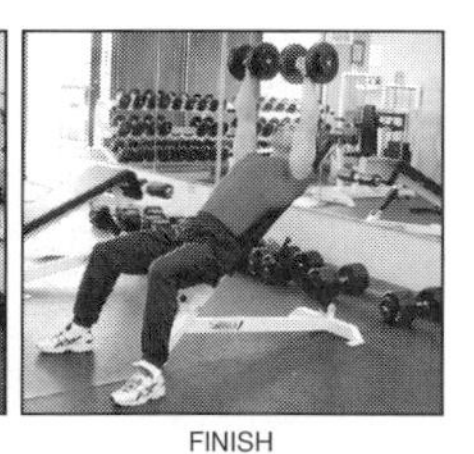

START FINISH

Incline Dumbbell Press

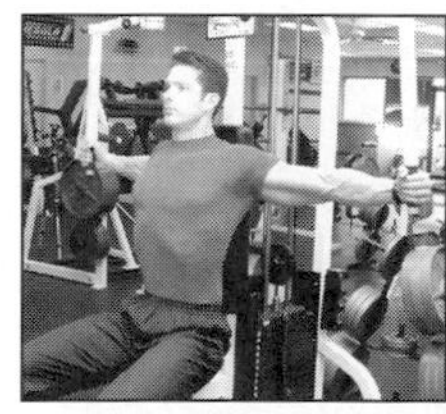
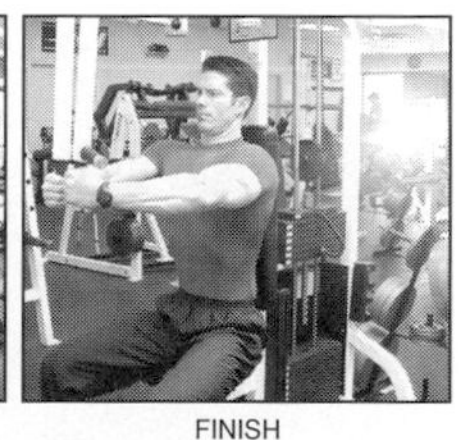

START FINISH

Pec Dec Fly Machine

PHASE FOUR - TRICEP EXERCISES

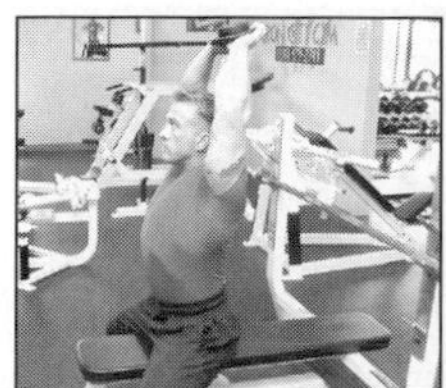
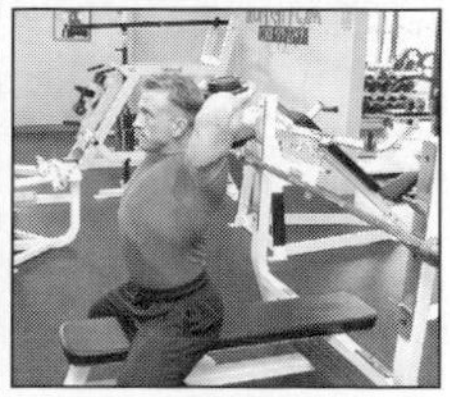

START FINISH

Overhead Dumbbell Tricep Extension

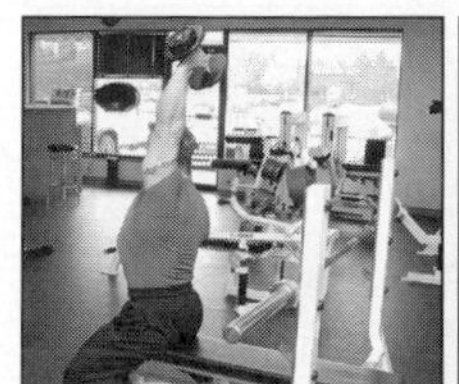
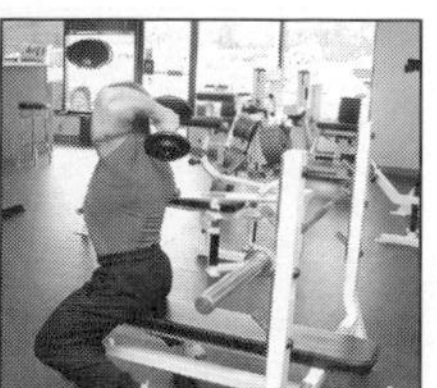

START FINISH

Overhead One Hand Tricep Extension

PHASE FOUR - TRICEP EXERCISES (continued)

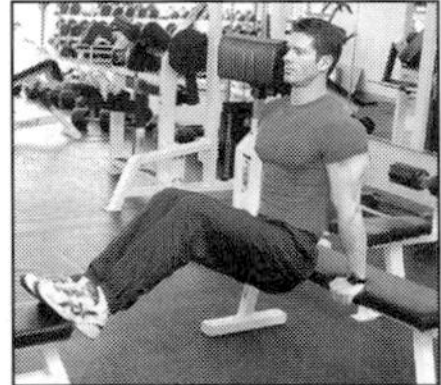

START FINISH

Bench Dip

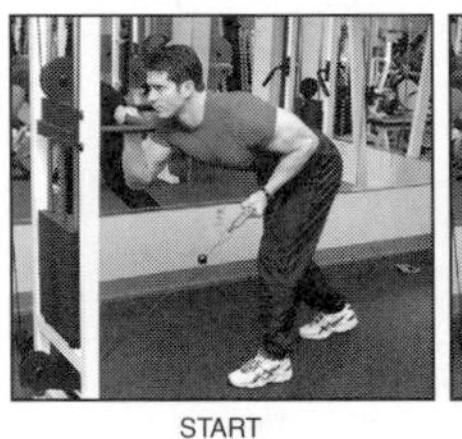
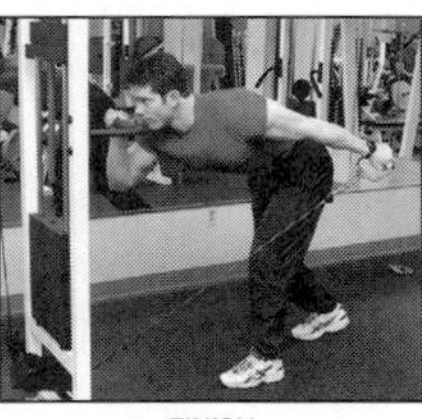

START FINISH

Cable Tricep Kickback

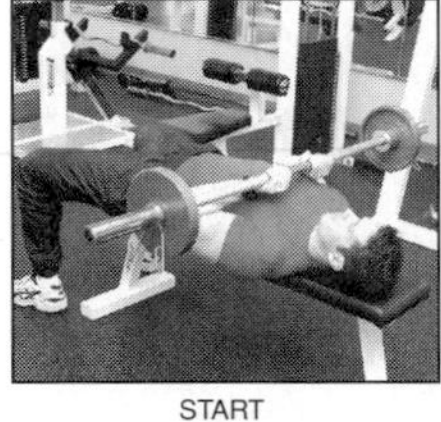
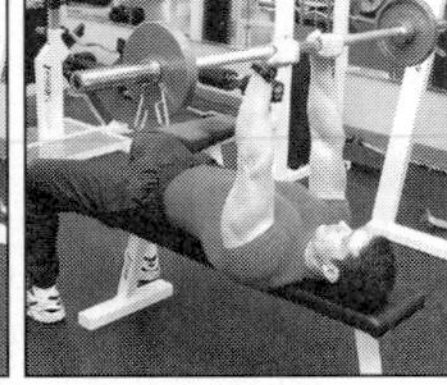

START FINISH

Close Grip Bench Press

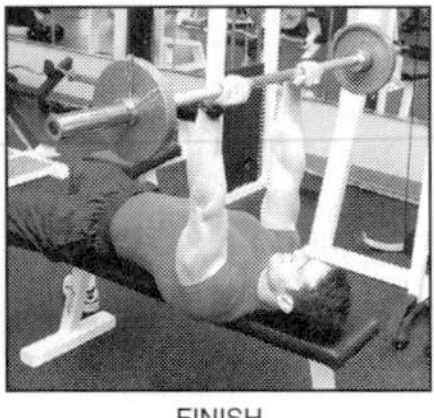

START FINISH

Lying Barbell Extension

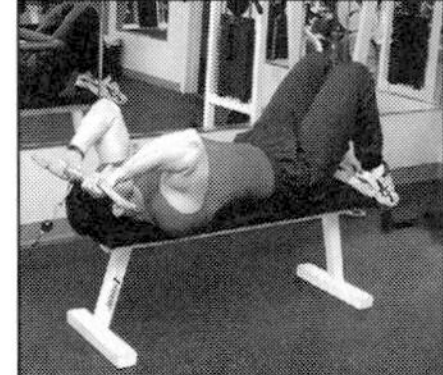
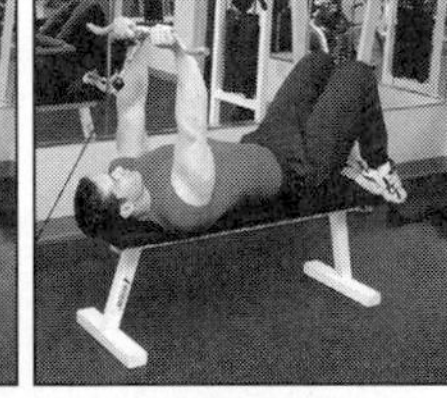

START FINISH

Lying Cable Tricep Extension

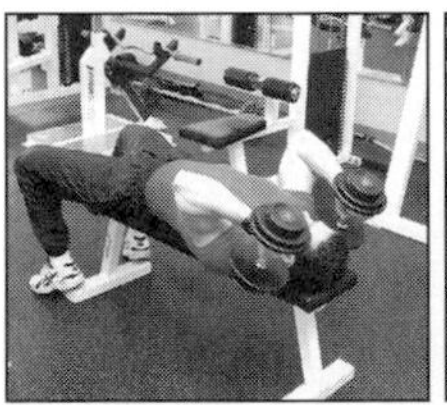
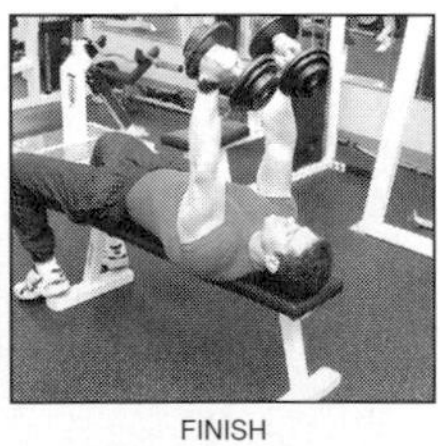

START FINISH

Lying Dumbbell Tricep Extension

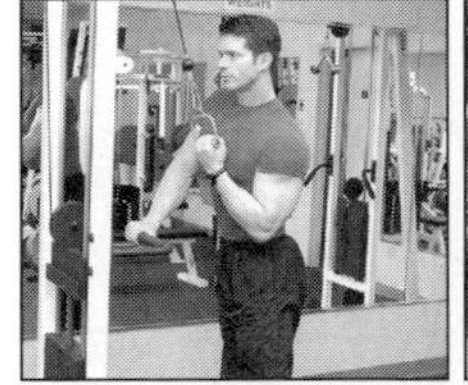
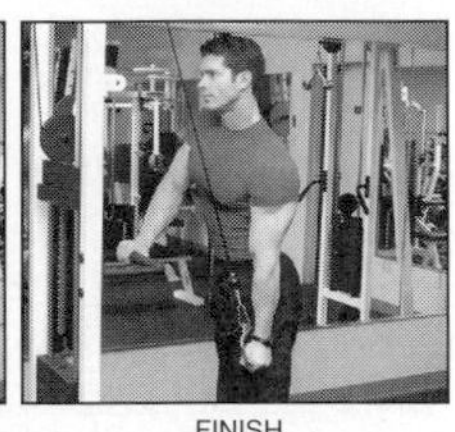

START FINISH

One Arm Cable Extension

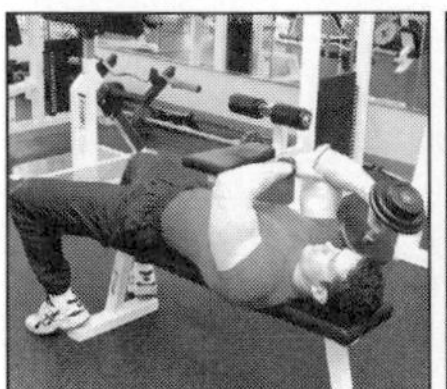
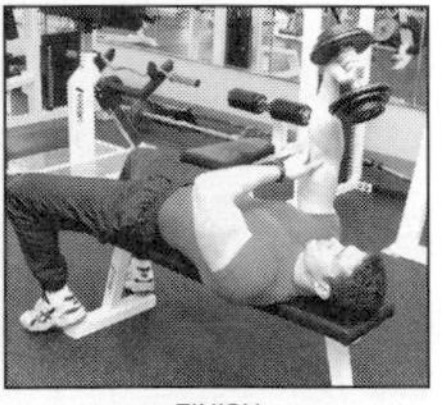

START FINISH

One Arm Lying Tricep Extension

PHASE FOUR - TRICEP EXERCISES (continued)

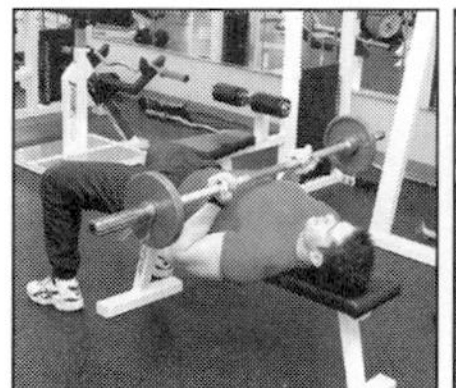

START FINISH

Reverse Bench Press

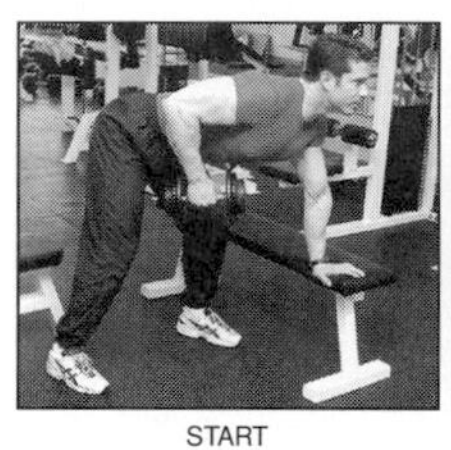
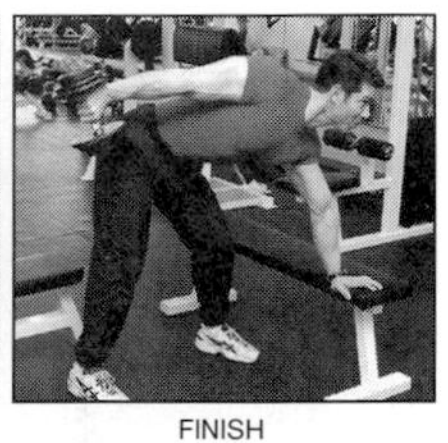

START FINISH

Tricep Kickback

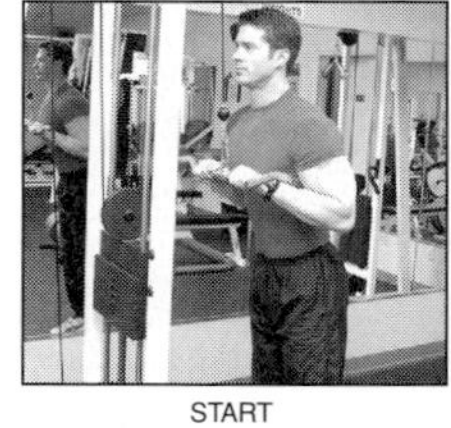
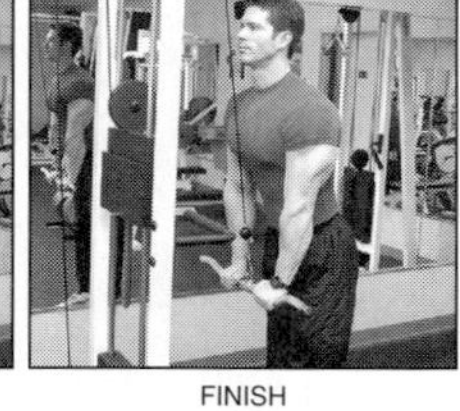

START FINISH

Tricep Pushdown

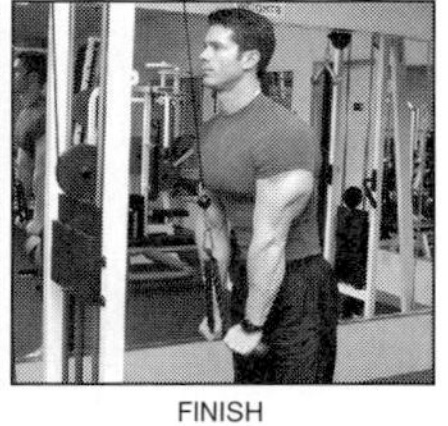

START FINISH

Tricep Rope Pushdown

PHASE FOUR - BICEP EXERCISES

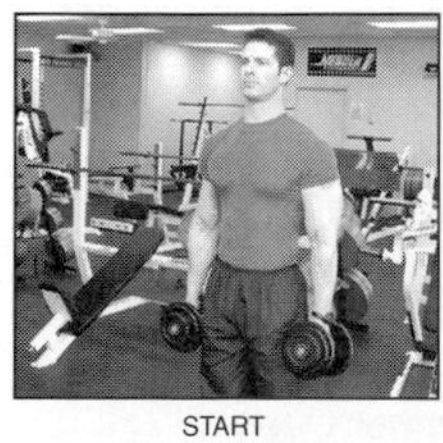
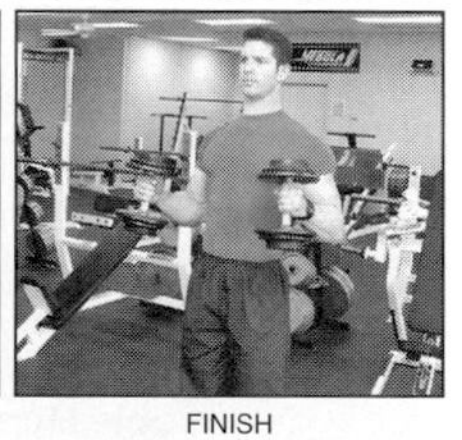

START FINISH

Double Hammer Curl

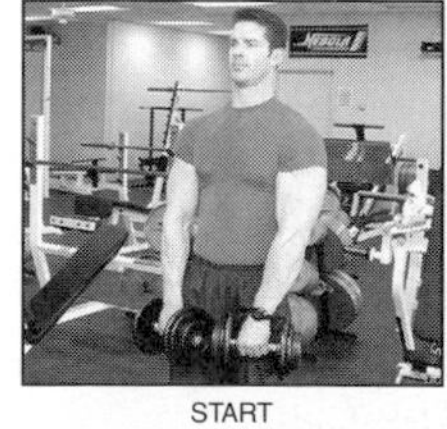
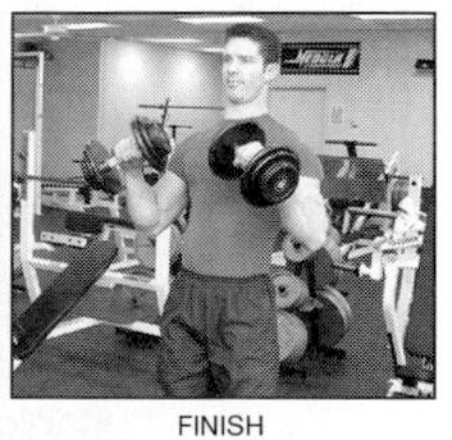

START FINISH

Dumbbell Reverse Curl

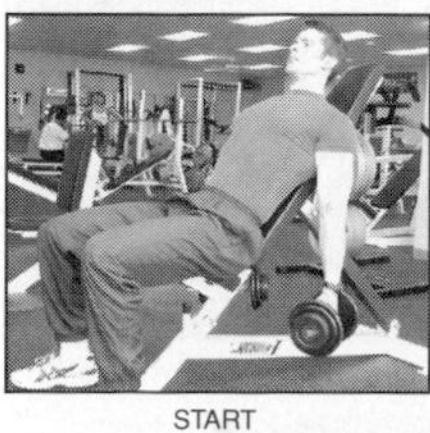
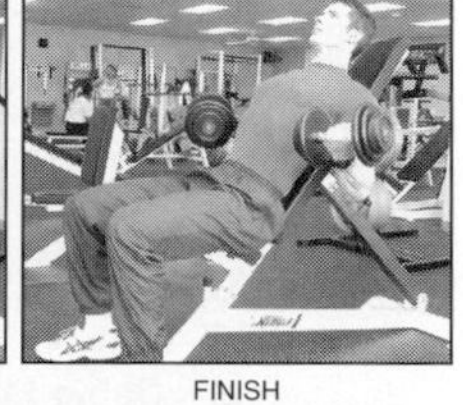

START FINISH

Incline Dumbbell Curl

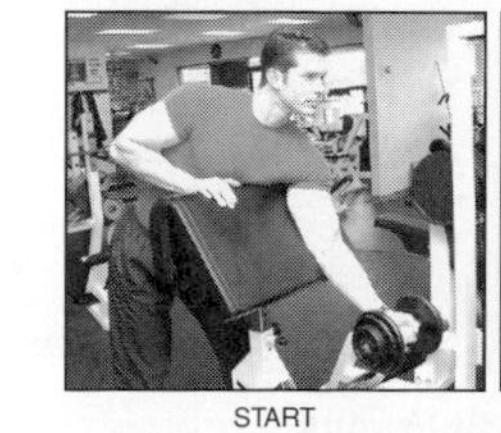
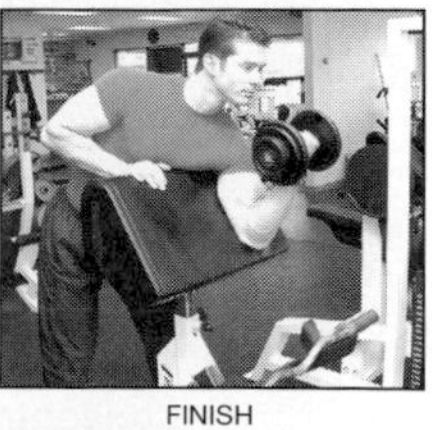

START FINISH

One Arm Preacher Curl

PHASE FOUR - BICEP EXERCISES (continued)

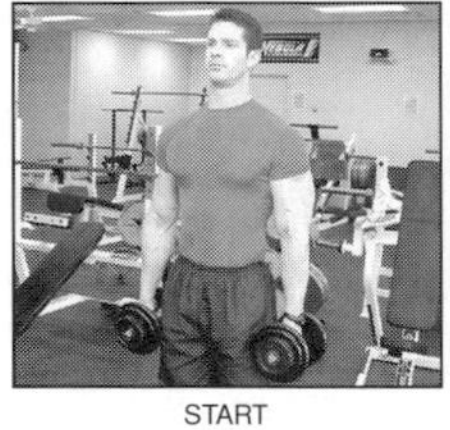

START FINISH

Alternating Dumbbell Curl

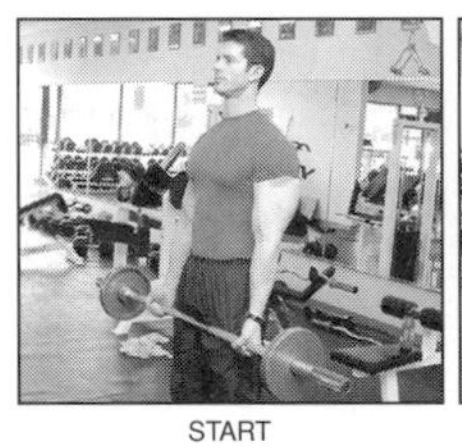
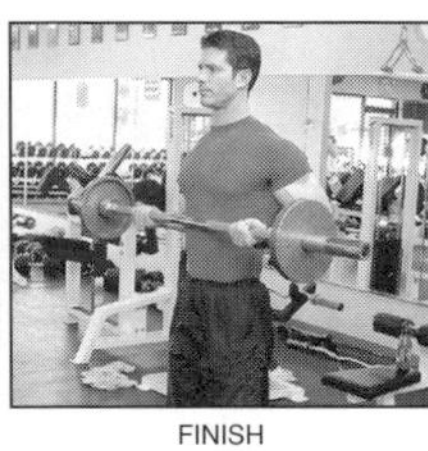

START FINISH

Barbell Drag Curl

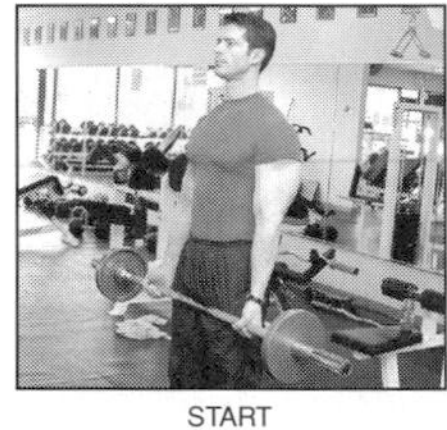
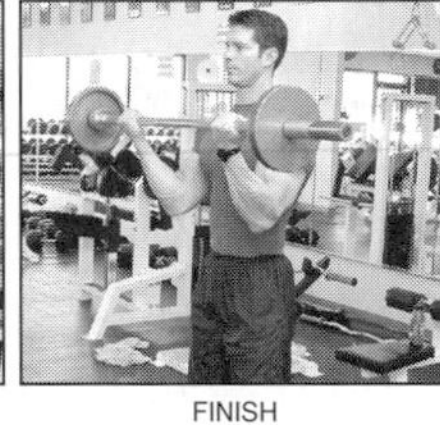

START FINISH

Barbell Curl

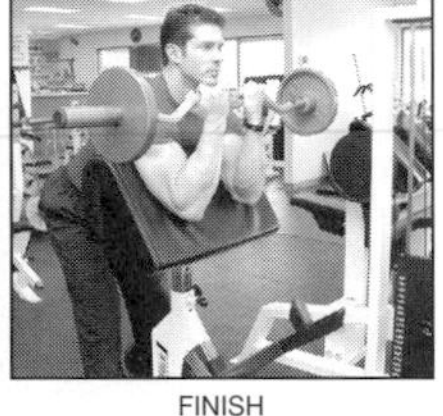

START FINISH

Barbell Preacher Curl

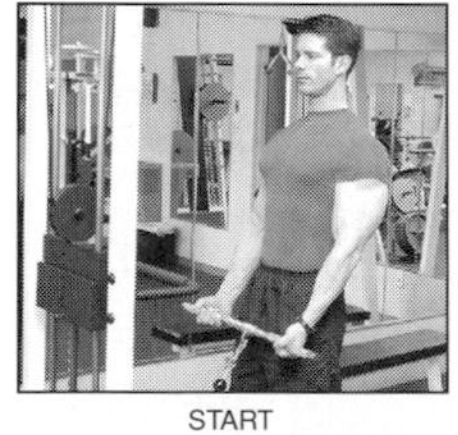
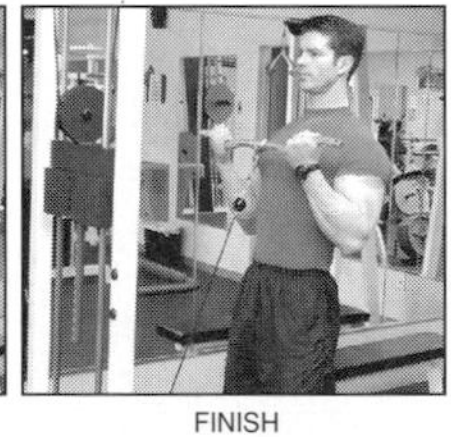

START FINISH

Cable Curl

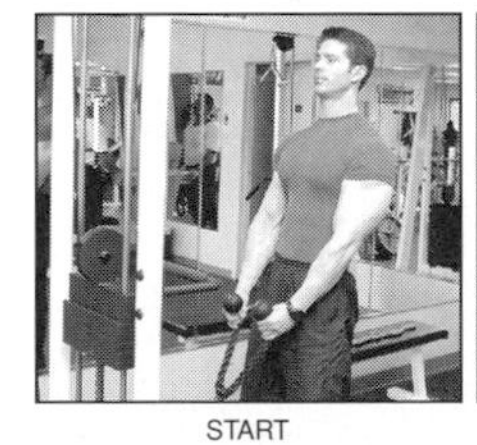
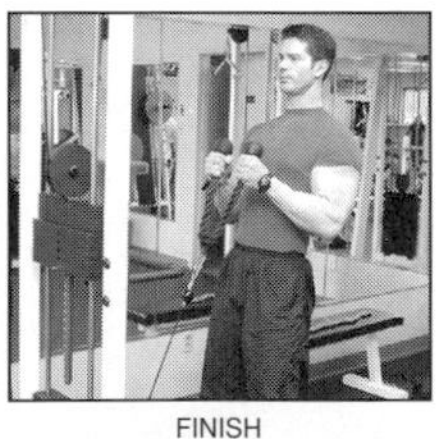

START FINISH

Cable Hammer Curl

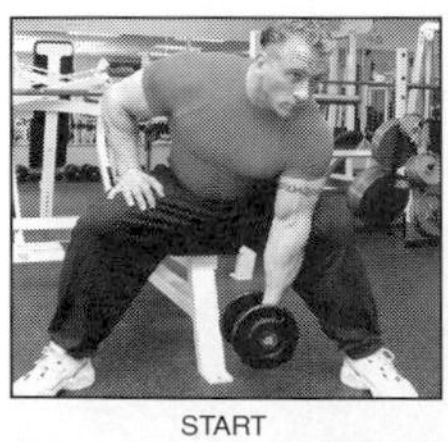
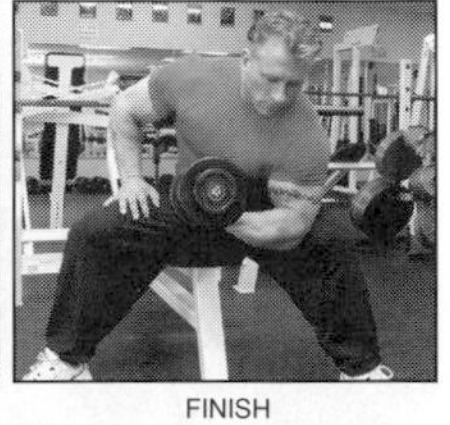

START FINISH

Concentration Curl

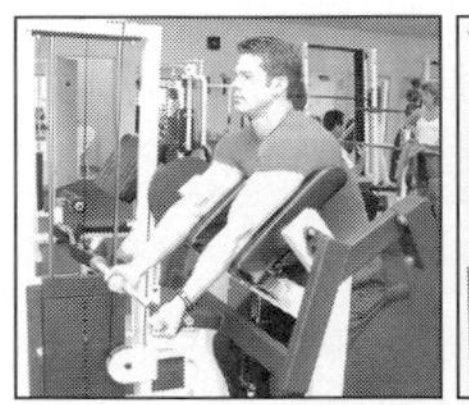
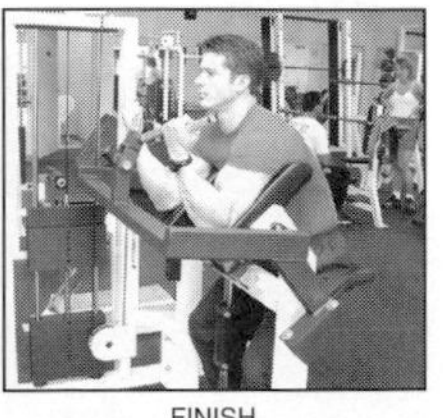

START FINISH

Cable Machine

PHASE FOUR - LEG EXERCISES

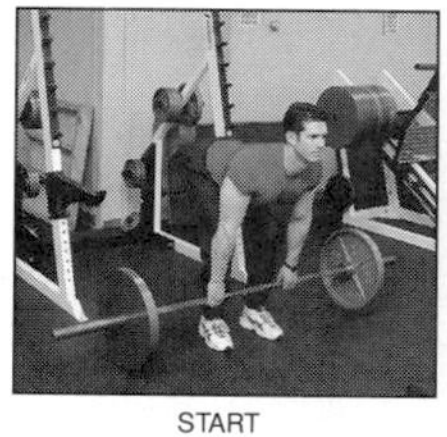

START FINISH

Barbell Deadlift

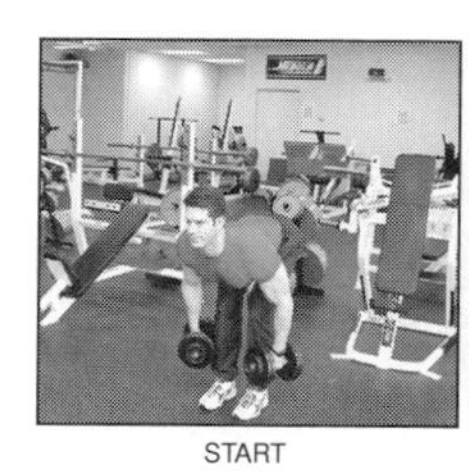
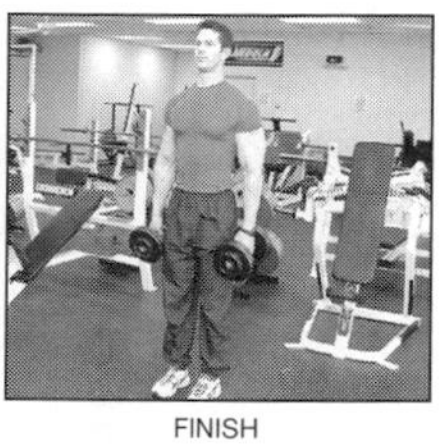

START FINISH

Dumbbell Deadlift

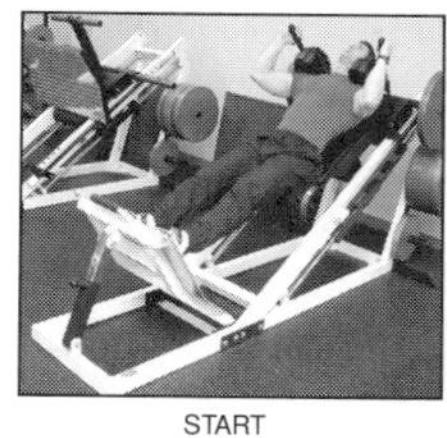
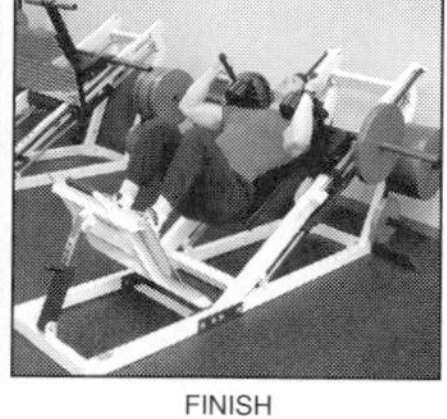

START FINISH

Hack Squats

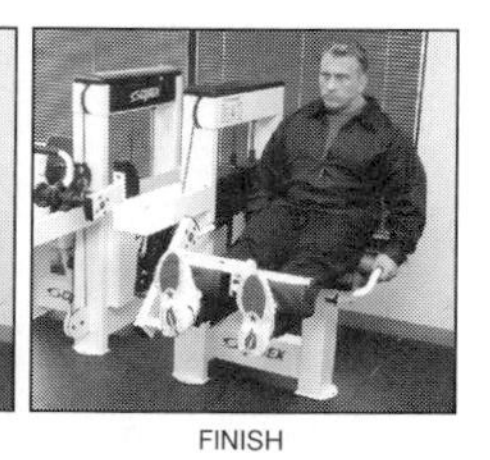

START FINISH

Leg Extension

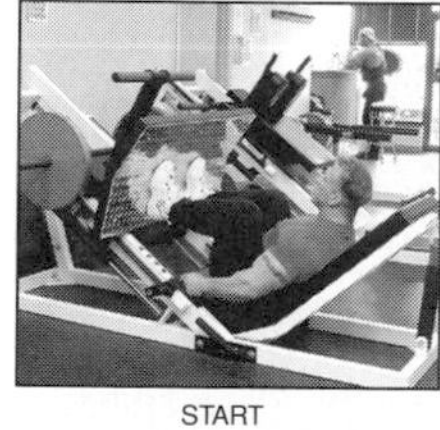
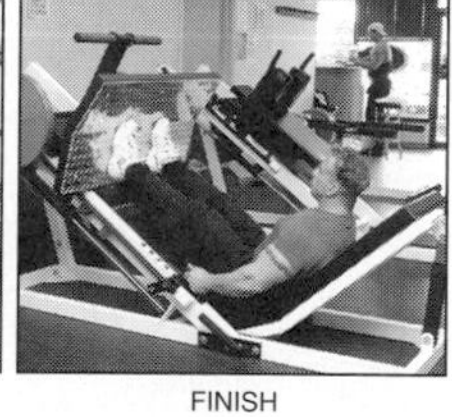

START FINISH

Leg Press

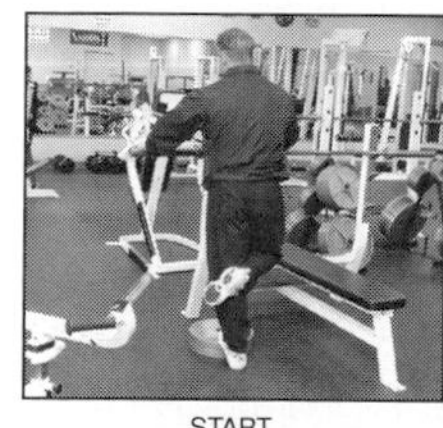
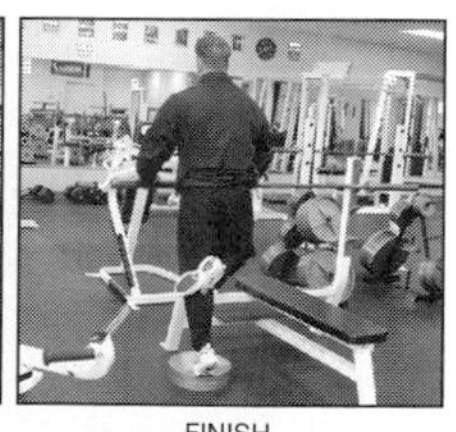

START FINISH

One Legged Calf Raise

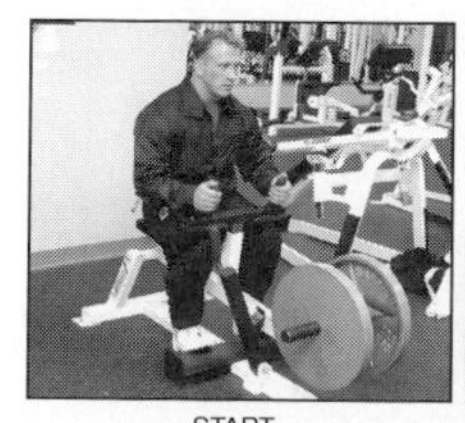
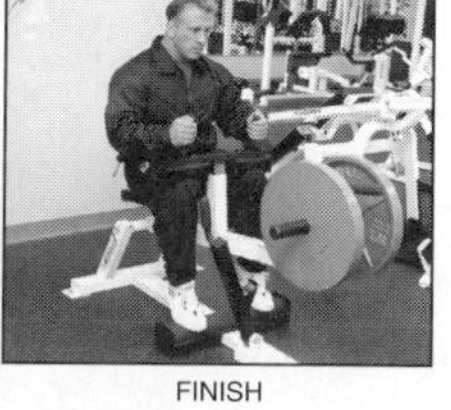

START FINISH

Seated Calf Raise

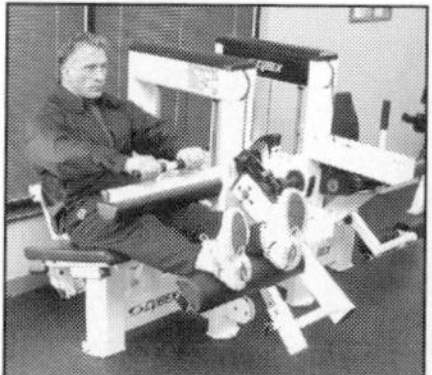
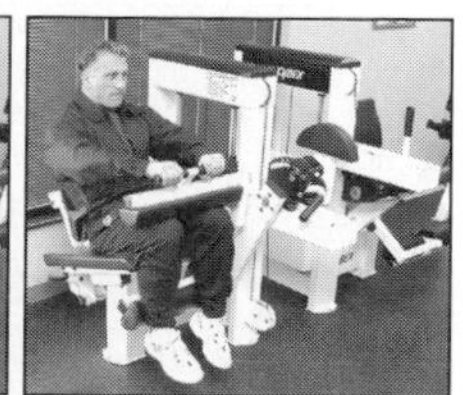

START FINISH

Seated Leg Curl

PHASE FOUR - LEG EXERCISES (continued)

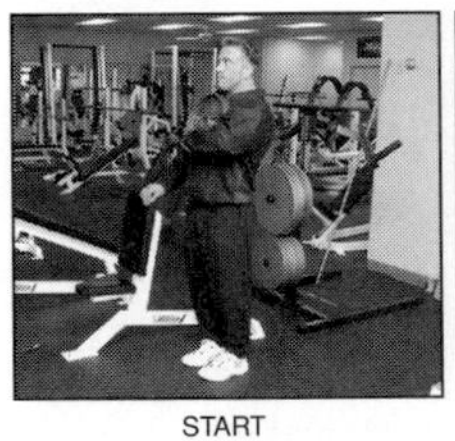
START

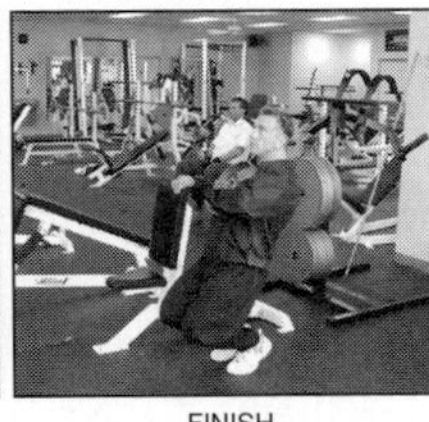
FINISH

Sissy Squat

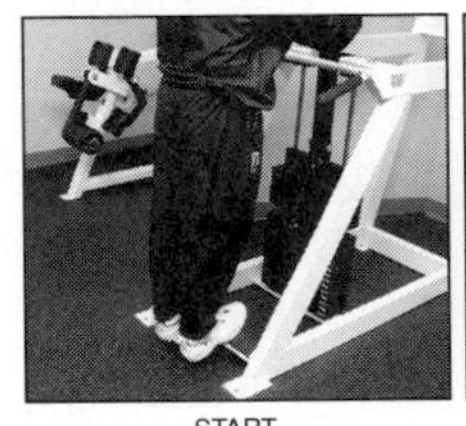
START

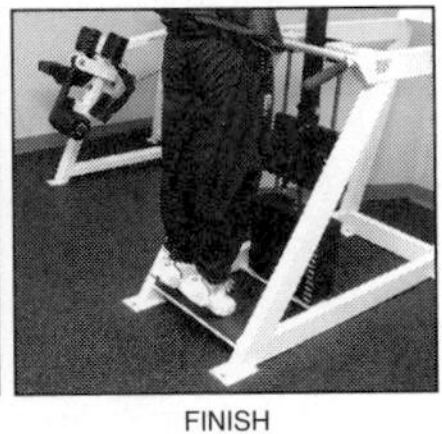
FINISH

Standing Calf Raise

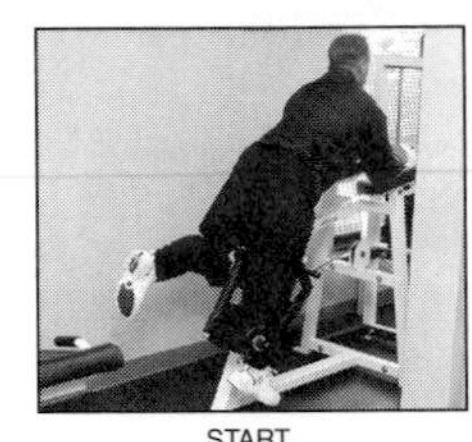
START

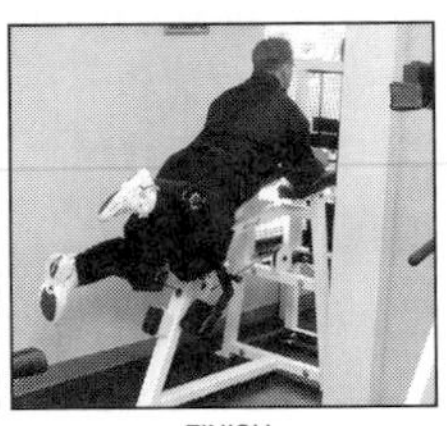
FINISH

Standing Leg Curl

APPENDIX A

A First-Ever From Biogenesis:

The Food Table

Ranking Foods By Fat And Calories

This exclusive food chart represents a comparison of fat grams and calories based on a proprietary formula developed by Biogenesis researchers in our test kitchen.

This is the first ranking of foods by fat grams and calories that use a common unit of measure for all the foods. All food values listed are for an 8 ounce serving. If you eat more or less than this amount, use the 8 ounce value and simply multiply or divide according to your individual serving size.

Use this table as a guide for choosing foods to eat. The first table is in ascending order by fat grams. The second table is an alphabetical listing of foods with Zone A, B, or C noted for each individual food.

Zone A foods should form the basis for most of your daily food intake. They are low in both fat and calories.

Zone B foods should be eaten in moderation. The caloric content of Zone B foods is still rather low, but in most cases the fat grams are noticeably higher than Zone A foods.

Zone C foods should be eaten very sparingly. For these foods, the fat grams and calories are at much higher levels when compared to Zone A or Zone B foods. We suggest using these foods only for those special occasions, such as a special dinner at your favorite restaurant on your birthday or anniversary, or family gatherings at home on holidays.

EAT ZONE A FOODS MOST OFTEN

Food	Per 8 ozs. Fat grams	Calories
Soft drink, 7-Up, diet	0.0	0
Soft drink, club soda	0.0	0
Spinach, cooked	0.0	0
Spinach, fresh	0.0	1
Celery, fresh	0.0	2
Soft drink, Fresca	0.0	4
Endive	0.0	4
Cabbage, cooked	0.0	4
Coffee, regular	0.0	4
Cabbage, fresh, grated	0.0	5
Alfalfa sprouts	0.0	5
Bamboo shoots, LaChoy	0.0	6
Gravy, brown mix	0.0	8
Chinese cabbage	0.0	10
Coffee, instant	0.0	11
Pear, Balsam, raw	0.0	15
Chicory	0.0	15
Chives	0.0	16
Vinegar, Whitehouse apple cider	0.0	16
Radish, fresh	0.0	17
Celery, diced, cooked	0.0	20
Mustard greens, fresh, boiled	0.0	22
Broccoli, fresh	0.0	24
Collards	0.0	24
Tomato, fresh	0.0	26
Green beans, snapped, canned	0.0	26
Dandelion greens, raw, chopped	0.0	26
Eggplant, fresh, boiled	0.0	26
Zucchini squash, fresh	0.0	28
Zucchini squash, cooked	0.0	28
Mushrooms, fresh	0.0	29
Iceberg lettuce, shredded	0.0	30
Pumpkin, raw, cubed	0.0	30
Cauliflower, cooked	0.0	30
Mung beans, sprouted seeds, raw	0.0	32
Cucumber	0.0	32
Pickles, zesty dill spears	0.0	32
Pokeberry shoots, fresh, cooked	0.0	32
Vinegar, Regina, red wine	0.0	32
Dandelion greens, cooked	0.0	34
Sharps non-alcoholic beer	0.0	34

EAT ZONE A FOODS MOST OFTEN

Food	Per 8 ozs. Fat grams	Calories
Cauliflower, fresh	0.0	38
Grapefruit, fresh	0.0	38
Kohlrabi, raw	0.0	38
Green peppers, fresh	0.0	38
Brussels sprouts, cooked	0.0	40
Brussels sprouts, fresh	0.0	40
Broccoli, cooked	0.0	44
Yellow beans	0.0	44
Strawberries, fresh	0.0	45
Dock, cooked	0.0	45
Carrots, fresh, shredded	0.0	48
Turnip greens, cooked	0.0	48
Onions, fresh green	0.0	48
Onions, fresh white	0.0	50
Rutabaga, raw	0.0	50
Cardoon	0.0	51
Watermelon	0.0	52
Cranberries, fresh	0.0	54
Mandarin orange-flavored drink, Koala	0.0	55
Sauerkraut, canned	0.0	56
Asparagus, fresh	0.0	60
Honeydew, fresh, cubed	0.0	60
Raspberries, red, fresh	0.0	60
Pimientos	0.0	60
Asparagus, cooked	0.0	60
Boysenberries, fresh	0.0	62
Celeriac root (wild celery)	0.0	62
Leeks, raw	0.0	64
Ale, brown, bottled	0.0	66
Lime juice	0.0	66
Bok Choy	0.0	68
Okra, fresh cooked	0.0	68
Peas, snow	0.0	68
Pumpkin, canned	0.0	70
Pomelo, raw	0.0	71
Currants, raw	0.0	72
Beer, Budweiser lite	0.0	73
Grapes, fresh	0.0	74
Figs, fresh	0.0	74
Blackberries, fresh	0.0	74
Shell beans	0.0	74
Pineapple, fresh	0.0	76
Fruit salad, water packed	0.0	80

EAT ZONE A FOODS MOST OFTEN

Food	Per 8 ozs. Fat grams	Calories
Casaba melon	0.0	80
Cherries, fresh sweet	0.0	80
Juice, body quencher, All Sport	0.0	80
Mixed vegetables, Libby's	0.0	80
Ginger beer	0.0	80
Papaya, fresh pulp	0.0	80
Fruit cocktail, mixed	0.0	80
Apple, fresh	0.0	81
Blueberries, fresh	0.0	82
Tonic water	0.0	85
Loganberries	0.0	90
Yogurt, Weight Watchers, all flavors	0.0	90
Collins mix, Schweppes	0.0	93
Coca Cola	0.0	93
Orange, fresh	0.0	96
Baking powder	0.0	96
Paprika seasoning	0.0	96
Salsa, Ortega medium green chili	0.0	96
Sugar Twin, white and brown	0.0	96
Beer, regular	0.0	96
Pears, fresh	0.0	97
Popped corncakes, cheddar	0.0	100
Eggbeaters egg substitute	0.0	100
Lemon sour mix, Schweppes	0.0	100
Parsnips, raw	0.0	100
Pineapple juice, Bluebird, 100% pure juice	0.0	100
Caramel corn cakes	0.0	100
Applesauce, unsweetened	0.0	104
Yogurt, blueberry, non-fat lite, Dannon	0.0	109
Yambean, boiled	0.0	110
Orange juice, Minute Maid	0.0	110
Mixed fruit, water packed	0.0	112
Orange drink, powder, prepared with water	0.0	115
Cider, 6.9% alcohol	0.0	116
Ice pop, lime, Hershey's	0.0	120
Soy sauce	0.0	120
Cream soda	0.0	120
Jello-O, regular	0.0	122
Ketchup, low salt, Heinz	0.0	128
Basil seasoning	0.0	144
Basil, French's	0.0	144
Croutons, Kellogg's	0.0	144

EAT ZONE A FOODS MOST OFTEN

Food	Per 8 ozs. Fat grams	Calories
Cranapple juice, Oceanspray	0.0	160
Butter beans	0.0	160
Figs, canned in light syrup	0.0	174
Kidney beans, canned	0.0	180
Cantaloupe, fresh	0.0	180
Peaches, Del Monte, heavy syrup	0.0	180
Champagne	0.0	180
Blackeyed peas, cooked	0.0	180
Baby lima beans	0.0	186
Broad beans	0.0	186
Mung beans, boiled	0.0	190
Bananas, fresh, whole	0.0	190
Garlic powder seasoning	0.0	192
Concord grape jelly, S&W	0.0	192
Orange marmalade, S&W	0.0	192
Strawberry jam, S&W	0.0	192
Cannellini beans	0.0	192
Applesauce, sweetened	0.0	194
Chocolate mocha, Ultra Slim Fast, skim milk	0.0	200
Yardlong beans	0.0	204
Corn, canned	0.0	206
Lemon ice, Ben & Jerry's	0.0	208
Kidney beans	0.0	218
Potato, plain baked	0.0	218
Lobster, northern, cooked	0.0	220
Mixed vegetables, canned, Hanover	0.0	220
Raspberry sorbet, Dole	0.0	220
Red beans, cooked	0.0	224
Cow peas, frozen, cooked	0.0	224
Black beans	0.0	228
Lentils	0.0	232
Baking soda	0.0	240
Rice Chex cereal, Ralston	0.0	240
Bread & butter pickles, Vlasic	0.0	240
Relish, sweet, Vlasic	0.0	240
Bay leaf seasoning	0.0	240
Bay leaf	0.0	240
Daiquiri (2)	0.0	248
Prunes, canned, heavy syrup	0.0	248
Beans, pink, boiled	0.0	248
Dressing, fat-free, whipped, Weight Watchers	0.0	258
Raspberries, red, frozen	0.0	258
Refried beans	0.0	260

EAT ZONE A FOODS MOST OFTEN

Food	Per 8 ozs. Fat grams	Calories
Ranch, free salad dressing, Kraft	0.0	260
Poi	0.0	268
Plums, whole, canned	0.0	270
Cassava root, raw	0.0	274
Sherry	0.0	280
Garlic powder	0.0	288
Allspice	0.0	288
Ketchup, Heinz	0.0	288
Ginger seasoning	0.0	288
Wine, dessert, dry 18.8% alcohol	0.0	299
Miracle Whip, fat-free	0.0	320
Pretzels, Shearer's	0.0	320
Waffles, Special K	0.0	320
Wine, sweet	0.0	356
Wine, dessert sweet, 18.8% alcohol	0.0	363
Cream of tartar	0.0	368
Pancake/waffle syrup, lite, Aunt Jemima	0.0	400
Cornmeal, white or yellow	0.0	400
Cracker meal	0.0	400
Syrup, Weight Watchers	0.0	400
Pinto beans, frozen, cooked	0.0	405
Currants, dried	0.0	408
Flour, arrowroot	0.0	464
Cinnamon, ground	0.0	480
Flour, bread	0.0	495
Lemon curd	0.0	528
Gin, rum, vodka, 80 proof	0.0	549
Applebutter, Smucker's	0.0	560
Marshmallows, Kraft	0.0	560
Gin, rum, vodka, 90 proof	0.0	624
Triple Sec	0.0	632
Molasses, blackstrap	0.0	640
Chutney, apple	0.0	656
Sloe gin	0.0	661
Peppermint Schnapps, liqueur	0.0	661
Brandy, fruit flavor	0.0	688
Gin, rum, vodka, 100 proof	0.0	698
Breading frying mix	0.0	720
Sugar, white, granulated	0.0	770
Honey	0.0	773
Anisette, liqueur	0.0	789
Onion ring mix	0.0	800
Quaker puffed wheat (8 cups)	0.0	800

EAT ZONE A FOODS MOST OFTEN

Food	Per 8 ozs. Fat grams	Calories
Sugar, brown, packed	0.0	821
Candy corn	0.0	824
Jelly, concord grape, Welch's	0.0	840
Jam, Smucker's, all flavors	0.0	864
Pancake and waffle syrup, Aunt Jemima	0.0	880
Drambuie liqueur	0.0	880
Pancake and waffle syrup, Golden Griddle	0.0	885
Dates, dried	0.0	912
Karo syrup, lite corn	0.0	928
Karo syrup	0.0	960
Molasses, Brer Rabbit, black and white	0.0	960
Creme de menthe liqueur	0.0	992
Tea, cinnamon stick, regular, Bigelow	Tr.	1
Tea, orange, spice, herbal, Bigelow	Tr.	1
Watercress, chopped	Tr.	2
Tea, amaretto, Celestial regular tea	Tr.	3
Tea, cinnamon, apple spice, Celestial	Tr.	3
Sesbania flowers	Tr.	5
Purslane, raw	Tr.	7
Cabbage, swamp, raw, chopped	Tr.	11
Purslane, cooked	Tr.	21
Sesbania flowers, cooked	Tr.	23
Turnip greens, raw, frozen	Tr.	34
Turnip greens, raw	Tr.	36
Melon balls, frozen	Tr.	55
Java plum	Tr.	82
Kellogg's Special K cereal	Tr.	83
Tangerine, fresh	Tr.	86
Kellogg's Corn Flakes cereal	Tr.	88
Clams, chopped, canned	Tr.	110
Passion fruit juice	Tr.	126
Jackfruit	Tr.	160
Sweet potato, canned in syrup	Tr.	183
Ultra Slim Fast, French vanilla, skim milk	Tr.	190
Ultra Slim Fast, French vanilla, prepared	Tr.	220
Tequila Sunrise	0.1	252
Pasta shell, dried, Mueller's	0.1	840
Tomato juice	0.2	41
Artichoke, plain	0.2	53
V-8 Juice	0.2	53
Apple juice, Mott's	0.2	117
Milk, skim	0.4	86
Orange juice, fresh squeezed	0.4	112

EAT ZONE A FOODS MOST OFTEN

Food	Per 8 ozs. Fat grams	Calories
Yogurt, non-fat	0.4	127
Angel food cake	0.4	166
Enchilada, chicken, frozen, Banquet	0.4	247
Chestnuts, roasted	0.4	560
Pitanga	0.6	57
Soup, clam chowder, Manhattan	0.6	66
Salsa, Chi Chi's mild	0.6	72
Mango, fruit, diced	0.6	109
Strawberry sorbet	0.6	142
Barley, cooked	0.6	193
Rice, white, cooked	0.6	264
Pierogi, onion	0.6	480
Apple fruit snack, Weight Watchers	0.6	800
Jellybeans	0.6	832
Log Cabin syrup, buttered	0.6	848
Cloves, seasoning	0.7	110
Gooseberries, raw	0.8	67
Elderberries, raw	0.8	105
Dates, chopped	0.8	489
Watercress, chopped	0.9	4
Swiss chard, fresh	0.9	6
Postum, instant, prepared	0.9	14
Cabbage, swamp, cooked	0.9	16
Chinese vegetables, LaChoy	0.9	20
Zucchini squash, raw sliced	0.9	28
Zucchini squash, Italian style	0.9	28
Swiss chard, cooked	0.9	36
Kale	0.9	40
Tomatillo, fresh	0.9	42
Tree fern, chopped, cooked	0.9	56
Mulberries	0.9	61
Chinese water chestnuts	0.9	70
Rose apple, fresh	0.9	73
Ground cherries, fresh	0.9	74
Bloody Mary mix, with Tabasco	0.9	75
Mixed vegetables, homemade	0.9	78
Burdock root, raw	0.9	85
Guava sauce	0.9	86
Sunkist funfruit	0.9	89
Plums, fresh sliced	0.9	91
Peas and carrots, homemade	0.9	96
Sage	0.9	96
Burdock root, cooked	0.9	110

EAT ZONE A FOODS MOST OFTEN

Food	Per 8 ozs. Fat grams	Calories
Taro, raw sliced	0.9	112
Feijoa, fresh	0.9	114
Rhubarb, frozen	0.9	120
Yam, cubed, cooked	0.9	158
Jujube, raw	0.9	184
Taro, cooked	0.9	188
Rosemary, dried	0.9	192
Macaroni, cooked	0.9	197
Ultra Slim chocolate pudding, prepared	0.9	200
Cranberry beans	0.9	216
Chocolate Instant Breakfast with skim milk	0.9	220
French beans, dried	0.9	228
Pepper	0.9	240
Ginkgo nuts, canned	0.9	256
Navy beans, boiled	0.9	258
Tamarind, fresh, cut up	0.9	287
Curry seasoning	0.9	288
Poultry seasoning	0.9	288
Pumpkin pie spice	0.9	288
Pickles, sweet gerkin	0.9	320
Sweet potato, fresh, mashed	0.9	344
Yams, candied, canned	0.9	360
Cumin seasoning	0.9	384
Flour, cake	0.9	395
Yeast, brewer's dried	0.9	400
Ginkgo nuts, raw	0.9	416
Coffeemate powder	0.9	480
Log Cabin syrup, lite	0.9	488
Molasses, Grandma's Green or Gold label	0.9	1120
Rhubarb	1.0	60
Shrimp creole dinner, Amour	1.0	185
Bran, Miller's processed	1.0	186
Salt seasoning	1.0	192
White beans	1.0	254
Prunes, dried	1.0	380
Zucchini squash, cooked	1.3	20
Kelp, raw	1.3	49
Chow mein, beef, LaChoy	1.3	93
Bread crumbs, soft	1.3	122
Salsa, chunky mild, Rosarita	1.3	133
Garlic salt	1.3	144
Cocoa, Swiss Miss prepared with milk	1.3	147
Borage, raw	2.0	18

	Food	Per 8 ozs. Fat grams	Calories
EAT MOST OFTEN	Borage, cooked	2.0	50
	Vegetable soup, Campbell's condensed	2.0	90
	Feijoa puree	2.0	119
	Quaker oatmeal, cooked	2.0	145
	Adzuki beans, boiled	2.0	149
	Beans, Great Northern, canned	2.0	180
	Pinto beans, Green Giant, canned	2.0	180
	Corn pudding, homemade	2.0	194
	Succotash, homemade	2.0	204
	Succotash, S&W country style	2.0	204
	Egg noodles, cooked	2.0	208
	Pollack, raw	2.0	208
	Vega burger, Loma Linda	2.0	220
	Yogurt, frozen, TCBY	2.0	220
	Cod, canned	2.0	237
	Corn dogs, Loma Linda	2.0	251
	Sherbet, lime	2.0	260
	Chinese noodles, dried	2.0	585
	Pink beans, raw	2.0	720
EAT IN MODERATION	Cottage cheese, 1% fat	2.2	162
	Chicken noodle soup, Campbell's	2.4	72
	Shrimp, steamed	2.4	224
	Jujube, dried	2.4	640
	Clam chowder, New England	2.5	87
	Chocolate milk, 1% fat	2.5	102
	Milk, 1%	2.5	158
	Stuffing, Brownberry	2.5	200
	Cod, frozen	2.5	293
	Coconut, angel flake	2.6	110
	Breadsticks, traditional, whole wheat	2.6	160
	Frogs' legs, raw	2.6	168
	Scallops	2.6	185
	Beef tenderloin, raw	2.6	187
	Crab, raw	2.6	189
	Sole, raw	2.6	205
	Beef flank steak, lean, raw	2.6	213
	Beef top round, raw	2.6	213
	Alaskan crab, canned	2.6	219
	Yogurt, low-fat, fruit	2.6	225
	Perch, cooked	2.6	264
	Seaweed, dried, Agar	2.6	693
	Ameranth, box mix	2.8	149
	Moth beans, cooked	3.0	70

EAT ZONE B FOODS IN MODERATION

Food	Per 8 ozs. Fat grams	Calories
Yogurt, all flavors, Cabot	3.0	110
Baked beans	3.0	120
Chinese fried rice, homemade	3.0	206
Sugar apple, fresh, cut up	3.0	236
Bluefish, raw	3.0	240
Baked beans, Campbell's	3.0	240
Pina colada	3.0	349
Popcorn, hot-air popped	3.0	369
Pizza, French bread and cheese, Healthy Choice	3.0	408
Cole slaw	3.2	82
Chicken noodles dinner, Banquet	3.2	136
Chocolate, Slender	3.2	176
Yogurt, frozen, all flavors, Bressler's	3.2	216
Yogurt, frozen, all flavors, Bressler's gourmet	3.2	232
Beef pepper steak, Healthy Choice	3.4	211
Roll, submarine	3.4	263
Sole, cooked	3.4	264
Flounder, cooked	3.4	266
Buttermilk	3.5	125
Peas, pigeon, fresh cooked	3.5	125
Flatfish, cooked	3.5	266
Beans, French, raw	4.0	52
Tomato soup, Campbell's condensed	4.0	140
Sirloin strip style dinner, Jaclyn's	4.0	172
Dynatrim, chocolate, prepared with 1% milk	4.0	220
Chick peas	4.0	268
Orange sherbet	4.0	270
Ritz crackers	4.0	476
Bread, white, regular (8 slices)	4.0	480
English muffins, sourdough	4.0	480
Yogurt, apple, Yoplait original	4.0	480
Lasagna	4.0	840
Macaroni	4.0	840
Spaghetti	4.0	840
Vermicelli	4.0	840
Beef stroganoff lite dinner, Armour	4.2	178
Enchilada, beef, frozen, Weight Watchers	4.4	167
Cottage cheese, 2% fat	4.4	204
Tofu, Mori-Nu extra firm	4.6	137
Chicken, Le Menu, Empress, lite	4.8	203
Evaporated milk, Carnation low-fat	4.8	216
Lotus seed	4.8	752
Crab, Dungeness canned	4.9	199

Food	Per 8 ozs. Fat grams	Calories
Chicken a la King dinner, Armour	4.9	200
Milk, Vitamite, Deihl	5.0	100
Chocolate milk, homemade, 2% milk	5.0	179
Chocolate milk, commercial, 2% fat	5.0	179
Milk, 2%	5.0	180
Nestle's Quik chocolate with 2% milk	5.0	210
Gizzards, chicken, simmered	5.0	222
Pike, northern, cooked	5.0	261
Pigs' feet	5.0	395
Beef, chuck roast, lean, raw	5.3	213
Beef, eye of the round, raw	5.3	213
Beef, ribeye, raw	5.3	240
Pierogi, cheese	5.3	583
Gravy, beef, canned	5.6	120
Tofu, Mori-Nu soft	6.0	122
Tofu, Mori-Nu firm	6.0	137
Strawberry ice cream, Bryers	6.0	220
Turkey gizzards, simmered	6.0	236
Pasta salad, Lite Italian, with dressing, Kraft	6.0	260
Evaporated milk, regular	6.0	338
Pheasant	6.4	235
Chocolate milkshake	6.4	282
Enchilada, cheese, frozen, Banquet	6.5	249
Lamb stew, takeout	6.7	165
Hot cocoa mix, Nestle's, 2% milk	6.7	280
Beef noodles and gravy, Banquet	6.9	206
Acerola juice	7.0	51
Mushrooms, sautéed with 1 Tbls. margarine	7.0	60
Carob	7.0	140
Lamb stew, homemade	7.0	165
Milkshake, vanilla	7.1	265
Chicken, light meat, skinless, roasted	7.2	357
Yogurt, plain, regular	7.4	138
Bran, Quaker Oat	7.6	330
Kidney, simmered	7.7	325
Asparagus soup with milk	7.9	161
Milk, imitation	8.0	150
Homemade chocolate milk	8.0	208
Chocolate milk, Land o' Lakes	8.0	210
Chicken dumpling dinner, Banquet	8.0	216
Cool Whip cream topping	8.0	224
Beef sirloin tip, raw	8.0	240
Yogurt, blueberry, Yoplait original	8.0	240

EAT ZONE B FOODS IN MODERATION

Food	Per 8 ozs. Fat grams	Calories
Oyster crackers	8.0	240
Quail breast, no skin	8.0	276
Chocolate Instant Breakfast with whole milk	8.0	280
Tapioca	8.0	290
Custard, flan, Spanish style with milk	8.0	296
Chocolate pudding, regular	8.0	300
Rice pudding	8.0	310
Breadsticks, Stella Dora	8.0	320
Eggnog, Carnation lite	8.0	320
Tuna, packed in water	8.0	360
Shoestring potatoes, Ore Ida	8.0	400
Egg Pro, regular	8.0	440
White bread, Schwebel's (6 slices)	8.0	560
Breadsticks, Italian soft	8.0	640
Fettuccine, prepared	8.0	693
Noodles, egg/spinach	8.0	836
Ravioli with beef	8.0	900
Milk, whole, 3.3% fat	8.1	14
Swedish meatballs with sauce, Dining Delight	8.8	249
Chocolate milk, Hershey's whole milk	9.0	210
Chocolate malted milk	9.0	229
Nestle's ready-to-drink Quik	9.0	230
Swordfish, raw	9.0	275
Beef, New York strip	9.1	304
Pasta salad with vegetables	9.1	320
Ham steak dinner, Armour	9.5	255
Goose liver	9.6	303
Yogurt, Ben & Jerry's frozen cherry	9.6	320
Spaghetti sauce, Ragu, meatless	10.0	180
Strawberry ice cream	10.0	232
Winged beans, cooked	10.0	252
Spaghetti sauce, Prego	10.0	260
Pudding, Jell-O instant butterscotch	10.0	336
Rigatoni, prepared	10.4	533
Saltine crackers (64)	10.6	132
Beef liver	10.6	365
Pork liver	10.6	376
French toast, Aunt Jemima	10.6	442
Nestle's Quik chocolate powder	10.6	960
Beans and Franks dinner, Banquet	11.2	280
Bluefin fish, fresh	11.2	325
Turkey giblets	11.2	389
Macaroni salad, take out	11.4	366

Food	Per 8 ozs. Fat grams	Calories
Turkey pastrami, thin sliced	11.6	276
Chocolate mocha pie, Weight Watchers	11.6	524
Chicken and dumplings, Swanson frozen	11.7	235
Glazed chicken dinner, Armour	11.9	238
Tofu, regular	12.0	176
Buttermilk biscuits	12.0	240
Tempeh	12.0	320
Yellowtail	12.0	330
Pudding, Swiss Miss chocolate prepared	12.0	60
Nutra shake, chocolate	12.0	400
Handy Pocket cheese sauce/ham, Weight Watchers	12.0	400
Wheat germ, plain, toasted	12.0	431
Egg noodles	12.0	880
Fettuccine	12.0	880
Egg noodles, Creamette	12.0	884
Mexican style dinner, Banquet	12.4	298
Trout	12.5	312
Carp, fresh	12.8	288
Giblets, capon	12.8	381
Beef heart, simmered	12.8	397
Tamales, beef, frozen, Banquet	13.0	305
French Fries	13.2	274
Flavor Tree fruit bears	13.0	891
Chicken gravy, canned	13.6	192
French toast, home recipe	14.0	310
Croissant, Pepperidge Farm	14.0	340
Pizza, cheese, Kid Cuisine	14.0	444
Vanilla ice cream, regular	14.4	268
Chocolate ice cream	14.4	310
Jack mackerel, canned, drained	14.4	354
Salmon	14.4	833
Enchilada frozen beef dinner, Patio	14.5	314
Baked custard, homemade	14.6	305
Beef stew, Chef Boyardee	14.9	251
Canadian bacon	15.8	356
Hershey's Orange Blossom ice cream bar	16.0	293
Tamales with sauce, Van Camps	16.0	293
Vanilla ice cream, Bryers	16.0	300
Chocolate ice cream, Bryers	16.0	320
Italian pasta salad, take-home	16.0	320
Turkey, ground, fried	16.0	320
Turkey, ground, fresh	16.0	320
Tofu, Spring Creek barbecue baked	16.0	352

EAT ZONE B FOODS IN MODERATION

EAT IN MODERATION

Food	Per 8 ozs. Fat grams	Calories
Nutri Balance frozen chocolate pudding	16.0	450
Rykrisp	16.0	540
Miso paste	16.0	570
Honey butter, Downey's original	16.0	800
Breadsticks, Oro Wheat cheese	16.0	880
Graham crackers (16 crackers)	16.0	960
Hot roll mix, Pillsbury	16.0	960
Shake and Bake, fish	16.0	1184
Shake and Bake, pork	16.0	1280
Chicken, dark meat, no skin, roasted	16.3	424
Oysters, eastern, canned	16.8	157
Phyllo dough	17.0	815
Chicken and noodles, home recipe	18.0	365
Beef chili beans, Chef Boyardee	18.1	352
Tuna salad, take-out	19.0	383
Leg o' lamb, lean, roasted	19.0	432
Waffles, buttermilk, frozen, Aunt Jemima	19.2	573
Natto	19.4	374
Evaporated milk, regular	20.0	338
Burrito, crisp fried, Van de Camp	20.0	487
Rolls, home recipe	20.0	800
Pound cake	20.1	351

EAT VERY RARELY

Food	Per 8 ozs. Fat grams	Calories
Herring, raw	20.2	357
Biscuits, mixed with milk	20.8	728
Zucchini squash, breaded, Ore Ida	21.0	400
Hummus, homemade	21.0	420
Corn muffins, Dromedary	21.3	640
Waffles, frozen, Multi-Grain, Weight Watchers	21.3	640
Salisbury steak with gravy, Banquet	21.7	297
Beef, extra lean ground	22.0	404
Franks, big meatless, Loma Linda	22.2	444
Hershey's Neo Wave ice cream bar	22.4	512
Tuna melt, Chefwich	22.4	576
Lamb curry, homemade	23.0	460
Brazil nuts	23.2	230
Vanilla ice cream, rich	23.6	350
Spaghetti sauce, Ragu thick and zesty	23.8	222
Vanilla wafers, Murray	24.0	64
Mayonnaise, home recipe	24.0	100
Olives, ripe	24.0	240
Franks, turkey links	24.0	360
Turkey pot pie, Swanson's	24.0	434
Croissant, home recipe	24.0	470
Olive loaf, Loma Linda	24.0	476

WATCH OUT — EAT ZONE C FOODS VERY RARELY

Food	Per 8 ozs. Fat grams	Calories
Cheese, Weight Watchers sharp cheddar	24.0	560
Mozzarella cheese substitute	24.0	560
Lemon Fi-Bar	24.0	720
Bacon bits, Betty Crocker	24.0	600
Macaroni and cheese, takeout	24.1	406
Ham, picnic	24.2	312
Meatless swiss steak with gravy, Loma Linda	24.6	431
Waffles, mix prepared with egg and milk	24.6	631
Eggs, raw, medium	24.9	369
Chicken potpie, Swanson's	25.1	434
Pigs' ears	25.9	396
Chocolate ice cream, Baskin Robbins	26.0	528
Cherry pie, Sara Lee homestyle	26.0	540
Sardines	26.2	457
Apple pie, Banquet	26.6	606
Tamales, Wolf brand	27.0	350
Blueberry pie, Banquet	27.0	655
Chicken ravioli, prepared	27.0	693
Muffins, blueberry, home recipe	27.0	720
Omelette, Chefwich cheese	27.2	608
Vanilla ice cream, Baskin Robbins	28.0	480
Beef brains, simmered	28.2	363
Goose, skinless	28.8	544
Hershey's Ice cream sandwich (3)	28.8	672
Ham, country cured	29.0	461
Waffles, Eggo frozen buttermilk	29.0	756
Waffles, Eggo frozen homestyle	29.0	756
Avocado, California, fresh	29.8	306
Cornbread, prepared from mix	30.0	987
Three Musketeers, chocolate bar	30.5	990
Pistachio nuts, dry roasted	30.8	368
Nutri Grain apple breakfast bar	30.8	923
Half and Half, Land o' Lakes	32.0	320
Avocado guacomole dip, Kraft	32.0	400
Nacho cheese dip, Kraft	32.0	440
French onion dip, Hormel	32.0	440
Homestyle pasta salad with dressing, Kraft	32.0	480
Vegetable with chicken potpie, Morton's	32.0	480
Bacon bits, Hormel	32.0	480
Chicken cacciatore, takeout	32.0	525
Ground round	32.0	573
Sweetbreads, veal, braised	32.0	581
Bran muffins, homemade	32.0	667

WATCH OUT — EAT ZONE C FOODS VERY RARELY

Food	Per 8 ozs. Fat grams	Calories
Bacon bits, Oscar Mayer	32.0	672
Corn muffins	32.0	773
Scone, plain	32.0	827
Hot fudge topping, Kraft	32.0	1,120
Cheese curls, Weight Watchers	32.0	1,120
Shake and Bake, chicken	32.0	1,200
Paté, chicken liver, canned	32.0	1,904
Scrambled eggs, Kid Cuisine	33.1	527
Popcorn with oil and salt (17 cups)	34.0	697
Veal parmigiana	34.2	531
Pork chop, lean with fat	34.3	619
Pepperoni pizza, Celeste	34.3	640
Lamb sweetbreads, braised	34.6	534
Pizza, Celeste supreme	34.6	613
Hershey's choc. eclair crunch ice cream bar (2 1/2)	34.6	640
Polish kielbasa, Mr. Turkey	35.0	472
Nibbles, cherry and chocolate	35.0	1,028
Beef potpie, Morton's	35.4	494
Ham croquettes, home recipe	36.0	560
Fondu, takeout	36.0	606
Lobster Newburg	37.0	464
Italian sausage roll, frozen, Ovenstuffs	37.0	857
Quail breast, with skin	37.1	442
Beef chuck arm roast, braised	37.8	635
French vanilla ice cream, Baskin Robbins	38.0	580
Apple pie, Sara Lee homestyle	38.0	653
Meatless patties, frozen, Morningstar	38.8	549
Hot dog, turkey links	39.0	495
Sweetbreads, beef, braised	40.0	613
Cheese, Ched-R-Low, Alpine Lace	40.0	640
Combos, cheddar	40.0	1,066
Herring, pickled	40.8	595
Bacon, cooked, crumbled	42.0	408
Danish pastry, apple, Sara Lee	42.0	800
Corned beef brisket, cooked	42.6	568
Tongue, pork	42.7	613
Chili, plain, Gebhardt	43.0	530
Sour cream non-dairy substitute	45.0	479
Doughnuts, Hostess Old Fashioned (5)	45.0	850
Tongue, lamb	45.3	624
Frogs' legs, floured, fried	45.3	667
Cheese Whiz	45.6	640
Akee, fresh	46.0	510

WATCH OUT — EAT ZONE C FOODS VERY RARELY

Food	Per 8 ozs. Fat grams	Calories
Ham salad, homemade	46.0	574
Lamb loin, lean, broiled	46.0	672
Carnation Chocolate Crunch breakfast bar	46.0	869
Mustard, French's prepared	48.0	288
Sour cream	48.0	496
Cremora, original	48.0	576
Feta cheese, Sargento	48.0	600
Tongue, beef	48.0	642
Beef, T-bone, lean 1/4" charbroiled	48.0	675
Quiche, mushroom, takeout	48.0	683
Cheese Twin, Delicia	48.0	720
Chocolate, Baker's semi-sweet chips	48.0	824
Mustard, Gray Poupon	48.0	864
Falafel	48.0	920
Doughnuts, powdered sugar, Drake's	48.0	960
Shake & Bake, country mild recipe	48.0	1,040
Doo Dads	48.0	1,120
Tortilla chips, Doritos	48.0	1,120
M & Ms	48.0	1,144
Pork chop, center loin, broiled	49.0	709
Goose, with skin, roasted	49.6	696
Sweet and sour pork	50.0	940
Mousse, Sara Lee	50.3	770
Beef porterhouse, fat trimmed, broiled	50.6	693
Biscuits, homemade	51.2	1,016
Tuna, packed in oil, Starkist	52.0	600
Doughnuts, glazed	52.0	940
Chicken and noodle dinner, Armour	53.0	167
Quiche, cheese, takeout	53.0	755
Doughnuts, cake type	53.0	933
Caramel bar, Little Debbie	55.0	1,162
Egg salad, takeout	56.0	614
Egg salad, homemade	57.0	615
Chef's salad, with ham and turkey	58.4	1,040
Andes creme de menthe thins	58.5	945
Bratwurst, pork, cooked	59.0	683
Chocolate chip cookies	59.0	987
Beef, ground, regular	60.0	702
Carnation peanut butter/chocolate chip breakfast bar	63.3	1,151
Pork sausage, country style, cooked	64.0	384
Sausage, Oscar Mayer	64.0	664
Bologna, beef, Oscar Mayer	64.0	720
Miracle Whip, lite	64.0	720

WATCH OUT — EAT ZONE C FOODS VERY RARELY

Food	Per 8 ozs.	
	Fat grams	Calories
Paté, liver	64.0	720
Cheese, Romano	64.0	880
Tostada, Lance	64.0	1,200
Chitterlings pork skins, simmered	65.0	688
Pastrami, beef, thin sliced	66.0	792
Peanut butter cookies	66.0	1,153
Quiche Lorraine, takeout	67.0	939
Franks, jumbo cheese, Eckrich	68.0	720
Pie crust, Pillsbury (2 cups)	68.8	1,082
Pork spareribs, braised	69.3	901
Hershey's Kisses (48 pieces)	69.6	1,224
Peanuts in oil, Planters	70.0	900
Walnuts, black, chopped, Planters	71.0	759
Nestle's semi-sweet chocolate candy	71.2	1,192
Cheese, baby Swiss, Cracker Barrel	72.0	880
Colby cheese, Golden Image cheese substitute	72.0	880
Cheese, blue, Kraft	72.0	880
Cheese, mild cheddar	72.0	912
Chocolate, semi-sweet, baking	72.0	1,088
Hershey's chocolate bar	72.3	1,239
Walnuts, English halves, Planters	74.0	770
Sesame seeds, dried	75.0	825
Whipped cream	80.0	720
Whipping cream, Land o' Lakes	80.0	720
Cream cheese, Philadelphia	80.0	800
Hot dog, beef links	80.0	880
Mayonnaise type salad dressing	80.0	912
Pork skins, Lance	80.0	1,120
Potato chips, Lay's	80.0	1,200
Frito's	80.0	1,280
Cheeto's puff balls	80.0	1,280
Sausage roll, takeout	82.4	1,082
Sausage, pork, Armour	88.0	880
Dressing, Kraft French regular	91.2	944
Touch of Butter, tub	96.0	800
Paté, goose liver, canned	96.0	1,048
Cashew nuts, dry-roasted	104.0	1,304
Miracle Whip, regular	112.0	1,120
Peanuts, dry-roasted in the shell	112.0	1,280
Spanish peanuts, dry-roasted	112.0	1,280
Cashew nuts, oil-roasted	112.0	1,360
Peanut butter, Skippy super chunky	119.0	1,330
Almonds	119.2	1,326

Food	Per 8 ozs. Fat grams	Calories
EAT VERY RARELY		
Chocolate, Baker's unsweetened	120.0	1,136
Blue cheese dressing, Kraft	121.6	1,216
Nuts, mixed, Eagle	128.0	1,440
Pinyon nuts, dried	136.0	1,288
Filbert nuts, dried	142.4	1,432
Filbert nuts, dry-roasted	150.4	1,504
Margarine spread, Parkay (16 Tbls.)	155.2	1,408
Pecans, Planters	160.0	1,520
Macadamia nuts	168.0	1,680
Blue Bonnet better butter blend, regular	176.0	1,440
Butter, stick	184.0	1,632
Chicken fat	205.0	1,846
Lard (16 Tbls.)	205.0	1,849
Olive oil (16 Tbls.)	216.0	1,909
Peanut oil (16 Tbls.)	216.0	1,909
Canola oil	218.0	1,927
Crisco (16 Tbls.)	224.0	1,920
Corn oil (16 Tbls.)	224.0	1,920
Crisco oil (16 Tbls.)	224.0	1,920

BIOTECH ALPHABETICAL LISTING OF FOODS

Food	Fat grams	Per 8 ozs. Calories	Zone
Acerola juice	7.0	51	B
Adzuki beans, boiled	2.0	149	A
Akee, fresh	46.0	510	C
Alaskan crab, canned	2.6	219	B
Ale, brown, bottled	0.0	66	A
Alfalfa sprouts	0.0	5	A
Allspice	0.0	288	A
Almonds	119.2	1,326	C
Ameranth, box mix	2.8	149	B
Andes creme de menthe thins	58.5	945	C
Angelfood cake	0.4	166	A
Anisette, liqueur	0.0	789	A
Apple fruit snack, Weight Watchers	0.6	800	A
Apple juice, Mott's	0.2	117	A
Apple pie, Banquet	26.6	606	C
Apple pie, Sara Lee homestyle	38.0	653	C
Apple, fresh	0.0	81	A
Applebutter, Smucker's	0.0	560	A
Applesauce, sweetened	0.0	194	A
Applesauce, unsweetened	0.0	104	A
Artichoke, plain	0.2	53	A
Asparagus soup with milk	7.9	161	B
Asparagus, cooked	0.0	60	A
Asparagus, fresh	0.0	60	A
Avocado guacamole dip, Kraft	32.0	400	C
Avocado, California, fresh	29.8	306	C
Baby lima beans	0.0	186	A
Bacon bits, Betty Crocker	24.0	600	C
Bacon bits, Hormel	32.0	480	C
Bacon bits, Oscar Mayer	32.0	672	C
Bacon, cooked, crumbled	42.0	408	C
Baked beans	3.0	120	B
Baked beans, Campbell's	3.0	240	B
Baked custard, homemade	14.6	305	B
Baking powder	0.0	96	A
Baking soda	0.0	240	A
Bamboo shoots, LaChoy	0.0	6	A
Bananas, fresh, whole	0.0	190	A
Barley, cooked	0.6	193	A
Basil seasoning	0.0	144	A
Basil, French's	0.0	144	A
Bay leaf seasoning	0.0	240	A
Bay leaf	0.0	240	A

Food	Per 8 ozs. Fat grams	Calories	Zone
Beans and Franks dinner, Banquet	11.2	280	B
Beans, French, raw	4.0	52	B
Beans, Great Northern, canned	2.0	180	A
Beans, pink, boiled	0.0	248	A
Beef brains, simmered	28.2	363	C
Beef chili beans, Chef Boyardee	18.1	352	B
Beef chuck arm roast, braised	37.8	635	C
Beef flank steak, lean, raw	2.6	213	B
Beef heart, simmered	12.8	397	B
Beef liver	10.6	365	B
Beef noodles and gravy, Banquet	6.9	206	B
Beef pepper steak, Healthy Choice	3.4	211	B
Beef porterhouse, fat trimmed, broiled	50.6	693	C
Beef potpie, Morton's	35.4	494	C
Beef sirloin tip, raw	8.0	240	B
Beef stew, Chef Boyardee	14.9	251	B
Beef stroganoff lite dinner, Armour	4.2	178	B
Beef tenderloin, raw	2.6	187	B
Beef top round, raw	2.6	213	B
Beef, chuck roast, lean, raw	5.3	213	B
Beef, extra lean ground	22.0	404	C
Beef, eye of the round, raw	5.3	213	B
Beef, ground, regular	60.0	702	C
Beef, New York strip	9.1	304	B
Beef, ribeye, raw	5.3	240	B
Beef, T-bone, lean 1/4" charbroiled	48.0	675	C
Beer, Budweiser lite	0.0	73	A
Beer, regular	0.0	96	A
Biscuits, homemade	51.2	1,016	C
Biscuits, mixed with milk	20.8	728	C
Black beans	0.0	228	A
Blackberries, fresh	0.0	74	A
Blackeyed peas, cooked	0.0	180	A
Bloody Mary mix, with Tabasco	0.9	75	A
Blue Bonnet better butter blend, regular	176.0	1,440	C
Blue cheese dressing, Kraft	121.6	1,216	C
Blueberries, fresh	0.0	82	A
Blueberry pie, Banquet	27.0	655	C
Bluefin fish, fresh	11.2	325	B
Bluefish, raw	3.0	240	B
Bok Choy	0.0	68	A
Bologna, beef, Oscar Mayer	64.0	720	C
Borage, cooked	2.0	50	A

Food	Fat grams	Per 8 ozs. Calorics	Zone
Borage, raw	2.0	18	A
Boysenberries, fresh	0.0	62	A
Bran muffins, homemade	32.0	667	C
Bran, Miller's processed	1.0	186	A
Bran, Quaker Oat	7.6	330	B
Brandy, fruit flavor	0.0	688	A
Bratwurst, pork, cooked	59.0	683	C
Brazil nuts	23.2	230	C
Bread & butter pickles, Vlasic	0.0	240	A
Bread crumbs, soft	1.3	122	A
Bread, white, regular (8 slices)	4.0	480	B
Breading frying mix	0.0	720	A
Breadsticks, Italian soft	8.0	640	B
Breadsticks, Oro Wheat cheese	16.0	880	B
Breadsticks, Stella Dora	8.0	320	B
Breadsticks, traditional, whole wheat	2.6	160	B
Broad beans	0.0	186	A
Broccoli, cooked	0.0	44	A
Broccoli, fresh	0.0	24	A
Brussells sprouts, cooked	0.0	40	A
Brussells sprouts, fresh	0.0	40	A
Burdock root, cooked	0.9	110	A
Burdock root, raw	0.9	85	A
Burrito, crisp fried, Van de Camp	20.0	487	B
Butter beans	0.0	160	A
Butter, stick	184.0	1,632	C
Buttermilk biscuits	12.0	240	B
Buttermilk	3.5	125	B
Cabbage, cooked	0.0	4	A
Cabbage, fresh, grated	0.0	5	A
Cabbage, swamp, cooked	0.9	16	A
Cabbage, swamp, raw, chopped	Tr	11	A
Canadian bacon	15.8	356	B
Candy corn	0.0	824	A
Cannellini beans	0.0	192	A
Canola oil	218.0	1,927	C
Cantaloupe, fresh	0.0	180	A
Caramel bar, Little Debbie	55.0	1,162	C
Caramel corn cakes	0.0	100	A
Cardoon	0.0	51	A
Carnation Chocolate Crunch breakfast bar	46.0	869	C
Carnation peanut butter/chocolate chip, breakfast	63.3	1,151	C
Carob	7.0	140	B

Food	Fat grams	Per 8 ozs. Calories	Zone
Carp, fresh	12.8	288	B
Carrots, fresh, shredded	0.0	48	A
Casaba melon	0.0	80	A
Cashew nuts, dry-roasted	104.0	1,304	C
Cashew nuts, oil-roasted	112.0	1,360	C
Cassava root, raw	0.0	274	A
Cauliflower, cooked	0.0	30	A
Cauliflower, fresh	0.0	38	A
Celeriac root (wild celery)	0.0	62	A
Celery, diced, cooked	0.0	20	A
Celery, fresh	0.0	2	A
Champagne	0.0	180	A
Cheese curls, Weight Watchers	32.0	1,120	C
Cheese Twin, Delicia	48.0	720	C
Cheese Whiz	45.6	640	C
Cheese, baby Swiss, Cracker Barrel	72.0	880	C
Cheese, blue, Kraft	72.0	880	C
Cheese, Ched-R-Low, Alpine Lace	40.0	640	C
Cheese, mild cheddar	72.0	912	C
Cheese, Romano	64.0	880	C
Cheese, Weight Watchers sharp cheddar	24.0	560	C
Chef's salad, with ham and turkey	58.4	1,040	C
Cherries, fresh sweet	0.0	80	A
Cherry pie, Sara Lee homestyle	26.0	540	C
Chestnuts, roasted	0.4	560	A
Chick peas	4.0	268	B
Chicken a la King dinner, Armour	4.9	200	B
Chicken and dumplings, Swanson frozen	11.7	235	B
Chicken and noodle dinner, Armour	53.0	167	C
Chicken and noodles, home recipe	18.0	365	B
Chicken cacciatore, takeout	32.0	525	C
Chicken dumpling dinner, Banquet	8.0	216	B
Chicken fat	205.0	1,846	C
Chicken gravy, canned	13.6	192	B
Chicken noodle soup, Campbell's	2.4	72	B
Chicken noodles dinner, Banquet	3.2	136	B
Chicken potpie, Swanson's	25.1	434	C
Chicken ravioli, prepared	27.0	693	C
Chicken, dark meat, no skin, roasted	16.3	424	B
Chicken, Le Menu, Empress, lite	4.8	203	B
Chicken, light meat, skinless, roasted	7.2	357	B
Chicory	0.0	15	A
Chili, plain, Gebhardt	43.0	530	C

Food	Per 8 ozs.		
	Fat grams	Calories	Zone
Chinese cabbage	0.0	10	A
Chinese fried rice, homemade	3.0	206	B
Chinese noodles, dried	2.0	585	A
Chinese vegetables, LaChoy	0.9	20	A
Chinese water chestnuts	0.9	70	A
Chito's puff balls	80.0	1,280	C
Chitterlings pork skins, simmered	65.0	688	C
Chives	0.0	16	A
Chocolate chip cookies	59.0	987	C
Chocolate ice cream	14.4	310	B
Chocolate ice cream, Baskin Robbins	26.0	528	C
Chocolate ice cream, Bryers	16.0	320	B
Chocolate Instant Breakfast with skim milk	0.9	220	A
Chocolate Instant Breakfast with whole milk	8.0	280	B
Chocolate malted milk	9.0	229	B
Chocolate milk, 1% fat	2.5	102	B
Chocolate milk, commercial, 2% fat	5.0	179	B
Chocolate milk, Hershey's whole milk	9.0	210	B
Chocolate milk, homemade, 2% milk	5.0	179	B
Chocolate milk, Land o' Lakes	8.0	210	B
Chocolate milkshake	6.4	282	B
Chocolate mocha pie, Weight Watchers	11.6	524	B
Chocolate mocha, Ultra Slim Fast, skim milk	0.0	200	A
Chocolate pudding, regular	8.0	300	B
Chocolate, Baker's semi-sweet chips	48.0	824	C
Chocolate, Baker's unsweetened	120.0	1,136	C
Chocolate, semi-sweet, baking	72.0	1,088	C
Chocolate, Slender	3.2	176	B
Chow mein, beef, LaChoy	1.3	93	A
Chutney, apple	0.0	656	A
Cider, 6.9% alcohol	0.0	116	A
Cinnamon, ground	0.0	480	A
Clam chowder, New England	2.5	87	B
Clams, chopped, canned	Tr	110	A
Cloves, seasoning	0.7	110	A
Coca Cola	0.0	93	A
Cocoa, Swiss Miss prepared with milk	1.3	147	A
Coconut, angel flake	2.6	110	B
Cod, canned	2.0	237	A
Cod, frozen	2.5	293	B
Coffee, instant	0.0	11	A
Coffee, regular	0.0	4	A
Coffeemate powder	0.9	480	A

Food	Fat grams	Per 8 ozs. Calories	Zone
Colby cheese, Golden Image cheese substitute	72.0	880	C
Cole slaw	3.2	82	B
Collards	0.0	24	A
Collins mix, Schweppes	0.0	93	A
Combos, cheddar	40.0	1,066	C
Concord grape jelly, S&W	0.0	192	A
Cool Whip cream topping	8.0	224	B
Corn dogs, Loma Linda	2.0	251	A
Corn muffins	32.0	773	C
Corn muffins, Dromedary	21.3	640	C
Corn oil (16 Tbls.)	224.0	1,920	C
Corn pudding, homemade	2.0	194	A
Corn, canned	0.0	206	A
Cornbread, prepared from mix	30.0	987	C
Corned beef brisket, cooked	42.6	568	C
Cornmeal, white or yellow	0.0	400	A
Cottage cheese, 1% fat	2.2	162	B
Cottage cheese, 2% fat	4.4	204	B
Cow peas, frozen, cooked	0.0	224	A
Crab, Dungeness canned	4.9	199	B
Crab, raw	2.6	189	B
Cracker meal	0.0	400	A
Cranapple juice, Oceanspray	0.0	160	A
Cranberries, fresh	0.0	54	A
Cranberry beans	0.9	216	A
Cream cheese, Philadelphia	80.0	800	C
Cream of tartar	0.0	368	A
Cream soda	0.0	120	A
Creme de menthe liqueur	0.0	992	A
Cremora, original	48.0	576	C
Crisco (16 Tbls.)	224.0	1,920	C
Croissant, home recipe	24.0	470	C
Croissant, Pepperidge Farm	14.0	340	B
Croutons, Kellogg's	0.0	144	A
Cucumber	0.0	32	A
Cumin seasoning	0.9	384	A
Currants, dried	0.0	408	A
Currants, raw	0.0	72	A
Curry seasoning	0.9	288	A
Custard, flan, Spanish style with milk	8.0	296	B
Daiquiri (2)	0.0	248	A
Dandelion greens, cooked	0.0	34	A
Dandelion greens, raw, chopped	0.0	26	A

Food	Fat grams	Per 8 ozs. Calories	Zone
Danish pastry, apple, Sara Lee	42.0	800	C
Dates, chopped	0.8	489	A
Dates, dried	0.0	912	A
Dock, cooked	0.0	45	A
Doo Dads	48.0	1,120	C
Doughnuts, cake type	53.0	933	C
Doughnuts, glazed	52.0	940	C
Doughnuts, Hostess Old Fashioned (5)	45.0	850	C
Doughnuts, powdered sugar, Drake's	48.0	960	C
Drambuie liqueur	0.0	880	A
Dressing, fat-free, whipped, Weight Watchers	0.0	258	A
Dressing, Kraft French regular	91.2	944	C
Dynatrim, chocolate, prepared with 1% milk	4.0	220	B
Egg noodles	12.0	880	B
Egg noodles, cooked	2.0	208	A
Egg noodles, Creamette	12.0	884	B
Egg Pro, regular	8.0	440	B
Egg salad, homemade	57.0	615	C
Egg salad, takeout	56.0	614	C
Eggbeaters egg substitute	0.0	100	A
Eggnog, Carnation lite	8.0	320	B
Eggplant, fresh, boiled	0.0	26	A
Eggs, raw, medium	24.9	369	C
Elderberries, raw	0.8	105	A
Enchilada frozen beef dinner, Patio	14.5	314	B
Enchilada, beef, frozen, Weight Watchers	4.4	167	B
Enchilada, cheese, frozen, Banquet	6.5	249	B
Enchilada, chicken, frozen, Banquet	0.4	247	A
Endive	0.0	4	A
English muffins, sourdough	4.0	480	B
Evaporated milk, Carnation low-fat	4.8	216	B
Evaporated milk, regular	20.0	338	B
Evaporated milk, regular	6.0	338	B
Falafel	48.0	920	C
Feijoa puree	2.0	119	A
Feijoa, fresh	0.9	114	A
Feta cheese, Sargento	48.0	600	C
Fettuccine	12.0	880	B
Fettuccine, prepared	8.0	693	B
Figs, canned in light syrup	0.0	174	A
Figs, fresh	0.0	74	A
Filbert nuts, dried	142.4	1,432	C
Filbert nuts, dry-roasted	150.4	1,504	C

Food	Fat grams	Per 8 ozs. Calories	Zone
Flatfish, cooked	3.5	266	B
Flavor Tree fruit bears	13.0	891	B
Flounder, cooked	3.4	266	B
Flour, arrowroot	0.0	464	A
Flour, bread	0.0	495	A
Flour, cake	0.9	395	A
Fondu, takeout	36.0	606	C
Franks, big meatless, Loma Linda	22.2	444	C
Franks, jumbo cheese, Eckrich	68.0	720	C
Franks, turkey links	24.0	360	C
French beans, dried	0.9	228	A
French Fries	13.2	274	B
French onion dip, Hormel	32.0	440	C
French toast, Aunt Jemima	10.6	442	B
French toast, home recipe	14.0	310	B
French vanilla ice cream, Baskin Robbins	38.0	580	C
Frito's	80.0	1,280	C
Frogs' legs, floured, fried	45.3	667	C
Frogs' legs, raw	2.6	168	B
Fruit cocktail, mixed	0.0	80	A
Fruit salad, water packed	0.0	80	A
Garlic powder seasoning	0.0	192	A
Garlic powder	0.0	288	A
Garlic salt	1.3	144	A
Giblets, capon	12.8	381	B
Gin, rum, vodka, 100 proof	0.0	698	A
Gin, rum, vodka, 80 proof	0.0	549	A
Gin, rum, vodka, 90 proof	0.0	624	A
Ginger beer	0.0	80	A
Ginger seasoning	0.0	288	A
Ginkgo nuts, canned	0.9	256	A
Ginkgo nuts, raw	0.9	416	A
Gizzards, chicken, simmered	5.0	222	B
Glazed chicken dinner, Armour	11.9	238	B
Goose liver	9.6	303	B
Goose, skinless	28.8	544	C
Goose, with skin, roasted	49.6	696	C
Gooseberries, raw	0.8	67	A
Graham crackers (16 crackers)	16.0	960	B
Grapefruit, fresh	0.0	38	A
Grapes, fresh	0.0	74	A
Gravy, beef, canned	5.6	120	B
Gravy, brown mix	0.0	8	A

Food	Per 8 ozs. Fat grams	Calories	Zone
Green beans, snapped, canned	0.0	26	A
Green peppers, fresh	0.0	38	A
Ground cherries, fresh	0.9	74	A
Ground round	32.0	573	C
Guava sauce	0.9	86	A
Half and Half, Land o' Lakes	32.0	320	C
Ham croquettes, home recipe	36.0	560	C
Ham salad, homemade	46.0	574	C
Ham steak dinner, Armour	9.5	255	B
Ham, country cured	29.0	461	C
Ham, picnic	24.2	312	C
Handy Pocket cheese sauce/ham, Weight Watchers	12.0	400	B
Herring, pickled	40.8	595	C
Herring, raw	20.2	357	C
Hershey's choc. eclair crunch ice cream bar (2 1/2)	34.6	640	C
Hershey's chocolate bar	72.3	1,239	C
Hershey's Ice cream sandwich (3)	28.8	672	C
Hershey's Kisses (48 pieces)	69.6	1,224	C
Hershey's Neo Wave ice cream bar	22.4	512	C
Hershey's Orange Blossom ice cream bar	16.0	293	B
Homemade chocolate milk	8.0	208	B
Homestyle pasta salad with dressing, Kraft	32.0	480	C
Honey butter, Downey's original	16.0	800	B
Honey	0.0	773	A
Honeydew, fresh, cubed	0.0	60	A
Hot cocoa mix, Nestle's, 2% milk	6.7	280	B
Hot dog, beef links	80.0	880	C
Hot dog, turkey links	39.0	495	C
Hot fudge topping, Kraft	32.0	1,120	C
Hot roll mix, Pillsbury	16.0	960	B
Hummus, homemade	21.0	420	C
Ice pop, lime, Hershey's	0.0	120	A
Iceberg lettuce, shredded	0.0	30	A
Italian pasta salad, takehome	16.0	320	B
Italian sausage roll, frozen, Ovenstuffs	37.0	857	C
Jack mackerel, canned, drained	14.4	354	B
Jackfruit	Tr	160	A
Jam, Smucker's, all flavors	0.0	864	A
Java plum	Tr	82	A
Jell-O, regular	0.0	122	A
Jellybeans	0.6	832	A
Jelly, concord grape, Welch's	0.0	840	A
Juice, body quencher, All Sport	0.0	80	A

Food	Fat grams	Per 8 ozs. Calories	Zone
Jujube, dried	2.4	640	B
Jujube, raw	0.9	184	A
Kale	0.9	40	A
Karo syrup	0.0	960	A
Karo syrup, lite corn	0.0	928	A
Kellogg's Corn Flakes cereal	Tr	88	A
Kellogg's Special K cereal	Tr	83	A
Kelp, raw	1.3	49	A
Ketchup, Heinz	0.0	288	A
Ketchup, low salt, Heinz	0.0	128	A
Kidney beans	0.0	218	A
Kidney beans, canned	0.0	180	A
Kidney, simmered	7.7	325	B
Kohlrabi, raw	0.0	38	A
Lamb curry, homemade	23.0	460	C
Lamb loin, lean, broiled	46.0	672	C
Lamb stew, homemade	7.0	165	B
Lamb stew, takeout	6.7	165	B
Lamb sweetbreads, braised	34.6	534	C
Lard (16 Tbls.)	205.0	1,849	C
Lasagna	4.0	840	B
Leeks, raw	0.0	64	A
Leg o' lamb, lean, roasted	19.0	432	B
Lemon curd	0.0	528	A
Lemon Fi-Bar	24.0	720	C
Lemon ice, Ben & Jerry's	0.0	208	A
Lemon sour mix, Schweppes	0.0	100	A
Lentils	0.0	232	A
Lime juice	0.0	66	A
Lobster Newburg	37.0	464	C
Lobster, northern, cooked	0.0	220	A
Log Cabin syrup, buttered	0.6	848	A
Log Cabin syrup, lite	0.9	488	A
Loganberries	0.0	90	A
Lotus seed	4.8	752	B
M & Ms	48.0	1,144	C
Macadamia nuts	168.0	1,680	C
Macaroni and cheese, take out	24.1	406	C
Macaroni salad, take out	11.4	366	B
Macaroni	4.0	840	B
Macaroni, cooked	0.9	197	A
Mandarin orange-flavored drink, Koala	0.0	55	A
Mango, fruit, diced	0.6	109	A

Food	Fat grams	Per 8 ozs. Calories	Zone
Margarine spread, Parkay (16 Tbls.)	155.2	1,408	C
Marshmallows, Kraft	0.0	560	A
Mayonnaise type salad dressing	80.0	912	C
Mayonnaise, home recipe	24.0	100	C
Meatless patties, frozen, Morningstar	38.8	549	C
Meatless swiss steak with gravy, Loma Linda	24.6	431	C
Melon balls, frozen	Tr	55	A
Mexican style dinner, Banquet	12.4	298	B
Milk, 1%	2.5	158	B
Milk, 2%	5.0	180	B
Milk, imitation	8.0	150	B
Milk, skim	0.4	86	A
Milk, Vitamite, Deihl	5.0	100	B
Milk, whole, 3.3% fat	8.1	14	B
Milkshake, vanilla	7.1	265	B
Miracle Whip, fat-free	0.0	320	A
Miracle Whip, lite	64.0	720	C
Miracle Whip, regular	112.0	1,120	C
Miso paste	16.0	570	B
Mixed fruit, water packed	0.0	112	A
Mixed vegetables, canned, Hanover	0.0	220	A
Mixed vegetables, homemade	0.9	78	A
Mixed vegetables, Libby's	0.0	80	A
Molasses, blackstrap	0.0	640	A
Molasses, Brer Rabbit, black and white	0.0	960	A
Molasses, Grandma's Green or Gold label	0.9	1,120	A
Moth beans, cooked	3.0	70	B
Mousse, Sara Lee	50.3	770	C
Mozzarella cheese substitute	24.0	560	C
Muffins, blueberry, home recipe	27.0	720	C
Mulberries	0.9	61	A
Mungo beans, boiled	0.0	190	A
Mungo beans, sprouted seeds, raw	0.0	32	A
Mushrooms, fresh	0.0	29	A
Mushrooms, sauteed with 1 Tbsp. margarine	7.0	60	B
Mustard greens, fresh, boiled	0.0	22	A
Mustard, French's prepared	48.0	288	C
Mustard, Gray Poupon	48.0	864	C
Nacho cheese dip, Kraft	32.0	440	C
Natto	19.4	374	B
Navy beans, boiled	0.9	258	A
Nestle's Quik chocolate powder	10.6	960	B
Nestle's Quik chocolate with 2% milk	5.0	210	B

Food	Fat grams	Per 8 ozs. Calories	Zone
Nestle's ready-to-drink Quik	9.0	230	B
Nestle's semi-sweet chocolate candy	71.2	1,192	C
Nibbles, cherry and chocolate	35.0	1,028	C
Noodles, egg/spinach	8.0	836	B
Nutra shake, chocolate	12.0	400	B
Nutri Balance frozen chocolate pudding	16.0	450	B
Nutri Grain apple breakfast bar	30.8	923	C
Nuts, mixed, Eagle	128.0	1,440	C
Okra, fresh cooked	0.0	68	A
Olive loaf, Loma Linda	24.0	476	C
Olive oil (16 Tbsp.)	216.0	1,909	C
Olives, ripe	24.0	240	C
Omelette, Chefwich cheese	27.2	608	C
Onion ring mix	0.0	800	A
Onions, fresh green	0.0	48	A
Onions, fresh white	0.0	50	A
Orange drink, powder, prepared with water	0.0	115	A
Orange juice, fresh squeezed	0.4	112	A
Orange juice, Minute Maid	0.0	110	A
Orange marmalade, S&W	0.0	192	A
Orange sherbet	4.0	270	B
Orange, fresh	0.0	96	A
Oyster crackers	8.0	240	B
Oysters, eastern, canned	16.8	157	B
Pancake and waffle syrup, Aunt Jemima	0.0	880	A
Pancake and waffle syrup, Golden Griddle	0.0	885	A
Pancake/waffle syrup, lite, Aunt Jemima	0.0	400	A
Papaya, fresh pulp	0.0	80	A
Paprika seasoning	0.0	96	A
Parsnips, raw	0.0	100	A
Passion fruit juice	Tr	126	A
Pasta salad with vegetables	9.1	320	B
Pasta salad, Lite Italian, with dressing, Kraft	6.0	260	B
Pasta shell, dried, Mueller's	0.1	840	A
Pastromi, beef, thin sliced	66.0	792	C
Paté, goose liver, canned	96.0	1,048	C
Paté, liver	64.0	720	C
Paté, chicken liver, canned	32.0	1,904	C
Peaches, Del Monte, heavy syrup	0.0	180	A
Peanut butter cookies	66.0	1,153	C
Peanut butter, Skippy super chunky	119.0	1,330	C
Peanut oil (16 Tbls.)	216.0	1,909	C
Peanuts, dry-roasted in the shell	112.0	1,280	C

Food	Per 8 ozs. Fat grams	Calories	Zone
Peanuts in oil, Planters	70.0	900	C
Pear, Balsam, raw	0.0	15	A
Pears, fresh	0.0	97	A
Peas and carrots, homemade	0.9	96	A
Peas, pigeon, fresh cooked	3.5	125	B
Peas, snow	0.0	68	A
Pecans, Planters	160.0	1,520	C
Pepper	0.9	240	A
Peppermint Schnapps, liqueur	0.0	661	A
Pepperoni pizza, Celeste	34.3	640	C
Perch, cooked	2.6	264	B
Pheasant	6.4	235	B
Phyllo dough	17.0	815	B
Pickles, sweet gerkin	0.9	320	A
Pickles, zesty dill spears	0.0	32	A
Pie crust, Pillsbury (2 cups)	68.8	1,082	C
Pierogi, cheese	5.3	583	B
Pierogi, onion	0.6	480	A
Pigs' ears	25.9	396	C
Pigs' feet	5.0	395	B
Pike, northern, cooked	5.0	261	B
Pimientos	0.0	60	A
Pina colada	3.0	349	B
Pineapple juice, Bluebird, 100% pure juice	0.0	100	A
Pineapple, fresh	0.0	76	A
Pinto beans, frozen, cooked	0.0	405	A
Pinto beans, Green Giant, canned	2.0	180	A
Pinyon nuts, dried	136.0	1,288	C
Pistachio nuts, dry-roasted	30.8	368	C
Pitanga	0.6	57	A
Pizza, Celeste supreme	34.6	613	C
Pizza, cheese, Kid Cuisine	14.0	444	B
Pizza, French bread and cheese, Healthy Choice	3.0	408	B
Plums, fresh sliced	0.9	91	A
Plums, whole, canned	0.0	270	A
Poi	0.0	268	A
Pokeberry shoots, fresh, cooked	0.0	32	A
Polish kielbasa, Mr. Turkey	35.0	472	C
Pollack, raw	2.0	208	A
Pomelo, raw	0.0	71	A
Popcorn with oil and salt (17 cups)	34.0	697	C
Popcorn, hot-air popped	3.0	369	B
Popped corncakes, cheddar	0.0	100	A

Food	Fat grams	Per 8 ozs. Calories	Zone
Pork chop, center loin, broiled	49.0	709	C
Pork chop, lean with fat	34.3	619	C
Pork liver	10.6	376	B
Pork sausage, country style, cooked	64.0	384	C
Pork skins, Lance	80.0	1,120	C
Pork spareribs, braised	69.3	901	C
Postum, instant, prepared	0.9	14	A
Potato chips, Lay's	80.0	1,200	C
Potato, plain baked	0.0	218	A
Poultry seasoning	0.9	288	A
Pound cake	20.1	351	C
Pretzels, Shearer's	0.0	320	A
Prunes, canned, heavy syrup	0.0	248	A
Prunes, dried	1.0	380	A
Pudding, Jell-O instant butterscotch	10.0	336	B
Pudding, Swiss Miss chocolate prepared	12.0	60	B
Pumpkin pie spice	0.9	288	A
Pumpkin, canned	0.0	70	A
Pumpkin, raw, cubed	0.0	30	A
Purslane, cooked	Tr	21	A
Purslane, raw	Tr	7	A
Quail breast, no skin	8.0	276	B
Quail breast, with skin	37.1	442	C
Quaker oatmeal, cooked	2.0	145	A
Quaker puffed wheat (8 cups)	0.0	800	A
Quiche Lorraine, takeout	67.0	939	C
Quiche, cheese, takeout	53.0	755	C
Quiche, mushroom, takeout	48.0	683	C
Radish, fresh	0.0	17	A
Ranch, free salad dressing, Kraft	0.0	260	A
Raspberries, red, fresh	0.0	60	A
Raspberries, red, frozen	0.0	258	A
Raspberry sorbet, Dole	0.0	220	A
Ravioli with beef	8.0	900	B
Red beans, cooked	0.0	224	A
Refried beans	0.0	260	A
Relish, sweet, Vlasic	0.0	240	A
Rhubarb	1.0	60	A
Rhubarb, frozen	0.9	120	A
Rice Chex cereal, Ralston	0.0	240	A
Rice pudding	8.0	310	B
Rice, white, cooked	0.6	264	A
Rigatoni, prepared	10.4	533	B

Food	Per 8 ozs. Fat grams	Calories	Zone
Ritz crackers	4.0	476	B
Roll, submarine	3.4	263	B
Rose apple, fresh	0.9	73	A
Rosemary, dried	0.9	192	A
Rutabaga, raw	0.0	50	A
Rykrisp	16.0	540	B
Sage	0.9	96	A
Salisbury steak with gravy, Banquet	21.7	297	C
Salmon	14.4	833	B
Salsa, Chi Chi's mild	0.6	72	A
Salsa, chunky mild, Rosarita	1.3	133	A
Salsa, Ortega medium green chili	0.0	96	A
Salt seasoning	1.0	192	A
Saltine crackers (64)	10.6	132	B
Sardines	26.2	457	C
Sauerkraut, canned	0.0	56	A
Sausage roll, takeout	82.4	1,082	C
Sausage, Oscar Mayer	64.0	664	C
Sausage, pork, Armour	88.0	880	C
Scallops	2.6	185	B
Scone, plain	32.0	827	C
Scrambled eggs, Kid Cuisine	33.1	527	C
Seaweed, dried, Agar	2.6	693	B
Sesame seeds, dried	75.0	825	C
Sesbania flowers	Tr	5	A
Sesbania flowers, cooked	Tr	23	A
Shake & Bake, country mild recipe	48.0	1,040	C
Shake and Bake, chicken	32.0	1,200	C
Shake and Bake, fish	16.0	1,184	B
Shake and Bake, pork	16.0	1,280	B
Sharps non-alcoholic beer	0.0	34	A
Shellie beans	0.0	74	A
Sherbet, lime	2.0	260	A
Sherry	0.0	280	A
Shoestring potatoes, Ore Ida	8.0	400	B
Shrimp creole dinner, Amour	1.0	185	A
Shrimp, steamed	2.4	224	B
Sirloin strip style dinner, Jaclyn's	4.0	172	B
Sloe gin	0.0	661	A
Soft drink, 7-Up, diet	0.0	0	A
Soft drink, club soda	0.0	0	A
Soft drink, Fresca	0.0	4	A
Sole, cooked	3.4	264	B

Food	Fat grams	Per 8 ozs. Calories	Zone
Sole, raw	2.6	205	B
Soup, clam chowder, Manhattan	0.6	66	A
Sour cream non-dairy substitute	45.0	479	C
Sour cream	48.0	496	C
Soy sauce	0.0	120	A
Spaghetti sauce, Prego	10.0	260	B
Spaghetti sauce, Ragu thick and zesty	23.8	222	C
Spaghetti sauce, Ragu, meatless	10.0	180	B
Spaghetti	4.0	840	B
Spanish peanuts, dry-roasted	112.0	1,280	C
Spinach, cooked	0.0	0	A
Spinach, fresh	0.0	1	A
Strawberries, fresh	0.0	45	A
Strawberry ice cream	10.0	232	B
Strawberry ice cream, Bryers	6.0	220	B
Strawberry jam, S&W	0.0	192	A
Strawberry sorbet	0.6	142	A
Stuffing, Brownberry	2.5	200	B
Succotash, homemade	2.0	204	A
Succotash, S&W country style	2.0	204	A
Sugar apple, fresh, cut up	3.0	236	B
Sugar Twin, white and brown	0.0	96	A
Sugar, brown, packed	0.0	821	A
Sugar, white, granulated	0.0	770	A
Sunkist funfruit	0.9	89	A
Swedish meatballs with sauce, Dining Delight	8.8	249	B
Sweet and sour pork	50.0	940	C
Sweet potato, canned in syrup	Tr	183	A
Sweet potato, fresh, mashed	0.9	344	A
Sweetbreads, beef, braised	40.0	613	C
Sweetbreads, veal, braised	32.0	581	C
Swiss chard, cooked	0.9	36	A
Swiss chard, fresh	0.9	6	A
Swordfish, raw	9.0	275	B
Syrup, Weight Watchers	0.0	400	A
Tamales with sauce, Van Camps	16.0	293	B
Tamales, beef, frozen, Banquet	13.0	305	B
Tamales, Wolf brand	27.0	350	C
Tamarind, fresh, cut up	0.9	287	A
Tangerine, fresh	Tr	86	A
Tapioca	8.0	290	B
Taro, cooked	0.9	188	A
Taro, raw sliced	0.9	112	A

Food	Fat grams	Per 8 ozs. Calories	Zone
Tea, amaretto, Celestial regular tea	Tr	3	A
Tea, cinnamon stick, regular, Bigelow	Tr	1	A
Tea, cinnamon, apple spice, Celestial	Tr	3	A
Tea, orange, spice, herbal, Bigelow	Tr	1	A
Tempeh	12.0	320	B
Tequilla Sunrise	0.1	252	A
Three Musketeers, chocolate bar	30.5	990	C
Tofu, Mori-Nu extra firm	4.6	137	B
Tofu, Mori-Nu firm	6.0	137	B
Tofu, Mori-Nu soft	6.0	122	B
Tofu, regular	12.0	176	B
Tofu, Spring Creek barbecue baked	16.0	352	B
Tomatillo, fresh	0.9	42	A
Tomato juice	0.2	41	A
Tomato soup, Campbell's condensed	4.0	140	B
Tomato, fresh	0.0	26	A
Tongue, beef	48.0	642	C
Tongue, lamb	45.3	624	C
Tongue, pork	42.7	613	C
Tonic water	0.0	85	A
Tortilla chips, Doritos	48.0	1,120	C
Tostada, Lance	64.0	1,200	C
Touch of Butter, tub	96.0	800	C
Tree fern, chopped, cooked	0.9	56	A
Triple Sec	0.0	632	A
Trout	12.5	312	B
Tuna melt, Chefwich	22.4	576	C
Tuna salad, takeout	19.0	383	B
Tuna, packed in oil, Starkist	52.0	600	C
Tuna, packed in water	8.0	360	B
Turkey giblets	11.2	389	B
Turkey gizzards, simmered	6.0	236	B
Turkey pastrami, thin sliced	11.6	276	B
Turkey potpie, Swanson's	24.0	434	C
Turkey, ground, fresh	16.0	320	B
Turkey, ground, fried	16.0	320	B
Turnip greens, cooked	0.0	48	A
Turnip greens, raw	Tr	36	A
Turnip greens, raw, frozen	Tr	34	A
Ultra Slim chocolate pudding, prepared	0.9	200	A
Ultra Slim Fast, French vanilla, prepared	Tr	220	A
Ultra Slim Fast, French vanilla, skim milk	Tr	190	A
V-8 Juice	0.2	53	A

Food	Fat grams	Per 8 ozs. Calories	Zone
Vanilla ice cream, Baskin Robbins	28.0	480	C
Vanilla ice cream, Bryers	16.0	300	B
Vanilla ice cream, regular	14.4	268	B
Vanilla ice cream, rich	23.6	350	C
Vanilla wafers, Murray	24.0	64	C
Veal parmigiana	34.2	531	C
Vega burger, Loma Linda	2.0	220	A
Vegetable soup, Campbell's condensed	2.0	90	A
Vegetable with chicken potpie, Morton's	32.0	480	C
Vermicelli	4.0	840	B
Vinegar, Regina, red wine	0.0	32	A
Vinegar, Whitehouse apple cider	0.0	16	A
Waffles, buttermilk, frozen, Aunt Jemima	19.2	573	B
Waffles, Eggo frozen buttermilk	29.0	756	C
Waffles, Eggo frozen homestyle	29.0	756	C
Waffles, frozen, Multi-Grain, Weight Watchers	21.3	640	C
Waffles, mix prepared with egg and milk	24.6	631	C
Waffles, Special K	0.0	320	A
Walnuts, black, chopped, Planters	71.0	759	C
Walnuts, English halves, Planters	74.0	770	C
Watercress, chopped	Tr	2	A
Watercress, chopped	0.9	4	A
Watermelon	0.0	52	A
Wheat germ, plain, toasted	12.0	431	B
Whipped cream	80.0	720	C
Whipping cream, Land o' Lakes	80.0	720	C
White beans	1.0	254	A
White bread, Schwebel's (6 slices)	8.0	560	B
Wine, dessert sweet, 18.8% alcohol	0.0	363	A
Wine, dessert, dry 18.8% alcohol	0.0	299	A
Wine, sweet	0.0	356	A
Winged beans, cooked	10.0	252	B
Yam, cubed, cooked	0.9	158	A
Yambean, boiled	0.0	110	A
Yams, candied, canned	0.9	360	A
Yardlong beans	0.0	204	A
Yeast, brewer's dried	0.9	400	A
Yellow beans	0.0	44	A
Yellowtail	12.0	330	B
Yogurt, all flavors, Cabot	3.0	110	B
Yogurt, apple, Yoplait original	4.0	480	B
Yogurt, Ben & Jerry's frozen cherry	9.6	320	B
Yogurt, blueberry, non-fat lite, Dannon	0.0	109	A

Food	Fat grams	Per 8 ozs. Calories	Zone
Yogurt, blueberry, Yoplait original	8.0	240	B
Yogurt, frozen, all flavors, Bressler's gourmet	3.2	232	B
Yogurt, frozen, all flavors, Bressler's	3.2	216	B
Yogurt, frozen, TCBY	2.0	220	A
Yogurt, low-fat, fruit	2.6	225	B
Yogurt, non-fat	0.4	127	A
Yogurt, plain, regular	7.4	138	B
Yogurt, Weight Watchers, all flavors	0.0	90	A
Zucchini squash, breaded, Ore Ida	21.0	400	C
Zucchini squash, cooked	1.3	20	A
Zucchini squash, cooked	0.0	28	A
Zucchini squash, fresh	0.0	28	A
Zucchini squash, Italian style	0.9	28	A
Zucchini squash, raw sliced	0.9	28	A

LOW-FAT FOODS TO SUBSTITUTE FOR HIGH-FAT FOODS

The following chart will help you make good low-fat food choices. Be sure to follow these guidelines when dining out or preparing meals at home. Just following these suggestions will likely give you a good start on a weight management program.

Instead of this:	Fat grams	Try this:	Fat grams	
Dark meat chicken	16	White meat chicken	5	
Dark meat turkey	12	White meat turkey	3	
Lamb chop	14	Veal cutlet (3 oz.)	4	
Tuna, oil packed	7	Tuna, water packed	1/2	
Salmon	9	Halibut	3	or
		Crab	1	or
		Lobster	1/2	or
		Clams	2	or
		Scallops	1	or
		Shrimp, boiled	1	

Instead of this:	Fat grams	Try this:	Fat grams	
Ground beef	20	Vegetarian burger	2	
Chuck roast	19	Braised brisket	10	or
		Bottom round roast	6	
Sirloin	17	T-bone	10	or
		Top Round	4	
Eggs with yolks	5	Eggs, whites only (or Egg Beater-type product)	0	
Beef or chicken liver	8	Simmered kidney	3	
Pork chops	14	Pork tenderloin	5	
Pork roast	28			
Pork shoulder	26			
Pork spareribs	30			
Whole milk	9	Skim milk	1/2	
Whole milk yogurt	4	Skim milk yogurt	0	
Pork sausage	8	Beef or vegetarian bacon	2	or
		ground turkey	2	
Hot dogs	16	Turkey dogs	8	or
		Vegetarian dogs	3	
Luncheon meats	8	95% fat-free luncheon meats	1	
Butter	12	Sunflower or low-fat margarine	4	
Sauces	27	Vegetable or fruit juices	0	
Oils	13	Stock pot flavorings, vegetable oil sprays	0	
Chocolate	13	Carob flavor mix powder	0	
Cream soups	12	Chicken noodle soup	3	
Sour cream	3	Light sour cream	1	or
		low-fat yogurt	0	
Chocolate chips	14	Raisins	1/2	
Cheddar cheese	12	Part-skim mozzarella	5	
Ice cream	15	Sherbet, ice milk, frozen low-fat yogurt	2	
Baked potato with butter & sour cream	15	Baked potato with stone ground mustard &/or salsa	0	
Cream	4	Skim milk	0	or
		Low-fat, non-dairy substitute	1	

Instead of this:	Fat grams	Try this:	Fat grams
Bacon bits	10	Fresh chives	0
Cottage cheese	5	Low-fat cottage cheese	2
Potato chips	10	Air popped popcorn	0
Cream cheese	10	Fat-free ricotta cheese	1
Nuts	15	Water chestnuts	0
		Roasted chestnuts	0
Mayonnaise	11	Non-fat mayonnaise or non-fat yogurt with mustard or vinegar	0
Oil-type salad dressing	9	Fat-free dressing	1

APPENDIX B

Foods You Can Eat As Much As You Want

Yes, it's true. There are many foods that you can eat whenever you like, and as much as you want. (Within reason, please. Nobody really needs to eat 20 baked potatoes.)

While it sounds illogical, the best way to lose weight is to eat whenever you are genuinely hungry, as long as you eat the right foods.

Let's face it — severe hunger, such as when counting calories or otherwise reducing food intake, leads one to binge eating. After a while, hunger becomes so strong that a person eats larger amounts of food. And usually, the food is the wrong kind, such as fat-laden snack foods, pizza or some other high-fat food.

The way to lose weight is this — eat food when you get hungry, but eat the right foods. Eat small snacks throughout the day. A constant supply of food keeps the metabolism high and actually accelerates a weight management program.

If you need a snack, reach for those carrots, celery, apples or oranges. You'll feel satisfied; you'll look great and you'll feel supercharged with energy.

To help you pick the right foods, here's a list of what you should eat between meals throughout the day if you get hungry. If you center your main meals around these foods, you'll absolutely power-charge your weight program and feel great at the same time!

FOODS TO EAT WHEN YOU GET HUNGRY

VEGETABLES

Artichoke
Asparagus *
Bamboo shoots *
Beets *
Broccoli *
Cabbage *
Carrots *
Cauliflower *
Celery *
Chives *
Cucumber *
Eggplant *
Endive *
Fennel *
Green Beans *
Horseradish *
Kale *
Leeks *
Lettuce *
Mung beans *
Mushrooms *
Okra *
Onion *
Parsley *
Parsnips *
Peas
Peppers, green, sweet or hot *
Pickles, dill or sour *
Pumpkin *
Red Radish *
Rhubarb *
Sauerkraut *
Shallots *
Snap Beans *
Spinach *
Squash *
Swiss Chard *

VEGETABLES (continued)

Watercress *
Wax beans *
Zucchini *
Tomatoes or tomato juice *
Turnip *
Water chestnuts *

CARBOHYDRATES

Corn
Black beans
Kidney beans
Grains
Potatoes
Rice

FRUITS

Apples
Bananas
Grapefruit
Lemon
Mandarin
Mango
Oranges
Papaya
Pineapple
Raspberries
Strawberries

MISCELLANEOUS

Coffee *
Tea *
Noodle soup *

NEGATIVE CALORIE FOODS

The foods listed with an asterisk are very low-calorie foods. They contain less than 30 calories per serving. As you can see, almost all the low-calorie foods are vegetables, and almost all vegetables are low-calorie foods.

These low-calorie foods are sometimes called "negative calorie" foods. The reasoning for calling them this is simple. The physical act of eating burns up 1.5 calories per minute. Since a serving of one of the above foods contains less than 30 calories, all of the calories in the food will be burned up by the body within 20 minutes. Assuming that the time spent eating a meal averages 30 minutes or so, it is actually possible to eat a serving of any of the low-calorie foods and burn up more calories than the food contains before the meal is over!

A person could eat several servings of these low-calorie foods at every meal and not gain weight. The calories would be completely used up long before the next meal. They would likely lose weight rather quickly since all of the low-calorie foods are also very low in fat content.

An additional benefit of the low-calorie foods is that they are nutritionally dense. These foods are low in calories, yet high in nutrition. They are loaded with vitamins, minerals and antioxidants, such as beta carotene. High-fat foods, on the other hand, are not nutritionally dense. They are high in calories but low in nutrition. Eating the low-calorie, nutritionally dense foods not only superpowers your weight management program, it can also boost your immune system and help you feel healthier.

Important — normal daily activity burns up 2.6 calories per minute, while any active sport or exercise burns up 5–15 calories per minute. So if a large portion of your daily food intake is composed of the nutrient-dense, 1.5-calorie-per-minute foods, your weight management plan will be greatly improved. This is because your body will need to rely on stored fat for fuel since you are eating low–calorie, low–fat foods. The end result — you will lose weight more easily, quickly and permanently than with most other "diet" plans.

HOW TO CALCULATE YOUR OWN METABOLISM

It is possible to calculate your own individual metabolic rate. This daily metabolic rate, called the basal metabolism, is the number of calories burned up by your body for normal body functions. These are the calories required every day to keep your heart, lungs, muscles, organs and autonomic system functioning. It is also quite easy to factor in the additional calories you burn based on your physical activity.

Knowing your own basal metabolism will enable you to custom-design a weight management program specifically for you. Your weight loss will then likely be greatly accelerated without the drastic lifestyle changes required by most diets.

The formula, called the Harris–Benedict formula, has been used by professional nutritionists for years as the most authoritative way to calculate basal metabolism.

THE HARRIS–BENEDICT FORMULA FOR MEN

1. Multiply height in inches by 2.5 to determine height in centimeters.
2. Multiply height in centimeters by 5.0 to determine the calories needed for body height.
3. Divide weight in pounds by 2.2 to determine weight in kilograms.
4. Multiply weight in kilograms by 13.5 to determine the calories needed for body weight.
5. Multiply age by 6.75 to determine the age factor number.
6. Total Basal Metabolism = 66 + calories needed for height + calories needed for weight — age factor number.

Let's work through a real-life example to see how it works. Let's calculate the basal metabolism for a 35 year old man, 6'0" tall, weighing 200 pounds.

1. 72 inches x 2.5 = 180 centimeters
2. 180 x 5.0 = 900 calories needed for height
3. 200 pounds divided by 2.2 = 90.9 kilograms
4. 90.9 kilograms x 13.5 = 1227 calories needed for weight
5. 35 years x 6.75 = 236 age factor
6. 66 + 900 + 1227 - 236 = 1957 calories needed per day

If this man centers his meals around low-fat foods, his weight management program will be successful, and he will be able to eat large quantities of satisfying, good-tasting food.

THE HARRIS–BENEDICT FORMULA FOR WOMEN

1. Multiply height in inches by 2.5 to determine height in centimeters.
2. Multiply height in centimeters by 1.8 to determine the calories needed for body height.
3. Divide weight in pounds by 2.2 to determine weight in kilograms.
4. Multiply weight in kilograms by 9.56 to determine the calories needed for body weight.
5. Multiply age by 4.68 to determine the age factor number.
6. Total Basal Metabolism = 65 + calories needed for height + calories needed for weight — age factor number.

Now let's calculate the basal metabolism for a 35 year-old woman, 5'2" tall, weighing 125 pounds.

1. 62 inches x 2.5 = 155 centimeters
2. 155 x 1.8 = 279 calories needed for height
3. 125 pounds divided by 2.2 = 56.82 kilograms

4. 56.82 x 9.56 = 543 calories needed for weight
5. 35 years x 4.68 = 164 age factor
6. 65 + 279 + 543 – 164 = 723 calories needed per day

The woman in our example needs to eat 723 calories per day just to maintain her present weight.

Neither of these formulas take into account calorie expenditure from physical activity. You may add calories every day based on your own personal activity and exercise regimen. (See chart on next page for calories and activity.)

An even easier, but slightly less accurate method is called the Body Weight Method. For this calculation, your body needs 1 calorie per kilogram per hour to maintain itself.

Example: Let's use the same 200 pound man as previously mentioned.

1. Weight in pounds divided by 2.2 equals weight in kilograms.
2. Kilograms times 1 equals calories needed per hour.
3. Calories per hour times 24 equals calories needed per day.

So, our 200 pound man calculates as follows:

1. 200 divided by 2.2 = 90.9 kilograms.
2. 90.9 kilogram x 1 = 90.9 calories per hour.
3. 90.9 x 24 = 2181 calories per day.

You can also use this method to figure out how many calories per day to eat to get to your goal weight.

Example: Goal weight (in kilograms) x 1 x 24 = calories to eat per day to reach goal weight.

Take the time right now to calculate your own basal metabolism using the Harris-Benedict Formula or Body Weight Method. Knowing your personal basal metabolism may give you an indication why previous "diets" have not worked for you. As we've already discussed, fat calories are not the same as protein or carbohydrate calories. Fat calories are not nutritionally dense and contain about twice the calories per gram of protein or carbohydrates. This is why many diets fail for many people time and time again – the diets do not take into account the difference between fat and other calories.

An especially appealing aspect of the Biogenesis Program is that you do not need to count calories to achieve maximum weight loss. The entire program has been designed around the low-fat method. Rather than counting calories, learn to concentrate instead on eating low-fat foods. Most low-fat foods will also be nutritionally dense, thus giving you good nutrition. They will also contain more fiber than fatty foods. The combination of high fiber and needed nutrients will fill you up and help you stay healthier.

The effort that you spend learning to eat the Biogenesis low-fat way will be far surpassed by its many benefits. And your body will love you for it. Happy Eating!

ACTIVITIES AND THE CALORIES THEY CONSUME

(for a person weighing approximately 150 pounds)

Activity	Calories expended per hour
Rest and light activity	**50-200**
Lying down or sleeping	80
Sitting	100
Typing	110
Driving	120
Standing	140
Housework	180
Shining shoes	185
Moderate activity	**200-350**
Bicycling (5 1/2 mph)	210
Walking (2 1/2)	210
Gardening	220
Canoeing (2 1/2 mph)	230
Golf (foursome)	250
Lawn-mowing (power mower)	250
Fencing	300
Rowing a boat (2 1/2 mph)	300
Swimming (1/4 mph)	300
Calisthenics	300
Walking (3 1/4 mph)	300
Badminton	350
Horseback riding (trotting)	350
Square dancing	350
Volleyball	350
Roller skating	350

Stacking heavy objects (boxes, logs)	350
Vigorous activity	**over 350**
Baseball pitching	360
Ditch-digging (hand shovel)	400
Ice-skating (10 mph)	400
Chopping or sawing wood	400
Bowling (continuous)	400
Tennis	420
Water-skiing	480
Hill-climbing (100 feet per hour)	490
Basketball	500
Football	500
Skiing (10 mph)	600
Squash and handball	600
Bicycling (13 mph)	660
Rowing (machine)	720
Scull-rowing (race)	840
Running (10 mph)	900
Resistance weight training	**over 900**

(From the New York Public Library Desk Reference, Webster's, New York, 1989.)

BIBLIOGRAPHY

Antonello, Jean, *How to Become Naturally Thin by Eating More*, Avon Books, New York, NY, 1989.

Bailey, Covert, *Smart Exercise*, Houghton Mifflin Company, Boston, MA, 1994.

Balch, Dr. James F., M.D. and Balch, Phyllis, *Prescription for Nutritional Healing*, Avery Publishing, Garden City Park, NY, 1990.

Basmajian, Dr. John, *The Human Body: Muscles, The Magic of Motion*, Torstar Books, New York, NY, 1985.

Bean, Constance, *The Better Back Book*, William Morrow, New York, NY, 1989.

Bragg, Paul, *The Natural Way to Reduce*, Health Science Publishers, Santa Barbara, CA, 1984.

Bricklin, Mark, *Lose Weight Naturally*, Rodale Press, Emmaus, PA, 1989.

Brody, Jane, *Jane Brody's Nutrition Book*, W.W. Norton & Company, New York, NY, 1981.

Concoby, Robert, *Discovered: Nature's Secret Fountains of Youth*, Hanford Press, Canton, OH, 1993.

Craig, Jenny, *What Have You Got to Lose*, Villard Books, New York, NY, 1992.

Feldenkrais, Moshe, *The Potent Self*, Harper and Row, San Francisco, CA, 1985.

Franks, B. Don and Howley, Edward T., *Fitness Facts: The Healthy Living Handbook*, Human Kinetics Books, Champaign, IL, 1989.

Good Food and Fitness, Better Homes and Garden Books, Des Moines, IA, 1981.

Gutfeld, Greg, *Banish your Potbelly: A Man's Guide to Fighting Fat*, Rodale Press, Emmaus, PA, 1993.

Jackson, Ian, *The Breathplay Approach to Whole Life Fitness*, Doubleday & Company, New York, NY, 1986.

Katahn, Martin, *Beyond Diet*, W.W. Norton & Company, New York, NY, 1984.

Logue, A.W., *The Psychology of Eating and Drinking*, W. H. Freeman & Company, New York, NY, 1986.

Mayer, Jean, *A Diet for Living*, David McKay Company, New York, NY, 1975.

McDougall, Dr. John A., M.D., *The McDougall Program for Maximum Weight Loss*, Penguin Books, New York, NY, 1994.

Netzer, Corinne, *The Complete Book of Food Counts*, Dell Publishing, 1994.

Ornish, Dr. Dean, M.D., *Eat More, Weigh Less*, Harper Collins, New York, N.Y., 1993.

Pennington, Jean A.T., *Bowes and Church's Food Values of Portions Commonly Used*, 16th ed., J.B. Lippincott Company, Philadelphia, PA, 1994.

Speads, Carola H., *Breathing: The ABC's*, Harper Colophon Books, New York, NY, 1978.

Stare, Frederick J., and Whelan, Elizabeth M., *Eat OK-Feel OK*, North Quincy, MA, Christopher Co., 1978.

Stare, Frederick J., and McWilliams, Margaret, *Living Nutrition*, 3rd ed., John Wiley & Sons, New York, NY, 1981.

Todd, Mabel Ellsworth, *The Thinking Body*, Dance Horizons, New York, NY, 1937.

Tver, David F. and Russell, Percy, Ph.D., *The Nutrition and Health Encyclopedia*, Van Nostrand Reinhold Company, New York, NY, 1981.